Directory of Schools for Alternative and Complementary Health Care

2nd Edition

Edited by Karen Rappaport

Oryx Press
1999

The rare Arabian Oryx is believed to have inspired the myth of the unicorn. This desert antelope became virtually extinct in the early 1960s. At that time several groups of international conservationists arranged to have 9 animals sent to the Phoenix Zoo to be the nucleus of a captive breeding herd. Today the Oryx population is over 800 and nearly 400 have been returned to reserves in the Middle East.

ISSN pending
ISBN 1-57356-294-7

To Bill

TABLE OF CONTENTS

FOREWORD

By Andrew Weil, M.D.

In the late 1970s, when the holistic medical movement was gaining ground, I began lecturing to first- and second-year medical students at the University of Arizona about alternative medicine in a required course called Human Behavior and Development. These were among the first lectures on this subject given at an American medical school. In 1983, I started an elective course in alternative medicine for fourth-year medical students, placing them with practitioners in southern Arizona so that they could observe firsthand such therapies as chiropractic, osteopathic manipulation, homeopathy, acupuncture, biofeedback, and others.

I continue to give the introductory lectures to beginning students and to supervise the elective course, but I now direct an extensive program in Integrative Medicine at the University of Arizona, and the whole landscape of healthcare has changed. Alternative and complementary therapies are now big business. To their credit, a great many medical students and physicians in practice now realize that they are not trained to provide services that patients want.

Training in some therapies is more readily available than others. If you want to learn massage therapy or acupuncture, there are a number of schools specializing in them, many of which are covered in this book. But how do you learn herbal medicine, Feldenkrais, or therapeutic touch? What if you are not a medical student or have not yet enrolled in college? The *Directory of Schools for Alternative and Complementary Health Care* fills the need for a comprehensive listing of educational opportunities for all in a wide range of modalities.

In coming years, there are certain to be new possibilities for providing these therapies to clients. Not only will hospitals, clinics, and health maintenance organizations be seeking practitioners and counselors to round out their offerings, I can envision the appearance of healing centers in which integrative care will be delivered by teams of conventional and alternative practitioners working together, not only for the relief of illness but for its prevention. The demand for such services can only increase along with opportunities for practice by those with the right skills. It is wonderful to watch this ideal of Integrative Medicine coming into being.

Tucson, Arizona

INTRODUCTION

Opportunities continue to grow for practitioners of alternative and complementary health care. Hospitals and health care networks around the country are making alternative and complementary therapies available. Research reported in *The Journal of the American Medical Association* found a substantial increase in the use of alternative medicine between 1990 and 1997.[1] The former Office of Alternative Medicine of the National Institutes of Health is now the National Center for Complementary and Alternative Medicine, with a significantly increased budget and greater autonomy to facilitate research and provide information to the public. Also mandated in 1999 is the establishment of a White House Commission on Complementary and Alternative Medicine Policy, to address issues of training, licensing, and insurance coverage.

As interest in and exposure to alternative and complementary health care increase, there is a greater demand for practitioners and for alternative medical education. This book provides information on schools and programs in the United States and Canada that offer professional training in alternative and complementary therapies, including acupressure, acupuncture and oriental medicine, Alexander Technique, aromatherapy, ayurvedic medicine, biofeed-

back, chiropractic, Feldenkrais, herbal medicine, homeopathy, hypnotherapy, massage therapy and bodywork, midwifery, naturopathic medicine, polarity therapy, reflexology, Reiki, shiatsu, and yoga.

Professional standards in these fields are developing as well. The status of alternative and complementary medical practice continues to change as associations and practitioners lobby for recognition and legislation. There is a wide range of standards and requirements, varying from state to state, that schools and practitioners must meet. Professional associations can provide information on modalities and their practice and treatment; the current status of the profession on state and national levels, including which practices are approved, certified, or licensed in which states; national standards that a school should meet; and other requirements that prospective practitioners need to fulfill.

To determine which school best suits your career goals and philosophy, research and evaluate several programs. Use this book to identify schools in your field of interest, and then write or call for catalogs and curriculum descriptions to review; visit schools to assess programs, faculty, and facilities; and interview graduates of the school. Consider whether the school is li-

[1]Eisenberg, David M., MD, et al., "Trends in Alternative Medicine Use in the United States, 1990-1997: Results of a Follow-Up National Survey," *JAMA, The Journal of the American Medical Association*, 280, no. 19 (November 11, 1998): 1569.

censed, approved, or accredited. Accreditation is a voluntary procedure overseen by nongovernmental agencies; however, the Accreditation and Eligibility Determination Division of the U.S. Department of Education and the Council on Higher Education Accreditation recognize only accrediting agencies that comply with their eligibility standards. Eligibility standards required of schools are available from their accrediting or approving agencies.

For schools that offer certification programs, determine what certification means in each instance: is it a designation conferred by the school, or is it recognized by the state or a national organization? National certification does not guarantee acceptance or approval in each state. To prepare for a career as a practitioner of alternative or complementary medicine, investigate qualifications required by the municipality where you intend to practice.[2]

About This Book

This book fills the need for a truly comprehensive resource by providing detailed information about 877 schools and professional training programs for alternative and complementary health care in the United States and Canada. Schools are indexed by program of study, and so this book is useful for students with interest in a particular modality, as well as for those with a general interest in alternative medical education but who are unfamiliar with the wide range of educational options available. The book is also beneficial to those in need of, or already receiving, alternative health care. This reference will help individuals to learn more about their healing partnership by understanding their practitioner's educational background and training.

School names were gathered from professional organizations, advertising, and word of mouth. Some screening was done before sending questionnaires. Entries in this book provide data gathered from schools that responded to questionnaires between December, 1998, and April, 1999. Inclusion in this *Directory* is free of charge to schools, and does not signify endorsement by the editor or publisher. All entries from the previous edition of the *Directory* have been updated, verified, or deleted (if no longer operating), and more than 250 new entries have been added.

This *Directory* focuses on schools that offer entire programs in a particular field of study. Readers should also check the Richard and Hinda Rosenthal Center for Complementary and Alternative Medicine at Columbia University College of Physicians and Surgeons for their list of medical schools offering courses in alternative medicine.

How to Use This Book

The directory section of this book consists of listings of schools in the United States and Canada. Schools are arranged alphabetically by state, with schools in the United States appearing first, followed by Canadian schools. All entries contain the school's name, address, and phone number and, where available, fax, e-mail, and Web page address. Entries may also include

- name of program administrator
- name of admissions contact
- year school was established
- staff (full- or part-time, and number)

---

[2]Bianco, David P., ed., *Professional and Occupational Licensing Directory: A Descriptive Guide to State and Federal Licensing, Registration & Certification Requirements*, 2nd ed. Detroit, MI: Gale Research Inc., 1996.

- average enrollment (per year)
- average class size (average number of students in the classroom)
- average number of graduates (per year)
- availability of wheelchair access
- accreditation, approval, or licensing by an association or accrediting body
- field of study (asterisks have been used to denote main programs of study—those in which the school specializes and has comprehensive expertise.)
- name and/or length of program of study (how many hours, weeks, or months required for completion of the program)
- degrees offered (i.e., certification, MD, PhD, license)
- license/certification preparation (licensing/certification exams for which the program prepares students, if any)
- admission requirements (specific requirements that must be met by students before enrolling)
- application deadlines (students should also contact schools for specific starting dates and deadlines)
- tuition and fees (tuition/fee amount is per program unless otherwise specified)
- financial aid (government aid, aid provided by the school, etc. Contact each program directly for more information)
- career placement (availability of career counseling, internships, etc.)

The directory section is followed by an expanded section of organizations, books, periodicals, and Web sites with information on alternative medicine and various modalities. The list of organizations provides addresses and phone numbers for organizations and accrediting bodies for selected modalities. The bibliography lists books, periodicals, and Web sites for further research on alternative health care training.

The directory portion of the book has two indexes: an index of schools arranged by name, which lists schools alphabetically, and a fields of study index, which lists schools alphabetically under the fields of study they offer.

Acknowledgements

I would like to thank the many individuals at the schools, organizations, and associations who provided information on their programs and professions. I also want to thank Jennifer Ashley at The Oryx Press, and the Sarasota County Libraries. I am grateful to my parents, Gertrude and Marvin Rappaport, for their support and assistance. Thanks to my sister, Linda Rappaport, and to Sandra Fallon, Kathleen O'Toole, and Frances Riemer for their encouragement and friendship. I especially thank my husband, Bill Stokes, consultant and sweetheart.

SAMPLE ENTRY

180. Yo San University of Traditional Chinese Medicine — SCHOOL NAME

ADDRESS —— 1314 2nd St, Santa Monica, CA 90401

(310) 917-2202; Fax: (310) 917-2203 — E-MAIL/INTERNET

E-mail: info@yosan.edu *Internet:* http://www. yosan.edu

CONTACTS —— *Program Administrator:* Dr. Richard Hammerschlag, Academic Dean/Research Dir. *Admissions Contact:* Curt Duffy, Dir of Admissions and Mktg.

YEAR ESTABLISHED — *Year Established:* 1989.

AVERAGE NUMBER OF STUDENTS IN THE CLASSROOM

NUMBER OF STAFF —— *Staff:* Full-time 3; Part-time 35.

AVERAGE ENROLLMENT PER YEAR —— *Avg Enrollment:* 55. *Avg Class Size:* 25. *Number of Graduates per Year:* 18. — AVERAGE NUMBER OF GRADUATES PER YEAR

Wheelchair Access? Yes.

WHEELCHAIR ACCESS —— *Accreditation/Approval/Licensing:* State board: CA Acupuncture Board; Accreditation Commission for Acupuncture and Oriental Medicine.

ACCREDITATION/ APPROVAL FROM LISTED ORGANIZATIONS (pending accreditation or candidacy is listed at the end of entries)

SCHOOL'S SPECIALIZATIONS AND LENGTH OF PROGRAMS —— *Field of Study:* Acupuncture*; Herbal Medicine*; Qigong*; Traditional Chinese Medicine; Life Style Counseling. **Program Name/Length:** Master of Acupuncture & Traditional Chinese Medicine, 4 yrs.

PREPARATION OFFERED FOR CERTIFICATION OR LICENSING

DEGREES OFFERED —— *Degree(s) Offered:* MAcTCM

License/Certification Preparation: State: CA Licensed Acupuncturist; National Certification Commission for Acupuncture and Oriental Medicine.

ADMISSION REQUIREMENTS —— *Admission Requirements:* Some college (2 yrs).

APPLICATION DEADLINES

Application Deadline(s): Fall: Aug; Winter: Dec.

Tuition and Fees: $7500 per yr. — TUITION

Financial Aid: Loans; Tutorships. —— FINANCIAL AID

CAREER PLACEMENT SERVICES —— *Career Placement:* Career counseling; Career information; Internships.

*Denotes a main program of study.

ABBREVIATIONS

AA	Associate of Arts	DN	Doctor of Naprapathy
AAS	Associate of Applied Science	DNSc	Doctor of Nursing Science
Admin	Administrator/Administration	DO	Doctor of Osteopathy
AMTA	American Massage Therapy Association	DOM	Doctor of Oriental Medicine
		DONA	Doulas of North America
AOS	Associate of Occupational Studies	DrPH	Doctor of Public Health
AP	Acupuncture Physician	DVM	Doctor of Veterinary Medicine
APP	Associate Polarity Practitioner	Ed	Education
AS	Associate of Science	EdD	Doctor of Education
Asst	Assistant	Exec	Executive
Avg	Average	FACCE	Fellow, Academy of Certified Childbirth Educators
BPS	Bachelor of Professional Studies		
BScPharm	Bachelor of Science in Pharmacy	FACNM	Fellow of the American College of Nurse-Midwives
BSIS	Bachelor of Science in Interdisciplinary Sciences		
		FNP	Family Nurse Practitioner
BSN	Bachelor of Science in Nursing	HD	Doctor of Homeopathic Medicine
BSW	Bachelor of Social Work	HNC	Holistic Nursing Certification
Bus	Business	hrs	hours
CCH	Certified in Classical Homeopathy	Instr	Instructor
CCHT	Certified Clinical Hypnotherapist	LAc	Licensed Acupuncturist
CD	Certified Doula	LCH	Licensed Colon Hydrotherapist
CEU	Continuing Education Unit	LCSW	Licensed Clinical Social Worker
CHom	Certified in Homeopathy	LDEM	Licensed Direct Entry Midwife
CHt	Certified Hypnotherapist	LM	Licensed Midwife
CM	Certified Midwife	LMP	Licensed Massage Practitioner
CMT	Certified Massage Therapist	LMT	Licensed Massage Therapist
CNM	Certified Nurse-Midwife	LPC	Licensed Professional Counselor
Coord	Coordinator	LPN	Licensed Practical Nurse
CRM	Certified Reiki Master	MA	Master of Arts
DC	Doctor of Chiropractic	MAc	Master of Acupuncture
DCH	Doctor of Clinical Hypnotherapy	MAcOM	Master of Acupuncture and Oriental Medicine
Dept	Department		
DHANP	Diplomate, Homeopathic Academy of Naturopathic Physicians	MAcTCM	Master of Acupuncture and Traditional Chinese Medicine
		MD	Doctor of Medicine
DHMS	Doctor of Homeopathic Medicine and Science	MEd	Master of Education
		MFCC	Marriage, Family, and Child Counselor
DHt	Diplomate in Homeotherapeutics		
DiplAc	Diplomate in Acupuncture	Mgmt	Management
Dir	Director	Mgr	Manager
Div	Division	MH	Master Herbalist

MHt	Master of Hypnotherapy		**NCTMB**	Nationally Certified in Therapeutic Massage & Bodywork
Mktg	Marketing			
min	minimum			
MN	Master of Nursing		**ND**	Doctor of Naturopathic Medicine
MOM	Master of Oriental Medicine		**OMD**	Doctor of Oriental Medicine
mos	months		**PA**	Physician Assistant
MPH	Master of Public Health		**Pres**	President
MPS	Master of Professional Studies		**Prog**	Program
MS	Master of Science		**PsyD**	Doctor of Psychology
MSN	Master of Science in Nursing		**qtrs**	quarters
MSOM	Master of Science in Oriental Medicine		**RMT**	Registered Massage Therapist
			RN	Registered Nurse
MSTCM	Master of Science in Traditional Chinese Medicine		**RPP**	Registered Polarity Practitioner
			RS Hom (NA)	Registered, Society of Homeopathy (North America)
MSW	Master of Social Work		**ScD**	Doctor of Science
MT	Massage Therapist		**Sec**	Secretary
MTCM	Master of Traditional Chinese Medicine		**Sr**	Senior
			Svcs	Services
MTI	Massage Therapist Instructor		**wks**	weeks
MTOM	Master of Traditional Oriental Medicine		**yrs**	years

GLOSSARY

For additional information on alternative and complementary therapies, consult the resource section, especially the books subsection. For specific descriptions of the programs offered by the individual schools, contact the schools directly.

Acupressure: pressure to points along the body's energy pathways, or meridians, to balance energy and promote healing; believed to be beneficial in the treatment of allergies, arthritis, back and shoulder pain, headaches, gastrointestinal problems, and stress.

Acupuncture: the insertion of fine needles to points along meridians (energy pathways) to stimulate the vital life force, or chi, and restore energy balance; used in the treatment of addictions, anxiety, depression, fatigue, menstrual imbalances, pain, shock and trauma, sinus problems, and ulcers.

Alexander Technique: an educational method developed by Frederick Matthias Alexander to identify and change inefficient physical habits and postures.

Animal Therapy: general term for therapies used in the treatment of animals, such as equine massage and holistic veterinary approaches that include acupuncture, chiroptractic, and homeopathy.

Applied Kinesiology: muscle testing to evaluate areas of weakness or dysfunction, combined with massage to pressure points to detoxify and revitalize.

Aromatherapy: the use of essential oils of herbs and flowers for healing, to relax and rejuvenate, improve circulation and digestion, and stimulate the immune system; used in treating asthma, colds, coughs, skin disorders, tension, and stress.

Ayurvedic Medicine: ancient Indian medicine meaning "science of life," considers a range of dietary and lifestyle factors in treatment of mind, body, and spirit; uses natural therapies to remove imbalances and restore health.

Biofeedback: the use of electronic instruments to feed back information about body processes to develop awareness and ability to influence processes such as blood pressure, pulse rate, temperature, and muscle tension.

Bodywork: general term for a wide range of manipulative therapies including acupressure, Alexander Technique, applied kinesiology, Aston-Patterning, Breema, Cranio-Sacral therapy, Feldenkrais, Hellerwork, Jin Shin Do, Jin Shin Jyutsu, massage therapy, myofascial release, polarity therapy, reflexology, Rosen Method, shiatsu, structural integration, Trager, tui na, and Zero Balancing.

Breathwork: the use of breathing techniques to free the breath and release energy.

Chi (or qi): pronounced "chee," the energy or life force that flows through the body in regular pathways along channels or meridians.

Chiropractic: developed by Dr. Daniel David Palmer in 1895; used to treat disturbances of the nervous system, spine, and musculoskeletal system through manipulation and corrective structural adjustment to normalize bodily structure and function.

Colon Hydrotherapy: cleansing the colon with water; used to detoxify, improve digestion and elimination, and enhance the immune system.

CranioSacral Therapy: developed by John Upledger, DO; a gentle manipulative technique used to evaluate the craniosacral system that surrounds and protects the brain and spinal cord, remove restrictions, and improve functioning of the central nervous system.

Doula: labor support caregiver; works with physicians, nurses, and midwives to provide physical, emotional, and informational support to women throughout childbirth.

Energy Work: stimulating healing on an energetic level, to unblock and balance energy; examples include use of flower essences, healing touch, homeopathy, polarity therapy, Reiki, therapeutic touch, and vibrational healing.

Esalen Massage: developed at the Esalen Institute in the 1960s; gentle massage combining Oriental and Swedish techniques used to reduce stress, relieve pain, and promote healing.

Feldenkrais: movement training developed by Moshe Feldenkrais to encourage freer movement and increase awareness, flexibility, and coordination.

Guided Imagery: *see* Visualization

Hellerwork: developed by Joseph Heller, deep tissue bodywork and movement education to align the body and release tension.

Herbal Medicine: practiced since earliest times in all civilizations and cultures; uses the healing properties of medicinal herbs, plants, and flowers to prevent and treat disease and enhance health and vitality.

Homeopathy: developed by physician Samuel Hahnemann; considers the whole person in prescribing minute doses of natural medicines according to the "law of similars," meaning that a symptom that can be produced by large quantities of a substance can be remedied by the same substance when used in very small and diluted quantities.

Hydrotherapy: the therapeutic use of water for healing, used since ancient times to improve circulation, detoxify, and relieve muscle strain, fever, congestion, and pain.

Hypnotherapy: the use of hypnosis, a state of deep relaxation and altered consciousness, for therapeutic purposes; used in the treatment of addiction, allergies, anxiety, colitis, migraines, pain, phobias, skin disorders, and stress.

Iridology: the study of the eye's iris to diagnose illness or weakness in the body.

Jin Shin Do: a body-mind acupressure method developed by Iona Marsaa Teeguarden; focuses on a particular network of acupoints to release physical and emotional tensions.

Jin Shin Jyutsu: ancient Japanese art brought to the United States in the 1950s by Mary Burmeister; gentle touch of "safety energy locks" along energy pathways used to harmonize body, mind, and spirit.

Kinesiology: the mechanics and principles of human movement and use of muscles.

LomiLomi Massage: Hawaiian massage; uses loving touch to stimulate mana, or life energy.

Lymphatic Massage: *see* Manual Lymph Drainage

Maharishi Vedic Medicine: *see* Ayurvedic Medicine

Manual Lymph Drainage: a massage technique developed by Dr. Emil Vodder to stimulate flow of lymphatic fluid, remove toxins, and enhance the immune system.

Massage: the use of touch for relaxation, stress reduction, pain relief, and rehabilitation of muscular injuries; believed to be beneficial to the musculoskeletal, circulatory, respiratory, digestive, and craniosacral systems.

Midwifery: health care for pregnancy and childbirth, from preconception through pregnancy, labor and delivery, and postpartum and infant care; emphasizes nonintervention in natural processes.

Myofascial Release: gentle pressure to relieve restrictions or dysfunction of the fascia, a network of connective tissue throughout the body surrounding organs, nerves, blood vessels, muscles, and bones.

Myotherapy: see Trigger Point Therapy

Naprapathy: developed by Dr. Oakly Smith, includes evaluation and manipulation of connective tissues to relieve tension and restrictions, therapeutic exercise, and dietary counseling.

Naturopathic Medicine: primary health care that treats the whole person and promotes optimal health; employs a wide variety of natural therapies to prevent disease and support the body's inherent healing abilities.

Neuromuscular Therapy: see Trigger Point Therapy

Oriental Medicine: encompasses a range of modalities including acupuncture, qigong, shiatsu, Thai massage, traditional Chinese medicine, and tui na.

Polarity Therapy: developed by Randolph Stone, DC, DO, ND; uses bodywork, diet, exercise, and self-awareness to balance polarity (the electromagnetic force field of the body) and renew vitality.

Qigong: uses breath, movement, and meditation to cleanse, strengthen, and circulate the life energy called qi or chi.

Rebirthing: a gentle breathing technique to develop self-awareness and release trauma.

Reflexology: pressure on reflex points on the hands and feet to stimulate energy flow to organs and other parts of the body, relax tension, and improve circulation.

Reiki: translates from Japanese as "universal life energy"; a hands-on healing technique used to transmit and balance energy.

Rolfing: see Structural Integration

Russian Massage: medical and sports massage to improve functioning and facilitate healing.

Shiatsu: Japanese pressure-point massage along energy meridians to balance and release energy, increase circulation, benefit the nervous and immune systems, enhance natural healing powers, and restore harmony; used in the treatment of headache, fatigue, high blood pressure, insomnia, and tension.

Somatic Education: movement education to relieve muscle tension, improve posture and coordination, and increase flexibility.

Sports Massage: focuses on three components to help athletes achieve optimal performance: maintenance (regular massage treatments incorporating a variety of massage techniques); event massage (before, during, and after); and rehabilitation (treatment and management of injuries) to improve range of motion and muscle flexibility, reduce chance of injury, and enhance the body's recovery process.

Structural Integration: developed by Dr. Ida Rolf; deep pressure to the fascia, or connective tissue, surrounding the muscles used to restructure the nervous and musculoskeletal systems and restore proper alignment.

Swedish Massage: uses long strokes, friction, and kneading techniques to promote relaxation, relieve muscle tension, and improve circulation.

Thai Massage: combines pressure along the sens, or energy lines, with stretching of joints.

Therapeutic Touch: developed by Dolores Krieger, PhD, RN, and Dora Kunz, RN; uses the hands on and above the body to transmit healing energy; used to accelerate wound healing and recovery from surgery and to relieve anxiety and pain.

Touch for Health: *see* Applied Kinesiology

Traditional Chinese Medicine: practiced for 3,000 years to treat mind, body, and spirit with herbal medicine, acupuncture, diet and lifestyle awareness, body movement, massage, and breathing exercises to maintain a balanced energy system and the free flow of chi along pathways of energy.

Trager: developed by Milton Trager, MD; gentle movements to loosen and release restrictions in joints and muscles; facilitates deep relaxation and flexibility.

Trigger Point Therapy: specific pressure to trigger points, extremely sensitive areas of pain or muscle spasm; used to release muscle tension and restore circulation.

Tui Na: Chinese massage to harmonize energy and treat injuries, disease, and dysfunction.

Visualization: the use of mental images for deep relaxation, to stimulate the immune system, and to influence positive physiological and psychological well-being.

Yoga: Sanskrit word meaning "union," promotes the flow of life energy, or prana, through breathing exercises (pranayama), movement and physical postures (asanas), and meditation to unite body, mind, and spirit.

Zero Balancing: developed by Fritz Smith, MD; integrates gentle manipulative techniques with movement to balance body energy with body structure.

U.S. SCHOOLS

ALABAMA

Birmingham

1. The PATH Foundation, Birmingham
1207 18th Ave S, Birmingham, AL 35205
Phone: (205) 322-7284; *Fax:* (281) 359-5700
E-mail: email@pathfoundation.com *Internet:* http:/
/www.pathfoundation.com
Program Administrator: Ed R. Martin, PhD, Dir.
  Admissions Contact: Cheryl W. Martin, CHt,
  Admissions Dir.
Year Established: 1989.
Staff: Full-time: 2.
Avg Enrollment: 24. *Avg Class Size:* 12. *Number
  of Graduates per Year:* 24.
Wheelchair Access: No.
Accreditation/Approval/Licensing: International
  Medical and Dental Hypnotherapy Association.
Field of Study: Hypnotherapy*. *Program
  Name/Length:* Hypnotherapy and Cell Com-
  mand Therapy Certification, 1 yr; Forensic Hyp-
  nosis Certification, 50 hrs.
Degrees Offered: Certificate.
License/Certification Preparation: American
  Board of Clinical Hypnosis; American Council
  of Hypnotist Examiners; International Medical
  and Dental Hypnotherapy Association; National
  Guild of Hypnotists.
Admission Requirements: Min age: 18; High
  school diploma/GED.

Application Deadline(s): Fall: Sep; Winter: Feb.

2. Red Mountain Institute for the Healing Arts, Inc
1900 20th Ave S, Ste 220, Birmingham, AL 35209
Phone: (205) 836-2024; *Fax:* (205) 278-8802
Program Administrator: Kitty Flewelling, Dir. *Ad-
  missions Contact:* Kitty Flewelling.
Year Established: 1994.
Staff: Full-time: 4; Part-time: 6.
Avg Enrollment: 25. *Avg Class Size:* 15. *Number
  of Graduates per Year:* 25.
Wheelchair Access: Yes.
Accreditation/Approval/Licensing: State board: AL
  Board of Ed.
Field of Study: Ayurvedic Medicine; Deep Tissue
  Massage; Massage Therapy*; Neuromuscular
  Therapy; Swedish Massage*. *Program
  Name/Length:* Clinical Massage Therapy
  Training, 1 yr.
Degrees Offered: Certificate.
License/Certification Preparation: National Certif-
  ication Board for Therapeutic Massage and
  Bodywork.
Tuition and Fees: $5800.
Financial Aid: Payment plan; State government
  aid; Vocational rehabilitation.
Career Services: Career counseling; Career infor-
  mation; Internships.

ALASKA

Anchorage

3. Gatekey School of Mind-Body Integration Studies
Massage Apprentice Program
4041 B St, Fl 300, Anchorage, AK 99503-5945
Phone: (907) 561-7327; *Fax:* (907) 561-6582
Program Administrator: Nancy Reeve, Carol
  Stiles, Co-owners. *Admissions Contact:* Carol
  Stiles.
Year Established: 1982.
Staff: Full-time: 2; Part-time: 15.
Avg Enrollment: 100. *Avg Class Size:* 10-20. *Num-
  ber of Graduates per Year:* 50.
Wheelchair Access: Yes.

Field of Study: Body-Mind Integration; Energy
  Work*; Massage Therapy*; Reiki. *Program
  Name/Length:* Massage I (with Human Sci-
  ences), 2.5 mos; Massage II (with Anatomy and
  Physiology), 2.5 mos; Massage Apprentice Pro-
  gram, 1 or 2 yrs; Medical-Centered Massage
  Therapy, 2.5 mos.
Degrees Offered: Certificate.
License/Certification Preparation: National Certif-
  ication Board for Therapeutic Massage and
  Bodywork.
Admission Requirements: Min age: 18; High
  school diploma/GED Min GPA: 2.0; Some col-
  lege preferred.
Application Deadline(s): Winter: Dec.

Tuition and Fees: $600 + $65 books (Massage I, II); $6000-$8000 + $500 books (Massage Apprentice); $300 + $25 books (Medical-Centered Massage Therapy).
Financial Aid: State government aid.
Career Services: Career counseling; Community Business Project.

Juneau

4. Acupressure Institute of Alaska
119 Second St, Juneau, AK 99801
Phone: (907) 463-5560
Program Administrator: Alexander Majewski, Dir.
   Admissions Contact: Alexander Majewski.
Year Established: 1988.
Staff: Full-time: 1; Part-time: 3.
Avg Enrollment: 12. *Avg Class Size:* 12. *Number of Graduates per Year:* 7.
Wheelchair Access: Yes.

Accreditation/Approval/Licensing: American Oriental Bodywork Therapy Association; Jin Shin Do Foundation.
Field of Study: Acupressure*; Aromatherapy; CranioSacral Therapy; Jin Shin Do*; Qigong; Shiatsu*. *Program Name/Length:* Jin Shin Do Body-Mind Acupressure, 330 hrs, 8-12 mos; Oriental Bodywork Therapy, 500 hrs, 1 yr.
Degrees Offered: Certificate.
License/Certification Preparation: National Certification Commission for Acupuncture and Oriental Medicine; American Oriental Bodywork Therapy Association.
Admission Requirements: Min age: 18; High school diploma/GED.
Application Deadline(s): Summer.
Tuition and Fees: $2400.
Financial Aid: Work study.
Career Services: Career counseling; Interview set up; Internships.

ARIZONA

Cottonwood

5. Arizona School of Integrative Studies
753 N Main St, Cottonwood, AZ 86326
Phone: (520) 639-3455; *Fax:* (520) 639-3694
E-mail: nmatthews@sedona.net
Program Administrator: Jamie Rongo, Co-Dir; Joseph Rongo, Co-Dir; Nancy Matthews, Co-Dir.
   Admissions Contact: Jamie Rongo; Joseph Rongo; Nancy Matthews.
Year Established: 1995.
Staff: Full-time: 3; Part-time: 8.
Avg Enrollment: 36. *Avg Class Size:* 18. *Number of Graduates per Year:* 36.
Wheelchair Access: Yes.
Accreditation/Approval/Licensing: State board: AZ Board for Private Postsecondary Ed; Accrediting Council for Continuing Education and Training; National Certification Board for Therapeutic Massage and Bodywork (CEUs).
Field of Study: Acupressure; Aromatherapy; CranioSacral Therapy; Energy Work; Homeopathy; Hydrotherapy*; Massage Therapy*; Polarity Therapy; Qigong; Reflexology; Shiatsu; Sports Massage*; Structural Integration*. *Program Name/Length:* Massage and Hydrotherapy, 750 hrs, 6 mos; Structural Integration, 200 hrs, 5 wks; Sports Massage Certification, 100 hrs, 3 mos; Massage and Movement Workshops, weekends.
Degrees Offered: CEUs; Certificate.

License/Certification Preparation: National Certification Board for Therapeutic Massage and Bodywork.
Admission Requirements: Min age: 18; High school diploma/GED; Specific course prerequisites: Massage experience required for Sports Massage and Structural Integration.
Application Deadline(s): Fall: Sep; Spring: Mar.
Tuition and Fees: $5500 (Massage and Hydrotherapy); $1700 (Structural Integration); $500 (Sports Massage).
Financial Aid: Vocational rehabilitation; Job Training Partnership Act.
Career Services: Career information.

Mesa

6. Institute for Natural Therapeutics, Inc
Massage Therapy Certification
217 W University Dr, Mesa, AZ 85201
Phone: (602) 844-2255; *Fax:* (602) 962-9907
Program Administrator: Rhonda J. Marinakis, Dir.
   Admissions Contact: Amy K. Hatch, Admin.
Year Established: 1988.
Staff: Part-time: 14.
Avg Enrollment: 60. *Avg Class Size:* 10. *Number of Graduates per Year:* 40.
Wheelchair Access: No.
Field of Study: Aromatherapy; CranioSacral Therapy; Deep Tissue Massage; Massage Therapy*; Reflexology; Reiki; Shiatsu. *Program*

Name/Length: Level I, 200 hrs; Level II, 500 hrs, 9 mos; Level III, 1000 hrs, 13-16 mos.
Degrees Offered: Certificate.
Admission Requirements: High school diploma/GED.
Application Deadline(s): Fall: Sep; Winter: Jan; Spring: Mar; Summer: Jul.
Tuition and Fees: $1600 (Level I); $3600 (Level II); $5500 (Level III); includes books.
Financial Aid: School financing.
Career Services: Career information; Job information.

Phoenix

7. International Yoga Studies
Yoga Teacher Training and Certification Program
13833 S 31st Pl, Phoenix, AZ 85048
Phone: (602) 759-1972; *Fax:* (602) 704-9656
E-mail: iysusa@aol.com
Program Administrator: Terry Ganem, Prog Admin. *Admissions Contact:* Sandra Summerfield Kozak, Dir.
Year Established: 1996.
Avg Class Size: 20.
Field of Study: Ayurvedic Medicine; Yoga Teacher Training*. *Program Name/Length:* 4 yrs, with Intensive course taken each yr.
Degrees Offered: Diploma; Certificate.
Admission Requirements: Min age: 18; High school diploma/GED; Specific course prerequisites: Intensive course; 2 yrs yoga training.
Tuition and Fees: $500 per yr + $500 per Intensive.
Financial Aid: Work study.
Career Services: Internships.

Scottsdale

8. Jin Shin Jyutsu, Inc
8719 E San Alberto Dr, Scottsdale, AZ 85258
Phone: (602) 998-9331; *Fax:* (602) 998-9335
Internet: http://www.jinshinjyutsu.com
Program Administrator: David Burmeister, Dir.
   Admissions Contact: Karen Moore, Office Mgr.
Year Established: 1974.
Staff: Full-time: 8.
Avg Enrollment: 1500. *Avg Class Size:* 25. *Number of Graduates per Year:* 500.
Accreditation/Approval/Licensing: National Certification Board for Therapeutic Massage and Bodywork (CEUs).
Field of Study: Jin Shin Jyutsu*. *Program Name/Length:* Basic Training, 5 days (repeat 3 times for certification); Now Know Myself Advanced Training, 5 days; Seminars given in various locations.
Degrees Offered: Certificate.
Admission Requirements: Specific course prerequisites: Basic Training required for Advanced Training.

Tuition and Fees: $300-$600 per course.

9. Phoenix Institute of Herbal Medicine and Acupuncture
7501 E Oak, Ste 114-115, Scottsdale, AZ 85257
Mailing Address: PO Box 2659, Scottsdale, AZ 85252
Phone: (602) 994-3648; *Fax:* (602) 439-1511
E-mail: contactus@pihma.com *Internet:* http://www.pihma.com
Program Administrator: Catherine Niemiec, Dir.
   Admissions Contact: Mary Beth Madden, Admissions.
Year Established: 1996.
Staff: Full-time: 3; Part-time: 7.
Avg Enrollment: 15. *Avg Class Size:* 15. *Number of Graduates per Year:* 10.
Wheelchair Access: Yes.
Accreditation/Approval/Licensing: State board: AZ Board for Private Postsecondary Ed; Candidate: Accreditation Commission for Acupuncture and Oriental Medicine.
Field of Study: Acupuncture*; Herbal Medicine*; Traditional Chinese Medicine*. *Program Name/Length:* Master of Science in Acupuncture and Oriental Medicine, 3-4 yrs; Seminars given in various locations; Master of Science in Chinese Herbology; Home study/Correspondence.
Degrees Offered: MS.
License/Certification Preparation: National Certification Commission for Acupuncture and Oriental Medicine.
Admission Requirements: High school diploma/GED; Some college (2 yrs).
Application Deadline(s): Winter: Jan; Summer: May.
Tuition and Fees: $2000 per semester.
Financial Aid: Loans; Scholarships; Work study; Payment plan.
Career Services: Career counseling; Internships.

10. Phoenix Therapeutic Massage College
609 N Scottsdale Rd, Scottsdale, AZ 85257
Phone: (480) 945-9461; *Fax:* (480) 425-8247
Program Administrator: Jean Murphy, Dir. *Admissions Contact:* Rose Taylor, Dir of Admissions.
Year Established: 1981.
Staff: Part-time: 22.
Avg Enrollment: 200. *Avg Class Size:* 21.
Wheelchair Access: Yes.
Accreditation/Approval/Licensing: State board: AZ Board for Private Postsecondary Ed; Accrediting Council for Continuing Education and Training.
Field of Study: Massage Therapy*; Swedish Massage*. *Program Name/Length:* Therapeutic Massage, 750 hrs, 38 wks/days or 48 wks/evenings; Professional Certification, 1125 hrs, 57-62 wks.
Degrees Offered: Diploma; Certificate.
Admission Requirements: Min age: 17; High school diploma/GED; Min GPA: 2.0.

Tuition and Fees: $6506 (Therapeutic Massage); $9316 (Professional Certification); includes books, table, supplies.

Financial Aid: Federal government aid; Grants; Loans; Payment plan; Scholarships; State government aid.

Career Services: Career development class; Externships.

11. RainStar College
4130 N Goldwater Blvd, Scottsdale, AZ 85251
Phone: (602) 423-0375; *Fax:* (602) 945-9824
Program Administrator: Edvard R. Richards, Dir. *Admissions Contact:* Denise Willey, Dir of Admissions.
Year Established: 1994.
Staff: Full-time: 6; Part-time: 30.
Avg Enrollment: 300. *Avg Class Size:* 20. *Number of Graduates per Year:* 200.
Wheelchair Access: Yes.
Accreditation/Approval/Licensing: State board: AZ Board for Private Postsecondary Ed; International Massage and Somatic Therapies Accreditation Council.
Field of Study: Acupressure; Aromatherapy; Breathwork; Chinese Herbal Medicine; CranioSacral Therapy; Geriatric Massage; Herbal Medicine; Homeopathy; Hydrotherapy; Hypnotherapy; Iridology; Lymphatic Massage; Massage Therapy*; Myofascial Release; On-Site Massage; Oriental Medicine; Pediatric Massage; Pregnancy Massage; Qigong; Reflexology; Reiki; Shiatsu; Spa Therapies; Sports Massage; Traditional Chinese Medicine; Trigger Point Therapy. *Program Name/Length:* Massage Therapist: Basic, 200 hrs, 2 mos; Advanced, 750 hrs, 5-10 mos; Masters, 500 hrs, 4-7 mos; Masters Graduate, 1000 hrs, 7-14 mos.
Admission Requirements: Min age: 18; High school diploma/GED.
Tuition and Fees: $1495-$6495.
Financial Aid: Loans; Scholarships; State government aid; VA approved; Vocational rehabilitation; Payment plan.
Career Services: Career counseling; Career information.

12. Southwest Institute of Healing Arts
1402 N Miller Rd, Ste D-2, Scottsdale, AZ 85257
Phone: (602) 994-9244; *Fax:* (602) 994-3228
E-mail: doyourdream@swiha.org *Internet:* http://www.swiha.org
Program Administrator: K.C. Miller, Dir. *Admissions Contact:* Carol Pilote, Student Svcs Rep.
Year Established: 1992.
Staff: Full-time: 4; Part-time: 30.
Avg Enrollment: 350. *Avg Class Size:* 16. *Number of Graduates per Year:* 350.
Accreditation/Approval/Licensing: State board: AZ Board for Private Postsecondary Ed; American Polarity Therapy Association; National Certification Board for Therapeutic Massage and Bodywork (CEUs).
Field of Study: Acupressure; Acupuncture; Aromatherapy; Ayurvedic Medicine; Body-Mind Psychology*; Childbirth Educator*; CranioSacral Therapy; Doula*; Energy Work; Equine Massage*; Herbal Medicine*; Holistic Health*; Hypnotherapy*; Massage Therapy*; Oriental Medicine; Polarity Therapy*; Qigong; Reflexology*; Reiki; Shiatsu*; Sports Massage; Traditional Chinese Medicine; Yoga Teacher Training. *Program Name/Length:* Massage Therapy, 200 hrs or 500 hrs, 3-9 mos; Oriental Bodywork Practitioner, 500 hrs; Equine Massage, 300 hrs; Holistic Health Care Practitioner, 1200 hrs; Western Herbalism, 500 hrs; Childbirth Educator, 200 hrs; Doula: Labor Support Professional, 100 hrs; Hypnotherapy, 100 hrs; Body-Mind Psychology, 1200 hrs.
Degrees Offered: CEUs; Diploma; Certificate; Associate of Occupational Studies.
License/Certification Preparation: American Council of Hypnotist Examiners; American Oriental Bodywork Therapy Association; National Certification Board for Therapeutic Massage and Bodywork; American Polarity Therapy Association.
Admission Requirements: Min age: 18; High school diploma/GED.
Tuition and Fees: $7.50-$10 per hr.
Financial Aid: Loans; Scholarships; Work study; Vocational rehabilitation; Job Training Partnership Act.
Career Services: Career counseling; Career information.

Sedona

13. The Foundation for Holistic Health Therapy
School of Lymphatic Massage
80 Farmer Brothers Dr, Sedona, AZ 86336
Mailing Address: PO Box 256, Sedona, AZ 86339
Phone: (520) 204-1968, (800) 578-7312; *Fax:* (520) 204-1968
E-mail: drbrown@cybertrails.com *Internet:* http://www.sedona-web.com/Lymphatic
Program Administrator: William N. Brown, PhD, Dir. *Admissions Contact:* William N. Brown.
Year Established: 1988.
Staff: Full-time: 2.
Avg Enrollment: 16. *Avg Class Size:* 8. *Number of Graduates per Year:* 16.
Wheelchair Access: Yes.
Field of Study: Energy Work; Lymphatic Massage*. *Program Name/Length:* Basic Course, 25 hrs, 3 days; Intermediate Course, 25 hrs, 3 days; Advanced Course, 25 hrs, 3 days.
Degrees Offered: Certificate.
Admission Requirements: Min age: 18.
Tuition and Fees: $550 per course.

Career Services: Career counseling; Career information; Internships.

Tempe

14. Southwest College of Naturopathic Medicine and Health Sciences

2140 E Broadway Rd, Tempe, AZ 85282
Phone: (602) 858-9100; *Fax:* (602) 858-9116
E-mail: admissions@scnm.edu *Internet:* http://www.scnm.edu
Program Administrator: Kareen O'Brien, ND, Dean of Naturopathic Medicine. *Admissions Contact:* Melissa Winquist, Dir of Recruitment and Admissions.
Year Established: 1994.
Staff: Full-time: 18; Part-time: 21.
Avg Enrollment: 90. *Number of Graduates per Year:* 50.
Wheelchair Access: Yes.
Accreditation/Approval/Licensing: State board: AZ Board of Private and Postsecondary Ed; Candidacy, Council on Naturopathic Medical Education.
Field of Study: Acupuncture*; Naturopathic Medicine*. *Program Name/Length:* Master's Level Certificate in Acupuncture, 3 yrs; Naturopathic Medicine, 4 yrs.
Degrees Offered: ND; Certificate.
License/Certification Preparation: State: AZ Naturopathic Medical Board Exam; National Certification Commission for Acupuncture and Oriental Medicine; Naturopathic Physicians Licensing Exam.
Admission Requirements: Some college (2 yrs) for Acupuncture; Bachelor's degree; Min GPA: 2.5, for ND; Specific course prerequisites: English, psychology, biology, chemistry; 3 letters of recommendation.
Application Deadline(s): Fall: Jul 1; Spring: Jan 1.
Financial Aid: Federal government aid; Loans; Work study.
Career Services: Residencies; Vacancy listings posted.

Tucson

15. Desert Institute of the Healing Arts

639 N 6th Ave, Tucson, AZ 87505-8330
Phone: (520) 882-0899, (800) 733-8098; *Fax:* (520) 624-2996
E-mail: diha@azstarnet.com *Internet:* http://www.diha.com
Program Administrator: Margaret Avery Moon, Owner/Dir. *Admissions Contact:* Dave Shahan, Admissions Dir.
Year Established: 1982.
Staff: Part-time: 40.
Avg Enrollment: 136. *Avg Class Size:* 25. *Number of Graduates per Year:* 128.

Wheelchair Access: No.
Accreditation/Approval/Licensing: State board: AZ Board for Private Postsecondary Ed; Commission on Massage Therapy Accreditation; Accrediting Commission of Career Schools and Colleges of Technology; National Certification Board for Therapeutic Massage and Bodywork (CEUs).
Field of Study: Aromatherapy; Hydrotherapy; Massage Therapy*; Reflexology; Shiatsu*; Sports Massage. *Program Name/Length:* Zen Shiatsu, 650 hrs, 10 mos; Massage Therapy, 1000 hrs, 10 mos.
Degrees Offered: Certificate.
License/Certification Preparation: National Certification Board for Therapeutic Massage and Bodywork.
Admission Requirements: Min age: 21 or parental consent; High school diploma/GED.
Application Deadline(s): Fall: Aug 1; Winter: Dec 1; Spring: Apr 1.
Tuition and Fees: $5655-$8700 per yr.
Financial Aid: Federal government aid; Grants; Loans; State government aid.
Career Services: Career counseling; Career information.

16. International Foundation of Bio-Magnetics

Bio-Magnetic Touch Healing
5447 E 5th St, Ste 111, Tucson, AZ 85711
Phone: (520) 751-7751; *Fax:* (520) 751-7751
E-mail: greet@flash.net *Internet:* http://www.planet-hawaii.com/bio-magnetics
Program Administrator: Paul Bucky, Pres. *Admissions Contact:* John Munno, Dir.
Year Established: 1991.
Staff: Part-time: 24.
Avg Enrollment: 50. *Avg Class Size:* 12. *Number of Graduates per Year:* 50.
Wheelchair Access: Yes.
Accreditation/Approval/Licensing: State board: HI Nurses Association.
Field of Study: Bio-Magnetic Touch Healing*; Energy Work*. *Program Name/Length:* Practitioner Training, 12 hrs; Certification, 24 hrs classroom + 60 hrs hands on; Seminars given in various locations.
Degrees Offered: CEUs; Certificate.
Tuition and Fees: $450 (Certification).
Career Services: Internships.

17. Bonnie Prudden School of Physical Fitness and Myotherapy, LLC

4725 E Sunrise Dr, Ste 346, Tucson, AZ 85718
Phone: (520) 529-3979, (800) 221-4634; *Fax:* (520) 529-6679
E-mail: info@bonnieprudden.com *Internet:* http://www.bonnieprudden.com
Program Administrator: Bonnie Prudden, Dir.
Year Established: 1979.
Staff: Full-time: 3; Part-time: 11.

Avg Enrollment: 15. *Avg Class Size:* 15. *Number of Graduates per Year:* 15.
Wheelchair Access: Yes.
Accreditation/Approval/Licensing: State board: AZ Board for Private Postsecondary Ed.
Field of Study: Exercise Therapy; Myotherapy*. *Program Name/Length:* Bonnie Prudden Myotherapy and Exercise Therapy, 1300 hrs, 9 mos.
Degrees Offered: Diploma; Certificate.
License/Certification Preparation: National Certification Board for Therapeutic Massage and Bodywork.
Admission Requirements: Min age: 18; High school diploma/GED.

18. University of Arizona, College of Medicine

Program in Integrative Medicine
1249 N Mountain, Tucson, AZ 85724-5153
Mailing Address: PO Box 245153, Tucson, AZ 85724-5153
Phone: (520) 626-7222; *Fax:* (520) 626-6484
Internet: http://www.ahsc.arizona.edu/ integrative_medicine
Program Administrator: Andrew Weil, MD. *Admissions Contact:* Colleen O. Grochowski, MA, Asst Dir.
Year Established: 1996.
Staff: Part-time: 25.
Avg Enrollment: 8. *Avg Class Size:* 4. *Number of Graduates per Year:* 4.
Wheelchair Access: Yes.
Field of Study: Integrative Medicine*. *Program Name/Length:* Fellowship (2 yrs).

Admission Requirements: Medical degree; Completed residency in primary care.
Application Deadline(s): Summer: Sep.
Comments: The Program in Integrated Medicine contains exposure to most areas of alternative health care and medicine.

19. Wesland Institute

Clinical Hypnotherapy; Neuro-Linguistic Programming
3367 N Country Club Rd, Tucson, AZ 85716-1349
Phone: (520) 881-1530; *Fax:* (520) 881-1530
E-mail: info@weslandinstitute.com *Internet:* http:/ /www.weslandinstitute.com
Program Administrator: Richard Corvino, MA, Dir of Ed. *Admissions Contact:* Richard Corvino.
Year Established: 1988.
Staff: Full-time: 1.
Avg Enrollment: 50. *Avg Class Size:* 10. *Number of Graduates per Year:* 45.
Wheelchair Access: No.
Accreditation/Approval/Licensing: State board: AZ Board for Private Postsecondary Ed.
Field of Study: Hypnotherapy*; Neuro-Linguistic Programming*. *Program Name/Length:* Hypnotherapy, 150 hrs, 1-3 mos; Neuro-Linguistic Programming, 50 hrs.
Degrees Offered: Diploma; Certificate.
Admission Requirements: Min age: 18; High school diploma/GED; Min GPA: 2.0.
Application Deadline(s): Fall: Sep; Winter: Feb; Spring: Apr; Summer: Jun.
Tuition and Fees: $1200.
Financial Aid: State government aid; Vocational rehabilitation; Payment plan.

ARKANSAS

Fayetteville

20. Center for Wellbeing

Polarity Therapy Training; Somatic Experiencing Training
101 W Mountain, Ste 107 GCM Bldg, Fayetteville, AR 72701
Mailing Address: PO Box 3698, Fayetteville, AR 72702
Phone: (501) 442-2026; *Fax:* (501) 442-2897
E-mail: cbeckerphd@aol.com
Program Administrator: Chandana Becker, PhD, Dir/Instr. *Admissions Contact:* Chandana Becker.
Year Established: 1992.
Staff: Full-time: 1; Part-time: 2.
Avg Enrollment: 35. *Avg Class Size:* 12. *Number of Graduates per Year:* 10.

Wheelchair Access: Yes.
Accreditation/Approval/Licensing: American Polarity Therapy Association; Foundation For Human Enrichment.
Field of Study: Polarity Therapy*; Somatic Experiencing (Shock Trauma Renegotiation Therapy)*. *Program Name/Length:* Associate Polarity Practitioner, 6 mos; Registered Polarity Practitioner, 2 yrs; Somatic Experiencing Practitioner, 3 yrs.
Degrees Offered: Diploma; Certificate.
License/Certification Preparation: APP and RPP; American Polarity Therapy Association; SEP certification; Foundation For Human Enrichment.
Admission Requirements: Min age: 18; High school diploma/GED; Specific course prerequisites: APP required for RPP training; Health or

helping professional prior to entering Somatic Experiencing training.

Tuition and Fees: $1500 (APP); $3000 per yr (RPP); $1500+ per yr (Somatic).

Financial Aid: Work study.

Career Services: Career counseling; Career information; Clinical supervision and professional consultation.

21. White River School of Massage

Professional Training Program
48 Colt Square Dr, Fayetteville, AR 72703
Phone: (501) 521-2550; *Fax:* (501) 521-2558
Internet: http://www.wrsm.com
Program Administrator: Ellen May, MTI, Dir. *Admissions Contact:* Denise Stramel, Office Mgr.
Year Established: 1991.
Staff: Full-time: 2; Part-time: 10.
Avg Enrollment: 96. *Avg Class Size:* 24. *Number of Graduates per Year:* 90.
Wheelchair Access: Yes.
Accreditation/Approval/Licensing: State board: AR Board of Massage Therapy; National Certification Board for Therapeutic Massage and Bodywork (CEUs).
Field of Study: Aromatherapy; CranioSacral Therapy; Energy Work; Massage Therapy*; Myofascial Release; Neuromuscular Therapy; Reflexology; Shiatsu; Sports Massage. *Program Name/Length:* 500 hrs, 7 mos/days, 10 mos/weekends, or 4 mos/summer intensive.
Degrees Offered: CEUs; Diploma.
License/Certification Preparation: State: AR Licensed Massage Therapist; National Certification Board for Therapeutic Massage and Bodywork.
Application Deadline(s): Fall: Aug 1; Winter: Dec 1; Summer: Apr 1.
Tuition and Fees: $3600.
Financial Aid: State government aid; VA approved; Vocational rehabilitation; Payment plans; discount for prepayment.
Career Services: Career counseling; Career information; Internships.

Fort Smith

22. A Healing Touch, Inc, Clinic and School of Massage Therapy

2201 Rogers Ave, Ste F, Fort Smith, AR 72901
Phone: (501) 783-7566
E-mail: touchwlm@gte.net
Program Administrator: Wendy L. Morgan, Pres. *Admissions Contact:* Wendy L. Morgan.
Year Established: 1997.
Staff: Full-time: 3.
Avg Enrollment: 20. *Avg Class Size:* 7. *Number of Graduates per Year:* 20.
Wheelchair Access: Yes.
Accreditation/Approval/Licensing: State board:.

Field of Study: Acupressure; Aromatherapy; CranioSacral Therapy; Deep Tissue Massage; Energy Work; Herbal Medicine; Hypnotherapy; Massage Therapy*; Shiatsu; Traditional Chinese Medicine. *Program Name/Length:* 525 hrs.
Degrees Offered: Diploma.
License/Certification Preparation: State: AR Licensed Massage Therapist.
Admission Requirements: Min age: 18; High school diploma/GED.
Application Deadline(s): Fall; Spring.
Tuition and Fees: $3200 (includes books).
Financial Aid: Loans.
Career Services: Career counseling; Career information.

Hot Springs

23. Jean's School of Therapy Technology, Inc

Massage Therapy
655 Park Ave, Hot Springs, AR 71901
Phone: (501) 623-9686; *Fax:* (501) 623-0070
Program Administrator: Jean R. Miller, Pres. *Admissions Contact:* Jean R. Miller.
Year Established: 1984.
Staff: Full-time: 2.
Avg Enrollment: 45. *Avg Class Size:* 15. *Number of Graduates per Year:* 45.
Wheelchair Access: Yes.
Accreditation/Approval/Licensing: State board: AR Board of Massage Therapy.
Field of Study: Acupressure; Deep Tissue Massage; Massage Therapy*; Reflexology; Reiki; Shiatsu. *Program Name/Length:* 500 hrs, 4-6 mos; Seminars given in various locations.
Degrees Offered: Diploma.
License/Certification Preparation: State: AR Licensed Massage Therapist.
Admission Requirements: Min age: 18; High school diploma/GED.
Tuition and Fees: $3000.
Financial Aid: State government aid; VA approved.
Career Services: Career counseling; Career information.

Little Rock

24. American Academy of Healing Arts

School of Massage Therapy
1501 N University, Ste 570, Little Rock, AR 72207
Phone: (501) 666-9100, (888) 666-9101; *Fax:* (501) 666-3133
Program Administrator: Martha Kimbrough, MTI, Dir. *Admissions Contact:* Eileen Joyce, LMT, Admissions Counselor.
Year Established: 1996.
Staff: Full-time: 2; Part-time: 12.

Avg Enrollment: 26. *Avg Class Size:* 10. *Number of Graduates per Year:* 26.
Wheelchair Access: Yes.
Accreditation/Approval/Licensing: State board: AR Board of Massage Therapy.
Field of Study: CranioSacral Therapy; Deep Tissue Massage; Energy Work; Hydrotherapy*; Massage Therapy*; Polarity Therapy; Reflexology*; Shiatsu. *Program Name/Length:* Licensed Massage Therapy, 500 hrs.
Degrees Offered: Diploma.
License/Certification Preparation: State: AR Licensed Massage Therapist; National Certification Board for Therapeutic Massage and Bodywork.
Admission Requirements: Min age: 18; Negative TB test; signed physician's statement of good health.
Tuition and Fees: $3400.
Financial Aid: Loans; Work study; Vocational rehabilitation.
Career Services: Career counseling; Career information; Internships.

25. Body Wellness Therapeutic Massage Academy

11323 Arcade Dr, Ste D, Little Rock, AR 72212
Phone: (501) 219-BODY (2639); *Fax:* (501) 221-7626
E-mail: bodywellness@aristotle.net
Program Administrator: Donna McGriff, Dir. *Admissions Contact:* Renate Paul, Office Mgr.
Year Established: 1995.
Staff: Full-time: 2; Part-time: 8.
Avg Enrollment: 40. *Avg Class Size:* 12. *Number of Graduates per Year:* 40.
Wheelchair Access: Yes.
Accreditation/Approval/Licensing: State board: AR Board of Massage Therapy.
Field of Study: Acupressure; Aromatherapy; Ayurvedic Medicine; Deep Muscle Massage*; Energy Work; Massage Therapy*; Myofascial Release; Polarity Therapy; Reflexology; Reiki; Sports Massage; Swedish Massage*. *Program Name/Length:* Massage Therapy, 5 mos.

Degrees Offered: Diploma.
License/Certification Preparation: State: AR Licensed Massage Therapist; National Certification Board for Therapeutic Massage and Bodywork.
Admission Requirements: Min age: 18; High school diploma/GED.
Application Deadline(s): Fall: Sep 25; Winter: Dec 28; Spring: Mar 25; Summer: Jun 25.
Tuition and Fees: $3150.
Financial Aid: Loans; Work study; VA approved; Vocational rehabilitation.
Career Services: Career counseling; Career information; Resume service.

26. Hot Springs School of Therapy Technology

3000 Kavanaugh, Ste A, Little Rock, AR 72205
Mailing Address: 1415 N Moore Rd, Hot Springs, AR 71913
Phone: (800) 844-0667
Program Administrator: Ronald L. Wallace, Dir. *Admissions Contact:* Ronald L. Wallace.
Year Established: 1951.
Staff: Full-time: 4.
Avg Enrollment: 40. *Avg Class Size:* 15. *Number of Graduates per Year:* 30.
Wheelchair Access: Yes.
Accreditation/Approval/Licensing: State board: AR Board of Massage Therapy.
Field of Study: Acupressure; Aromatherapy; Herbal Medicine; Hydrotherapy; Massage Therapy*; Reflexology; Shiatsu. *Program Name/Length:* Massage Therapy, 500 hrs, 6 mos.
Degrees Offered: Diploma.
License/Certification Preparation: State: AR Licensed Massage Therapist.
Admission Requirements: Min age: 18; High school diploma/GED.
Application Deadline(s): Fall: Aug 15; Spring: Jan 1.
Tuition and Fees: $3250.
Career Services: Referral service.

CALIFORNIA

Anaheim

27. South Baylo University

1126 N Brookhurst St, Anaheim, CA 92801
Phone: (714) 533-1495; *Fax:* (714) 533-6040
E-mail: ron@sbu.edu *Internet:* http://www.sbu.edu

Program Administrator: Ronald Sokolsky, DiplAc, Prog Dir/Registrar. *Admissions Contact:* Ronald Sokolsky.
Year Established: 1977.
Staff: Full-time: 46.
Avg Enrollment: 280. *Avg Class Size:* 27. *Number of Graduates per Year:* 120.
Wheelchair Access: Yes.

Accreditation/Approval/Licensing: State board: CA Acupuncture Board; Accreditation Commission for Acupuncture and Oriental Medicine.
Field of Study: Acupuncture*; Herbal Medicine*; Qigong; Shiatsu; Traditional Chinese Medicine*; Tui Na. *Program Name/Length:* Master of Science in Traditional Oriental Medicine, 12 qtrs, 3 yrs.
Degrees Offered: BS; MS.
License/Certification Preparation: State: CA Licensed Acupuncturist; National Certification Commission for Acupuncture and Oriental Medicine.
Admission Requirements: Min age: 18; High school diploma/GED; Some college (60 units from accredited college or university, 2 yrs), Min GPA 2.25.
Application Deadline(s): Fall: Oct; Winter: Jan; Spring: Apr; Summer: Jul.
Tuition and Fees: $1360 per qtr.
Financial Aid: Federal government aid; Grants; State government aid; Work study; Vocational rehabilitation.
Career Services: Career counseling; Career information.
Comments: Branch campus located at 2727 W 6th St, Los Angeles, CA 90015; (213) 738-0712; Fax: (213) 480-1332.

28. West Pacific

Massage
434 N Lakeview Ave, Anaheim, CA 92807
Phone: (714) 998-8079; *Fax:* (714) 998-8079
Program Administrator: Joel Doti, Owner. *Admissions Contact:* Joel Doti.
Year Established: 1996.
Staff: Full-time: 2; Part-time: 1.
Avg Enrollment: 100. *Number of Graduates per Year:* 98.
Wheelchair Access: No.
Accreditation/Approval/Licensing: State board: CA Bureau of Private Postsecondary and Vocational Ed.
Field of Study: Deep Tissue Massage; Massage Therapy*; Sports Massage. *Program Name/Length:* 100-500 hrs; Seminars given in various locations; Home study/Correspondence.
Degrees Offered: Certificate.
License/Certification Preparation: City licensing.
Admission Requirements: Min age: 18.
Tuition and Fees: $450 (100 hrs).
Financial Aid: Loans.
Career Services: Internships; Interview set up.

Auburn

29. Dry Creek Herb Farm and Learning Center

13935 Dry Creek Rd, Auburn, CA 95602
Phone: (530) 878-2441; *Fax:* (530) 878-0613

Program Administrator: Shatoiya de la Tour, Dir of Ed. *Admissions Contact:* Rick de la Tour, Admissions Dir.
Year Established: 1988.
Staff: Full-time: 3; Part-time: 8.
Avg Enrollment: 100. *Avg Class Size:* 20. *Number of Graduates per Year:* 70.
Wheelchair Access: Yes.
Accreditation/Approval/Licensing: State board: CA Board of Registered Nursing; Accrediting Council for Continuing Education and Training.
Field of Study: Aromatherapy*; Ayurvedic Medicine; Energy Work; Herbal Medicine*; Qigong; Traditional Chinese Medicine. *Program Name/Length:* Internship, 4 mos; Apprenticeship, 9 mos (1 weekend/mo); Home study/Correspondence.
Degrees Offered: Certificate.
Tuition and Fees: $3800 (Internship); $1350 (Apprenticeship).
Financial Aid: Work study.
Career Services: Career counseling; Career information.

Berkeley

30. Acupressure Institute

Shiatsu, Massage and Asian Bodywork Trainings
1533 Shattuck Ave, Berkeley, CA 94709
Phone: (510) 845-1059; *Fax:* (510) 845-1496
E-mail: colburn@acupressure.com *Internet:* http://www.acupressure.com
Program Administrator: Pat Colburn, Admin. *Admissions Contact:* Peggy Vittovia, Admissions/Student Affairs.
Year Established: 1976.
Staff: Full-time: 6; Part-time: 24.
Avg Enrollment: 300. *Avg Class Size:* 16. *Number of Graduates per Year:* 200.
Wheelchair Access: No.
Accreditation/Approval/Licensing: Accrediting Council for Continuing Education and Training.
Field of Study: Acupressure*; Emotional Balancing; Energy Work; Massage Therapy*; Oriental Medicine; Shiatsu*; Sports Massage; Thai Massage*; Traditional Chinese Medicine; Yoga Teacher Training. *Program Name/Length:* Acupressure Basic Training Program, 150 hrs, 1-12 mos; Acupressure Specialization, 200 hrs, 1-24 mos; Acupressure Therapy, 850 hrs, 1-4 yrs.
Degrees Offered: Diploma; Certificate.
License/Certification Preparation: American Oriental Bodywork Therapy Association.
Admission Requirements: Min age: 18.
Tuition and Fees: $1250-$5600.
Financial Aid: Work study.
Career Services: Career information; Apprenticeship Trainings.

31. The Alexander Educational Center

St. John Presbyterian Church, 2727 College Ave, Rm 207, Berkeley, CA 94705
Mailing Address: 90 Island Ct, Walnut Creek, CA 94595
Phone: (925) 937-5746
Program Administrator: Giora Pinkas, Co-Dir; John Baron, Co-Dir. *Admissions Contact:* Giora Pinkas; John Baron.
Year Established: 1974.
Accreditation/Approval/Licensing: American Society for the Alexander Technique.
Field of Study: Alexander Technique. *Program Name/Length:* Teacher Training, 3 yrs.
License/Certification Preparation: American Society for the Alexander Technique.
Admission Requirements: Prior experience in the Alexander Technique; Lessons with directors recommended; 3 mo trial term.
Tuition and Fees: $1777 per term.

32. Feldenkrais Resources

Feldenkrais Professional Training Program
830 Bancroft Way, Ste 112, Berkeley, CA 94710
Phone: (510) 540-7600; *Fax:* (510) 540-7683
E-mail: feldenres@aol.com *Internet:* http://www.feldenkrais-resources.com
Program Administrator: Carol Kress, Admin. *Admissions Contact:* Carol Kress.
Year Established: 1983.
Staff: Full-time: 2; Part-time: 5.
Avg Enrollment: 50. *Avg Class Size:* 50. *Number of Graduates per Year:* 44.
Wheelchair Access: Yes.
Accreditation/Approval/Licensing: Feldenkrais Guild.
Field of Study: Feldenkrais*. *Program Name/Length:* Professional Training, 4 yrs.
Degrees Offered: Certificate.
License/Certification Preparation: Certified Feldenkrais Practitioner, Feldenkrais Guild.
Admission Requirements: Min age: 18.
Tuition and Fees: $3600 per yr.
Financial Aid: Work study; Vocational rehabilitation; Payment plan.

33. Meiji College of Oriental Medicine

Master of Science in Oriental Medicine
2550 Shattuck Ave, Berkeley, CA 94704
Phone: (510) 666-8248; *Fax:* (510) 666-0111
E-mail: meiji@pacbell.net
Program Administrator: Hirohisa Oda, Pres. *Admissions Contact:* Laura Pitre, Admissions Officer.
Year Established: 1990.
Staff: Full-time: 5; Part-time: 11.
Avg Enrollment: 60. *Avg Class Size:* 20. *Number of Graduates per Year:* 12.
Wheelchair Access: Yes.
Accreditation/Approval/Licensing: State board: CA Acupuncture Board; CA Bureau of Private Postsecondary and Vocational Ed; Accreditation Commission for Acupuncture and Oriental Medicine.
Field of Study: Acupuncture*; Herbal Medicine; Oriental Medicine*; Traditional Chinese Medicine. *Program Name/Length:* Master of Science in Oriental Medicine (includes Western Sciences), 3 yrs (maximum 6 yrs).
Degrees Offered: MSOM.
License/Certification Preparation: State: CA Licensed Acupuncturist; National Certification Commission for Acupuncture and Oriental Medicine.
Admission Requirements: Bachelor's degree; Min GPA: 2.5; Specific course prerequisites: general biology; chemistry, physics, psychology.
Application Deadline(s): Fall: Jul 31.
Tuition and Fees: $8200 per yr.
Financial Aid: Loans.
Career Services: Career information.

34. Movement Studies Institute

1832 Second St, Berkeley, CA 94710
Phone: (800) 342-3424; *Fax:* (510) 548-4349
E-mail: info@movementstudies.com *Internet:* http://www.movementstudies.com
Program Administrator: Dr. Frank Wildman, Dir. *Admissions Contact:* Kaellyn Moss, Prog Coord/Admin.
Year Established: 1984.
Avg Enrollment: 50. *Avg Class Size:* 40.
Accreditation/Approval/Licensing: Feldenkrais Guild.
Field of Study: Feldenkrais*. *Program Name/Length:* Practitioner Training, 4 yrs; Seminars given in various locations.
Degrees Offered: Diploma; Certificate.
License/Certification Preparation: Certified Feldenkrais Practitioner, Feldenkrais Guild; International Somatic Movement and Education Therapy Association.
Admission Requirements: High school diploma/GED.
Tuition and Fees: $3700+ per yr depending on location.
Financial Aid: Scholarships; Work study.

35. Pacific School of Herbal Medicine

PO Box 2194, Berkeley, CA 94702
Phone: (510) 845-4028
Admissions Contact: Adam Seller, Dir.
Year Established: 1987.
Staff: Full-time: 1; Part-time: 5.
Avg Class Size: 10. *Number of Graduates per Year:* 10.
Field of Study: Aromatherapy*; Ayurvedic Medicine; Herbal Medicine*. *Program Name/Length:* Clinical Herbal Medicine, 5-8 semesters.
Admission Requirements: Min age: 15.
Financial Aid: Scholarships.

Career Services: Career counseling; Career information.

36. reSource
825 Bancroft Way, Berkeley, CA 94702
Mailing Address: PO Box 5398, Berkeley, CA 94705
Phone: (510) 433-7917; *Fax:* (510) 841-3258
Program Administrator: Gail Stewart, Dir. *Admissions Contact:* Gail Stewart.
Year Established: 1982.
Staff: Part-time: 6.
Avg Enrollment: 20. *Avg Class Size:* 12. *Number of Graduates per Year:* 15.
Wheelchair Access: Yes.
Accreditation/Approval/Licensing: State board: CA Bureau of Private Postsecondary and Vocational Ed; Accrediting Council for Continuing Education and Training.
Field of Study: Deep Tissue Massage; Massage Therapy*; Ortho-Bionomy; Trager. *Program Name/Length:* Massage Practitioner, 1 yr; Bodywork Practitioner, 1-2 yrs; Advanced Bodywork Practitioner, 3-4 yrs.
Degrees Offered: Certificate.
Admission Requirements: Min age: 18.
Application Deadline(s): Fall: Sep 15.
Career Services: Career counseling; Career information.

37. Rosen Method: The Berkeley Center
Rosen Method Bodywork and Movement
825 Bancroft Way, Berkeley, CA 94710
Phone: (510) 845-6606; *Fax:* (510) 845-8114
E-mail: rosenmethod@batnet.com *Internet:* http://www.mcn.org/b/rosen/berkeley/Berkmm.htm
Program Administrator: Sara Webb, Exec Dir; Gloria Hessellund, Dir of Teaching. *Admissions Contact:* Abby Paige, Office Mgr.
Year Established: 1983.
Staff: Part-time: 9.
Avg Enrollment: 50. *Avg Class Size:* 18. *Number of Graduates per Year:* 20.
Wheelchair Access: Yes.
Accreditation/Approval/Licensing: State board: CA Bureau of Private Postsecondary and Vocational Ed; Rosen Institute.
Field of Study: Rosen Method Bodywork*. *Program Name/Length:* Rosen Method Bodywork Training, 3 yrs; Seminars given in various locations; Rosen Method Movement Training, 1 1/2 yrs.
Degrees Offered: Certificate.
Admission Requirements: Specific course prerequisites: Rosen Method introductory workshop.
Tuition and Fees: $2150 per yr.
Financial Aid: Scholarships.
Career Services: Referral service; Practice building seminar.

38. The School of Homeopathy
Homeopathic Educational Services (Correspondence Courses)
2124 Kittredge St, Berkeley, CA 94704
Phone: (510) 649-0294; *Fax:* (510) 649-1955
E-mail: mail@homeopathic.com *Internet:* http://www. homeopathic.com
Program Administrator: Stuart Gracie, Admin.
Year Established: 1985.
Accreditation/Approval/Licensing: Council on Homeopathic Education.
Field of Study: Homeopathy*. *Program Name/Length:* Foundation Course; Advanced Course; Home study/Correspondence.
Degrees Offered: Diploma.
License/Certification Preparation: Council for Homeopathic Certification; North American Society of Homeopaths.
Tuition and Fees: $1595 (1st yr); $1595 (2nd yr); $1095 (3rd yr); $3695 (Advance Payment); $100 registration fee.
Financial Aid: Payment plan.

Beverly Hills

39. International College of Homeopathy
600 Hour Classical Homeopathic Training
8306 Wilshire Blvd, Ste 728, Beverly Hills, CA 90211
Phone: (310) 645-0443; *Fax:* (310) 645-1814
E-mail: registrar@qvius.edu *Internet:* http://www. qvius.edu
Program Administrator: Cornella Franz, MD, Dean. *Admissions Contact:* Cherrie DeWonder, Registrar.
Year Established: 1990.
Staff: Part-time: 7.
Avg Enrollment: 100. *Avg Class Size:* 20. *Number of Graduates per Year:* 40.
Accreditation/Approval/Licensing: Candidate, Council on Homeopathic Education; National Board of Homeopathic Examiners.
Field of Study: Energy Work; Homeopathy*; Oriental Medicine. *Program Name/Length:* Classical Homeopathy, Level I, 2 yrs; Classical Homeopathy, Level II, 2 yrs.
Degrees Offered: CEUs; Certificate.
License/Certification Preparation: National Board of Homeopathic Examiners.
Admission Requirements: Medical degree or RN.
Application Deadline(s): Fall: Sep; Winter: Jan; Spring: Mar.
Tuition and Fees: $6600 per program.
Career Services: Referral service.

40. Quantum-Veritas International University Systems
8306 Wilshire Blvd, Ste 728, Beverly Hills, CA 90211
Phone: (310) 645-0443; *Fax:* (310) 645-1814

E-mail: registrar@qvius.edu Internet: http://www.
  qvius.edu
Program Administrator: Edwin C. Floyd, MS,
  Chancellor; Abbas Qutab, PhD, Dir of
  Ayurvedic Medicine; Roger Johansen, DC,
  Somiatry Prog Dir. Admissions Contact: Cherie
  DeWonder, Registrar.
Year Established: 1998.
Staff: Part-time: 25.
Avg Enrollment: 100. Avg Class Size: 25. Number
  of Graduates per Year: 50.
Wheelchair Access: Yes.
Field of Study: Acupressure; Aromatherapy;
  Ayurvedic Medicine*; CranioSacral Therapy;
  Deep Tissue Massage; Energy Work; Herbal
  Medicine*; Kinesiology; Massage Therapy*;
  Oriental Medicine; Polarity Therapy; Qigong;
  Reflexology*; Shiatsu*; Sports Massage; Tradi-
  tional Chinese Medicine; Yoga Teacher
  Training. Program Name/Length: Introduction
  to Somiatry, 100 hrs, 1 yr; Applied Clinical
  Somiatry, 100 hrs, 1 yr; Postgraduate Ayurvedic
  Medical Program, 60 hrs; Seminars given in var-
  ious locations; Seminar in Ayurvedic Medicine,
  216 hrs; Home study in Ayurvedic Medicine,
  384 hrs; Bio-Functional Medicine, 36 hrs-2 yrs.
Degrees Offered: Diploma; Certificate.
License/Certification Preparation: American Ori-
  ental Bodywork Therapy Association; American
  Reflexology Certification Board; National Cer-
  tification Board for Therapeutic Massage and
  Bodywork.
Admission Requirements: Min age: 18; High
  school diploma/GED; Medical degree required
  for Ayurvedic Medicine.
Application Deadline(s): Fall: Sep; Winter: Jan;
  Spring: Mar.

Big Sur

41. Esalen Institute
Hwy 1, Big Sur, CA 93920
Phone: (408) 667-3000; Fax: (408) 667-2724
Field of Study: Esalen Massage*.

Burbank

42. American Academy of Reflexology
606 E Magnolia Blvd, Ste B, Burbank, CA
  91501-2618
Phone: (818) 841-7741; Fax: (818) 841-2346
Program Administrator: Bill Flocco, Dir.
Year Established: 1981.
Staff: Full-time: 1; Part-time: 2.
Avg Enrollment: 48. Avg Class Size: 12. Number
  of Graduates per Year: 40.
Wheelchair Access: Yes.
Accreditation/Approval/Licensing: State board: CA
  Bureau of Private Postsecondary and Vocational
  Ed.

Field of Study: Reflexology*. Program
  Name/Length: Integrated Foot, Hand and Ear
  Reflexology, 200 hrs, 9 mos.
Degrees Offered: Certificate.
License/Certification Preparation: American
  Reflexology Certification Board; City and
  county licensing.
Admission Requirements: Min age: 18; Conversa-
  tional English.
Application Deadline(s): Fall: Aug; Winter: Jan.
Tuition and Fees: $1575.
Financial Aid: Work study.
Career Services: Career counseling; Career infor-
  mation.

Capitola

43. Zero Balancing Association
PO Box 1727, Capitola, CA 95010
Phone: (408) 476-0665; Fax: (408) 476-0665
E-mail: zbaoffice@aol.com Internet: http://www.
  zerobalancing.com
Program Administrator: Fritz Smith, MD, Curricu-
  lum Head; Bhasa Markman, Admin. Admissions
  Contact: Bhasa Markman, Admin.
Year Established: 1973.
Staff: Part-time: 34.
Avg Enrollment: 1000. Avg Class Size: 25. Num-
  ber of Graduates per Year: 30.
Accreditation/Approval/Licensing: State board: CA
  Acupuncture Board; CA Nurses Association;
  Accrediting Council for Continuing Education
  and Training; National Certification Board for
  Therapeutic Massage and Bodywork (CEUs).
Field of Study: Zero Balancing*. Program
  Name/Length: Core Zero Balancing I, 25 hrs, 4
  days; Core Zero Balancing II, 25 hrs, 4 days;
  Certification, 150 hrs, 18 mos-2 yrs; Seminars
  given in various locations.
Degrees Offered: Certificate.
Admission Requirements: Certified or licensed
  health care professional.
Financial Aid: Scholarships.

Cardiff

44. Reese Movement Institute, Inc
2187 Newcastle, Cardiff, CA 92007
Phone: (760) 436-9087; Fax: (760) 436-9141
E-mail: rmiinc@aol.com
Program Administrator: Mark Reese, Educational
  Dir. Admissions Contact: Donna Ray-Reese,
  Admin Dir.
Year Established: 1990.
Staff: Full-time: 3; Part-time visiting trainers and
  assistants.
Avg Enrollment: 45. Avg Class Size: 45. Number
  of Graduates per Year: 14.
Accreditation/Approval/Licensing: Feldenkrais
  Guild.

Field of Study: Feldenkrais*. *Program Name/Length:* Professional Training, 4 yrs.
Degrees Offered: Certificate.
License/Certification Preparation: Certified Feldenkrais Practitioner, Feldenkrais Guild.
Admission Requirements: Min age: 18; Specific course prerequisites: Feldenkrais Functional Integration and Awareness through Movement classes.
Tuition and Fees: $3600 per yr.

Carmel

45. Monterey Institute of Touch
27820 Dorris Dr, Carmel, CA 93923
Phone: (831) 624-1006; *Fax:* (831) 626-6916
E-mail: mit@redshift.com
Program Administrator: Birgit Ball-Eisner, Owner/Admin. *Admissions Contact:* Birgit Ball-Eisner.
Year Established: 1983.
Staff: Part-time: 15.
Avg Enrollment: 100. *Avg Class Size:* 20. *Number of Graduates per Year:* 75.
Wheelchair Access: Yes.
Accreditation/Approval/Licensing: Accrediting Council for Continuing Education and Training; National Certification Board for Therapeutic Massage and Bodywork (CEUs).
Field of Study: Acupressure; Aromatherapy; CranioSacral Therapy; Massage Therapy*; Polarity Therapy; Reflexology; Shiatsu; Sports Massage. *Program Name/Length:* Massage, 200 hrs, 5 wks (summer intensive), 14 wks (3 days/wk), or 5 mos (weekends or 2 evenings/wk); Intermediate Massage, 100 hrs; Advanced Massage, 100 hrs; Massage Therapist, 500 hrs.
Degrees Offered: Certificate.
Admission Requirements: Min age: 18; High school diploma/GED; Specific course prerequisites: basic math; Reading comprehension.
Tuition and Fees: $1000.
Career Services: Career information.

Chico

46. Chico Therapy: Wellness Center
State Certified Massage Program
1215 Mangrove Ave, Ste B, Chico, CA 95926
Phone: (530) 891-4301; *Fax:* (530) 891-4359
E-mail: chicothrpy@aol.com *Internet:* http://www.chicotherapy.com
Program Administrator: Mike L. Metzger, NMT, Dir. *Admissions Contact:* Mike L. Metzger.
Year Established: 1989.
Staff: Part-time: 5.
Avg Enrollment: 150. *Avg Class Size:* 12. *Number of Graduates per Year:* 150.
Wheelchair Access: Yes.

Accreditation/Approval/Licensing: State board: CA Bureau of Private Postsecondary and Vocational Ed.
Field of Study: Acupressure; Aromatherapy; Ayurvedic Medicine; Deep Tissue Massage; Herbal Medicine; Infant Massage*; Manual Lymph Drainage*; Massage Therapy*; Neuromuscular Therapy*; Prenatal Massage*; Reflexology; Shiatsu; Traditional Chinese Medicine. *Program Name/Length:* 100-500 hrs, weekends; Seminars given in various locations; Home study/Correspondence.
Degrees Offered: Certificate.
Admission Requirements: Min age: 16 with parental consent; High school diploma/GED; Must be Certified Massage Therapist for advanced classes.
Application Deadline(s): Fall: Sep 1; Winter: Jan 1; Spring: May 1.
Tuition and Fees: $8-$12 per hr.
Financial Aid: Discount for prepayment.
Career Services: Career counseling; Career information; Internships; Interview set up; Job placement.

Corte Madera

47. Diamond Light School of Massage and Healing Arts
45 San Clemente Dr, Corte Madera, CA 94928
Mailing Address: PO Box 5443, Mill Valley, CA 94942
Phone: (415) 454-6651
Program Administrator: Vajra Matusow, Dir. *Admissions Contact:* Vajra Matusow.
Year Established: 1987.
Staff: Full-time: 3; Part-time: 2.
Avg Enrollment: 50. *Avg Class Size:* 16. *Number of Graduates per Year:* 50.
Wheelchair Access: No.
Accreditation/Approval/Licensing: State board: CA Bureau of Private Postsecondary and Vocational Ed.
Field of Study: Acupressure; Energy Work; Hypnotherapy*; Massage Therapy*; Reflexology; Reiki; Swedish Massage*. *Program Name/Length:* Massage Therapist, 3 mos; Deep Bodywork Specialist, 3 mos; Hypnotherapist, 6 mos; Advanced Bodyworker, 1 yr.
Degrees Offered: Certificate.
License/Certification Preparation: National Certification Board for Therapeutic Massage and Bodywork.
Admission Requirements: Min age: 18 or parental consent.
Application Deadline(s): Fall: Sep 1; Winter: Jan 1; Spring: Mar 1.
Tuition and Fees: $600-$1495.
Financial Aid: Work study.

Career Services: Career counseling; Career information.

Costa Mesa

48. American Institute of Massage Therapy, Costa Mesa
2156 Newport Blvd, Costa Mesa, CA 92627
Phone: (949) 642-0735, 655-5555; *Fax:* (949) 642-1729
Program Administrator: M. K. Hungerford, PhD, Dean/Chancellor. *Admissions Contact:* M. K. Hungerford.
Year Established: 1989.
Staff: Full-time: 2; Part-time: 2.
Avg Enrollment: 50. *Avg Class Size:* 12. *Number of Graduates per Year:* 36.
Wheelchair Access: Yes.
Accreditation/Approval/Licensing: Commission on Massage Therapy Accreditation.
Field of Study: Acupressure; Aromatherapy; CranioSacral Therapy; Massage Therapy*; Neuromuscular Therapy; Reflexology; Reiki; Shiatsu; Sports Massage*; Thai Massage. *Program Name/Length:* Massage and Sports Therapy, 11 mos.
Degrees Offered: Diploma; Certificate; AA.
License/Certification Preparation: National Certification Board for Therapeutic Massage and Bodywork.
Admission Requirements: Min age: 18; High school diploma/GED.
Tuition and Fees: $5600.
Financial Aid: Scholarships; Work study; Payment plan.
Career Services: Career counseling; Career information; Internships; Referral service.

49. Pacific College
Physical Medicine Assistant
3160 Redhill Ave, Costa Mesa, CA 92626
Phone: (714) 662-4402; *Fax:* (714) 662-1702
Program Administrator: Dr. Ronda Wimmer. *Admissions Contact:* Betty Gross, Dir of Admin.
Year Established: 1994.
Staff: Full-time: 2.
Avg Class Size: 18.
Accreditation/Approval/Licensing: State board: CA Bureau of Private Postsecondary and Vocational Ed; Accrediting Commission of Career Schools and Colleges of Technology.
Field of Study: Acupressure; Aromatherapy; Massage Therapy*; Reflexology; Shiatsu; Sports Massage. *Program Name/Length:* Physical Medicine Assistant, 1200 hrs.
Degrees Offered: Diploma.
Admission Requirements: Min age: 18; High school diploma/GED; Entrance exam.
Tuition and Fees: $8790.

Financial Aid: Federal government aid; Grants; Loans; VA approved; Vocational rehabilitation; Payment plan.
Career Services: Career counseling; Career information; Internships; Resume service; Job information; Referral service.

Culver City

50. Biofeedback Institute of Los Angeles
3710 S Robertson Blvd, Ste 216, Culver City, CA 90232-2351
Phone: (310) 841-4970, (800) 246-3526; *Fax:* (310) 840-0923
Program Administrator: Marjorie K. Toomim, PhD, Dir. *Admissions Contact:* Maria Bercier-Weir, Admin.
Year Established: 1973.
Staff: Full-time: 2; Part-time: 1.
Avg Enrollment: 30. *Avg Class Size:* 10. *Number of Graduates per Year:* 30.
Wheelchair Access: Yes.
Accreditation/Approval/Licensing: State board: Biofeedback Society of CA; CA Psychological Association; CA Board of Registered Nursing; CA Postsecondary Educational Institute; Biofeedback Certification Institute of America; American Psychological Association; American Dental Association.
Field of Study: Biofeedback*; Neuromuscular Therapy. *Program Name/Length:* Comprehensive Professional Biofeedback Training, 5 mos; Intensive course, 9 or 14 days; Neuromuscular Reeducation, 1 wk; Weekend training; Individual tutorials; Home study/Correspondence.
Degrees Offered: Certificate.
License/Certification Preparation: Biofeedback Certification Institute of America.
Admission Requirements: Min age: 18; High school diploma/GED; Bachelor's degree in health-related field required for Biofeedback Certification Institute of America certification.
Application Deadline(s): Fall: Oct; Winter: Feb; Summer: Jun.
Tuition and Fees: $2450 (comprehensive); $1550 (9-day intensive); $1850 (14-day intensive); $1500 (Neuromuscular Re-education); $425 (correspondence); $295 (weekends).
Financial Aid: Vocational rehabilitation.
Career Services: Career counseling; Career information; Internships; Referral service.

51. Touch for Health Kinesiology Association
11262 Washington Blvd, Culver City, CA 90230
Phone: (310) 313-5580, (800) 466-8342; *Fax:* (310) 313-9319
E-mail: tch4hlth@aol.com *Internet:* http://www.touch4health.org
Program Administrator: JacQueline, Exec Dir. *Admissions Contact:* Mark McCutcheon.

Year Established: 1991.
Staff: Part-time: 220.
Avg Class Size: 5. *Number of Graduates per Year:* 25.
Field of Study: Kinesiology*; Touch for Health*.
Program Name/Length: Touch for Health Levels I-IV, 60 hrs; Touch for Health Instructor Training, 60 hrs, 8 days; Professional Kinesiology Practitioner I-IV, 50 hrs.
Degrees Offered: Certificate.
Tuition and Fees: $200-$700 per course.
Financial Aid: Scholarships; Payment plan.
Career Services: Career information; Promotional assistance; Referral service.
Comments: Taught as seminars around the United States.

Cupertino

52. Pacific College of Alternative Therapies
19997 Stevens Creek Blvd, Ste 2, Cupertino, CA 95014
Phone: (408) 777-0102; *Fax:* (408) 777-0188
E-mail: pcollege-atherapies@juno.com
Program Administrator: Peter Hou, Dir. *Admissions Contact:* Peter Hou.
Year Established: 1993.
Staff: Full-time: 2; Part-time: 4.
Avg Enrollment: 60. *Avg Class Size:* 10. *Number of Graduates per Year:* 60.
Wheelchair Access: No.
Accreditation/Approval/Licensing: State board: CA Bureau of Private Postsecondary and Vocational Ed.
Field of Study: Acupressure*; Massage Therapy*; Qigong; Traditional Chinese Medicine; Tui Na*.
Program Name/Length: Fundamental Massage, 100 hrs; Intermediate Massage, 100 hrs; Acupressure, 100 hrs; Fundamental Tui Na, 100 hrs; Intermediate Tui Na, 100 hrs.
Degrees Offered: Certificate.
Admission Requirements: Min age: 18.
Tuition and Fees: $1700.
Career Services: Career counseling; Career information; Resume service.

Del Mar

53. California Naturopathic College
1228 Camino Del Mar, Del Mar, CA 92014
Phone: (619) 259-1222; *Fax:* (619) 259-0730
Program Administrator: Bettina Yelman, Dir.
Year Established: 1996.
Staff: Part-time: 35.
Avg Enrollment: 50. *Avg Class Size:* 10. *Number of Graduates per Year:* 20.
Accreditation/Approval/Licensing: State board: CA Bureau of Private Postsecondary and Vocational Ed.

Field of Study: Acupressure*; Aromatherapy; Ayurvedic Medicine; CranioSacral Therapy; Energy Work; Herbal Medicine*; Holistic Health*; Homeopathy*; Hypnotherapy*; Massage Therapy*; Naturopathic Medicine*; Nutrition; Oriental Medicine; Polarity Therapy; Reflexology; Reiki; Shiatsu; Sports Massage. *Program Name/Length:* Massage Technician, 100 hrs, 3 mos; Holistic Health Practitioner, 1000 hrs, 2 yrs; Naturopathic Physician, 2500 hrs, 4-5 yrs.
Degrees Offered: Diploma; Certificate.
License/Certification Preparation: American Board of Clinical Hypnosis; American Council of Hypnotist Examiners; American Oriental Bodywork Therapy Association; Council for Homeopathic Certification; Homeopathic Academy of Naturopathic Physicians; North American Society of Homeopaths; National Certification Board for Therapeutic Massage and Bodywork.
Admission Requirements: Min age: 18; High school diploma/GED; Min GPA: 3.0; Bachelor's degree; Min GPA: 3.0; Interview.
Application Deadline(s): Fall: May; Spring: Nov.
Tuition and Fees: $10,500 (Holistic Health Practitioner); $30,000 (Naturopathic Physician).
Financial Aid: Loans; Scholarships; Work study; Vocational rehabilitation; Payment plan.

Desert Hot Springs

54. Desert Resorts School of Somatherapy
13100 Palm Dr, Desert Hot Springs, CA 92240
Phone: (760) 329-1175; *Fax:* (760) 329-5925
E-mail: ramonam@somatherapy.com *Internet:* http://www.somatherapy.com
Program Administrator: Ramona Moody French, Dir. *Admissions Contact:* Rochelle Quitiquit, Registrar.
Year Established: 1991.
Staff: Part-time: 8.
Avg Enrollment: 140. *Avg Class Size:* 15. *Number of Graduates per Year:* 140.
Accreditation/Approval/Licensing: State board: CA Bureau of Private Postsecondary and Vocational Ed; National Certification Board for Therapeutic Massage and Bodywork (CEUs).
Field of Study: Acupressure; Aromatherapy; CranioSacral Therapy; Deep Tissue Massage; Holistic Health*; Manual Lymph Drainage*; Massage Therapy*; Polarity Therapy; Reflexology; Shiatsu; Sports Massage; Swedish Massage*. *Program Name/Length:* Comprehensive Decongestive Therapy (Lymph Drainage), 160 hrs; Massage Technician, 300 hrs; Massage Therapist, 600 hrs; Holistic Health Practitioner, 1000 hrs.
Degrees Offered: Certificate.
License/Certification Preparation: National Certification Board for Therapeutic Massage and Bodywork.

Admission Requirements: Min age: 18; Reading comprehension.
Application Deadline(s): Fall: Sep 15; Winter: Jan 2; Spring: Apr 1; Summer: Jul 1.
Tuition and Fees: $1995 (Comprehensive); $1815 (300 hr Massage); $3885 (600 hr Massage); $5790 (Holistic Health).
Financial Aid: VA approved; Vocational rehabilitation.
Career Services: Career counseling; Career information.

55. Desert Springs Therapy Center

Banning Massage School
66-705 E 6th St, Desert Hot Springs, CA 92240
Phone: (760) 329-5066; *Fax:* (760) 251-6206
E-mail: dstc@gnn.com
Program Administrator: Charles Thomas, Dir. *Admissions Contact:* Charles Thomas.
Year Established: 1987.
Staff: Full-time: 3.
Avg Enrollment: 38. *Avg Class Size:* 14. *Number of Graduates per Year:* 34.
Wheelchair Access: Yes.
Accreditation/Approval/Licensing: Accrediting Council for Continuing Education and Training.
Field of Study: Deep Tissue Massage; Hydrotherapy; Massage Therapy*; Sports Massage. *Program Name/Length:* Massage Technician, 100 hrs; Massage Specialist, 250 hrs; Therapeutic Massage, 250 hrs; Hydrotherapy, 2 wks.
Degrees Offered: Certificate.
License/Certification Preparation: National Certification Board for Therapeutic Massage and Bodywork.
Admission Requirements: High school diploma/GED; Min GPA: 2.5.
Application Deadline(s): Fall: Dec 1; Spring: Apr 1.
Tuition and Fees: $1300 (Massage Technician); $1918 (Massage Specialist); $3100 (Therapeutic Massage); $630 (Hydrotherapy).
Career Services: Career counseling; Career information.

Emeryville

56. National Holistic Institute

5900 Hollis St, Ste J, Emeryville, CA 94608
Phone: (510) 547-6442, (800) 315-3552; *Fax:* (510) 547-6621
E-mail: nhi@nhimassage.com *Internet:* http://www.nhimassage.com
Program Administrator: Philip Ayala, Dir. *Admissions Contact:* Nancy Seyfert, Admissions Mgr.
Year Established: 1978.
Staff: Full-time: 10; Part-time: 35.
Avg Enrollment: 500. *Avg Class Size:* 20. *Number of Graduates per Year:* 425.
Wheelchair Access: Yes.

Accreditation/Approval/Licensing: Accrediting Council for Continuing Education and Training; National Certification Board for Therapeutic Massage and Bodywork (CEUs).
Field of Study: Holistic Health; Massage Therapy*; Shiatsu; Sports Massage. *Program Name/Length:* 10 mos/days, 1 yr/evenings and weekends or 17 mos/weekends.
Degrees Offered: Certificate.
License/Certification Preparation: National Certification Board for Therapeutic Massage and Bodywork.
Tuition and Fees: $7900.
Financial Aid: Federal government aid; Grants; Loans; Scholarships; Work study; VA approved; Vocational rehabilitation; Payment plan.
Career Services: Career counseling; Career information; Internships; Resume service; Job information; Referral service.

Encinitas

57. Natural Healing Institute of Naturopathy, Inc

2146 Encinitas Blvd, Ste 105, Encinitas, CA 92024
Mailing Address: PO Box 230294, Encinitas, CA 92023-0294
Phone: (760) 943-8485; *Fax:* (760) 943-9477
E-mail: nhi@inetworld.net
Program Administrator: Steven Schechter, Dir. *Admissions Contact:* Patti Valentine, Admissions Dir.
Year Established: 1997.
Staff: Part-time: 8.
Avg Enrollment: 60. *Avg Class Size:* 16. *Number of Graduates per Year:* 40.
Wheelchair Access: Yes.
Field of Study: Acupressure; Aromatherapy; Ayurvedic Medicine; Deep Tissue Massage; Energy Work; Herbal Medicine*; Hypnotherapy*; Massage Therapy*; Naturopathic Medicine*; Nutrition; Oriental Medicine; Reflexology; Shiatsu; Traditional Chinese Medicine. *Program Name/Length:* Residential College, 100-1000 hrs; Distance Learning College, 100-2500 hrs; Home study/Correspondence.
Admission Requirements: Min age: 18; High school diploma/GED.
Financial Aid: Work study; Vocational rehabilitation.
Career Services: Career information.

58. The Yoga Room

953-957 2nd St, Encinitas, CA 92024
Phone: (619) 753-1828; *Fax:* (619) 753-4639
Internet: http://www.synergy-yoga.com
Program Administrator: Peri Ness, Owner/Teacher Trainer. *Admissions Contact:* Wendy Bricker, Mgr.
Year Established: 1992.
Staff: Full-time: 6; Part-time: 22.

Avg Enrollment: 50. *Avg Class Size:* 25. *Number of Graduates per Year:* 25.
Wheelchair Access: Yes.
Field of Study: Yoga Teacher Training*. *Program Name/Length:* Synergy Yoga Teacher Training, 1 yr.
Degrees Offered: Certificate.
Admission Requirements: Min age: 18.
Application Deadline(s): Fall: Oct 14; Spring: Apr 14; Summer: Jul 14.
Tuition and Fees: $895.
Financial Aid: Payment plan.
Career Services: Apprenticeships.

Encino

59. Reiki Center of Los Angeles

16161 Ventura Blvd, Ste 802, Encino, CA 91436
Phone: (818) 881-5959; *Fax:* (818) 881-1613
Program Administrator: Joyce Morris, MS, Reiki Master Teacher. *Admissions Contact:* Joyce Morris.
Year Established: 1982.
Staff: Full-time: 1; Part-time: 4.
Avg Enrollment: 300. *Avg Class Size:* 15.
Wheelchair Access: Yes.
Accreditation/Approval/Licensing: Accrediting Council for Continuing Education and Training.
Field of Study: Reiki. *Program Name/Length:* 1st Degree Reiki, 13 hrs; 2nd Degree Reiki, 7 hrs; Master's Level, 2 yrs+; Seminars given in various locations.
Degrees Offered: Certificate.
Admission Requirements: Min age: 18.
Tuition and Fees: $225 (1st Degree); $500 (2nd Degree); $10,000 (Master).
Financial Aid: Work study.

60. The Touch Therapy Institute

15720 Ventura Blvd, Ste 101, Encino, CA 91436
Phone: (818) 788-0824; *Fax:* (818) 788-0875
Internet: http://www.touchtherapyinstitute.com
Program Administrator: Maria Grove, MA, Founding Dir. *Admissions Contact:* Kate Campbell, Admin Asst.
Year Established: 1989.
Staff: Part-time: 35.
Avg Enrollment: 300. *Avg Class Size:* 15. *Number of Graduates per Year:* 300.
Wheelchair Access: Yes.
Accreditation/Approval/Licensing: State board: CA Bureau of Private Postsecondary and Vocational Ed; Accrediting Council for Continuing Education and Training.
Field of Study: Acupressure; Alexander Technique; Anatomy and Physiology; Aromatherapy; Chair Massage; CPR/First Aid; CranioSacral Therapy; Energy Work; LomiLomi Massage; Lymphatic Massage; Massage Therapy*; Myofascial Release; Pregnancy Massage; Qigong; Reflexology; Sports Massage; Swedish Mas-

sage*; Therapeutic Touch; Trager. *Program Name/Length:* Massage Therapist, 200 hrs, 3 mos/days or 4 1/2 mos/evenings; Advanced Massage Therapist: Level I, 500 hrs (includes 200 hr course); Advanced Massage Therapist: Level II, 1000 hrs (includes 200 and 500 hr courses).
Degrees Offered: Certificate.
License/Certification Preparation: National Certification Board for Therapeutic Massage and Bodywork; City license.
Admission Requirements: Min age: 18.
Tuition and Fees: $1675 (Massage Therapist); $2400-$4225 (Advanced: Level I); $2940-$6418 (Advanced: Level II).
Financial Aid: VA approved; Vocational rehabilitation; Payment plan.
Career Services: Career counseling; Career information; Internships; Instruction in business management.

Escondido

61. Healing Hands School of Holistic Health

125 W Mission, Ste 212, Escondido, CA 92025
Phone: (760) 746-9364, (800) 355-6463, CA only
Program Administrator: Paula Curtiss, Dir. *Admissions Contact:* Paula Curtiss.
Year Established: 1993.
Staff: Part-time: 15.
Avg Enrollment: 200. *Avg Class Size:* 15. *Number of Graduates per Year:* 20.
Wheelchair Access: No.
Accreditation/Approval/Licensing: State board: CA Bureau of Private Postsecondary and Vocational Ed.
Field of Study: Acupressure; Aromatherapy; CranioSacral Therapy; Deep Tissue Massage; Herbal Medicine; Holistic Health*; Homeopathy; Hypnotherapy*; Massage Therapy*; Reflexology; Reiki; Shiatsu; Sports Massage. *Program Name/Length:* Massage Technician, 3 mos; Massage Therapist, 1 yr; Holistic Health Practitioner, 2 yrs; Hypnotherapy, 4 mos.
Degrees Offered: Certificate.
License/Certification Preparation: American Board of Clinical Hypnosis.
Admission Requirements: Min age: 16.
Tuition and Fees: $440 (Massage Technician); $2750 (Massage Therapist); $5500 (Holistic Practitioner); $1320 (Hypnotherapy).
Career Services: Referral service.

Fairfax

62. Four Winds Seminars

187 Hillside Dr, Fairfax, CA 94930
Phone: (415) 457-2079; *Fax:* (415) 457-2079
E-mail: mfairbanks@igc.apc.org

Program Administrator: Melissa Fairbanks.
Year Established: 1991.
Accreditation/Approval/Licensing: Council on Homeopathic Education.
Field of Study: Homeopathy*. *Program Name/Length:* 3-10 day seminars.
Tuition and Fees: $300-$1800 per course.

Forestville

63. California School of Herbal Studies
9309 Hwy 116, Forestville, CA 95436
Mailing Address: PO Box 39, Forestville, CA 95436
Phone: (707) 887-7457
Internet: http://www.cshs.com
Program Administrator: James Green, Dir. *Admissions Contact:* Rebecca Maxfield, Co-Mgr.
Year Established: 1978.
Staff: Full-time: 5; Part-time: 10.
Avg Enrollment: 30. *Avg Class Size:* 28. *Number of Graduates per Year:* 25.
Wheelchair Access: Yes.
Field of Study: Aromatherapy*; Herbal Medicine*. *Program Name/Length:* Foundations of Herbalism, 4 1/2 mos; Therapeutics, 4 1/2 mos; Clinical Program, 6 mos.
Degrees Offered: Certificate.
Admission Requirements: Min age: 18.
Tuition and Fees: $4995 (entire program).
Financial Aid: Work study.

Fortuna

64. Loving Hands Institute of Healing Arts
639 11th St, Fortuna, CA 95540-2346
Phone: (707) 725-9627; *Fax:* (707) 725-2471
E-mail: skyhawk@northcoast.com *Internet:* http://www.springville.com/lovinghands
Program Administrator: Dr. Rosalind Skyhawk Ojala, Admin Dir. *Admissions Contact:* Amanda Biesen, Admin Sec.
Year Established: 1979.
Staff: Full-time: 2.
Avg Enrollment: 50. *Avg Class Size:* 10. *Number of Graduates per Year:* 45.
Wheelchair Access: Yes.
Accreditation/Approval/Licensing: State board: CA Bureau of Private Postsecondary and Vocational Ed; CA Board of Registered Nursing.
Field of Study: Acupressure; Deep Tissue Massage; Esalen Massage*; Holistic Health*; Lymphatic Massage; Massage Therapy*; Reflexology; Swedish Massage*; Trigger Point Therapy. *Program Name/Length:* Holistic Massage Therapy (HMT), 120 hrs, 2 mos; Advanced Holistic Massage Therapy (AHMT), 100 hrs, 2 mos; Universal Concepts of Health and Holism (UCHH), 140 hrs, 2 wk intensive; Teacher Training Certif-

icate (TTC), 120 hrs, 2 mos; Holistic Health Educator (HHE), 140 hrs, 2 wk intensive.
Degrees Offered: Certificate.
License/Certification Preparation: National Certification Board for Therapeutic Massage and Bodywork.
Admission Requirements: Min age: 18; High school diploma/GED; Min GPA: 2.0; Specific course prerequisites: HMT required for AHMT; AHMT for TTC; UCHH and TTC for HHE.
Application Deadline(s): Fall: Sep; Winter: Jan; Spring: Mar; Summer: Jun.
Tuition and Fees: $1050 (HMT); $1300 (AHMT); $600 (UCHH; TTC); $400 (HHE).
Career Services: Career counseling; Career information; Internships.

Fresno

65. Therapeutic Learning Center
Massage School
3636 N First St, Ste 154, Fresno, CA 93727
Phone: (559) 225-7772; *Fax:* (559) 252-5313
Program Administrator: Evangeline K. Hentrich, Owner/Dir. *Admissions Contact:* Evangeline K. Hentrich.
Year Established: 1986.
Staff: Full-time: 10.
Avg Enrollment: 80. *Avg Class Size:* 20. *Number of Graduates per Year:* 80.
Wheelchair Access: Yes.
Accreditation/Approval/Licensing: State board: CA Bureau of Private Postsecondary and Vocational Ed.
Field of Study: Energy Work; Massage Therapy*; Reflexology*; Shiatsu*; Swedish Massage*. *Program Name/Length:* Swedish Massage, 200 hrs, 3 1/2 mos; Reflexology and Shiatsu, 100 hrs, 3 mos.
Degrees Offered: Certificate.
Admission Requirements: Min age: 19; High school diploma/GED.
Application Deadline(s): Fall: Sep; Winter: Jan; Summer: Apr.
Tuition and Fees: $1600 (200 hrs); $800 (100 hrs).
Career Services: Job information; Referral service.

Garberville

66. Heartwood Institute
Massage Therapy; Oriental Healing Arts; Somatic Therapy
220 Harmony Ln, Garberville, CA 95542
Phone: (707) 923-5000; *Fax:* (707) 923-5010
E-mail: enroll@heartwoodinstitute.com *Internet:* http://www.heartwoodinstitute.com
Program Administrator: Chela Burger, Dir of Ed. *Admissions Contact:* Eve Carroll, Admissions Dir (3-12 mo progs); Cindy Robbins, Intensive Coord (1-3 wk intensives).

Year Established: 1978.
Staff: Full-time: 10; Part-time: 25.
Avg Enrollment: 300. *Avg Class Size:* 24. *Number of Graduates per Year:* 280.
Wheelchair Access: No.
Accreditation/Approval/Licensing: State board: CA Board of Registered Nursing; CA Council of Private Postsecondary and Vocational Ed; OR, WA, and IA Boards of Massage; Accrediting Council for Continuing Education and Training; American Polarity Therapy Association; National Certification Board for Therapeutic Massage and Bodywork (CEUs); American Oriental Bodywork Therapy Association.
Field of Study: Acupressure; CranioSacral Therapy; Deep Tissue Massage; Energy Work; Holistic Health*; Hypnotherapy; Massage Therapy*; Neuromuscular Therapy; Oriental Medicine; Polarity Therapy*; Shiatsu*; Sports Massage; Swedish Massage*; Traditional Chinese Medicine. *Program Name/Length:* Massage Practitioner, 3 mos; Massage Therapist, 6 mos; Advanced Massage Therapist, 9 mos; Somatic Therapist, 9 mos; Holistic Health Practitioner, 1 yr; Intensives, 1-3 wks.
Degrees Offered: Diploma; Certificate.
License/Certification Preparation: American Oriental Bodywork Therapy Association; National Certification Board for Therapeutic Massage and Bodywork; American Polarity Therapy Association.
Admission Requirements: Min age: 21; High school diploma/GED.
Application Deadline(s): Fall: Aug; Winter: Nov; Spring: Feb; Summer: May.
Tuition and Fees: $2450 per qtr.
Financial Aid: VA approved; Vocational rehabilitation.
Career Services: Career counseling; Career information.

Garden Grove

67. Inner Quest Awareness Center
Hypnotherapy and Reiki Training
13924 Taft St, Ste 3, Garden Grove, CA 92843
Phone: (800) 769-1230; *Fax:* (714) 539-2977
E-mail: iqac-jans@webtv.net
Program Administrator: Jeanne A. Neher-Schurz, PhD, Dir. *Admissions Contact:* Jeanne A. Neher-Schurz.
Year Established: 1992.
Staff: Part-time: 2.
Avg Enrollment: 45. *Avg Class Size:* 8. *Number of Graduates per Year:* 40.
Wheelchair Access: Yes.
Accreditation/Approval/Licensing: State board: CA Bureau of Private Postsecondary and Vocational Ed; Accrediting Council for Continuing Education and Training; International Medical and Dental Hypnotherapy Association.

Field of Study: Hypnotherapy*; Reiki*. *Program Name/Length:* Basic Hypnosis, 50 hrs; Intermediate Hypnosis, 50 hrs; Advanced Hypnosis, 5 programs, 20-30 hrs each; Reiki: Level I, 8-16 hrs; Reiki: Level II, 8-16 hrs; Reiki: Level III, 16 hrs.
Degrees Offered: American Board of Hypnotherapy; International Medical and Dental Hypnotherapy Association.
License/Certification Preparation: American Board of Clinical Hypnosis.
Admission Requirements: Min age: 18; High school diploma/GED.
Tuition and Fees: $450-$595 (Basic; Intermediate); $225-$325 (Advanced); $150 (Reiki I); $250 (Reiki II); $1250 (Reiki III).
Financial Aid: Payment plan.
Career Services: Career information.

Garden Grove City

68. Kyung San University USA School of Oriental Medicine
8322 Garden Grove, Garden Grove City, CA 92844
Phone: (714) 636-0337; *Fax:* (714) 636-8459
E-mail: admin@kyungsan.edu *Internet:* http://www.kyungsan.edu/~kyungsan
Program Administrator: Han Kwang Ohm, Pres. *Admissions Contact:* Eun Suk Lee, Admissions Dir.
Year Established: 1994.
Staff: Full-time: 8; Part-time: 12.
Avg Enrollment: 40. *Avg Class Size:* 15. *Number of Graduates per Year:* 15.
Wheelchair Access: Yes.
Accreditation/Approval/Licensing: State board: CA Acupuncture Board; Pending, Accreditation Commission for Acupuncture and Oriental Medicine; Pending, Accreditation Commission for Acupuncture and Medicine.
Field of Study: Acupressure; Acupuncture*; CranioSacral Therapy; Herbal Medicine; Oriental Medicine*; Qigong; Reflexology; Shiatsu; Traditional Chinese Medicine*. *Program Name/Length:* Master of Science in Oriental Medicine, 3-4 yrs.
Degrees Offered: MS; Diploma.
License/Certification Preparation: State: CA Licensed Acupuncturist; National Certification Commission for Acupuncture and Oriental Medicine.
Admission Requirements: Min age: 30; High school diploma/GED; Min GPA: 2.0; 4 yrs college; Min GPA: 2.7; Specific course prerequisites: acupuncture, herbology.
Tuition and Fees: $8000 per yr.
Financial Aid: Loans; Scholarships; Work study.
Career Services: Career counseling; Career information; Internships; Interview set up; Resume service.

Comments: Candidacy, Accreditation Commission for Acupuncture and Oriental Medicine.

Glendale

69. Hypnotism Training Institute of Los Angeles

700 S Central Ave, Glendale, CA 91204
Phone: (818) 242-1159; *Fax:* (818) 247-9379
Internet: http://www.gilboyne.com
Program Administrator: Gil Boyne, Dir. *Admissions Contact:* Jon Young, Mgr.
Year Established: 1957.
Staff: Full-time: 1.
Avg Enrollment: 100. *Avg Class Size:* 15. *Number of Graduates per Year:* 100.
Wheelchair Access: No.
Accreditation/Approval/Licensing: State board: CA Bureau of Private Postsecondary and Vocational Ed.
Field of Study: Hypnotherapy*. *Program Name/Length:* Basic Hypnotism, 50 hrs; Hypnotherapy, 50 hrs; Advanced Hypnotherapy, 50 hrs; Healing and Pain Control, 50 hrs.
Degrees Offered: Diploma; Certificate.
License/Certification Preparation: American Council of Hypnotist Examiners.
Admission Requirements: Min age: 18; High school diploma/GED.
Tuition and Fees: $750 per course.

Grass Valley

70. California College of Ayurveda

1117A E Main St, Grass Valley, CA 95945
Phone: (530) 274-9100; *Fax:* (530) 274-7350
E-mail: info@ayurvedacollege.com *Internet:* http://www.ayurvedacollege.com
Program Administrator: Dr. Marc Halpern, Dir. *Admissions Contact:* Dr. Marc Halpern.
Year Established: 1995.
Staff: Part-time: 4.
Avg Enrollment: 90. *Avg Class Size:* 20. *Number of Graduates per Year:* 40.
Wheelchair Access: Yes.
Accreditation/Approval/Licensing: State board: CA Bureau of Private Postsecondary and Vocational Ed.
Field of Study: Aromatherapy; Ayurvedic Medicine*; Herbal Medicine. *Program Name/Length:* Clinical Ayurvedic Specialist, 2 yrs.
Degrees Offered: Certificate.
Admission Requirements: High school diploma/GED.
Application Deadline(s): Fall: Oct; Winter: Jan; Spring: Apr.
Tuition and Fees: $5775.
Career Services: Internships.

71. International Sivananda Yoga Vedanta Center

14651 Ballantree Ln, Grass Valley, CA 95949
Mailing Address: 1200 Arguello Blvd, San Francisco, CA 94122
Phone: (415) 681-2731, (800) 469-YOGA (9642); *Fax:* (415) 681-5162, (916) 477-6054
E-mail: swsita@ix.netcom.com *Internet:* http://www.sivananda.org
Program Administrator: Swami Sitaramananda, Dir. *Admissions Contact:* Swami Pranavananda, Asst Dir.
Year Established: 1971.
Staff: Full-time: 8; Part-time: 16.
Avg Enrollment: 50. *Avg Class Size:* 10. *Number of Graduates per Year:* 50.
Wheelchair Access: No.
Field of Study: Yoga Teacher Training*. *Program Name/Length:* Teachers Training Course, 1 mo; Intensive Residential, 1 mo; Work Study, 1 mo or 3 mos.
Degrees Offered: Certificate.
License/Certification Preparation: Sivananda Yoga Vedanta Forest Academy.
Admission Requirements: Yoga practice.
Application Deadline(s): Spring: Apr.
Tuition and Fees: $1450 per mo.
Financial Aid: Work study.
Career Services: Career counseling; Career information; Internships.

Gualala

72. Pacific School of Massage and Healing Arts

44800 Fish Rock Rd, Gualala, CA 95445
Phone: (707) 884-3138; *Fax:* (707) 884-4106
E-mail: mitouer@mcn.org *Internet:* http://www.bodyworkmassage.com
Program Administrator: Cheryl Mitouer, Co-Dir; Fred Mitouer, Co-Dir. *Admissions Contact:* Cheryl Mitouer; Fred Mitouer.
Year Established: 1978.
Staff: Full-time: 2; Part-time: guest teachers.
Avg Enrollment: 36. *Avg Class Size:* 12. *Number of Graduates per Year:* 36.
Wheelchair Access: Yes.
Accreditation/Approval/Licensing: State board: CA Bureau of Private Postsecondary and Vocational Ed.
Field of Study: Massage Therapy*; Transformational Bodywork. *Program Name/Length:* Massage and Healing Arts, 110 hrs.
Degrees Offered: Certificate.
Admission Requirements: Min age: 18; High school diploma/GED.
Tuition and Fees: $1700.
Career Services: Career information.

Huntington Beach

73. California College of Physical Arts, Inc

18582 Beach Blvd, Ste 11, Huntington Beach, CA 92648

Phone: (714) 964-7744; *Fax:* (714) 962-3934

E-mail: calcopa@gte.net *Internet:* http://www.fyi.com

Program Administrator: Deborah S. Mulholland, Dir. *Admissions Contact:* Deborah S. Mulholland.

Year Established: 1980.

Staff: Full-time: 3; Part-time: 5.

Avg Enrollment: 600. *Avg Class Size:* 10. *Number of Graduates per Year:* 500.

Wheelchair Access: Yes.

Accreditation/Approval/Licensing: State board: CA Bureau of Private Postsecondary and Vocational Ed.

Field of Study: Acupressure; Alexander Technique; Aromatherapy; Herbal Medicine; Holistic Health*; Massage Therapy*; Oriental Medicine; Reflexology; Reiki; Shiatsu; Sports Massage. *Program Name/Length:* Massage Therapist, 300 hrs, 3 mos/full-time or 6 mos/part-time; Massage Practitioner, 500 hrs, 5 mos/full-time or 10 mos/part-time; Holistic Health Practitioner, 1000 hrs, 11 mos/full-time or 2 yrs/part-time.

Degrees Offered: Certificate.

License/Certification Preparation: National Certification Board for Therapeutic Massage and Bodywork; City license.

Admission Requirements: Min age: 18; High school diploma/GED.

Tuition and Fees: $2625 (Massage Therapist); $4125 (Massage Practitioner); $8250 (Holistic Practitioner).

Career Services: Career counseling; Career information; Job information.

Irvine

74. American Institute of Hypnotherapy

16842 Von Karman Ave, Ste 475, Irvine, CA 92606

Phone: (949) 261-6400, (800) 872-9996; *Fax:* (949) 251-4632

E-mail: aih@hypnosis.com *Internet:* http://www.hypnosis.com

Program Administrator: Tad James, Dir. *Admissions Contact:* Guy Robert, Admissions Dir.

Accreditation/Approval/Licensing: State board: CA Bureau of Private Postsecondary and Vocational Ed; American Board of Hypnotherapy.

Field of Study: Hypnotherapy*. *Program Name/Length:* Bachelor of Clinical Hypnotherapy, 4 modules; Doctor of Clinical Hypnotherapy, 3 modules; Seminars given in various locations.

Degrees Offered: Bachelor of Clinical Hypnotherapy; DCH.

Admission Requirements: Some college (60 semester units—30 general ed—or equivalent); Bachelor's degree for Doctor of Clinical Hypnotherapy.

Tuition and Fees: $1150 per module (Bachelor); $1650 per module (Doctor).

Financial Aid: Payment plan.

Kensington

75. Institute of Orthopedic Massage

406 Berkeley Park Blvd, Kensington, CA 94706

Phone: (510) 524-8256; *Fax:* (510) 524-8242

E-mail: iom@dnai.com

Program Administrator: Thomas Hendrickson, DC, Dir. *Admissions Contact:* Claudia Moore, Admin.

Year Established: 1982.

Staff: Full-time: 3; Part-time: 2.

Avg Enrollment: 30. *Avg Class Size:* 30. *Number of Graduates per Year:* 30.

Wheelchair Access: No.

Field of Study: Massage Therapy*; Orthopedic Massage*. *Program Name/Length:* Orthopedic Massage Training, 200 hrs, 8 mos.

Degrees Offered: Certificate.

Admission Requirements: Licensed or certified health care professional.

Application Deadline(s): Fall: Sep 1.

Tuition and Fees: $3200.

Kneeland

76. Dandelion Herbal Center

4803 Greenwood Hts Dr, Kneeland, CA 95549

Phone: (707) 442-8157

Program Administrator: Jane Bothwell, Dir. *Admissions Contact:* Jane Bothwell.

Year Established: 1987.

Staff: Full-time: 1; Part-time: 10.

Avg Enrollment: 150. *Avg Class Size:* 25. *Number of Graduates per Year:* 148.

Wheelchair Access: No.

Field of Study: Herbal Medicine*. *Program Name/Length:* Beginning with Herbs, 2 mos; Herbs for Common Imbalances, 2 mos; Festival of Herbs, 8 mos; Herbal Apprenticeship, 10 mos.

Degrees Offered: Certificate.

Tuition and Fees: $200 (2 mo programs); $1000 (8-10 mo programs).

Financial Aid: Work study.

La Jolla

77. Chopra Center for Well-Being

7630 Fay Ave, La Jolla, CA 92037

Phone: (619) 551-7788; *Fax:* (619) 551-9570

Internet: http://www.chopra.com

Program Administrator: David Simon, MD, Medical Dir.
Year Established: 1993.
Staff: Full-time: 1.
Avg Enrollment: 125. *Avg Class Size:* 30. *Number of Graduates per Year:* 100.
Wheelchair Access: Yes.
Field of Study: Ayurvedic Medicine*; Childbirth Education*; Herbal Medicine*; Meditation*; Mind-Body Medicine*. *Program Name/Length:* Meditation Instructor Certification, 1 yr; Mind-Body Instructor Certification, 1 yr; Childbirth Education Instructor Certification, 6 mos; Classroom and home study.
Degrees Offered: Certificate.
Admission Requirements: Min age: 21; Bachelor's degree.
Tuition and Fees: $100-$2500.

78. Kate Jordan Seminars
Bodywork for the Childbearing Year
8950 Villa La Jolla Dr, Ste 2162, La Jolla, CA 92037
Phone: (619) 436-0418, (888) 287-6860; *Fax:* (619) 457-3615
E-mail: pregmassge@aol.com
Program Administrator: Kathy Sartain, Prog Dir. *Admissions Contact:* Kathy Sartain.
Year Established: 1984.
Staff: Full-time: 1; Part-time: 3.
Avg Enrollment: 300. *Avg Class Size:* 25. *Number of Graduates per Year:* 300.
Wheelchair Access: Yes.
Accreditation/Approval/Licensing: National Certification Board for Therapeutic Massage and Bodywork (CEUs); National Association of Pregnancy Massage Therapists.
Field of Study: Postpartum Massage*; Pregnancy Massage*. *Program Name/Length:* Certification, 34 hrs.
Degrees Offered: Certificate.
License/Certification Preparation: National Certification Board for Therapeutic Massage and Bodywork.
Admission Requirements: Graduate of massage therapy program or 5 yrs experience in therapeutic massage; RN or Childbirth Educator with instructor's permission.
Tuition and Fees: $525 (enrollment 1 mo before course) or $575.
Financial Aid: Work study.
Career Services: Career information; Referral service.

79. Master Yoga Academy
Yoga Teacher Training
7592 Fay Ave, La Jolla, CA 92037
Phone: (619) 454-6978; *Fax:* (619) 454-5541
E-mail: info@masteryoga.org *Internet:* http://www.masteryoga.org

Program Administrator: Rama Berch, Dir/Master Teacher. *Admissions Contact:* Sandy Joubert, Enrollment Coord.
Year Established: 1992.
Staff: Full-time: 1; Part-time: 2.
Avg Enrollment: 75. *Avg Class Size:* 16. *Number of Graduates per Year:* 75.
Wheelchair Access: Yes.
Field of Study: Yoga Teacher Training*. *Program Name/Length:* Hatha Yoga Teacher Training, 500 hrs, 9 mos; Hatha Yoga Teacher Training Summer Intensive, 4 wks.
Degrees Offered: Certificate.
Admission Requirements: Interview.
Tuition and Fees: $2300-$3500.
Financial Aid: Scholarships.
Career Services: Career information; Internships; Referral service.

80. University of California at San Diego, School of Medicine
Nurse-Midwifery Program, Division of Graduate Nursing Education
9500 Gilman Dr, La Jolla, CA 92093-0809
Phone: (619) 543-5480; *Fax:* (619) 543-7757
Program Administrator: Lauren Hunter, MS, Dir.
Year Established: 1976.
Staff: Full-time: 2.
Avg Enrollment: 8. *Avg Class Size:* 8. *Number of Graduates per Year:* 8.
Wheelchair Access: Yes.
Accreditation/Approval/Licensing: American College of Nurse-Midwives, Division of Accreditation.
Field of Study: Midwifery*. *Program Name/Length:* 2 yrs.
Degrees Offered: MS.
License/Certification Preparation: Certified Nurse-Midwife, American College of Nurse-Midwives.
Admission Requirements: Bachelor's degree; RN.

La Mesa

81. Academy of Professional Careers
Massage Therapy; Holistic Health Practitioner
8376 Hercules St, La Mesa, CA 91942
Phone: (619) 461-5100; *Fax:* (619) 461-1401
Program Administrator: Beth Knottly, Prog Coord. *Admissions Contact:* Juanita Cherry, Admissions Advisor.
Year Established: 1995.
Staff: Part-time: 10-12.
Avg Enrollment: 100. *Avg Class Size:* 30. *Number of Graduates per Year:* 75.
Wheelchair Access: Yes.
Accreditation/Approval/Licensing: Accrediting Council for Continuing Education and Training.
Field of Study: Energy Work; Holistic Health*; Massage Therapy*; Neuromuscular Therapy; Reflexology; Reiki; Shiatsu; Sports Massage.

Program Name/Length: Massage Therapy, 730 hrs; Holistic Health Practitioner, 1000 hrs.
Degrees Offered: Certificate.
Admission Requirements: Min age: 18; High school diploma/GED.
Tuition and Fees: $8225-$10,661.
Financial Aid: Federal government aid; Grants; Loans; Scholarships; State government aid; Work study; VA approved; Vocational rehabilitation; Payment plan.
Career Services: Career counseling; Career information; Internships; Interview set up; Resume service; Job information; Referral service.

Lafayette

82. Hypnosis Clearing House
Hypnotherapy Training
3702 Mount Diablo Blvd, Lafayette, CA 94549
Phone: (510) 283-3941; *Fax:* (510) 283-9044
E-mail: hch@hypnotherapytraining.com *Internet:* http://www.hypnotherapytraining.com
Program Administrator: Holly Holmes-Meredith, MFCC, Owner/Clinical Dir. *Admissions Contact:* Roxanne Vasconcellos, Admin.
Year Established: 1977.
Staff: Part-time: 4.
Avg Enrollment: 50. *Avg Class Size:* 13. *Number of Graduates per Year:* 40.
Wheelchair Access: No.
Accreditation/Approval/Licensing: State board: CA Bureau of Private Postsecondary and Vocational Ed; International Board of Regression Therapy.
Field of Study: Hypnotherapy*. *Program Name/Length:* Certification, 4 mos.
Degrees Offered: Diploma; Certificate.
License/Certification Preparation: American Board of Clinical Hypnosis; American Council of Hypnotist Examiners; International Board of Regression Therapy.
Admission Requirements: Min age: 18; High school diploma/GED; Entrance exam.
Application Deadline(s): Fall: Oct; Winter: Feb; Spring: Jun.
Tuition and Fees: $2700.
Financial Aid: Loans.
Career Services: Internships.

Laguna Beach

83. The Belavi Institute for Facial Massage
1500 N Coast Hwy, Laguna Beach, CA 92651
Phone: (714) 443-1954, (800) 235-2844; *Fax:* (714) 443-2292
E-mail: info@belavi.com *Internet:* http://www.belavi.com
Program Administrator: Belle Tuckerman, Owner/Instr. *Admissions Contact:* Belle Tuckerman.
Year Established: 1989.

Staff: Full-time: 10.
Avg Enrollment: 85. *Avg Class Size:* 12. *Number of Graduates per Year:* 85.
Wheelchair Access: Yes.
Accreditation/Approval/Licensing: Accrediting Council for Continuing Education and Training; National Certification Board for Therapeutic Massage and Bodywork (CEUs).
Field of Study: Facial Massage*; Spa Therapies*. *Program Name/Length:* Workshop, 2-3 days; Home study/Correspondence; Seminars given in various locations.
Degrees Offered: Certificate.
License/Certification Preparation: State: CA Certificate, Belavi Specialist.
Admission Requirements: Licensed massage therapist or esthetician.
Tuition and Fees: $650 (Workshop); $299 (Correspondence).
Financial Aid: Loans; Scholarships.

84. Institute for Applied Iridology
PO Box 301, Laguna Beach, CA 92652
Phone: (888) 886-8985; *Fax:* (888) 886-8985
Program Administrator: Harri Wolf, MA, Dir.
Year Established: 1991.
Staff: Full-time: 1.
Avg Class Size: 10. *Number of Graduates per Year:* 4.
Field of Study: Iridology*. *Program Name/Length:* 2 yrs; Seminars given in various locations; Home study/Correspondence.
Degrees Offered: Certificate.
Admission Requirements: Anatomy and physiology courses.
Tuition and Fees: $350.

Laguna Hills

85. Western Institute of Neuromuscular Therapy
Professional Massage Therapist; Professional Therapeutic and Sports Massage
22981 Mill Creek Dr, Ste A, Laguna Hills, CA 92653
Phone: (714) 830-6151; *Fax:* (714) 830-1729
E-mail: director@wintherapy.com *Internet:* http://www.wintherapy.com
Program Administrator: Cynthia Ribeiro, Dir. *Admissions Contact:* Cynthia Ribeiro; Sandra Espino, Admin Asst.
Year Established: 1994.
Staff: Full-time: 1; Part-time: 5.
Avg Enrollment: 72. *Avg Class Size:* 24. *Number of Graduates per Year:* 70.
Wheelchair Access: Yes.
Accreditation/Approval/Licensing: State board: CA Bureau of Private Postsecondary and Vocational Ed; National Certification Board for Therapeutic Massage and Bodywork (CEUs).

Field of Study: Massage Therapy*; Neuromuscular Therapy*; Sports Massage*. *Program Name/Length:* Professional Massage Therapist, 500 hrs, 1 yr; Professional Therapeutic and Sports Massage Therapist, 1000 hrs, 16 mos.
Degrees Offered: Diploma.
License/Certification Preparation: National Certification Board for Therapeutic Massage and Bodywork.
Admission Requirements: Min age: 18; High school diploma/GED; 3 letters of recommendation; Health release.
Tuition and Fees: $5400 (500 hrs); $6200 (1000 hrs).
Financial Aid: State government aid; Vocational rehabilitation.
Career Services: Career counseling; Career information; Job information.

Leucadia

86. Circle of Friends
Yoga and Meditation Program
704 N Hwy 101, Leucadia, CA 92024
Phone: (800) 434-YOGA (9642); *Fax:* (619) 753-8823
E-mail: rudra@unit.edu
Program Administrator: Rudi M. Kadre, Prog Dir. *Admissions Contact:* Rudi M. Kadre.
Year Established: 1974.
Staff: Full-time: 4; Part-time: 4.
Avg Enrollment: 15. *Avg Class Size:* 6. *Number of Graduates per Year:* 10.
Wheelchair Access: Yes.
Field of Study: Meditation; Yoga Teacher Training*. *Program Name/Length:* Hatha Yoga, 144 hrs, 1 yr; Kundalini Yoga, 144 hrs, 1 yr; Tao Yoga, 144 hrs, 1 yr; Tibetan Yoga, 144 hrs, 1 yr; Womb of Passage (comprehensive course in all four yogas), 2 yrs; Seminars given in various locations; Home study/Correspondence.
Tuition and Fees: $1600 (1 yr); $3200 (2 yrs).
Career Services: Referral service.

Los Angeles

87. California Graduate Institute
1145 Gayley Ave, Ste 322, Los Angeles, CA 90024
Phone: (310) 208-4240; *Fax:* (310) 208-0684
Internet: http://www.cgi.edu
Program Administrator: Terry Oleson, PhD, Chair, Dept of Psych. *Admissions Contact:* Alan Cranis.
Year Established: 1968.
Staff: Full-time: 20; Part-time: 40.
Avg Enrollment: 350. *Avg Class Size:* 15. *Number of Graduates per Year:* 80.
Wheelchair Access: Yes.
Accreditation/Approval/Licensing: State board: CA Bureau of Private Postsecondary and Vocational Ed; Biofeedback Certification Institute of America.
Field of Study: Biofeedback*; Hypnotherapy. *Program Name/Length:* Master of Arts in Psychology, 51-67 units, 4 yrs; PsyD, 88-94 units.
Degrees Offered: MA; PsyD.
License/Certification Preparation: State: CA Board of Psychology; Biofeedback Certification Institute of America.
Admission Requirements: Min age: 21; Bachelor's degree; Min GPA: 2.5.
Tuition and Fees: $215 per unit + $80 registration.
Financial Aid: Loans.
Career Services: Internships.

88. Cleveland Chiropractic College, Los Angeles
590 N Vermont Ave, Los Angeles, CA 90004
Phone: (213) 660-6166, (800) 466-2252; *Fax:* (213) 660-5387
Internet: http://www.clevelandchiropractic.edu
Program Administrator: Carl S. Cleveland III, DC, Pres.
Accreditation/Approval/Licensing: Council on Chiropractic Education.
Field of Study: Chiropractic*.
Degrees Offered: DC.
Admission Requirements: Some college.

89. Curentur University
11543 Olympic Blvd, Los Angeles, CA 90064
Phone: (310) 914-4116; *Fax:* (310) 479-3376
E-mail: mail@curentur.org *Internet:* http://www.curentur.org
Program Administrator: John A. Zulli, Pres. *Admissions Contact:* Marlan Goodwin, Registrar.
Year Established: 1995.
Staff: Part-time: 16.
Avg Enrollment: 60. *Avg Class Size:* 20. *Number of Graduates per Year:* 40.
Wheelchair Access: No.
Field of Study: Biofeedback; Holistic Health*; Homeopathy*; Hypnotherapy*; Iridology. *Program Name/Length:* Master of Arts in Homeopathy, 4 trimesters; Master of Arts in Holistic Health Studies, 2 yrs; Master of Arts in Hypnotherapy, 4 trimesters.
Degrees Offered: MA; PhD.
License/Certification Preparation: State: NV State License; Council for Homeopathic Certification.
Admission Requirements: High school diploma/GED; Bachelor's degree.
Tuition and Fees: $215 per unit.
Financial Aid: Loans; Work study; Vocational rehabilitation.

90. Dongguk Royal University
Oriental Medicine
440 Shatto Pl, Los Angeles, CA 90020
Phone: (213) 487-0110, (800) 303-1800; *Fax:* (213) 487-0527
E-mail: dru@pdc.net *Internet:* http://www.dru.edu

Program Administrator: Jin-Soo Han, PhD, Pres; Samuel B. Kim, PhD, LAc, Dean of Academic Affairs. *Admissions Contact:* David Burciaga, LAc, Dir of English Programs.
Year Established: 1959.
Wheelchair Access: Yes.
Accreditation/Approval/Licensing: State board: CA Acupuncture Board; CA Bureau of Private Postsecondary and Vocational Ed; Accreditation Commission for Acupuncture and Oriental Medicine.
Field of Study: Acupressure; Acupuncture*; Herbal Medicine; Oriental Medicine*; Qigong; Traditional Chinese Medicine*. *Program Name/Length:* Master of Science in Oriental Medicine, 4 yrs.
Degrees Offered: MS.
License/Certification Preparation: State: CA Licensed Acupuncturist; National Certification Commission for Acupuncture and Oriental Medicine.
Admission Requirements: Some college (2 yrs), 60 semester credits or 90 qtr credits.
Application Deadline(s): Fall; Winter: Jan; Spring: Apr; Summer: Jul.
Tuition and Fees: $6250 per yr.
Financial Aid: Grants; Loans; Scholarships; Work study; VA approved.
Career Services: Career counseling; Internships.

91. Charles R. Drew University of Medicine and Science, College of Allied Health Sciences

Nurse-Midwifery Education Program
1621 E 120th St, Los Angeles, CA 90059
Phone: (213) 563-4951
Program Administrator: H. Frances Hayes-Cushenberry, CNM, Interim Prog Chair.
Accreditation/Approval/Licensing: American College of Nurse-Midwives, Division of Accreditation.
Field of Study: Midwifery*.
Degrees Offered: MS.
License/Certification Preparation: Certified Nurse-Midwife, American College of Nurse-Midwives.
Admission Requirements: RN.

92. The Institute of Professional Practical Therapy

Massage Therapy and Physical Therapy Aide
1835 S La Cienega Blvd, Ste 260, Los Angeles, CA 90035
Phone: (310) 836-8811; *Fax:* (310) 836-8857
E-mail: ippt@aol.com *Internet:* http://www.ippt.com
Program Administrator: Boris Prilutsky, Owner/Sr Instr. *Admissions Contact:* Victor Dence, Operations Dir.
Year Established: 1996.
Staff: Full-time: 2; Part-time: 1.

Avg Enrollment: 175. *Avg Class Size:* 18. *Number of Graduates per Year:* 100.
Wheelchair Access: No.
Accreditation/Approval/Licensing: State board: CA Bureau of Private Postsecondary and Vocational Ed.
Field of Study: Deep Tissue Massage*; Massage Therapy*. *Program Name/Length:* Massage Therapy and Physical Therapy Aide, 150 hrs, 6 mos.
Degrees Offered: Certificate.
Admission Requirements: Min age: 18.
Tuition and Fees: $1500.
Financial Aid: Payment plan.
Career Services: Internships; Interview set up; Resume service.

93. Institute of Psycho-Structural Balancing

3767 Overland Ave, Ste 103, Los Angeles, CA 90034
Phone: (310) 815-3675; *Fax:* (310) 815-3670
Internet: http://www.ipsb.com
Program Administrator: Eileen Hamsa Henry, OMD, Dir. *Admissions Contact:* Sue Heffner, Admissions Dir.
Year Established: 1980.
Staff: Full-time: 12; Part-time: 12.
Avg Enrollment: 500. *Avg Class Size:* 18. *Number of Graduates per Year:* 400.
Wheelchair Access: Yes.
Accreditation/Approval/Licensing: State board: CA Bureau of Private Postsecondary and Vocational Ed.
Field of Study: Acupressure; Aromatherapy; CranioSacral Therapy*; Energy Work; Massage Therapy*; Polarity Therapy*; Qigong; Reflexology; Sports Massage; Tai Chi. *Program Name/Length:* Massage Technician, 3 mos; Massage Therapist (includes Massage Technician), 12-18 mos; Polarity Associate, 1 yr; Cranial Balancing, 3-6 mos.
Degrees Offered: Certificate.
Admission Requirements: Min age: 18; Exam; Interview.
Tuition and Fees: $1275 (Massage Technician); $4312 (Massage Therapist); $1779 (Polarity); $939 (Cranial).
Career Services: Career information.

94. Internal Environment Institute

Colon Hydrotherapy Course
11739 Washington Blvd, Los Angeles, CA 90066
Phone: (310) 572-6223; *Fax:* (310) 572-6217
E-mail: allred@idt.net
Program Administrator: Conda J. Allred, Admin. *Admissions Contact:* Talya Meldy, Consultant/Teacher.
Year Established: 1995.
Staff: Full-time: 2; Part-time: 1.
Avg Enrollment: 25. *Avg Class Size:* 10. *Number of Graduates per Year:* 25.
Wheelchair Access: No.

Accreditation/Approval/Licensing: Accrediting Council for Continuing Education and Training; International Association for Colon Hydrotherapy.
Field of Study: Colon Hydrotherapy*. *Program Name/Length:* 125 hrs, 16 days.
Degrees Offered: Certificate.
License/Certification Preparation: International Association for Colon Hydrotherapy.
Admission Requirements: Min age: 18; High school diploma/GED; Specific course prerequisites: anatomy and physiology, massage; RN preferred; 10 colonics.
Application Deadline(s): Winter: Jan; Spring: May.
Tuition and Fees: $1695.
Career Services: Career counseling; Career information.

95. Linda Lack, Two-Snake Studios
Teacher Training: Hatha Yoga, Yoga Therapy, Movement Therapy
1637 S La Cienega Blvd, Los Angeles, CA 90035
Phone: (310) 273-4797; *Fax:* (323) 932-1441
Program Administrator: Linda Lack, MA, Dir. *Admissions Contact:* Linda Lack.
Year Established: 1975.
Staff: Full-time: 1; Part-time: 3.
Avg Enrollment: 10. *Avg Class Size:* 10. *Number of Graduates per Year:* 4.
Wheelchair Access: Yes.
Accreditation/Approval/Licensing: International Yoga Therapists Association.
Field of Study: Movement Therapy*; Yoga Teacher Training*; Yoga Therapy*. *Program Name/Length:* 1 yr (weekly technique classes and monthly workshops).
Degrees Offered: Certificate.
Admission Requirements: Min age: 21; High school diploma/GED; Specific course prerequisites: yoga or modern dance technique classes.
Tuition and Fees: $3300.
Career Services: Internships; Referral service.

96. Samra University of Oriental Medicine
Master of Science in Oriental Medicine
3000 S Robertson Blvd, 4th Fl, Los Angeles, CA 90034
Phone: (310) 202-6444; *Fax:* (310) 202-6007
E-mail: admissions@samra.edu *Internet:* http://www.samra.edu
Program Administrator: Kathryn P. White, PhD, Academic Dean. *Admissions Contact:* Aaron Sui, LAc, Dean of Enrollment Svcs.
Year Established: 1969.
Staff: Full-time: 6; Part-time: 68.
Avg Enrollment: 500. *Avg Class Size:* 15. *Number of Graduates per Year:* 95.
Wheelchair Access: Yes.
Accreditation/Approval/Licensing: State board: CA Acupuncture Board; Accrediting Council for Continuing Education and Training; Accredita-tion Commission for Acupuncture and Oriental Medicine.
Field of Study: Acupressure; Acupuncture*; Herbal Medicine; Oriental Medicine*; Qigong; Traditional Chinese Medicine*. *Program Name/Length:* Master of Science in Oriental Medicine, 3 yrs+.
Degrees Offered: MS.
License/Certification Preparation: State: CA Licensed Acupuncturist; National Certification Commission for Acupuncture and Oriental Medicine.
Admission Requirements: Some college (2 yrs); Min GPA: 2.0.
Application Deadline(s): Fall: Sep 15; Winter: Dec 15; Spring: Mar 15; Summer: Jun 15.
Tuition and Fees: $7760 per yr.
Financial Aid: Federal government aid; Pell grants.
Career Services: Career information; Internships.

97. Michael Scholes School for Aromatic Studies
117 N Robertson Blvd, Los Angeles, CA 90048
Phone: (310) 276-1191, (800) 677-2368; *Fax:* (310) 276-1156
E-mail: joanaroma@aol.com
Program Administrator: Michael Scholes, Joan Clark, Owners. *Admissions Contact:* Michael Scholes; Joan Clark.
Year Established: 1990.
Staff: Full-time: 7; Part-time: 2.
Avg Enrollment: 80. *Avg Class Size:* 30. *Number of Graduates per Year:* 75.
Wheelchair Access: No.
Field of Study: Aromatherapy*; Energy Work. *Program Name/Length:* Introduction to Aromatherapy, 5 days; Diploma Course, 1 yr; Seminars given in various locations; Home study/Correspondence.
Degrees Offered: Diploma; Certificate.
Admission Requirements: Min age: 18.
Financial Aid: Payment plan.

98. University of California at Los Angeles, Nurse-Midwifery Education Program
Primary Care Division
10833 LeConte Ave, Los Angeles, CA 90099-4973
Mailing Address: UCLA School of Nursing, Factor Bldg, Box 956919, Los Angeles, CA 90095-6919
Phone: (310) 794-4434; *Fax:* (310) 206-3241
E-mail: mday@sonnet.ucla.edu
Program Administrator: Mary Day, MSN, Dir. *Admissions Contact:* Mary Day.
Year Established: 1994.
Staff: Full-time: 5.
Avg Enrollment: 10. *Avg Class Size:* 10. *Number of Graduates per Year:* 8.
Wheelchair Access: Yes.
Accreditation/Approval/Licensing: State board: CA Board of Registered Nursing; American College of Nurse-Midwives, Division of Accreditation.

Field of Study: Midwifery*. *Program Name/Length:* Master of Science in Nursing, 6 qtrs, 2 academic yrs.
Degrees Offered: MSN.
License/Certification Preparation: State: CA CNM; Certified Nurse-Midwife, American College of Nurse-Midwives.
Admission Requirements: Bachelor's degree; Min GPA: 3.0; Specific course prerequisites: physiology, statistics, physical assessment.
Application Deadline(s): Fall: Dec 21; Spring: Mar 1.
Tuition and Fees: $2000 per qtr.
Financial Aid: Fellowships; Grants; Loans; Work study.
Career Services: Career information.

99. University of Southern California
Nurse-Midwifery Graduate Program
1540 E Alcazar St, CHP222, Los Angeles, CA 90033
Phone: (323) 442-2001; *Fax:* (323) 442-2090
E-mail: uscnurse@hsc.usc.edu *Internet:* http://uscnurse.usc.edu
Program Administrator: BJ Snell, PhD, Director. *Admissions Contact:* BJ Snell.
Year Established: 1997.
Staff: Full-time: 3; Part-time: 4.
Avg Enrollment: 6-10. *Avg Class Size:* 6-10. *Number of Graduates per Year:* 6-10.
Wheelchair Access: Yes.
Accreditation/Approval/Licensing: State board: California Board of Registered Nurses; American College of Nurse-Midwives, Division of Accreditation.
Field of Study: Midwifery. *Program Name/Length:* Certificate, 30 units, 12 mos (3 semesters); Masters degree, 38 units, 18 mos (4 semesters).
Degrees Offered: Certificate (Post-Masters); MSN.
License/Certification Preparation: State: CA Board of Registered Nurses; Certified Nurse-Midwife, American College of Nurse-Midwives.
Admission Requirements: Some college; Min GPA: 3.0; Bachelor's degree; Min GPA: 3.0; Master's degree; RN.
Tuition and Fees: $700 per unit.
Financial Aid: Federal government aid; Grants; Loans; Scholarships; State government aid; Work study.

Los Gatos

100. Lupin Massage Institute—Center for Conscious Touch
PO Box 1274, Los Gatos, CA 95031
Phone: (408) 353-4231
Program Administrator: Stuart Grace, Admin/Principal Instr. *Admissions Contact:* Stuart Grace.
Year Established: 1994.

Staff: Full-time: 1; Part-time: 2.
Avg Enrollment: 40. *Avg Class Size:* 8. *Number of Graduates per Year:* 30.
Wheelchair Access: Yes.
Accreditation/Approval/Licensing: State board: CA Bureau of Private Postsecondary and Vocational Ed.
Field of Study: Acupressure; Anatomy and Physiology; CranioSacral Therapy; Esalen Massage*; Manual Lymph Drainage; Massage Therapy*; Swedish Massage*; Visceral Massage;. *Program Name/Length:* Art of Conscious Touch Intensive, 2 wks; Art of Conscious Touch Series, 5 weekends.
Degrees Offered: Certificate.
Admission Requirements: Min age: 18.
Tuition and Fees: $1250 per course.
Financial Aid: Community service.
Career Services: Marketing and business practice information.

Manhattan Beach

101. South Bay Massage College
Massage Technician Program
3770 Highland Ave, Ste 204, Manhattan Beach, CA 90266
Phone: (310) 546-8774; *Fax:* (310) 546-8775
Program Administrator: Dr. Kevin Dobalian, College Dir. *Admissions Contact:* Betsy Anderson, Prog Dir.
Year Established: 1998.
Staff: Full-time: 7.
Avg Enrollment: 100. *Avg Class Size:* 12. *Number of Graduates per Year:* 100.
Wheelchair Access: No.
Accreditation/Approval/Licensing: State board: CA Bureau of Private Postsecondary and Vocational Ed.
Field of Study: Deep Tissue Massage*; Massage Therapy*; Reflexology; Sports Massage*. *Program Name/Length:* Massage Technician, 100 hrs, 6 wks; Deep Tissue Sports Massage, 50 hrs.
Degrees Offered: Certificate.
Admission Requirements: Min age: 18; High school diploma/GED.
Tuition and Fees: $1095 (Massage Technician).
Career Services: Career counseling; Career information; Internships.

Marina Del Rey

102. British Institute of Homeopathy and Complementary Medicine
520 Washington Blvd, Ste 423, Marina Del Rey, CA 90292
Phone: (310) 577-2235; *Fax:* (310) 577-0296
E-mail: bihus@thegrid.net
Program Administrator: Dr. Trevor Cook, Pres. *Admissions Contact:* Betty Lee, Registrar.

Year Established: 1987.
Staff: Full-time: 15.
Avg Enrollment: 1000. **Number of Graduates per Year:** 750.
Accreditation/Approval/Licensing: British Naturopathic and Osteopathic Association.
Field of Study: Animal Therapy*; Flower Essences; Herbal Medicine*; Homeopathy*. **Program Name/Length:** Diploma in Homeopathy, 1-2 yrs, home study; Diploma in Nutrition and Herbology, 1-2 yrs, home study; Diploma Course in Homeopathic Pharmacy, home study; Veterinary Diploma Course, home study.
Degrees Offered: Diploma; Certificate.
License/Certification Preparation: Council for Homeopathic Certification; Homeopathic Academy of Naturopathic Physicians; North American Society of Homeopaths.
Admission Requirements: Min age: 18; Pharmacy degree for Homeopathic Pharmacy.
Tuition and Fees: $1500-$1995.

103. Polarity Healing Arts of Santa Monica

4033 S Via Marina, Ste G315, Marina Del Rey, CA 90292
Phone: (310) 393-7329; **Fax:** (310) 301-3639
Program Administrator: Gary Strauss, Dir. **Admissions Contact:** Beth Hurewitz.
Year Established: 1987.
Staff: Full-time: 3; Part-time: 7.
Avg Enrollment: 200. **Avg Class Size:** 16. **Number of Graduates per Year:** 50.
Wheelchair Access: Yes.
Accreditation/Approval/Licensing: State board: CA Bureau of Private Postsecondary and Vocational Ed; American Polarity Therapy Association.
Field of Study: CranioSacral Therapy*; Energy Work; Polarity Therapy*. **Program Name/Length:** CranioSacral Unwinding, 2-6 mos; Associate Polarity Practitioner, 6 mos; Registered Polarity Practitioner, 12-18 mos.
Degrees Offered: Diploma; Certificate.
License/Certification Preparation: APP and RPP; American Polarity Therapy Association.
Admission Requirements: Specific course prerequisites: bodywork experience required for CranioSacral; APP required for RPP.
Tuition and Fees: $900 (CranioSacral); $1700 (APP); $3552 (RPP).

Menlo Park

104. Center for the Alexander Technique

714 Nash Ave, Menlo Park, CA 94025
Phone: (650) 328-4736
E-mail: edavak@worldnet.att.net
Program Administrator: Edward Avak, Co-Dir; Linda Avak, Co-Dir. **Admissions Contact:** Edward Avak; Linda Avak.
Year Established: 1982.
Staff: Full-time: 2.

Avg Enrollment: 5. **Avg Class Size:** 5. **Number of Graduates per Year:** 2.
Wheelchair Access: No.
Accreditation/Approval/Licensing: American Society for the Alexander Technique.
Field of Study: Alexander Technique*. **Program Name/Length:** Teacher Training, 3 yrs.
Degrees Offered: Certificate.
License/Certification Preparation: American Society for the Alexander Technique.
Admission Requirements: Min age: 18; High school diploma/GED; Specific course prerequisites: private course of Alexander lessons.
Tuition and Fees: $16,200.
Career Services: Career counseling; Career information.

Middletown

105. School of Shiatsu and Massage

18424 Harbin Springs Rd, Middletown, CA 95461
Mailing Address: PO Box 889, Middletown, CA 95461
Phone: (707) 987-3801; **Fax:** (707) 987-9638
E-mail: info@waba.edu **Internet:** http://www.waba.edu
Program Administrator: Harold Dull, Dir. **Admissions Contact:** Tatiana Geyman, Registrar.
Year Established: 1980.
Staff: Part-time: 15.
Avg Class Size: 15.
Wheelchair Access: Yes.
Accreditation/Approval/Licensing: State board: CA Board of Registered Nursing; CA Bureau of Private Postsecondary and Vocational Ed.
Field of Study: Acupressure*; Massage Therapy*; Shiatsu*; Watsu Aquatic Bodywork*. **Program Name/Length:** 50 hrs, 1 wk; Practitioner, 100 hrs, 2 wks; Therapist, 500 hrs; Advanced Body Therapist, 1000 hrs; Watsu Instructor, 650 hrs.
Degrees Offered: Certificate.
Admission Requirements: Min age: 18; High school diploma/GED.
Tuition and Fees: $600 (50 hrs); $1200 (Practitioner); $5400 (Therapist); $10,800 (Advanced Body Therapist).
Financial Aid: Vocational rehabilitation.

Mill Valley

106. Academy for Guided Imagery

311 Miller Ave, Ste E, Mill Valley, CA 94941
Mailing Address: PO Box 2070, Mill Valley, CA 94942
Phone: (800) 726-2070; **Fax:** (415) 389-9342
E-mail: agi1996@aol.com **Internet:** http://www.healthy.net/agi
Program Administrator: Martin Rossman, MD, Co-Dir; David Bresler, PhD, Co-Dir. **Admissions Contact:** Roy Johnston, Exec Dir.

Year Established: 1989.
Staff: Part-time: 57.
Accreditation/Approval/Licensing: State board: CA Alcoholism and Drug Counselors Ed Program; CA Board of Behavioral Sciences; CA Board of Registered Nursing.
Field of Study: Guided Imagery*. *Program Name/Length:* Interactive Guided Imagery Certification, 1-2 yrs.
Degrees Offered: Certificate.
Admission Requirements: Practicing health care professional or full-time student.
Tuition and Fees: $2995.
Financial Aid: Payment plan.

107. Grof Transpersonal Training
20 Sunnyside Ave, Ste A314, Mill Valley, CA 94941
Phone: (415) 383-8779; *Fax:* (415) 383-0965
E-mail: gtt@dnai.com *Internet:* http://www. holotropic.com
Program Administrator: Cary Sparks, Dir of Training. *Admissions Contact:* Maggie Bedord, Training Coord.
Year Established: 1991.
Staff: Full-time: 2; Part-time: 2.
Avg Enrollment: 300. *Avg Class Size:* 50. *Number of Graduates per Year:* 50.
Wheelchair Access: Yes.
Field of Study: Breathwork*. *Program Name/Length:* Holotropic Breathwork Practitioner Certification, 2 yrs+.
Degrees Offered: Certificate.
Tuition and Fees: $10,000.
Financial Aid: Work study.

108. The Trager Institute
21 Locust Ave, Mill Valley, CA 94941-2806
Phone: (415) 388-2688; *Fax:* (415) 388-2710
E-mail: admin@trager.com *Internet:* http://www. trager.com
Program Administrator: Don Schwartz, PhD, Exec Dir. *Admissions Contact:* Marcia Koski, Registrar.
Year Established: 1980.
Staff: Part-time: 17.
Avg Enrollment: 300. *Avg Class Size:* 8. *Number of Graduates per Year:* 300.
Wheelchair Access: Yes.
Accreditation/Approval/Licensing: National Certification Board for Therapeutic Massage and Bodywork (CEUs).
Field of Study: Trager*. *Program Name/Length:* Trager Psychophysical Integration Professional Certification, 18 mos.
Degrees Offered: Certificate.
Tuition and Fees: $2500.

Montebello

109. Montebello Career College
Therapeutic Massage
2465 W Whittier Blvd, Ste 201, Montebello, CA 90640
Phone: (323) 728-9636; *Fax:* (323) 728-0952
Program Administrator: Eric Babaoka, Massage Dept Head. *Admissions Contact:* Rosa Sanchez, Admin.
Staff: Part-time: 4.
Avg Class Size: 6. *Number of Graduates per Year:* 25.
Wheelchair Access: Yes.
Accreditation/Approval/Licensing: Accrediting Commission of Career Schools and Colleges of Technology.
Field of Study: Massage Therapy*. *Program Name/Length:* 150 hrs, 6 wks or 3 mos; 500 hrs, 3 mos or 6 mos.
Degrees Offered: Certificate.
Tuition and Fees: $1450 (150 hrs); $4000 (500 hrs).
Financial Aid: Vocational rehabilitation; Payment plan.
Career Services: Internships; Resume service; Job information; Referral service.

Monterey

110. Meridian Institute
Master of Science in Traditional Chinese Medicine
99 Pacific St, Heritage Harbor Bldg 375A, Monterey, CA 93940
Phone: (831) 649-6684; *Fax:* (831) 649-6688
E-mail: info@meridian.edu *Internet:* http://www. meridian.edu
Program Administrator: Bruce Robinson, MD, Pres. *Admissions Contact:* Andy Seplow, LAc, Admissions Dir.
Year Established: 1997.
Staff: Part-time: 12.
Avg Enrollment: 40. *Avg Class Size:* 20.
Wheelchair Access: Yes.
Accreditation/Approval/Licensing: State board: CA Bureau of Private Postsecondary and Vocational Ed.
Field of Study: Acupuncture*; Herbal Medicine*; Massage Therapy; Traditional Chinese Medicine*. *Program Name/Length:* Master of Science in Traditional Chinese Medicine, 3 1/3 yrs.
Degrees Offered: CEUs; MS; Certificate in Chinese Herbal Medicine; Certificate in Chinese Therapeutic Massage.
License/Certification Preparation: National Certification Commission for Acupuncture and Oriental Medicine.
Admission Requirements: Some college (2 yrs, 60 semester units); Min GPA: 2.7.
Application Deadline(s): Fall: Jul; Spring: Nov.
Tuition and Fees: $3000 per trimester.

Financial Aid: Loans; Scholarships.
Career Services: Career counseling; Career information; Internships.

111. Monterey Peninsula College

Massage Therapy Program/Physical Fitness
980 Fremont St, Monterey, CA 93940
Phone: (831) 646-4220; *Fax:* (831) 645-1334
E-mail: paultuff@redshift.com *Internet:* http://www.mpc.edu
Program Administrator: Dawn Sare, Faculty Advisor.
Year Established: 1994.
Staff: Part-time: 2.
Avg Enrollment: 75. *Avg Class Size:* 20. *Number of Graduates per Year:* 15.
Wheelchair Access: Yes.
Accreditation/Approval/Licensing: State board: CA Bureau of Private Postsecondary Vocational Ed.
Field of Study: Acupressure; Massage Therapy*; Polarity Therapy; Reflexology; Shiatsu; Sports Massage*. *Program Name/Length:* Associate in Science in Massage Therapy, 2 yrs.
Degrees Offered: Certificate.
License/Certification Preparation: National Certification Board for Therapeutic Massage and Bodywork.
Tuition and Fees: $150 approx per semester for CA residents; $1500 approx for nonresidents.
Financial Aid: Federal government aid; Grants; Loans.
Career Services: Career counseling; Career information.

Mount Shasta

112. Hellerwork International LLC

Certified Hellerwork Training
406 Berry St, Mount Shasta, CA 96067
Phone: (800) 392-3900; *Fax:* (916) 926-6839
E-mail: hellerwork@hellerwork.com *Internet:* http://www.hellerwork.com
Program Administrator: Joseph Heller, Managing Member. *Admissions Contact:* Karen Finan, Office Mgr.
Year Established: 1979.
Staff: Full-time: 8; Part-time: 10.
Avg Enrollment: 50. *Avg Class Size:* 15. *Number of Graduates per Year:* 50.
Wheelchair Access: Yes.
Field of Study: Hellerwork*; Structural Integration*. *Program Name/Length:* Practitioner Training, 18 mos.
Degrees Offered: Certificate.
License/Certification Preparation: Certified Hellerwork Practitioner.
Admission Requirements: Min age: 21; High school diploma/GED.
Tuition and Fees: $12,000-$14,000.
Career Services: Career information.

Nevada City

113. The Expanding Light at Ananda

Ananda Yoga Teacher Training
14618 Tyler Foote Rd, Nevada City, CA 95959
Phone: (800) 346-5350; *Fax:* (530) 478-7519
E-mail: info@expandinglight.org *Internet:* http://www.expandinglight.org
Program Administrator: Richard McCord, Dir. *Admissions Contact:* Richard McCord.
Year Established: 1968.
Staff: Full-time: 6; Part-time: 6.
Avg Enrollment: 70. *Avg Class Size:* 20. *Number of Graduates per Year:* 70.
Wheelchair Access: Yes.
Field of Study: Yoga Teacher Training*. *Program Name/Length:* Ananda Yoga Teacher Training, 210 hrs.
Degrees Offered: Certificate.
Admission Requirements: Specific course prerequisites: near daily hatha yoga practice for at least 4 mos.
Tuition and Fees: $1770-$3804 depending on accommodations.
Financial Aid: Scholarships.
Career Services: Career information.

114. Flower Essence Society

Flower Essence Practitioner Training
13139 Daisey Blue Mine Rd, Nevada City, CA 95959
Mailing Address: PO Box 459, Nevada City, CA 95959
Phone: (800) 736-9222; *Fax:* (530) 265-0584
E-mail: mail@flowersociety.org *Internet:* http://www.flowersociety.org
Program Administrator: Patricia Kaminski, Exec Dir. *Admissions Contact:* Susan Amidon, Ed Admin.
Year Established: 1982.
Avg Enrollment: 100. *Avg Class Size:* 40. *Number of Graduates per Year:* 90.
Wheelchair Access: Yes.
Field of Study: Flower Essences*. *Program Name/Length:* Flower Essence Therapy Professional Certification, 7 days classroom and 7 mo case study program.
Degrees Offered: Certificate.
Admission Requirements: Basic understanding of flower essence therapy and holistic healing; professional degree and experience desirable.
Tuition and Fees: $1000.
Financial Aid: Third World scholarships.
Career Services: Referral service.

115. Phillips School of Massage

101 Broad St, Ste B, Nevada City, CA 95959
Mailing Address: PO Box 1999, Nevada City, CA 95959
Phone: (916) 265-4645; *Fax:* (916) 265-9485
E-mail: psm@jps.net *Internet:*

http://www.jps.net/psm/
Program Administrator: Judith Phillips, Owner/Instr. *Admissions Contact:* Kimberly Kenyon, Registrar.
Year Established: 1983.
Staff: Full-time: 1; Part-time: 7.
Avg Enrollment: 100. *Avg Class Size:* 20. *Number of Graduates per Year:* 100.
Wheelchair Access: No.
Accreditation/Approval/Licensing: State board: CA Board of Registered Nursing; CA Bureau of Private Postsecondary and Vocational Ed.
Field of Study: Massage Therapy*. *Program Name/Length:* Level I Massage Therapy Training, 230 hrs; Level II Certificate, 600 hrs; Continuing Education.
Degrees Offered: Certificate.
Application Deadline(s): Fall: Sep; Winter: Jan; Spring: Apr; Summer: Jun.
Tuition and Fees: $1700 (230 hrs); $3500-$4100 (600 hrs).
Financial Aid: Vocational rehabilitation; Payment plan.

North Hollywood

116. Taoist Institute
10630 Burbank Blvd, North Hollywood, CA 91601
Phone: (818) 760-4219
Program Administrator: Carl Totton, PsyD. *Admissions Contact:* Carl Totton.
Year Established: 1981.
Staff: Full-time: 1; Part-time: 4.
Avg Enrollment: 30. *Avg Class Size:* 15. *Number of Graduates per Year:* 30.
Wheelchair Access: No.
Field of Study: Acupressure*; Qigong*; Tui Na*. *Program Name/Length:* Tui Na and Medical Qigong, 2 mos.
Degrees Offered: Certificate.
Admission Requirements: Min age: 18.
Application Deadline(s): Fall: Sep 10; Spring: Feb 10.
Tuition and Fees: $300.
Career Services: Career information.

North San Juan

117. Foothills Massage School
Certified Massage Therapy Training
PO Box 826, North San Juan, CA 95960
Phone: (530) 292-3123; *Fax:* (530) 292-3123 on request
Program Administrator: Saria Farr, Dir. *Admissions Contact:* Saria Farr.
Year Established: 1997.
Staff: Full-time: 1; Part-time: 1.
Avg Enrollment: 80. *Avg Class Size:* 20. *Number of Graduates per Year:* 75.
Wheelchair Access: Yes.

Accreditation/Approval/Licensing: State board: CA Board of Registered Nursing; CA Bureau of Private Postsecondary and Vocational Ed.
Field of Study: Acupressure; Aromatherapy; Deep Tissue Massage; Energy Work; Herbal Medicine; Massage Therapy*; Polarity Therapy; Reflexology; Shiatsu; Yoga Teacher Training. *Program Name/Length:* 100 hrs, 10 wks.
Degrees Offered: Certificate; CMT.
Admission Requirements: Min age: 18.
Tuition and Fees: $520.
Financial Aid: Payment plan.

Oakland

118. Academy of Chinese Culture and Health Sciences
1601 Clay St, Oakland, CA 94612
Phone: (510) 763-7787; *Fax:* (510) 834-8646
E-mail: acchs@best.com *Internet:* http://www.acchs.edu
Year Established: 1984.
Staff: Full-time: 7; Part-time: 32.
Avg Enrollment: 45. *Avg Class Size:* 25. *Number of Graduates per Year:* 35.
Wheelchair Access: Yes.
Accreditation/Approval/Licensing: State board: CA Acupuncture Board; Accreditation Commission for Acupuncture and Oriental Medicine.
Field of Study: Acupuncture*; Herbal Medicine*; Traditional Chinese Medicine*. *Program Name/Length:* Master of Science in Traditional Chinese Medicine, 3 yrs.
Degrees Offered: MSTCM.
License/Certification Preparation: State: CA Licensed Acupuncturist; National Certification Commission for Acupuncture and Oriental Medicine.
Admission Requirements: Some college (60 units—2 yrs); Min GPA: 2.0.
Application Deadline(s): Fall: Aug 1.
Tuition and Fees: $8500 per yr.
Financial Aid: Loans.

119. The Biofeedback Training Institute, Stens Corporation
6451 Oakwood Dr, Oakland, CA 94611
Phone: (800) 257-8367; *Fax:* (510) 339-2222
E-mail: stensco@aol.com
Program Administrator: Wendy Kesseler, Operations Mgr. *Admissions Contact:* Steve Stern, Pres.
Year Established: 1979.
Staff: Full-time: 6.
Avg Enrollment: 350. *Avg Class Size:* 20. *Number of Graduates per Year:* 350.
Wheelchair Access: Yes.
Accreditation/Approval/Licensing: State board: CA Board of Registered Nursing; CA Psychological Association; American Psychological Association.

Field of Study: Biofeedback*. *Program Name/Length:* Professional Biofeedback Certificate, 9 days.
Degrees Offered: Certificate.
License/Certification Preparation: Biofeedback Certification Institute of America.
Admission Requirements: Min age: 21.
Tuition and Fees: $1990.

120. The Breema Center
6076 Claremont Ave, Oakland, CA 94618
Phone: (510) 428-0937; *Fax:* (510) 428-9235
E-mail: center@breema.com *Internet:* http://www.
breema.com
Program Administrator: Joh Schreiber, DC, Dir.
  Admissions Contact: Mary Cuneo, Prog Dir.
Year Established: 1980.
Wheelchair Access: Yes.
Accreditation/Approval/Licensing: State board: CA Bureau of Private Postsecondary and Vocational Ed; National Certification Board for Therapeutic Massage and Bodywork (CEUs).
Field of Study: Breema Bodywork. *Program Name/Length:* 165 hrs, 7 mos min.
Degrees Offered: Certificate.
Admission Requirements: Min age: 15.
Tuition and Fees: $1800 for certification.
Financial Aid: Work study.

121. Center for Hypnotherapy Certification
455 Newton Ave, Ste 1, Oakland, CA 94606
Phone: (510) 839-4800, (800) 398-0034; *Fax:* (510) 836-0477
E-mail: mgordon@hypnotherapycenter.com
Internet: http://www.hypnotherapycenter.com
Program Administrator: Marilyn Gordon, Clinical Hypnotherapist, Dir/Instr. *Admissions Contact:* Marilyn Gordon.
Year Established: 1996.
Staff: Part-time: 3.
Avg Enrollment: 75. *Avg Class Size:* 15. *Number of Graduates per Year:* 75.
Wheelchair Access: Yes.
Accreditation/Approval/Licensing: State board: CA Bureau of Private Postsecondary and Vocational Ed; National Guild of Hypnotists.
Field of Study: Hypnotherapy*. *Program Name/Length:* Core Training, 100 hrs; Advanced, 50 hrs; Clinic Internship, 50 hrs.
Degrees Offered: Certificate.
License/Certification Preparation: National Guild of Hypnotists.
Admission Requirements: High school diploma/GED.
Tuition and Fees: $1500 + $85 Certification (Core Training); $500 (Advanced).
Financial Aid: Payment plan.
Career Services: Career counseling; Internships; Career planning and development.

122. Friends Landing International Centers for Conscious Living, Oakland
Hypnotherapy Certification; Spherical Reality Certification
419 48th St, Oakland, CA 94609
Phone: (541) 484-6004 (Main office: Eugene, OR);
  Fax: (541) 741-1705
E-mail: office@friendslanding.net *Internet:* http://
  www.friendslanding.net
Program Administrator: Whitewind Swan Fisher, Exec Dir. *Admissions Contact:* Whitewind Swan Fisher.
Year Established: 1996.
Staff: Full-time: 2; Part-time: 7.
Avg Enrollment: 90. *Avg Class Size:* 20. *Number of Graduates per Year:* 60.
Wheelchair Access: Yes.
Accreditation/Approval/Licensing: American Association of Professional Hypnotherapists.
Field of Study: Hypnotherapy*. *Program Name/Length:* Hypnotherapy Certification, 100 hrs, 5 mos or intensive format; Seminars given in various locations; Spherical Reality Certification, 10 mos (1 weekend per month and retreats); Seminars given in various locations; Friends Practitioner Certification, 4 levels, up to 8 yrs.
Degrees Offered: Certificate.
Application Deadline(s): Fall: Aug 15 for Hypnotherapy and Spherical Reality; Spring: Feb 15 for Hypnotherapy; Summer: May 15 for Hypnotherapy.
Tuition and Fees: $1635 (Hypnotherapy); $7500 (Spherical Reality).
Financial Aid: Scholarships.
Career Services: Business support.

123. Institute of Chinese Herbology
3871 Piedmont Ave, Ste 363, Oakland, CA 94611
Phone: (510) 428-2061; *Fax:* (510) 428-2061
Program Administrator: Kenneth Morris, Managing Dir. *Admissions Contact:* Jamie Long, Admin.
Year Established: 1986.
Staff: Full-time: 2; Part-time: 2.
Avg Enrollment: 200.
Field of Study: Herbal Medicine*; Traditional Chinese Medicine*. *Program Name/Length:* Comprehensive Herbalist Training, 9 mos-1 yr; Home study/Correspondence; Advanced Certified Herbalist Training, 6 mos; Home study/Correspondence.
Degrees Offered: Certificate.
Tuition and Fees: $1215 (Comprehensive); $525 (Advanced).

124. McKinnon Institute of Professional Massage and Bodywork
2940 Webster St, Oakland, CA 94609-3407
Phone: (510) 465-3488; *Fax:* (510) 465-1533

Program Administrator: Judith McKinnon, Dir.
Admissions Contact: Tiffany Miller, Bus Mgr.
Year Established: 1973.
Staff: Part-time: 30.
Avg Enrollment: 550. *Avg Class Size:* 12. *Number of Graduates per Year:* 525.
Wheelchair Access: Yes.
Accreditation/Approval/Licensing: CA Board of Registered Nurses and Respiratory Care Practitioners (CE Credits); CA Bureau of Private Postsecondary and Vocational Ed; National Certification Board for Therapeutic Massage and Bodywork (CEUs).
Field of Study: Acupressure*; Anatomy and Physiology; CranioSacral Therapy; Deep Tissue Massage*; Massage Therapy*; On-Site Massage; Reflexology; Shiatsu*; Sports Massage*; Swedish Massage*. *Program Name/Length:* Swedish Massage, 100 hrs; Sports-Deep Tissue Massage Level I, 142 hrs; Subtle Systems, 142 hrs; Acupressure and Shiatsu Level I, 142 hrs; Sports-Deep Tissue Massage Level II, 142 hrs; Acupressure and Shiatsu Level II, 132 hrs; Advanced Modalities, 126 hrs.
Degrees Offered: Certificate.
License/Certification Preparation: National Certification Board for Therapeutic Massage and Bodywork.
Admission Requirements: Min age: 18; High school diploma/GED.
Tuition and Fees: $10 per hr.
Financial Aid: Vocational rehabilitation; Payment plan.
Career Services: Career information; Referral service.

Orange

125. Mesa Institute
Sports Massage Therapist; Holistic Health Practitioner
150 N Feldner, Orange, CA 92868
Phone: (714) 937-4161; *Fax:* (714) 937-6360
Program Administrator: Sadie Nichols, Dir. *Admissions Contact:* Chad Marta.
Year Established: 1996.
Staff: Part-time: 12.
Avg Class Size: 10. *Number of Graduates per Year:* 30.
Wheelchair Access: Yes.
Field of Study: Acupressure; Aromatherapy; Ayurvedic Medicine; CranioSacral Therapy; Deep Tissue Massage; Energy Work; Holistic Health*; Hypnotherapy; Massage Therapy*; Polarity Therapy; Reflexology; Reiki; Shiatsu; Sports Massage*. *Program Name/Length:* Sports Massage Therapist, 6-12 mos; Holistic Health Practitioner, 6-12 mos.
Degrees Offered: Certificate.

License/Certification Preparation: National Certification Board for Therapeutic Massage and Bodywork.
Admission Requirements: Min age: 18; High school diploma/GED.
Tuition and Fees: $860-$5200.
Financial Aid: Scholarships; Vocational rehabilitation.
Career Services: Career counseling; Career information; Internships.

Orinda

126. John F. Kennedy University
Graduate School for Holistic Studies
12 Altarinda Rd, Orinda, CA 94563
Phone: (925) 254-0105; *Fax:* (925) 254-3322
Internet: http://www.jfku.edu
Program Administrator: K. Sue Duncan, MA, Dean. *Admissions Contact:* Admissions and Records Office.
Year Established: 1964.
Staff: Full-time: 10; Part-time: 40.
Avg Enrollment: 400. *Avg Class Size:* 20. *Number of Graduates per Year:* 125.
Wheelchair Access: Yes.
Accreditation/Approval/Licensing: State board: CA Board of Behavioral Sciences; Western Association of Schools and Colleges.
Field of Study: Holistic Health*. *Program Name/Length:* Master of Arts in Holistic Health Education, 68 units; Master of Arts in Consciousness Studies, 55 units; Master of Arts in Counseling Psychology (specializations in somatic and transpersonal psychology), 92 units.
Degrees Offered: MA.
License/Certification Preparation: State: CA Marriage, Family, and Child Counselor.
Admission Requirements: Bachelor's degree; Min GPA: 2.0; Personal statement; Two sets of transcripts; Interview.
Application Deadline(s): Fall: Sep 1; Winter: Dec 1; Spring: Mar 1; Summer: Jun 1.
Tuition and Fees: $19,900-$30,000.
Financial Aid: Federal government aid; Loans; Scholarships; VA approved; Vocational rehabilitation.
Career Services: Career counseling; Career information; Internships.

Palm Springs

127. National Institute of Massage
Massage Technician/Therapist
1150 E Palm Canyon Dr, Ste 54, Palm Springs, CA 92264
Phone: (760) 323-3535
Program Administrator: A. Rutkoff, Founder. *Admissions Contact:* Sharon Leeds.
Year Established: 1985.

Staff: Full-time: 2; Part-time: 6.
Avg Enrollment: 50. *Avg Class Size:* 6-10. *Number of Graduates per Year:* 50.
Wheelchair Access: No.
Accreditation/Approval/Licensing: State board: CA Bureau of Private Postsecondary Vocational Ed.
Field of Study: Energy Work; Herbal Medicine; Massage Therapy*; Polarity Therapy; Yoga Teacher Training. *Program Name/Length:* 2 wks to 2 mos; Seminars given in various locations.
Degrees Offered: Certificate.
Application Deadline(s): Fall; Spring.
Tuition and Fees: $700 per course.
Financial Aid: Work study; Payment plan.

Palo Alto

128. Body Therapy Center

368 California Ave, Palo Alto, CA 94306
Phone: (650) 328-9400; *Fax:* (650) 328-9478
Internet: http://www.bodymindspirit.net
Program Administrator: Laura Skinner, Dir. *Admissions Contact:* Laura Skinner.
Year Established: 1983.
Staff: Part-time: 22.
Avg Enrollment: 320. *Avg Class Size:* 18. *Number of Graduates per Year:* 300.
Wheelchair Access: Yes.
Accreditation/Approval/Licensing: State board: CA Board of Registered Nursing; National Certification Board for Therapeutic Massage and Bodywork (CEUs).
Field of Study: CranioSacral Therapy; Deep Tissue Massage; Esalen Massage*; Massage Therapy*; On-Site Massage; Reflexology; Reiki; Shiatsu*; Sports Massage*; Swedish Massage*; Trager. *Program Name/Length:* Fundamentals of Massage, 125 hrs; Advanced Massage and Bodywork Training, 125 hrs; Fundamentals of Shiatsu, 125 hrs; Advanced Shiatsu, 125 hrs; Advanced Massage Symposium, 125 hrs; Clinical Deep Tissue Massage, 125 hrs; Sports Massage, 125 hrs; Continuing Education Workshops: Reiki, CranioSacral Therapy, On-Site Massage, Trager.
Degrees Offered: Certificate.
Admission Requirements: Min age: 18; Specific course prerequisites: Fundamentals of Massage required for Advanced Massage, Fluid Body, and Deep Tissue Massage; Fundamentals of Shiatsu or equivalent for Intermediate Shiatsu; Professional massage experience required for Continuing Ed.
Tuition and Fees: $1050 (Fundamentals programs); $1275 (all other 125 hr programs); $55-$385 (Continuing Ed).
Financial Aid: Payment plan.

129. Palo Alto School of Hypnotherapy

Professional Hypnotherapy

2443 Ash St, Ste D, Palo Alto, CA 94306
Phone: (415) 321-6419, (800) 774-9766; *Fax:* (650) 941-2485
E-mail: josie@deepideas.com *Internet:* http://www.pasoh.com
Program Administrator: Josie Hadley, Dir. *Admissions Contact:* Josie Hadley.
Year Established: 1977.
Staff: Full-time: 2; Part-time: 4.
Avg Class Size: 12. *Number of Graduates per Year:* 1000.
Wheelchair Access: No.
Accreditation/Approval/Licensing: State board: CA Board of Registered Nursing; CA Bureau of Private Postsecondary and Vocational Ed; Accrediting Council for Continuing Education and Training.
Field of Study: Hypnotherapy*; Qigong; Reiki. *Program Name/Length:* Hypnotherapy Certification, 50 hrs, 3 mos; Advanced Hypnotherapy, 50 hrs, 3 mos; Clinical Hypnotherapy, 50 hrs, 3 mos; Medical Hypnosis, 40 hrs, 6 wks; all programs day or evening classes.
Degrees Offered: CEUs; Certificate.
Admission Requirements: Min age: 18; High school diploma/GED.
Application Deadline(s): Fall; Winter; Spring; Summer.
Tuition and Fees: $725 + $350 materials (Hypnotherapy Certification); $675 (Advanced and Clinical).
Financial Aid: Federal government aid; Grants; Loans; Scholarships; Vocational rehabilitation.
Career Services: Career information; Internships.

Placerville

130. EverGreen Herb Garden and Learning Center

PO Box 1445, Placerville, CA 95667
Phone: (916) 626-9288; *Fax:* (916) 626-9288
Program Administrator: Candis Cantin Packard, ND, Ayurvedic Consultant, Herbalist. *Admissions Contact:* Candis Cantin Packard; Lonnie Packard.
Year Established: 1984.
Staff: Full-time: 2; Part-time: 1.
Avg Enrollment: 120. *Avg Class Size:* 20. *Number of Graduates per Year:* 100.
Wheelchair Access: No.
Field of Study: Ayurvedic Medicine*; Herbal Medicine*; Polarity Therapy. *Program Name/Length:* Beginning Program, 3 mos; Intermediate, 3 mos; Ayurvedic Lifestyle Counselor Training, 18 mos.
Degrees Offered: Certificate.
Admission Requirements: Specific course prerequisites: Beginning Program required for Intermediate; Intermediate for Ayurvedic Lifestyle.
Tuition and Fees: $450 (Beginning); $450 (Intermediate); $1500 + books (Ayurvedic Lifestyle).

Career Services: Internships.

Port Richmond

131. Hahnemann College of Homeopathy
80 Nicholl Ave, Port Richmond, CA 94801
Phone: (510) 232-2079; *Fax:* (510) 412-9044
E-mail: hahnemann@igc.apc.org *Internet:* http://
www.hahnemanncollege.com
Program Administrator: Roger Morrison, MD,
Co-Dir; Jonathan Shore, MD, Co-Dir; Nancy
Herrick, PA, Co-Dir. *Admissions Contact:*
Debra Callahan, Admin.
Year Established: 1984.
Staff: Full-time: 3; Part-time: 5.
Avg Enrollment: 70. *Avg Class Size:* 35.
Wheelchair Access: No.
Accreditation/Approval/Licensing: State board: CA
Bureau of Private Postsecondary and Vocational
Ed; Accrediting Council for Continuing Educa-
tion and Training.
Field of Study: Homeopathy*. *Program
Name/Length:* Comprehensive Professional
Course, 4 yrs.
Degrees Offered: Diploma.
Admission Requirements: Medical degree or RN.
Tuition and Fees: $4000 per yr.

Redding

132. Conscious Choice School of Massage and Integral Healing Arts
698 Azalea, Redding, CA 96002
Phone: (530) 224-0957
Program Administrator: Robert Newman, Dir. *Ad-
missions Contact:* Robert Newman.
Year Established: 1994.
Staff: Full-time: 1; Part-time: 1.
Avg Enrollment: 15. *Avg Class Size:* 5. *Number of
Graduates per Year:* 15.
Wheelchair Access: Yes.
Accreditation/Approval/Licensing: State board: CA
Bureau of Private Postsecondary and Vocational
Ed.
Field of Study: Acupressure; Ayurvedic Medicine;
CranioSacral Therapy; Deep Tissue Massage;
Energy Work; Hypnotherapy*; Massage Ther-
apy*; Polarity Therapy; Reflexology; Reiki*.
Program Name/Length: Massage Practitioner
Certification, 100 hrs; Massage Therapist Certif-
ication, 200 hrs; Advanced Massage Therapist
Certification, 150 hrs; Transpersonal
Hypnotherapist Certification, 150 hrs; Advanced
Transpersonal Hypnotherapist Certification, 50
hrs.
Degrees Offered: Certificate.
Admission Requirements: Min age: 18 or parental
consent; High school diploma/GED preferred.
Tuition and Fees: $900 (Massage Practitioner);
$1350 (Massage Therapist); $1100 (Advanced
Massage); $1700 (Transpersonal
Hypnotherapist); $625 (Advanced
Hynotherapist).

133. New Life Institute of Massage Therapy
1159 Hilltop Dr, Redding, CA 96002
Phone: (530) 222-1467; *Fax:* (530) 222-3489
E-mail: glatal@c-zone.net *Internet:* http://www.
newlifeinstitute.com
Program Administrator: Gerry Latal, Dir. *Admis-
sions Contact:* Shirley Latal.
Year Established: 1990.
Staff: Full-time: 2; Part-time: 3.
Avg Class Size: 12.
Wheelchair Access: No.
Accreditation/Approval/Licensing: State board:
CA Bureau of Private Postsecondary and Voca-
tional Ed.
Field of Study: CranioSacral Therapy*; Massage
Therapy*; Myofascial Release*; Reflexology*.
Program Name/Length: Certification Massage
Course, 180 hrs; Advanced Massage Program,
120 hrs.
Degrees Offered: Certificate; CMT.
Admission Requirements: Min age: 18; Specific
course prerequisites: 100 hrs massage therapy or
bodywork training required for Advanced Mas-
sage.
Application Deadline(s): Fall: Sep; Winter: Jan;
Spring: Apr; Summer: Jun.
Tuition and Fees: $1436 (Certification) includes
books; $973 (Advanced).
Financial Aid: Vocational rehabilitation; Payment
plan.
Career Services: Career counseling; Career infor-
mation; Job information.

Redwood Valley

134. Mendocino School of Holistic Massage and Advanced Healing Arts
2680 Rd B, Redwood Valley, CA 95470
Phone: (707) 485-8197
E-mail: rammpack@pacific.net
Program Administrator: Clark Ramm, Dir. *Admis-
sions Contact:* Clark Ramm.
Year Established: 1993.
Staff: Full-time: 1.
Avg Enrollment: 100. *Avg Class Size:* 10. *Number
of Graduates per Year:* 100.
Wheelchair Access: Yes.
Accreditation/Approval/Licensing: Accrediting
Council for Continuing Education and Training.
Field of Study: Aromatherapy; Ayurvedic Medi-
cine; Energy Work; Esalen Massage*; Herbal
Medicine; Holistic Health*; Homeopathy;
Hypnotherapy; Lymphatic Massage; Massage
Therapy*; Polarity Therapy; Rebirthing*;
Reflexology; Swedish Massage*. *Program
Name/Length:* Certified Holistic Massage Ther-
apist, 120 hrs, 3 mos/weekends; Certified Ad-

vanced Holistic Massage Therapist, 220 hrs, 6 mos/weekends; Certified Rebirther, 100 hrs, 8 mos/weekends; Holistic Health Practitioner, 500 hrs, 1 yr/weekends.
Degrees Offered: Diploma; Certificate.
Admission Requirements: Min age: 16; Specific course prerequisites: massage therapy, somatic psychology, and stress management required for Holistic Health Practitioner.
Tuition and Fees: $1380 (Holistic Massage); $1275 (Advanced Massage); $660 (Rebirther); $1100 (Holistic Practitioner).
Financial Aid: Scholarships.
Career Services: Career counseling; Career information.

Riverside

135. Southern California School of Massage

12702 Magnolia Ave, Ste 21, Riverside, CA 92503
Phone: (909) 340-3336; *Fax:* (909) 340-0154
Program Administrator: Elizabeth Kelly, Dir. *Admissions Contact:* Elizabeth Kelly.
Year Established: 1983.
Wheelchair Access: Yes.
Field of Study: Acupressure; Aromatherapy; Deep Tissue Massage; Energy Work; Holistic Health*; Hypnotherapy; Massage Therapy*; Polarity Therapy; Reflexology; Shiatsu; Sports Massage; Traditional Chinese Medicine. *Program Name/Length:* Massage Technician, 9 days, 5 weekends, or 10 wks; Massage Specialist, 3 mos; Massage Therapist, 6 mos; Holistic Health Practitioner, 1 yr.
Degrees Offered: CEUs; Certificate.
License/Certification Preparation: National Certification Board for Therapeutic Massage and Bodywork.
Admission Requirements: Min age: 18; High school reading level.
Career Services: Career counseling; Career information.

136. Valley Hypnosis Center

3705 Sunnyside Dr, Riverside, CA 92506
Phone: (909) 781-0282
E-mail: cernie@pe.net
Admissions Contact: Sally Cernie, PhD, Admin.
Year Established: 1982.
Staff: Full-time: 1; Part-time: 2.
Avg Enrollment: 50. *Avg Class Size:* 15. *Number of Graduates per Year:* 48.
Wheelchair Access: Yes.
Accreditation/Approval/Licensing: State board: CA Bureau of Private Postsecondary and Vocational Ed; Accrediting Council for Continuing Education and Training.
Field of Study: Hypnotherapy*; Pranic Healing*; Reflexology*; Reiki*. *Program Name/Length:*

Reiki, 2 mos; Reflexology, 2 mos; Pranic Healing, 3 mos; Hypnotherapy, 1 yr.
Degrees Offered: Diploma; Certificate.
Admission Requirements: Min age: 21; High school diploma/GED.
Application Deadline(s): Fall; Winter; Summer.
Financial Aid: Payment plan.

Rohnert Park

137. Calistoga Massage Therapy School

5959 Commerce Blvd, Ste 13, Rohnert Park, CA 94928
Phone: (707) 586-1953
Program Administrator: Dr. Steven L. Ticen, Owner/Dir. *Admissions Contact:* Dr. Steven L. Ticen.
Year Established: 1981.
Staff: Full-time: 2.
Avg Enrollment: 80. *Avg Class Size:* 10. *Number of Graduates per Year:* 80.
Wheelchair Access: Yes.
Accreditation/Approval/Licensing: State board: CA Bureau of Private Postsecondary and Vocational Ed.
Field of Study: Massage Therapy*. *Program Name/Length:* 7 wks and 10 wks.
Degrees Offered: Certificate.
Admission Requirements: Min age: 18 (or parental consent).
Tuition and Fees: $800.

Roseville

138. Healing Arts Institute, Roseville

Swedish Massage; Acupressure Therapy
112 Douglas Blvd, Roseville, CA 95678
Phone: (916) 782-1275, (800) 718-6824; *Fax:* (916) 783-4258
E-mail: jmally@usa.net *Internet:* http://www. abundanthealth.com
Program Administrator: Dr. James Mally, Dir. *Admissions Contact:* Joyce Meredith, Associate Dir.
Year Established: 1990.
Staff: Full-time: 1; Part-time: 3.
Avg Enrollment: 200. *Avg Class Size:* 24. *Number of Graduates per Year:* 180.
Wheelchair Access: Yes.
Accreditation/Approval/Licensing: State board: CA Bureau of Private Postsecondary and Vocational Ed.
Field of Study: Acupressure*; Alexander Technique; Aromatherapy; Deep Tissue Massage; Massage Therapy*; Reflexology; Reiki; Shiatsu; Soft Tissue Release; Sports Massage; Swedish Massage*. *Program Name/Length:* Swedish Massage, 126 hrs; Acupressure Therapy, 120 hrs; Workshops.
Degrees Offered: Diploma.

Admission Requirements: Min age: 18; High school diploma/GED.
Application Deadline(s): Winter: Jan, for Acupressure.
Tuition and Fees: $950 (Swedish); $1150 (Acupressure).
Financial Aid: Vocational rehabilitation.
Career Services: Job information.

Sacramento

139. Pacific Institute for the Alexander Technique

930 Alhambra Blvd, Ste 270, Sacramento, CA 95816
Phone: (916) 448-7424
E-mail: piat@sunset.net
Program Administrator: Sherry Berjeron-Oliver, Dir. *Admissions Contact:* Sherry Berjeron-Oliver.
Year Established: 1985.
Staff: Full-time: 1; Part-time: 1.
Avg Enrollment: 6. *Avg Class Size:* 6.
Wheelchair Access: Yes.
Accreditation/Approval/Licensing: Accrediting Council for Continuing Education and Training; American Society for the Alexander Technique.
Field of Study: Alexander Technique*. *Program Name/Length:* Teacher Training, 3 yrs.
Degrees Offered: Certificate.
License/Certification Preparation: American Society for the Alexander Technique.
Admission Requirements: 20-30 lessons in the Alexander Technique; Interview with director.
Tuition and Fees: $5700 per yr.
Career Services: Career information.

San Andreas

140. Calaveras College of Therapeutic Massage

96 Court St, San Andreas, CA 95249
Mailing Address: PO Box 274, San Andreas, CA 95249
Phone: (209) 754-4876
Program Administrator: Michelle Olkowski, Owner. *Admissions Contact:* Michelle Olkowski.
Year Established: 1996.
Staff: Part-time: 4.
Avg Enrollment: 100. *Avg Class Size:* 8. *Number of Graduates per Year:* 100.
Wheelchair Access: No.
Field of Study: Acupressure; Aromatherapy; CranioSacral Therapy; Massage Therapy*; Reflexology; Shiatsu; Swedish Massage*. *Program Name/Length:* 100 hrs.
Degrees Offered: Certificate.

License/Certification Preparation: National Certification Board for Therapeutic Massage and Bodywork.
Admission Requirements: Min age: 18.
Tuition and Fees: $750.

141. Oakendell School of Massage and Healing Arts

Japanese Restorative Massage
3585 Hawver Rd, San Andreas, CA 95249
Mailing Address: 1360 E Oak Park Dr, San Andreas, CA 95249
Phone: (209) 754-0244; *Fax:* (209) 754-1081
Program Administrator: Steve Mertens, Dir. *Admissions Contact:* Steve Mertens.
Year Established: 1994.
Staff: Full-time: 1; Part-time: 3.
Avg Enrollment: 5. *Avg Class Size:* 10. *Number of Graduates per Year:* 4.
Wheelchair Access: No.
Accreditation/Approval/Licensing: State board: CA Bureau of Private Postsecondary Vocational Ed.
Field of Study: Acupressure; Energy Work; Massage Therapy*; Neuromuscular Therapy; Oriental Medicine; Qigong; Traditional Chinese Medicine. *Program Name/Length:* 150 hrs (6 mos).
Degrees Offered: Certificate.
License/Certification Preparation: American Oriental Bodywork Therapy Association.
Admission Requirements: Min age: 18.
Tuition and Fees: $150 reg. fee, $800 tuition.

San Anselmo

142. Alive and Well! Institute of Conscious BodyWork

100 Shaw Dr, San Anselmo, CA 94960
Phone: (415) 258-0402; *Fax:* (415) 258-0635
E-mail: alivewel@aol.com
Program Administrator: Jocelyn Olivier, Dir.
Year Established: 1987.
Staff: Part-time: 32.
Avg Enrollment: 200. *Avg Class Size:* 20. *Number of Graduates per Year:* 150.
Wheelchair Access: Yes.
Accreditation/Approval/Licensing: State board: CA Bureau of Private Postsecondary and Vocational Ed; Accrediting Council for Continuing Education and Training; National Certification Board for Therapeutic Massage and Bodywork (CEUs).
Field of Study: Acupressure; Aromatherapy; CranioSacral Therapy; Massage Therapy*; Neuromuscular Reprogramming; Polarity Therapy; Qigong; Reflexology; Synergetic Studies. *Program Name/Length:* Certified Massage Technician, 3 mos-2 yrs; Advanced Bodyworker, 6 mos-2 yrs; Conscious Bodyworker, 1-3 yrs; Master Bodyworker, 2-5 yrs.

Degrees Offered: Certificate.
Admission Requirements: Min age: 18.
Tuition and Fees: $1300-$14,000.
Financial Aid: Work study; Local government programs.
Career Services: Career counseling; Career information.

San Diego

143. Academy of Health Professions
Massage Therapy; Holistic Health Practitioner
6784 El Cajon Blvd, Ste G, San Diego, CA 92115
Phone: (619) 464-3570, 461-5100; *Fax:* (619) 461-5375
Program Administrator: Karen Croft, Asst Dir. *Admissions Contact:* Karen Croft.
Year Established: 1986.
Staff: Part-time: 14.
Avg Enrollment: 100. *Avg Class Size:* 25. *Number of Graduates per Year:* 80.
Wheelchair Access: Yes.
Accreditation/Approval/Licensing: Accrediting Council for Continuing Education and Training.
Field of Study: Aromatherapy; Deep Tissue Massage; Energy Work; Hawaiian Massage; Herbal Medicine; Holistic Health*; Hypnotherapy; Massage Therapy*; Nutrition; Passive Joint Movement; Pregnancy Massage; Reflexology; Reiki; Shiatsu; Sports Massage; Structural Alignment; Swedish Massage; Tui Na. *Program Name/Length:* Massage Therapy, 730 hrs, 10 mos/evenings; Holistic Health Practitioner, 1000 hrs, 10 mos.
Degrees Offered: Certificate.
License/Certification Preparation: National Certification Board for Therapeutic Massage and Bodywork.
Admission Requirements: High school diploma/GED.
Tuition and Fees: $8231-$10,649.
Financial Aid: Federal government aid; Grants; Loans; Scholarships; Work study; VA approved; Vocational rehabilitation.
Career Services: Career counseling; Career information; Internships; Interview set up; Resume service.

144. International Professional School of Bodywork
1366 Hornblend St, San Diego, CA 92109
Phone: (619) 272-4142; *Fax:* (619) 272-4772
E-mail: beingipsb@aol.com *Internet:* http://www.webcom.com/ipsb
Program Administrator: Barbara Clark, Dir. *Admissions Contact:* Valerie Vaughan, Student Dir.
Year Established: 1977.
Staff: Part-time: 35.
Avg Enrollment: 250. *Avg Class Size:* 26.
Wheelchair Access: Yes.

Accreditation/Approval/Licensing: State board: CA Bureau of Private Postsecondary and Vocational Ed; CA Board of Registered Nursing; Commission on Massage Therapy Accreditation; National Certification Board for Therapeutic Massage and Bodywork (CEUs); American Oriental Bodywork Therapy Association.
Field of Study: Acupressure; Alexander Technique; CranioSacral Therapy; Feldenkrais; Herbal Medicine; Massage Therapy*; Neuromuscular Therapy; Qigong; Shiatsu; Sports Massage. *Program Name/Length:* Associate of Science in Massage and Bodywork, 2 yrs; Associate of Arts in Massage and Bodywork, 2-5 yrs; Bachelor of Arts in Massage and Bodywork, 4 yrs; Master in Somatics, 1 yr.
Degrees Offered: MS; Diploma; Certificate; AA; AS; BA.
License/Certification Preparation: American Oriental Bodywork Therapy Association; National Certification Board for Therapeutic Massage and Bodywork; City Massage Technician Permit.
Admission Requirements: Min age: 18; High school diploma/GED.
Tuition and Fees: $8704 (AS); $11,352 (AA); $21,300 (BA, includes AA); $6000 (MS).
Career Services: Career information.

145. Mueller College of Holistic Studies
4607 Park Blvd, San Diego, CA 92116
Phone: (619) 291-9811; *Fax:* (619) 543-1113
E-mail: info@muellercollege.com *Internet:* http://www.muellercollege.com
Program Administrator: Bill Mueller, Dir of Academics. *Admissions Contact:* Jan Freya, Admissions.
Year Established: 1976.
Staff: Full-time: 3; Part-time: 14.
Avg Enrollment: 450. *Avg Class Size:* 22. *Number of Graduates per Year:* 400.
Wheelchair Access: Yes.
Accreditation/Approval/Licensing: State board: CA Bureau of Private Postsecondary and Vocational Ed; Commission on Massage Therapy Accreditation; National Certification Board for Therapeutic Massage and Bodywork (CEUs); American Oriental Bodywork Therapy Association.
Field of Study: Acupressure*; Aromatherapy; Ayurvedic Medicine; CranioSacral Therapy; Herbal Medicine; Holistic Health*; Massage Therapy*; Oriental Medicine; Polarity Therapy; Qigong; Reflexology; Shiatsu; Traditional Chinese Medicine. *Program Name/Length:* Massage Technician, 100 hrs; Massage Therapist, 512 hrs (includes Tech); Acupressurist, 626 hrs (includes Tech); Holistic Health Practitioner, 1000 hrs (includes Therapist or Acupressurist).
Degrees Offered: Certificate.
License/Certification Preparation: American Oriental Bodywork Therapy Association; National Certification Board for Therapeutic Massage and Bodywork.

Admission Requirements: Min age: 18; Entrance exam.

Tuition and Fees: $770 (Massage Technician); $3600 (Massage Therapist); $4625 (Acupressurist); $1080 (Holistic Practitioner).

Financial Aid: VA approved; Vocational rehabilitation; Payment plan.

146. Pacific College of Oriental Medicine, San Diego

7445 Mission Valley Rd, Ste 105, San Diego, CA 92108

Phone: (619) 574-6909; *Fax:* (619) 574-6641

E-mail: jmiller@ormed.edu *Internet:* http://www.ormed.edu

Program Administrator: Jack Miller, LAc, Pres/Dean. *Admissions Contact:* Reine S. Deming, Admissions Dir.

Year Established: 1987.

Staff: Full-time: 2; Part-time: 28.

Avg Enrollment: 317. *Avg Class Size:* 20. *Number of Graduates per Year:* 50.

Wheelchair Access: Yes.

Accreditation/Approval/Licensing: State board: CA Acupuncture Board; CA Bureau of Private Postsecondary and Vocational Ed; Accreditation Commission for Acupuncture and Oriental Medicine; American Oriental Bodywork Therapy Association.

Field of Study: Acupressure*; Acupuncture*; Energy Work; Herbal Medicine; Holistic Health*; Massage Therapy*; Oriental Medicine*; Qigong; Reflexology; Shiatsu*; Sports Massage; Traditional Chinese Medicine*. *Program Name/Length:* Master of Traditional Oriental Medicine, 4 yrs; Massage Therapist, 2-14 wks; Oriental Bodywork Therapy, 1 2/3 yrs; Holistic Health Practitioner, 2 yrs.

Degrees Offered: Certificate; MTOM.

License/Certification Preparation: State: CA Licensed Acupuncturist; National Certification Commission for Acupuncture and Oriental Medicine; American Oriental Bodywork Therapy Association; National Certification Board for Therapeutic Massage and Bodywork.

Admission Requirements: For MTOM: High school diploma/GED; Some college (60 semester units); Min GPA: 2.25.

Application Deadline(s): Fall: Aug; Winter: Dec; Spring: Apr.

Financial Aid: MTOM only; Grants; Loans.

147. School of Healing Arts

1001 Garnet Ave, Ste 200, San Diego, CA 92109

Phone: (619) 581-9429; *Fax:* (619) 490-2555

E-mail: sha@adnc.com *Internet:* http://www.schoolhealingarts.com

Program Administrator: Seymour Koblin, Dir.

Year Established: 1984.

Staff: Full-time: 15; Part-time: 20.

Avg Enrollment: 1000. *Avg Class Size:* 20.

Accreditation/Approval/Licensing: Accrediting Council for Continuing Education and Training; National Certification Board for Therapeutic Massage and Bodywork (CEUs).

Field of Study: Acupressure; Holistic Health*; Hypnotherapy*; Massage Therapy*; Shiatsu*. *Program Name/Length:* Massage Technician, 2 mos; Clinical Massage Therapist, 1 yr; Whole Foods Nutritional Consultant, 9 mos; Holistic Health Practitioner, 2 yrs.

Degrees Offered: Certificate.

License/Certification Preparation: American Oriental Bodywork Therapy Association; National Certification Board for Therapeutic Massage and Bodywork; American Board of Hypnotherapy.

Admission Requirements: Min age: 18; High school diploma/GED.

Tuition and Fees: $750 (Massage Technician); $3750 (Massage Therapist); $2250 (Whole Foods Consultant); $7500 (Holistic Practitioner).

Financial Aid: Work study; VA approved; Vocational rehabilitation; Payment plan.

Career Services: Internships; Job board.

148. Wyrick Institute and Clinic

Manual Lymph Drainage: Basic and Advanced

PO Box 99745, San Diego, CA 92169

Phone: (619) 273-9764; *Fax:* (619) 277-7358

Program Administrator: Dana Wyrick, BA, Dir. *Admissions Contact:* Dana Wyrick, Dir.

Year Established: 1984.

Staff: Full-time: 1; Part-time: 1.

Avg Enrollment: 100. *Avg Class Size:* 12. *Number of Graduates per Year:* 100.

Accreditation/Approval/Licensing: National Certification Board for Therapeutic Massage and Bodywork (CEUs).

Field of Study: Manual Lymph Drainage*. *Program Name/Length:* Basic Body, 5 days; Advanced Body, 5 days; Basic Neck and Face, 2 days; Advanced Neck and Face, 2 days.

Degrees Offered: Certificate.

Admission Requirements: Min age: 18; Health care professional.

Tuition and Fees: $600 (5 days); $300 (2 days).

San Francisco

149. Alexander Training Institute of San Francisco

c/o ACT, 30 Grant Ave, 8th Fl, San Francisco, CA 94108

Mailing Address: 931 Elizabeth, San Francisco, CA 94114

Phone: (415) 439-2465

Program Administrator: Frank Ottiwell, Dir. *Admissions Contact:* Stella Moon, Admin.

Year Established: 1974.

Staff: Part-time: 6.

Avg Enrollment: 20. *Avg Class Size:* 16. *Number of Graduates per Year:* 5.
Wheelchair Access: Yes.
Accreditation/Approval/Licensing: State board: CA Bureau of Private Postsecondary and Vocational Ed; American Society for the Alexander Technique.
Field of Study: Alexander Technique. *Program Name/Length:* Teacher Training, 3 yrs.
Degrees Offered: Certificate.
Admission Requirements: Min age: 21; Specific course prerequisites: 30 private lessons with certified Alexander Technique teacher.
Application Deadline(s): Fall: Sep; Winter: Dec; Spring: Feb; Summer: May.
Tuition and Fees: $17,400.

150. American College of Traditional Chinese Medicine

455 Arkansas St, San Francisco, CA 94107
Phone: (415) 282-7600; *Fax:* (415) 282-0856
E-mail: lhuang@actcm.org *Internet:* http://www. actcm.org
Program Administrator: Lixin Huang, Pres. *Admissions Contact:* Wally Walker, Dir of Admin/Admissions.
Year Established: 1980.
Staff: Full-time: 4; Part-time: 16.
Avg Enrollment: 120. *Avg Class Size:* 22. *Number of Graduates per Year:* 15.
Wheelchair Access: Yes.
Accreditation/Approval/Licensing: State board: CA Bureau of Private Postsecondary and Vocational Ed; Accreditation Commission for Acupuncture and Oriental Medicine.
Field of Study: Acupuncture*; Herbal Medicine; Qigong; Traditional Chinese Medicine*. *Program Name/Length:* Master of Science in Traditional Chinese Medicine, 3 yrs/full-time or 4-5 yrs/part-time.
Degrees Offered: MSTCM.
License/Certification Preparation: State: CA Licensed Acupuncturist; National Certification Commission for Acupuncture and Oriental Medicine.
Admission Requirements: Bachelor's degree; Min GPA: 3.0.
Application Deadline(s): Fall: Sep; Winter: Dec; Spring: Mar; Summer: Jun.
Tuition and Fees: $30,000.
Financial Aid: Federal government aid; Loans.
Career Services: Career counseling; Career information.

151. California Institute of Integral Studies

Somatics Program
1453 Mission St, San Francisco, CA 94103
Phone: (415) 575-6126; *Fax:* (415) 575-1264
E-mail: iang@ciis.edu *Internet:* http://www.ciis. edu
Program Administrator: Ian Grand, Dir. *Admissions Contact:* Beth Bremer.

Year Established: 1964.
Staff: Full-time: 2; Part-time: 5.
Avg Enrollment: 50. *Avg Class Size:* 12. *Number of Graduates per Year:* 14.
Wheelchair Access: Yes.
Accreditation/Approval/Licensing: Western Association of Schools and Colleges.
Field of Study: Somatic Education*. *Program Name/Length:* Master of Arts in Health Education, 6 qtrs.
Degrees Offered: MA.
License/Certification Preparation: MFCC.
Admission Requirements: Bachelor's degree; Min GPA: 3.0; Background in movement or bodywork; 2 letters of recommendation.
Application Deadline(s): Spring: May 1.
Tuition and Fees: $275 per unit.
Financial Aid: Federal government aid; Loans; Scholarships; State government aid; Work study.
Career Services: Career counseling; Career information; Internships.

152. Institute for the Study of Somatic Education

1158 Naples St, San Francisco, CA 94112
Phone: (415) 333-6644; *Fax:* (415) 333-6644
E-mail: isse@aol.com
Program Administrator: Paul Rubin, Educational Dir. *Admissions Contact:* Paul Rubin.
Year Established: 1992.
Staff: Full-time: 2; Part-time: 15.
Avg Enrollment: 200. *Avg Class Size:* 50.
Wheelchair Access: Yes.
Accreditation/Approval/Licensing: Feldenkrais Guild.
Field of Study: Feldenkrais*; Somatic Education*. *Program Name/Length:* Professional Teachers' Training, 3 1/2-4 yrs; Seminars given in various locations.
Degrees Offered: Diploma.
License/Certification Preparation: Certified Feldenkrais Practitioner, Feldenkrais Guild.
Tuition and Fees: $3400 per yr.
Career Services: Career counseling; Career information.

153. Institute of Classical Homeopathy

Fort Mason Center, San Francisco, CA 94123
Mailing Address: 1336D Oak Ave, Saint Helena, CA 94574
Phone: (707) 963-7796; *Fax:* (707) 963-6131
E-mail: ichinfo@classicalhomoeopathy.org
Internet: http://www.classical homoeopathy.org
Program Administrator: Cara Landry, Prog Dir. *Admissions Contact:* Stephanie Bero, Office Mgr.
Year Established: 1991.
Staff: Full-time: 2.
Wheelchair Access: Yes.
Accreditation/Approval/Licensing: British Register of Complementary Practitioners.

Field of Study: Homeopathy*. *Program Name/Length:* Classical Hahnemannian Homeopathy Professional Training, 4 yrs.
Degrees Offered: Diploma; Certificate; Doctorate (application in process).
License/Certification Preparation: Council for Homeopathic Certification; North American Society of Homeopaths; British Register of Complementary Practitioners.
Admission Requirements: Min age: 18; High school diploma/GED; Interview; Specific course prerequisites: anatomy and physiology, may be taken during first year.
Application Deadline(s): Fall: May 15.
Tuition and Fees: $3400 per yr.
Financial Aid: Scholarships; Work study.
Career Services: Career counseling; Career information; Internships; Referral service.

154. Iyengar Yoga Institute

2404 27th Ave, San Francisco, CA 94116
Phone: (415) 753-0909; *Fax:* (415) 753-0913
E-mail: iyisf@sirius.com *Internet:* http://www. iyoga.com/iyisf
Admissions Contact: Janet MacLeod, Prog Dir.
Year Established: 1972.
Avg Enrollment: 35. *Avg Class Size:* 20. *Number of Graduates per Year:* 10.
Wheelchair Access: No.
Accreditation/Approval/Licensing: State board: CA Bureau of Private Postsecondary and Vocational Ed.
Field of Study: Yoga Teacher Training*. *Program Name/Length:* Teacher Training Certificate, 2 yrs.
Degrees Offered: Certificate.
License/Certification Preparation: Certification, Iyengar Yoga National Association.
Admission Requirements: Min age: 18; Specific course prerequisites: 2 yrs of Iyengar-style yoga study.
Tuition and Fees: $4215.
Financial Aid: Scholarships; Work study.
Career Services: Career counseling; Career information; Internships.

155. Midwifery Institute of California

3739 Balboa, Ste 179, San Francisco, CA 94121
Mailing Address: PO Box 128, Bristol, VT 05443
Phone: Voice mail: (415) 248-1671, administration office: (802) 453-3332
Program Administrator: Shannon Ariton, Elizabeth Davis, Co-Founders. *Admissions Contact:* Shannon Ariton, Elizabeth Davis.
Year Established: 1995.
Staff: Part-time: 4.
Avg Class Size: 10.
Wheelchair Access: Yes.
Accreditation/Approval/Licensing: Midwifery Education Accreditation Council.

Field of Study: Midwifery*. *Program Name/Length:* 84 semester units, 3 academic yrs; Distance Learning Program.
Degrees Offered: Certificate.
License/Certification Preparation: State: CA, approval pending; Certified Professional Midwife, North American Registry of Midwives.
Admission Requirements: Min age: 18; High school diploma/GED.
Tuition and Fees: $7500.
Career Services: Career information; Program prepares student to set up practice.
Comments: First year of program taught in San Francisco, remainder of program taught in the San Francisco Bay area.

156. Pacific Academy of Homeopathy

1199 Sanchez St, San Francisco, CA 94114
Phone: (415) 458-8238; *Fax:* (415) 695-8220
E-mail: pahm@slip.net
Program Administrator: Richard Pitt, Exec Dir.
Year Established: 1985.
Avg Enrollment: 25. *Avg Class Size:* 20. *Number of Graduates per Year:* 20.
Wheelchair Access: Yes.
Accreditation/Approval/Licensing: State board: CA Bureau of Private Postsecondary and Vocational Ed.
Field of Study: Homeopathy*. *Program Name/Length:* 2 yrs; Postgraduate course, 1 yr.
Degrees Offered: Certificate.
Admission Requirements: Specific course prerequisites: CPR/First Aid; anatomy and physiology, and acute care differential course by end of first year; pathology during program.
Tuition and Fees: $3500 per yr.
Financial Aid: Limited work study; Payment plan.
Career Services: Career counseling; Career information.

157. ROSA Institute of Aromatherapy

Aromatherapy and Herbal Studies
219 Carl St, San Francisco, CA 94117-3804
Phone: (415) 564-6785; *Fax:* (415) 564-6799
Internet: http://www.aromaticplantproject.com
Program Administrator: Jeanne Rose, MH, Head Tutor. *Admissions Contact:* Kimberly Neahr, Admissions.
Year Established: 1988.
Staff: Full-time: 1; Part-time: 5.
Avg Enrollment: 250. *Avg Class Size:* 25. *Number of Graduates per Year:* 25.
Accreditation/Approval/Licensing: State board: CA Board of Registered Nursing; Accrediting Council for Continuing Education and Training.
Field of Study: Aromatherapy*; Herbal Medicine*. *Program Name/Length:* Aromatherapy, 6-12 mos, home study; Herbal Studies, 2-3 yrs, home study; Aromatherapy and Herbal Study for Certification, 3 yrs, home study and intensives.
Degrees Offered: Diploma; Certificate.

License/Certification Preparation: National Association for Holistic Aromatherapy.
Admission Requirements: High school diploma/GED; Min GPA: 2.0.
Tuition and Fees: $350-$675 + $250-$400 for Certification intensives.
Career Services: Career information.

158. San Francisco School of Massage
1327 A Chestnut St, San Francisco, CA 94123
Phone: (415) 474-4600; *Fax:* (415) 474-4601
E-mail: sfsmschool@aol.com *Internet:* http://www.dharmanet.org/SFSM
Program Administrator: Richard Bergess, Co-Dir; Paulette Bergess, Co-Dir. *Admissions Contact:* Richard Bergess; Paulette Bergess.
Year Established: 1969.
Staff: Part-time: 7.
Avg Enrollment: 230. *Avg Class Size:* 14. *Number of Graduates per Year:* 160.
Wheelchair Access: No.
Accreditation/Approval/Licensing: State board: CA Board of Registered Nursing; CA Bureau of Private Postsecondary and Vocational Ed.
Field of Study: Acupressure; Aromatherapy; Breema Bodywork; CranioSacral Therapy; Deep Tissue Massage; Esalen Massage*; Lymphatic Massage; Massage Therapy*; Reflexology; Reiki; Shiatsu*; Sports Massage; Swedish Massage*; Trigger Point Therapy. *Program Name/Length:* Swedish/Esalen Massage, 102 hrs, ongoing or two week intensives; Advanced Swedish, 201 hrs, 5 mos; Shiatsu, 103 hrs, 13 wks; Advanced Shiatsu, 201 hrs, 5 mos.
Degrees Offered: Certificate.
License/Certification Preparation: American Oriental Bodywork Therapy Association; National Certification Board for Therapeutic Massage and Bodywork.
Admission Requirements: Min age: 18; Proficiency in English.
Tuition and Fees: $875.
Financial Aid: Payment plan.
Career Services: Job information.

159. TouchPro Institute of Chair Massage
584 Castro St, Ste 555, San Francisco, CA 94114
Phone: (800) 999-5026; *Fax:* (415) 621-1260
E-mail: info@touchpro.org *Internet:* http://www.touchpro.org
Program Administrator: David Palmer, Exec Dir. *Admissions Contact:* Douglas Hudson, Prog Coord.
Year Established: 1986.
Avg Enrollment: 600. *Avg Class Size:* 14. *Number of Graduates per Year:* 600.
Field of Study: Chair Massage*. *Program Name/Length:* TouchPro Technique; TouchPro Marketing; Seminars given in various locations; Home study/Correspondence.
Degrees Offered: Certificate.

Admission Requirements: Professional bodyworker or student.
Tuition and Fees: $330 (Technique); $100 (Marketing).

160. United States Yoga Association
Instructor Training Program
2159 Filbert St, San Francisco, CA 94123
Phone: (415) 931-YOGA (9642); *Fax:* (415) 921-6676
E-mail: tony@usyoga.org *Internet:* http://www.usyoga.org
Program Administrator: Tony Sanchez, Dir. *Admissions Contact:* Sandy Wong, Admissions.
Year Established: 1984.
Staff: Full-time: 1; Part-time: 5.
Avg Enrollment: 45. *Avg Class Size:* 12. *Number of Graduates per Year:* 40.
Wheelchair Access: Yes.
Field of Study: Yoga Teacher Training*. *Program Name/Length:* Yoga Challenge I System, 3 mos.
Degrees Offered: Certificate.
Tuition and Fees: $1200.
Financial Aid: Scholarships; Work study; Payment plan.
Career Services: Career counseling; Career information; Internships; Interview set up.

161. The World School of Massage and Advanced Healing Arts
401 32nd Ave, San Francisco, CA 94121
Phone: (415) 221-2533; *Fax:* (415) 221-0430
Program Administrator: Patricia Cramer, Owner/Founder; Edwin Niskanen, Dir. *Admissions Contact:* Karsta Jensen.
Year Established: 1982.
Staff: Full-time: 5; Part-time: 5.
Avg Enrollment: 120. *Avg Class Size:* 15. *Number of Graduates per Year:* 100.
Wheelchair Access: No.
Accreditation/Approval/Licensing: State board: CA Bureau of Private Postsecondary and Vocational Ed.
Field of Study: Aromatherapy; CranioSacral Therapy; Holistic Health*; Massage Therapy*; Reflexology; Vibrational Therapy. *Program Name/Length:* Holistic Massage Therapy, 3-4 mos; Advanced Massage Therapy, 4-5 mos; Holistic Health Counselor, 9 mos; Master Bodyworker/Holistic Health Educator, 12-14 mos.
Degrees Offered: Certificate.
Admission Requirements: Min age: 17; High school diploma/GED.
Tuition and Fees: $1300 (Holistic Massage); $2500 (Advanced Massage); $3950 (Holistic Counselor); $8200-$9950 (Master Bodyworker).
Financial Aid: Work study.
Career Services: Job information.

San Jose

162. Just for Your Health College of Massage
Massage Certification
2075 Lincoln Ave, Ste E, San Jose, CA 95125
Phone: (408) 723-2131; *Fax:* (408) 723-7389
Program Administrator: Tina Garcia, Owner/Dir.
   Admissions Contact: Tria Vangel, Mgr.
Year Established: 1986.
Staff: Full-time: 2; Part-time: 5.
Avg Enrollment: 180. *Avg Class Size:* 12. *Number of Graduates per Year:* 180.
Wheelchair Access: No.
Accreditation/Approval/Licensing: Accrediting Council for Continuing Education and Training.
Field of Study: Acupressure*; Aromatherapy; Deep Tissue Massage*; Energy Work; Massage Therapy*; Reflexology*; Shiatsu*; Sports Massage*; Tai Chi. *Program Name/Length:* Certified Massage Therapist, 100 hrs, 2 wks/full-time or 17 wks/part-time; Master Massage Therapist, 400 hrs, 6 mos/part-time.
Degrees Offered: Certificate.
Admission Requirements: Min age: 16.
Tuition and Fees: $925-$4375.
Financial Aid: Federal government aid; State government aid; VA approved; Vocational rehabilitation; Payment plan.
Career Services: Career information; Job information; Referral service.

163. Palmer College of Chiropractic West
90 E Tasman Dr, San Jose, CA 95134
Phone: (408) 944-6000, (800) 442-4476; *Fax:* (408) 944-6111
Internet: http://www.palmer.edu
Program Administrator: Peter A. Martin, DC, Pres.
Accreditation/Approval/Licensing: Council on Chiropractic Education.
Field of Study: Chiropractic*.
Degrees Offered: DC.
Admission Requirements: Some college.

San Lorenzo

164. Life Chiropractic College West
2005 Via Barrett, San Lorenzo, CA 94580
Phone: (800) 788-4476; *Fax:* (510) 276-4893
E-mail: info@lifewest.edu *Internet:* http://www.lifewest.edu
Program Administrator: Gerard W. Clum, DC, Pres. *Admissions Contact:* Jeffrey D. Cook, Admissions Dir.
Year Established: 1976.
Staff: Full-time: 25; Part-time: 75.
Avg Enrollment: 800. *Avg Class Size:* 50. *Number of Graduates per Year:* 200.
Wheelchair Access: Yes.
Accreditation/Approval/Licensing: Council on Chiropractic Education.

Field of Study: Chiropractic*. *Program Name/Length:* Doctor of Chiropractic, 12 qtrs.
Degrees Offered: DC.
Admission Requirements: Min age: 21 to graduate; Some college (2 yrs).
Application Deadline(s): Fall: Aug 1; Winter: Nov 1; Spring: Feb 1; Summer: May 1.
Tuition and Fees: $4100 per qtr.
Financial Aid: Federal government aid; Grants; Loans; Scholarships; State government aid; Work study; VA approved.
Career Services: Career information; Internships; Job information.

San Luis Obispo

165. Central California School of Body Therapy
1330 Southwood Dr, Ste 7, San Luis Obispo, CA 93401
Phone: (805) 783-2200; *Fax:* (805) 783-2200
E-mail: siouxsun1@aol.com
Program Administrator: Susan E. Stocks, MA, Owner/Admin. *Admissions Contact:* Susan E. Stocks.
Year Established: 1991.
Staff: Part-time: 9.
Avg Enrollment: 18. *Avg Class Size:* 18. *Number of Graduates per Year:* 18.
Accreditation/Approval/Licensing: State board: CA Bureau of Private Postsecondary and Vocational Ed; Commission on Massage Therapy Accreditation.
Field of Study: Acupressure; CranioSacral Therapy; Herbal Medicine; Homeopathy; Hypnotherapy; Massage Therapy*; Shiatsu. *Program Name/Length:* Massage Therapist, 10 mos.
Degrees Offered: Certificate.
License/Certification Preparation: City/county License.
Admission Requirements: Min age: 18; High school diploma/GED; Exam; Interview with clinical psychologist.
Application Deadline(s): Winter: Jan.
Tuition and Fees: $6000 includes books.

San Mateo

166. Vitality Sciences Institute
Reposturing Dynamics Certification
70-A N El Camino Real, San Mateo, CA 94401-2866
Phone: (650) 347-4565; *Fax:* (650) 344-7783
E-mail: vitality7@aol.com *Internet:* http://www.vitality7.com
Program Administrator: Aaron Ulysses Parnell, Exec Dir. *Admissions Contact:* Alicia Parnell, Dir of Admissions.
Year Established: 1994.

Staff: Part-time: 3.
Avg Enrollment: 8. *Avg Class Size:* 8. *Number of Graduates per Year:* 8.
Wheelchair Access: No.
Field of Study: Reposturing Dynamics*. *Program Name/Length:* 140 hrs, 4 mos (7 weekends).
Degrees Offered: Certificate.
Admission Requirements: Min age: 18; Proficiency in English.
Application Deadline(s): Fall: Sep 1; Spring: Jan 15.
Tuition and Fees: $1895 + $35 student insurance.
Career Services: Career counseling; Business training.

San Rafael

167. Pacific Institute of Aromatherapy
PO Box 6723, San Rafael, CA 94903
Phone: (415) 479-9121; *Fax:* (415) 479-0119
Program Administrator: Dr. Kurt Schnaubelt, Dir.
Field of Study: Aromatherapy*. *Program Name/Length:* Correspondence course, 12-14 wks.
Degrees Offered: Certificate.
Tuition and Fees: $365.

Santa Barbara

168. Body Therapy Institute of Santa Barbara
835 N Milpas St, Santa Barbara, CA 93103
Phone: (805) 966-5802
E-mail: bti@silcom.com *Internet:* http://www.silcom.com/~bti
Program Administrator: Katie Mickey, Dir. *Admissions Contact:* Gael Ashwood, Dir of Admissions.
Year Established: 1984.
Staff: Part-time: 12.
Avg Enrollment: 100. *Avg Class Size:* 12. *Number of Graduates per Year:* 60.
Wheelchair Access: No.
Accreditation/Approval/Licensing: State board: CA Bureau of Private Postsecondary and Vocational Ed.
Field of Study: Acupressure*; CranioSacral Therapy; Deep Tissue Massage; Energy Work*; Holistic Health*; Massage Therapy*; Polarity Therapy*; Qigong; Reflexology*; Reiki; Shiatsu. *Program Name/Length:* Massage Technician, 200 hrs, 3 mos; Massage Therapist, 650 hrs, 8-16 mos; Holistic Health Practitioner, 1000 hrs, 16-24 mos.
Degrees Offered: Certificate.
License/Certification Preparation: National Certification Board for Therapeutic Massage and Bodywork.
Admission Requirements: Min age: 18.

Application Deadline(s): Fall: Oct; Winter: Feb; Spring: May; Summer: Aug.
Tuition and Fees: $1100 (Massage Technician); $4600 (Massage Therapist); $6500 (Holistic Health Practitioner).
Financial Aid: Work study; Vocational rehabilitation; Payment plans.
Career Services: Career information.

169. Santa Barbara College of Oriental Medicine
Master's Degree in Chinese Oriental Medicine
1919 State St, Ste 204, Santa Barbara, CA 93101
Phone: (805) 898-1180; *Fax:* (805) 682-1864
E-mail: 76774.3507@compuserve.com *Internet:* http://www.sbcom.edu
Program Administrator: JoAnn Hickey, Pres. *Admissions Contact:* Lark Batteau Bailey, Registrar.
Year Established: 1986.
Staff: Part-time: 16.
Avg Enrollment: 30. *Avg Class Size:* 24. *Number of Graduates per Year:* 18.
Wheelchair Access: Yes.
Accreditation/Approval/Licensing: State board: CA Acupuncture Board; Accrediting Council for Continuing Education and Training; Accreditation Commission for Acupuncture and Oriental Medicine.
Field of Study: Acupressure; Acupuncture*; Chinese Herbal Medicine; Oriental Medicine*; Qigong; Shiatsu; Traditional Chinese Medicine*. *Program Name/Length:* Master of Science in Acupuncture and Oriental Medicine, 3 yrs.
Degrees Offered: MS.
License/Certification Preparation: State: CA Licensed Acupuncturist; National Certification Commission for Acupuncture and Oriental Medicine.
Admission Requirements: Min age: 20; Some college (2 yrs); Min GPA: 2.0; Specific course prerequisites: anatomy and physiology.
Application Deadline(s): Fall: Jun.
Tuition and Fees: $8000 per yr.
Financial Aid: Federal government aid; Loans.
Career Services: Career information.

170. Santa Barbara Yoga Center
32 E Micheltorena St, Santa Barbara, CA 93101
Phone: (805) 965-6045
Internet: http://www.santabarbarayogacenter.com
Program Administrator: Lais Da Silva, Owner/Dir. *Admissions Contact:* Lais Da Silva.
Year Established: 1992.
Staff: Part-time: 25.
Avg Enrollment: 100. *Avg Class Size:* 35. *Number of Graduates per Year:* 70.
Wheelchair Access: Yes.
Field of Study: Yoga Teacher Training*. *Program Name/Length:* Certification, 170 hrs.
Degrees Offered: Certificate.

Tuition and Fees: $1500-$2000.
Career Services: Internships.

171. School of Intuitive Massage and Healing

503 Foxen Dr, Santa Barbara, CA 93105
Phone: (805) 687-2917; *Fax:* (805) 563-0927
Program Administrator: Anne Parks, Dir. *Admissions Contact:* Anne Parks.
Year Established: 1984.
Staff: Part-time: 10.
Avg Enrollment: 100. *Avg Class Size:* 16. *Number of Graduates per Year:* 95.
Wheelchair Access: No.
Accreditation/Approval/Licensing: State board: CA Bureau of Private Postsecondary and Vocational Ed; Accrediting Council for Continuing Education and Training.
Field of Study: Energy Work*; Massage Therapy*. *Program Name/Length:* Massage Therapist Certification, 200 hrs, 3 1/2 mos; Massage Therapist II Certification, 200 hrs, 3 1/2 mos; Massage Program, 600 hrs, 9 mos; 1000 hrs, 15 mos; Intuitive Massage and Healing Certification, 200 hrs, 3 1/2-6 mos; Energy Work Healing Certification, 200 hrs, 4-8 mos; Awareness Skills Certification, 200 hrs, 3 1/2 mos; Professional Skills (Business) Certification, 200 hrs, 3 1/2 mos.
Degrees Offered: Certificate.
License/Certification Preparation: National Certification Board for Therapeutic Massage and Bodywork.
Admission Requirements: Min age: 18; Specific course prerequisites: 200 hr massage therapy course required for Energy Work and Intuitive Massage.
Tuition and Fees: $1100 (200 hrs).
Financial Aid: Fee waiver; Loans; Scholarships; Work study.
Career Services: Career counseling; Career information.

Santa Cruz

172. Cypress Health Institute

PO Box 2941, Santa Cruz, CA 95063
Phone: (831) 476-2115
Program Administrator: Larry Bernstein, Admin. *Admissions Contact:* Larry Bernstein.
Year Established: 1981.
Staff: Full-time: 4.
Avg Enrollment: 75. *Avg Class Size:* 15. *Number of Graduates per Year:* 75.
Wheelchair Access: Yes.
Accreditation/Approval/Licensing: State board: CA Bureau of Private Postsecondary and Vocational Ed; Accrediting Council for Continuing Education and Training.
Field of Study: Acupressure; CranioSacral Therapy; Deep Tissue Massage; Holistic Health*; Hypnotherapy; Massage Therapy*; Polarity Therapy; Reflexology; Sports Massage; Swedish Massage*; Thai Massage. *Program Name/Length:* Massage Therapy, 170 hrs, 3 mos; Holistic Health Educator, 500 hrs, 1 yr.
Degrees Offered: Certificate.
Admission Requirements: Min age: 18.
Application Deadline(s): Fall: Sep; Winter: Jan; Spring: Apr; Summer: Jun.
Tuition and Fees: $1150 (Massage); $2000-$3000 (Holistic Health).
Financial Aid: Payment plan.

173. East West School of Herbology

PO Box 712, Santa Cruz, CA 95061
Phone: (800) 717-5010; *Fax:* (831) 336-4548
E-mail: herbcourse@planetherbs.com *Internet:* http://www.planetherbs.com
Program Administrator: Michael Tierra. *Admissions Contact:* Jill Agnello, Admin.
Year Established: 1980.
Avg Enrollment: 500.
Accreditation/Approval/Licensing: State board: CA Board of Registered Nursing.
Field of Study: Herbal Medicine*. *Program Name/Length:* Correspondence, 12 or 36 lessons, 12-18 mos; Intensive Seminars.
Degrees Offered: Certificate.
Tuition and Fees: $225 (12 lessons); $575 (36 lessons).

174. Five Branches Institute of Traditional Chinese Medicine

200 7th Ave, Santa Cruz, CA 95062
Phone: (831) 476-9424; *Fax:* (831) 476-8928
E-mail: tcm@fivebranches.edu *Internet:* http://www.fivebranches.edu
Program Administrator: Kimberly Miller, Admin. *Admissions Contact:* Meredith Bigley, Admissions Dir.
Year Established: 1984.
Staff: Full-time: 17.
Avg Enrollment: 25. *Avg Class Size:* 20. *Number of Graduates per Year:* 20.
Wheelchair Access: Yes.
Accreditation/Approval/Licensing: State board: CA Acupuncture Board; Accreditation Commission for Acupuncture and Oriental Medicine.
Field of Study: Acupuncture*; Herbal Medicine*; Traditional Chinese Medicine*. *Program Name/Length:* Master of Traditional Chinese Medicine, 4 yrs.
Degrees Offered: MTCM.
License/Certification Preparation: State: CA Licensed Acupuncturist; National Certification Commission for Acupuncture and Oriental Medicine.
Admission Requirements: Some college (2 yrs).
Application Deadline(s): Fall: Jun; Spring: Dec.
Tuition and Fees: $6600 per yr.
Financial Aid: Loans; Student loan deferment.

175. Kali Ray Tri Yoga Center

PO Box 4287, Santa Cruz, CA 95063
Phone: (408) 464-8100; *Fax:* (408) 462-1945
E-mail: kaliji@aol.com *Internet:* http://www.
kaliraytriyoga.com
Program Administrator: Kali Ray, Founder/Pres.
  Admissions Contact: Leela Vani, Admin Asst.
Year Established: 1980.
Staff: Full-time: 10.
Avg Class Size: 11.
Wheelchair Access: Yes.
Field of Study: Yoga Teacher Training*.
Degrees Offered: Certificate.
Financial Aid: Work study.
Career Services: Internships; Interview set up; Resume service.

176. Twin Lakes College of the Healing Arts

1210 Brommer St, Santa Cruz, CA 95062
Phone: (831) 476-2152
Program Administrator: Becky Williams, Dir. *Admissions Contact:* Amber Sharman, Registrar.
Year Established: 1982.
Staff: Part-time: 18.
Avg Enrollment: 200. *Avg Class Size:* 14. *Number of Graduates per Year:* 180.
Wheelchair Access: No.
Accreditation/Approval/Licensing: State board: CA Bureau of Private Postsecondary and Vocational Ed.
Field of Study: Acupressure; Aromatherapy*; Energy Work; Hypnotherapy*; Massage Therapy*; Polarity Therapy; Reflexology; Reiki; Shiatsu. *Program Name/Length:* Integrative Massage Practitioner, 200 hrs, 3 mos/days or 6-9 mos/evenings; Massage Therapist and Natural Health Counselor, 500 hrs, 1 yr; Hypnosis Practitioner: Level I, 100 hrs, 4 mos; Hypnotherapist, 200 hrs (includes Level I), 9 mos.
Degrees Offered: CEUs; Certificate.
Admission Requirements: Min age: 17; High school diploma/GED.
Application Deadline(s): Fall: Sep; Winter: Jan; Spring: Apr; Summer: Jul.
Financial Aid: Vocational rehabilitation; Payment plan.
Career Services: Career information.

Santa Monica

177. The Alexander Training Institute of Los Angeles

1526 14th St, Ste 110, Santa Monica, CA 90404
Phone: (310) 395-9170
Program Administrator: Lyn Charlsen, Dir. *Admissions Contact:* Lyn Charlsen.
Year Established: 1987.
Staff: Part-time: 5.
Avg Class Size: 10.
Wheelchair Access: Yes.
Accreditation/Approval/Licensing: State board: CA Bureau of Private Postsecondary and Vocational Ed; American Society for the Alexander Technique.
Field of Study: Alexander Technique*. *Program Name/Length:* Teacher Training, 9 semesters, 3 yrs.
Degrees Offered: Certificate.
License/Certification Preparation: American Society for the Alexander Technique.
Admission Requirements: Specific course prerequisites: 30-40 lessons in the Alexander Technique (some with directors); References; School visit; Interview.
Application Deadline(s): Fall: Aug; Winter: Oct; Spring: Jan; Summer: Mar.
Tuition and Fees: $1833 per semester.

178. Emperor's College of Traditional Oriental Medicine

1807 Wilshire Blvd, Santa Monica, CA 90403
Phone: (310) 453-8300; *Fax:* (310) 829-3838
E-mail: dsl@emperors.edu *Internet:* http://www.
emperors.edu
Program Administrator: William R. Morris, LAc, Academic Dean. *Admissions Contact:* Leah McMahon, LAc, Admissions Dir.
Year Established: 1983.
Staff: Full-time: 3; Part-time: 35.
Avg Enrollment: 100. *Avg Class Size:* 25. *Number of Graduates per Year:* 70.
Wheelchair Access: Yes.
Accreditation/Approval/Licensing: State board: CA Acupuncture Board; Accreditation Commission for Acupuncture and Oriental Medicine.
Field of Study: Acupressure*; Acupuncture*; Herbal Medicine*; Massage Therapy*; Oriental Medicine*; Qigong; Reflexology; Reiki; Traditional Chinese Medicine*. *Program Name/Length:* Basic Acupressure/Massage, 3 mos; Acupressure/Massage Technician, 6 mos; Acupressure/Massage Therapist, 1 yr; Master of Traditional Oriental Medicine, 3-4 yrs.
Degrees Offered: CEUs; Certificate; (MTOM).
License/Certification Preparation: State: CA Licensed Acupuncturist; National Certification Commission for Acupuncture and Oriental Medicine.
Admission Requirements: High school diploma/GED for Massage; Some college (2 yrs) for MTOM.
Tuition and Fees: $7000-$8000 per yr.
Financial Aid: Loans; VA approved.
Career Services: Internships; Externships.

179. Massage School of Santa Monica

1453 Third St Promenade, Ste 340, Santa Monica, CA 90401
Phone: (310) 393-7461; *Fax:* (310) 453-2386
Program Administrator: Bernadette Gessner, Dir.
  Admissions Contact: Maryse Gessner, Asst Dir.

Year Established: 1979.
Staff: Part-time: 20.
Avg Enrollment: 350. *Avg Class Size:* 15. *Number of Graduates per Year:* 300.
Wheelchair Access: No.
Accreditation/Approval/Licensing: Accrediting Council for Continuing Education and Training; National Certification Board for Therapeutic Massage and Bodywork (CEUs).
Field of Study: Acupressure; Aromatherapy; CranioSacral Therapy; Energy Work; Massage Therapy*; Polarity Therapy; Qigong; Reflexology; Shiatsu; Sports Massage; Swedish Massage*. *Program Name/Length:* Massage Therapist, 3 mos; Massage Therapist Addendum, 1 mo; Continuing Education Program, 1 yr.
Degrees Offered: Diploma.
License/Certification Preparation: National Certification Board for Therapeutic Massage and Bodywork.
Admission Requirements: Min age: 18; High school diploma/GED.
Tuition and Fees: $1190 (Massage Therapist).
Financial Aid: Vocational rehabilitation.
Career Services: Career information.

180. Yo San University of Traditional Chinese Medicine

1314 2nd St, Santa Monica, CA 90401
Phone: (310) 917-2202; *Fax:* (310) 917-2203
E-mail: info@yosan.edu *Internet:* http://www.yosan.edu
Program Administrator: Dr. Richard Hammerschlag, Pres. *Admissions Contact:* Doris Johnson, Dir of Admissions and Mktg.
Year Established: 1989.
Staff: Full-time: 3; Part-time: 35.
Avg Enrollment: 55. *Avg Class Size:* 25. *Number of Graduates per Year:* 18.
Wheelchair Access: Yes.
Accreditation/Approval/Licensing: State board: CA Acupuncture Board; Accreditation Commission for Acupuncture and Oriental Medicine.
Field of Study: Acupuncture*; Herbal Medicine*; Lifestyle Counseling; Qigong*; Traditional Chinese Medicine*. *Program Name/Length:* Master of Acupuncture and Traditional Chinese Medicine, 4 yrs.
Degrees Offered: MAcTCM.
License/Certification Preparation: State: CA Licensed Acupuncturist; National Certification Commission for Acupuncture and Oriental Medicine.
Admission Requirements: Some college (2 yrs).
Application Deadline(s): Fall: Aug; Winter: Dec.
Tuition and Fees: $7500 per yr.
Financial Aid: Loans; Tutorships.
Career Services: Career counseling; Career information; Internships.

181. Yoga Works, Inc

1426 Montana Ave, 2nd Fl, Santa Monica, CA 90403
Phone: (310) 393-5150; *Fax:* (310) 656-5892
Program Administrator: Maty Ezraty, Pres. *Admissions Contact:* Julie Jacobs, Gen Mgr.
Year Established: 1987.
Staff: Part-time: 35.
Avg Enrollment: 60. *Avg Class Size:* 35.
Wheelchair Access: Yes.
Field of Study: Yoga Teacher Training*. *Program Name/Length:* 1-2 yrs.
Admission Requirements: 1 yr practice of basic yoga postures.
Application Deadline(s): Winter: Jan 5; Summer: Jun 15.
Tuition and Fees: $950.

Santa Rosa

182. Hypnotherapy Training Institute

4730 Alta Vista Ave, Santa Rosa, CA 95404
Phone: (707) 579-9023; *Fax:* (707) 578-1033
E-mail: hypno@sonic.net *Internet:* http://www.sonic.net/hypno
Program Administrator: Randal Churchill, Dir. *Admissions Contact:* Marleen Mulder, Dir.
Year Established: 1978.
Staff: Full-time: 2; Part-time: 1.
Avg Enrollment: 100. *Avg Class Size:* 26. *Number of Graduates per Year:* 85.
Wheelchair Access: Yes.
Accreditation/Approval/Licensing: State board: CA Bureau of Private Postsecondary and Vocational Ed.
Field of Study: Hypnotherapy*. *Program Name/Length:* Levels 1, 2, 3, and 4: 50 hrs each (1 wk or 1 mo).
Degrees Offered: Diploma.
License/Certification Preparation: American Council of Hypnotist Examiners.
Admission Requirements: Min age: 18; High school diploma/GED.
Application Deadline(s): Winter: Jan; Spring: Feb; Summer: May, Jul.
Tuition and Fees: $695 per course.
Financial Aid: Vocational rehabilitation.
Career Services: Career information.
Comments: Classes are held in Corte Madera, near San Francisco.

183. Polarity Wellness Center West

325 Shortt Rd, Santa Rosa, CA 95405
Phone: (707) 542-7966
E-mail: polaritywell@juno.com
Program Administrator: Jan Milthaler, MSW, Dir. *Admissions Contact:* Jan Milthaler.
Year Established: 1993.
Staff: Full-time: 2; Part-time: 4.
Avg Enrollment: 15. *Avg Class Size:* 7.

Wheelchair Access: No.
Accreditation/Approval/Licensing: American Polarity Therapy Association.
Field of Study: Polarity Therapy*. *Program Name/Length:* Associate Polarity Practitioner, 168 hrs, 6 mos.
Degrees Offered: Certificate.
License/Certification Preparation: APP; American Polarity Therapy Association.
Admission Requirements: Min age: 18.
Tuition and Fees: $1680.

184. Wellness Holistic School of Massage
345 South E St, Santa Rosa, CA 95404
Phone: (707) 546-8115, (800) 939-6837
Program Administrator: Virginia Romero, Dir. *Admissions Contact:* Virginia Romero.
Year Established: 1984.
Staff: Full-time: 1.
Avg Enrollment: 24. *Avg Class Size:* 12. *Number of Graduates per Year:* 24.
Wheelchair Access: No.
Accreditation/Approval/Licensing: State board: CA Bureau of Private Postsecondary and Vocational Ed.
Field of Study: Energy Work; Esalen Massage*; Kinesiology; Massage Therapy*; Polarity Therapy; Reflexology; Swedish Massage*; Touch for Health. *Program Name/Length:* Massage Practitioner, 3 mos; Natural Health Counselor, 3 mos; Certified Wellness Coach, 3 mos.
Degrees Offered: Certificate.
Admission Requirements: Min age: 18.
Application Deadline(s): Fall: Sep; Winter: Jan; Spring: Apr; Summer: Jun.
Tuition and Fees: $1040.
Financial Aid: Work study; Short-term loan.
Career Services: Internships.

Sebastopol

185. Ayurveda Institute of Massage and Spa Services
3140 Stone Station, Sebastopol, CA 95472
Phone: (707) 523-9923; *Fax:* (707) 824-4778
Program Administrator: Dharmini Zelin, Dir. *Admissions Contact:* Dharmini Zelin.
Year Established: 1998.
Staff: Full-time: 1.
Avg Enrollment: 150. *Avg Class Size:* 15.
Wheelchair Access: No.
Field of Study: Ayurvedic Medicine*; Energy Work; Massage Therapy*; Polarity Therapy; Reflexology; Spa Therapies*. *Program Name/Length:* 2-3 day seminars; Seminars given in various locations.
Degrees Offered: Certificate; Ayurvedic Aesthetician; Ayurvedic Rejuvenation Therapist.
Admission Requirements: Min age: 20; Massage or holistic training preferred.
Tuition and Fees: $325-$375 per course.

186. Day-Break Geriatric Massage Project
19091 N 5th St
216 Pleasant Hill Ave N, Sebastopol, CA 95472
Mailing Address: PO Box 1815, Sebastopol, CA 95473-1815
Phone: (707) 829-2798; *Fax:* (707) 829-2799
E-mail: daybreak@monitor.net *Internet:* http://www.daybreak-massage.com
Program Administrator: Dietrich Miesler, Dir. *Admissions Contact:* Felicity Doyle, Admin.
Year Established: 1991.
Staff: Part-time: 3.
Avg Enrollment: 320. *Avg Class Size:* 20. *Number of Graduates per Year:* 320.
Wheelchair Access: Yes.
Accreditation/Approval/Licensing: State board: CA Bureau of Private Postsecondary and Vocational Ed; FL Massage Therapy Association; National Certification Board for Therapeutic Massage and Bodywork (CEUs).
Field of Study: Geriatric Massage*. *Program Name/Length:* Geriatric Massage Techniques Workshop, 17 CEUs, 2 1/2 days; Advanced Geriatric Massage Techniques Workshop, 17 CEUs, 2 1/2 days; Correspondence course, 54 CEUs; Annual Symposium, 45 CEUs, 1 wk.
Degrees Offered: CEUs; Certificate.
Admission Requirements: Min age: 18; Minimum 150 hrs of massage training.
Tuition and Fees: $250 (Workshops); $265 (Correspondence); $950 (Symposium).
Career Services: Career counseling; Career information.

187. Sebastopol Massage Center
108 N Main, Ste 5, Sebastopol, CA 95472
Phone: (707) 823-3550
Program Administrator: Patricia Oberg, Dir. *Admissions Contact:* Patricia Oberg.
Year Established: 1983.
Staff: Full-time: 1.
Avg Enrollment: 100. *Avg Class Size:* 12. *Number of Graduates per Year:* 90.
Wheelchair Access: No.
Field of Study: Acupressure*; CranioSacral Therapy; Energy Work; Esalen Massage; Massage Therapy*; Ortho-Bionomy; Reflexology; Shiatsu; Swedish Massage*. *Program Name/Length:* Massage Therapist Certificate, 150 hrs.
Degrees Offered: Diploma; Certificate.
Tuition and Fees: $800.
Financial Aid: Payment plan.
Career Services: Career information; Job information; Referral service.

Solana Beach

188. Vitality Training Center
243 N Hwy 101, Ste 5, Solana Beach, CA 92075

Phone: (619) 259-9491; *Fax:* (619) 259-2008
Program Administrator: Annie Benefield, Dir. *Admissions Contact:* Vickie Mayheux.
Year Established: 1993.
Staff: Full-time: 10; Part-time: 4.
Avg Enrollment: 120. *Avg Class Size:* 8. *Number of Graduates per Year:* 80.
Wheelchair Access: Yes.
Accreditation/Approval/Licensing: Accrediting Council for Continuing Education and Training.
Field of Study: Acupressure; Aromatherapy*; CranioSacral Therapy; Energy Work; Herbal Medicine; Holistic Health*; Hypnotherapy; Massage Therapy*; Neuromuscular Therapy; Reflexology; Reiki; Shiatsu; Sports Massage; Yoga Teacher Training*. *Program Name/Length:* Massage Therapist, 500 hrs, 6-9 mos; Holistic Health Practitioner, 1000 hrs, 12-18 mos; Holistic Health Instructor, 1200 hrs, 18-24 mos; Therapeutic Yoga Teacher Training, 100 hrs, 10 wks; Reflexology Certification, 100 hrs, 2 wks + intensive or 11 wks; Aromatherapy Certification, 200 hrs, 3-6 mos.
Degrees Offered: Certificate.
License/Certification Preparation: American Council of Hypnotist Examiners; American Reflexology Certification Board; National Certification Board for Therapeutic Massage and Bodywork.
Admission Requirements: Min age: 18.
Tuition and Fees: $4250 (Massage Therapist); $8500 (Holistic Practitioner); $10,200 (Holistic Instructor); $850 (Therapeutic Yoga); $850 (Reflexology); $1700 (Aromatherapy).
Financial Aid: Loans; Work study; VA approved; Vocational rehabilitation.

Sonoma

189. California Institute of Massage and Spa Services
730 Broadway, Sonoma, CA 95476
Mailing Address: PO Box 673, Sonoma, CA 95476
Phone: (707) 939-9431
Program Administrator: Kate Alves, Dir. *Admissions Contact:* Kate Alves.
Year Established: 1991.
Staff: Full-time: 1; Part-time: 3.
Avg Enrollment: 60. *Avg Class Size:* 10. *Number of Graduates per Year:* 50.
Wheelchair Access: Yes.
Accreditation/Approval/Licensing: State board: CA Bureau of Private Postsecondary and Vocational Ed; CA Board of Registered Nursing.
Field of Study: Acupressure; Aromatherapy; CranioSacral Therapy; Energy Work; Massage Therapy*; Polarity Therapy; Reflexology; Shiatsu; Spa Therapies*; Swedish Massage*.
Program Name/Length: Massage Technician Certification, 3 1/2 mos; Advanced Massage I

and II, 3 1/2 mos; Massage Therapist Certification, 1 yr; Spa Services Certification, 3 1/2 mos.
Degrees Offered: Certificate.
Admission Requirements: Min age: 18; High school diploma/GED.
Application Deadline(s): Fall: Sep; Winter: Jan; Spring: Apr; Summer: Jun.
Tuition and Fees: $895-$1150.
Financial Aid: Vocational rehabilitation.
Career Services: Career counseling; Career information; Student clinic.

South Lake Tahoe

190. Lake Tahoe Massage School
1966 US Hwy 50, South Lake Tahoe, CA 96150
Mailing Address: 1034 Emerald Bay Rd, Ste 401, South Lake Tahoe, CA 96150
Phone: (530) 544-1227
E-mail: jet@oakweb.com
Program Administrator: Jeannette Cunniff, Dir. *Admissions Contact:* Jeannette Cunniff.
Year Established: 1996.
Staff: Full-time: 2; Part-time: 3.
Avg Enrollment: 85. *Avg Class Size:* 12. *Number of Graduates per Year:* 75.
Wheelchair Access: No.
Accreditation/Approval/Licensing: State board: CA Bureau of Private Postsecondary and Vocational Ed; Accrediting Council for Continuing Education and Training.
Field of Study: CranioSacral Therapy; Deep Tissue Massage; Massage Therapy*; Medical Massage; Polarity Therapy; Reflexology; Shiatsu; Sports Massage*. *Program Name/Length:* Massage Practitioner, 150 hrs; Sports Massage and Sports Injuries, 100 hrs.
Degrees Offered: CEUs; Certificate.
License/Certification Preparation: National Certification Board for Therapeutic Massage and Bodywork.
Admission Requirements: Min age: 18; High school diploma/GED.
Financial Aid: Work study; Vocational rehabilitation; Payment plan.

Stockton

191. College of Bio-Energetic Medicine
Bio-Energetic Bodywork and Energy Medicine
1955 Lucile, Ste D, Stockton, CA 95209
Phone: (209) 473-4993; *Fax:* (209) 473-4997
Program Administrator: A. R. Bordon, Dean; Michael J. Eakin, Academic Dir. *Admissions Contact:* Michael J. Eakin, Academic Dir; Kelly Graham, Admin.
Year Established: 1998.
Staff: Full-time: 3; Part-time: 6.
Avg Class Size: 12.
Wheelchair Access: Yes.

Accreditation/Approval/Licensing: State board: CA Bureau of Private Postsecondary and Vocational Ed.

Field of Study: Acupressure; Aromatherapy; Deep Tissue Massage; Energy Work*; Massage Therapy*; Qigong; Reflexology*; Reiki; Thai Massage*; Traditional Chinese Medicine. *Program Name/Length:* Clinical Bodywork Practitioner, 700 hrs; Master Bodywork Energetics Therapist, 600 hrs; Master Reflexology Energetics Therapist, 600 hrs; Traditional Chinese Energetic Bodywork, 600 hrs; Ancient and Traditional Thai Medical Bodywork, 600 hrs.

License/Certification Preparation: National Certification Board for Therapeutic Massage and Bodywork.

Admission Requirements: Min age: 18; High school diploma/GED.

Application Deadline(s): Fall: Jul; Winter: Nov; Summer: Mar.

Financial Aid: Federal government aid; Scholarships; State government aid; Vocational rehabilitation.

Career Services: Career counseling; Career information; Internships; Resume service; Referral service.

192. Touching for Health Center School of Professional Bodywork

628 Lincoln Ctr, Stockton, CA 95207-2640
Phone: (209) 474-9559; *Fax:* (209) 474-9559
E-mail: tfhc@familyinternet.net
Program Administrator: Roberta Dodie Baker, Dir/Sr Instr. *Admissions Contact:* Roberta Dodie Baker.
Year Established: 1990.
Staff: Full-time: 1; Part-time: 7.
Avg Enrollment: 75. *Avg Class Size:* 16. *Number of Graduates per Year:* 70.
Wheelchair Access: No.
Accreditation/Approval/Licensing: State board: CA Bureau of Private Postsecondary and Vocational Ed; Accrediting Council for Continuing Education and Training.
Field of Study: Acupressure*; Aromatherapy; CranioSacral Therapy; Deep Tissue Massage; Manual Lymph Drainage; Massage Therapy*; Myofascial Release; Polarity Therapy; Reflexology. *Program Name/Length:* Massage Technician, 105 hrs, 7-11 wks; Acupressure Certification, 100 hrs, 6 mos part-time; Holistic Health Massage Practitioner, 225 hrs, 3 mos; Therapeutic Massage Practitioner, 500 hrs, 1-3 yrs part-time.
Degrees Offered: Certificate.
License/Certification Preparation: National Certification Board for Therapeutic Massage and Bodywork.
Admission Requirements: Min age: 18.
Application Deadline(s): Fall: Oct; Winter: Jan; Spring: Apr; Summer: Jul.

Tuition and Fees: $900 (Massage Technician); $750 (Acupressure); $1025 (Holistic Health); $5000 (Therapeutic Massage).
Financial Aid: Payment plan.
Career Services: Resume service.

Tarzana

193. Hypnosis Motivation Institute

Clinical Hypnotherapy
18607 Ventura Blvd, Ste 310, Tarzana, CA 92670
Phone: (818) 758-2745
E-mail: geokappa@aol.com *Internet:* http://www.hypnosismotivation.com
Program Administrator: George Kappas, MA, Dir. *Admissions Contact:* Candace Coleman, Dir of Admissions.
Year Established: 1968.
Staff: Full-time: 6; Part-time: 13.
Avg Enrollment: 250. *Avg Class Size:* 25. *Number of Graduates per Year:* 200.
Wheelchair Access: Yes.
Accreditation/Approval/Licensing: State board: CA Bureau of Private Postsecondary and Vocational Ed; Accrediting Council for Continuing Education and Training.
Field of Study: Hypnotherapy*. *Program Name/Length:* Resident School, 1 yr; Home Study, 300 hrs.
Degrees Offered: Diploma.
Admission Requirements: High school diploma/GED.
Financial Aid: Federal government aid; Grants; Loans; Scholarships.

Temecula

194. Reflexology Institute

27636 Ynez Rd L-7, Ste 232, Temecula, CA 92591
Phone: (909) 694-0225; *Fax:* (909) 694-5910
E-mail: mrrfxology@aol.com
Program Administrator: Lynn Nelson, Dir.
Year Established: 1985.
Staff: Full-time: 1.
Avg Enrollment: 150. *Avg Class Size:* 10. *Number of Graduates per Year:* 150.
Wheelchair Access: Yes.
Accreditation/Approval/Licensing: State board: CA Bureau of Private Postsecondary and Vocational Ed.
Field of Study: Reflexology*. *Program Name/Length:* Reflexology Diploma, 100 hrs; Reflexology Certificate, 1-2 days; Seminars given in various locations; Home study/Correspondence.
Degrees Offered: Diploma; Certificate.
License/Certification Preparation: American Reflexology Certification Board.
Admission Requirements: Min age: 18; High school diploma/GED.

Tuition and Fees: $2995 (100 hrs).
Financial Aid: Grants; Loans.
Career Services: Career counseling; Career information; Interview set up; Resume service.

Thousand Oaks

195. Advanced School of Massage Therapy
1414 E Thousand Oaks Blvd, Ste 213, Thousand Oaks, CA 91362
Mailing Address: 1414 E Thousand Oaks Blvd, Ste 211, Thousand Oaks, CA 91362
Phone: (805) 495-1353; *Fax:* (805) 379-1408
Program Administrator: Jan Suckut, Owner/Dir. *Admissions Contact:* Jan Suckut.
Year Established: 1997.
Staff: Full-time: 2; Part-time: 6.
Avg Enrollment: 80. *Avg Class Size:* 10. *Number of Graduates per Year:* 75.
Wheelchair Access: Yes.
Accreditation/Approval/Licensing: State board: CA Bureau of Private Postsecondary and Vocational Ed.
Field of Study: CranioSacral Therapy; Energy Work; Facial Massage; Infant Massage; Massage Therapy*; Pregnancy Massage; Reflexology; Sports Massage; Trigger Point Therapy. *Program Name/Length:* Basic Massage Therapy, 200 hrs; Advanced Program, 500 hrs, 6-8 mos.
Degrees Offered: Certificate.
Admission Requirements: Min age: 18; High school diploma/GED.
Tuition and Fees: $1000 (Basic); $1750 (Advanced).
Financial Aid: Payment plan.
Career Services: Job information.

196. Thousand Oaks Healing Arts Institute
Massage Therapy
2955 Moorpark Rd, Thousand Oaks, CA 91360
Phone: (805) 241-4194; *Fax:* (805) 493-4039
Internet: http://www.a2z.health.com
Program Administrator: Cindy Herbert, Dir. *Admissions Contact:* Cindy Herbert.
Year Established: 1997.
Staff: Part-time: 15.
Avg Enrollment: 40. *Avg Class Size:* 10. *Number of Graduates per Year:* 10.
Wheelchair Access: Yes.
Accreditation/Approval/Licensing: State board: CA Bureau of Private Postsecondary and Vocational Ed.
Field of Study: Acupressure; Aromatherapy; Deep Tissue Massage* Swedish Massage*; Massage Therapy*; Reflexology; Shiatsu. *Program Name/Length:* Basic Swedish, 200 hrs; Seminars, 2-50 hrs.
Degrees Offered: Certificate.
Admission Requirements: Min age: 18.
Tuition and Fees: $1050 (200 hrs).
Career Services: Internships.

Tomales

197. Polarity Therapy Center of Marin
PO Box 23, Tomales, CA 94971
Phone: (707) 878-2278
Program Administrator: Hanna Hammerli, RPP, Dir. *Admissions Contact:* Hanna Hammerli.
Year Established: 1991.
Staff: Full-time: 1.
Avg Enrollment: 30. *Avg Class Size:* 6.
Wheelchair Access: No.
Accreditation/Approval/Licensing: American Polarity Therapy Association.
Field of Study: Polarity Therapy*. *Program Name/Length:* Associate Polarity Practitioner, 155 hrs, 6-12 mos; Registered Polarity Practitioner, 615 hrs, 2 yrs.
Degrees Offered: Certificate.
License/Certification Preparation: APP and RPP; American Polarity Therapy Association.
Admission Requirements: Min age: 18; Interview.
Tuition and Fees: $1650 (APP); $5400 (RPP).
Financial Aid: Work study.

Ventura

198. Caring Hands School of Massage
1484 E Main St, Ventura, CA 93001
Phone: (805) 643-3032
Year Established: 1993.
Staff: Part-time: 3.
Avg Enrollment: 85. *Avg Class Size:* 10.
Wheelchair Access: No.
Field of Study: Acupressure*; LomiLomi Massage*; Massage Therapy*; Shiatsu*. *Program Name/Length:* Therapeutic Massage, 14 wks; LomiLomi Massage, 6 wks; Shiatsu, 6 wks.
Degrees Offered: Diploma.
Career Services: Career counseling; Career information.

199. International Association of Infant Massage
1891 Goodyear Ave, Ste 622, Ventura, CA 93003
Mailing Address: PO Box 1045, Oak View, CA 93022
Phone: (805) 644-8524, (800) 248-5432; *Fax:* (805) 644-7699
E-mail: iaim4us@aol.com
Program Administrator: E. Riddle, Exec Dir. *Admissions Contact:* Susan Campbell, Bus Admin.
Year Established: 1986.
Staff: Full-time: 6.
Avg Class Size: 20. *Number of Graduates per Year:* 350.
Accreditation/Approval/Licensing: State board: CA and NY Nursing Associations; National Certification Board for Therapeutic Massage and Bodywork (CEUs).
Field of Study: Infant Massage*. *Program Name/Length:* Infant Massage Instructor Certif-

ication, 4 days; Seminars given in various locations.
Degrees Offered: CEUs; Certificate.
Admission Requirements: Min age: 18.
Tuition and Fees: $550.

200. Kali Institute for Massage and Somatic Therapies

746 E Main St, Ventura, CA 93001
Phone: (805) 648-6204
E-mail: kalind@gte.net *Internet:* http://www.
kaliinstitute.com
Program Administrator: Nancy DeLucrezia, Dir.
Admissions Contact: Nancy DeLucrezia.
Year Established: 1993.
Staff: Full-time: 4; Part-time: 12.
Avg Enrollment: 50. *Avg Class Size:* 14. *Number of Graduates per Year:* 50.
Wheelchair Access: No.
Accreditation/Approval/Licensing: State board: CA Bureau of Private Postsecondary and Vocational Ed.
Field of Study: Acupressure; Aromatherapy; CranioSacral Therapy; Energy Work*; Massage Therapy*; Neuro-Structural Bodywork*; Polarity Therapy; Reflexology; Somatic Education; Sports Massage. *Program Name/Length:* Massage Therapy, 200 hrs; Neuro-Structural Bodywork, 124 hrs; Oriental Studies, 100 hrs; Intuitive and Energy Healing, 100 hrs; Advanced Practitioner Training, 600 hrs.
Degrees Offered: Certificate.
Admission Requirements: Min age: 17; High school diploma/GED.
Tuition and Fees: $1650 (Massage Therapy); $1195 (Neuro-Structural); $995 (Oriental Studies; Intuitive Healing); $4990 (Advanced Practitioner).
Career Services: Career counseling; Career information; Resume service; Job information; Referral service.

201. Lu Ross Academy of Health and Beauty

470 E Thompson Blvd, Ventura, CA 93001
Phone: (805) 643-5690
Internet: http://www.lurossacademy.com
Program Administrator: Chrys Huynh, Dir. *Admissions Contact:* Debbie Johnson, Admin/Admissions and Financial Aid.
Year Established: 1954.
Staff: Full-time: 5; Part-time: 4.
Avg Enrollment: 200. *Avg Class Size:* 15. *Number of Graduates per Year:* 150.
Wheelchair Access: Yes.
Accreditation/Approval/Licensing: CA Bureau of Private Postsecondary and Vocational Ed; Accrediting Council for Continuing Education and Training; Accrediting Commission of Career Schools and Colleges of Technology.
Field of Study: Acupressure; Aromatherapy; CranioSacral Therapy; Energy Work; Herbal

Medicine; Massage Therapy*; Neuromuscular Therapy; Polarity Therapy; Qigong; Reflexology*; Reiki; Shiatsu; Sports Massage. *Program Name/Length:* Therapeutique Massage, 200 hrs, 3 mos; 600 hrs, 6 mos; 1000 hrs, 1 yr.
Degrees Offered: Certificate.
License/Certification Preparation: City license; American Reflexology Certification Board.
Admission Requirements: Min age: 17; High school diploma/GED.
Tuition and Fees: $1495 (200 hrs); $4500 (600 hrs).
Financial Aid: Loans; Scholarships; State government aid.
Career Services: Career counseling; Career information; Internships; Interview set up; Resume service.

202. Ventura Yoga Studio

110 N Olive St, Ste P, Ventura, CA 93001
Mailing Address: PO Box 2802, Ventura, CA 93002
Phone: (805) 643-5979; *Fax:* (805) 648-6964
Program Administrator: Bryan Legere, Dir. *Admissions Contact:* Bryan Legere.
Year Established: 1991.
Staff: Full-time: 1; Part-time: 5.
Avg Class Size: 10.
Wheelchair Access: No.
Accreditation/Approval/Licensing: Iyengar Yoga National Association.
Field of Study: Yoga Teacher Training*. *Program Name/Length:* 3 yrs.
Degrees Offered: Certificate.
License/Certification Preparation: Iyengar Yoga Certification.

Visalia

203. Life Skills Wellness Center and Valley Birthing Network

Doula Training Seminar
1220 W Center, Visalia, CA 93291
Phone: (559) 627-9983; *Fax:* (559) 627-5451
E-mail: lifeskills@mindinfo.com
Program Administrator: Jan Graham, Owner.
Year Established: 1997.
Staff: Full-time: 2.
Avg Class Size: 12.
Wheelchair Access: No.
Accreditation/Approval/Licensing: Doulas of North America.
Field of Study: Doula*. *Program Name/Length:* 16 hrs; Seminars given in various locations.
Degrees Offered: Certificate.
License/Certification Preparation: Certification, Doulas of North America.
Admission Requirements: High school diploma/GED; Specific course prerequisites: childbirth education.

Application Deadline(s): Winter: Nov; Summer: Aug.

Watsonville

204. Jin Shin Do Foundation for Bodymind Acupressure
1084G San Miguel Canyon Rd, Watsonville, CA 95076
Phone: (831) 763-7702; *Fax:* (831) 763-1151
Program Administrator: Iona Marsaa Teeguarden, MA, Dir. *Admissions Contact:* Iona Marsaa Teeguarden.
Year Established: 1982.
Staff: Part-time: 80.
Avg Enrollment: 1000. *Avg Class Size:* 15. *Number of Graduates per Year:* 100.
Accreditation/Approval/Licensing: State board: CA Board of Registered Nursing; National Certification Board for Therapeutic Massage and Bodywork (CEUs); American Oriental Bodywork Therapy Association.
Field of Study: Acupressure*; Jin Shin Do*. *Program Name/Length:* Jin Shin Do Acupressure, minimum 250 hrs + 135 experience hrs (intensives or weekly classes); Seminars given in various locations.
Degrees Offered: Certificate.
License/Certification Preparation: National Certification Commission for Acupuncture and Oriental Medicine; American Oriental Bodywork Therapy Association; Registered Acupressurist, Jin Shin Do Foundation.
Tuition and Fees: $2000-$3000.
Financial Aid: Work study; Payment plan.
Career Services: Jin Shin Do Foundation Directory of Authorized Teachers and Registered Acupressurists.
Comments: Jin Shin Do Foundation is a network of authorized teachers throughout the United States, Canada, and Europe.

205. Mount Madonna Center
445 Summit Rd, Watsonville, CA 95076
Phone: (408) 847-0406; *Fax:* (408) 847-2683
E-mail: programs@mountmadonna.org *Internet:* http://www.mountmadonna.org
Program Administrator: Gerald Friedberg, PhD, Prog Dir. *Admissions Contact:* Gerald Friedberg.
Year Established: 1978.
Staff: Full-time: 1; Part-time: 60.
Avg Enrollment: 130. *Avg Class Size:* 30. *Number of Graduates per Year:* 25.
Wheelchair Access: Yes.
Field of Study: Ayurvedic Medicine*; Yoga Teacher Training*. *Program Name/Length:* Ayurveda: Ancient Health Science of India, 5 wks; Yoga Teacher Training, 3 wks.
Degrees Offered: Certificate.
Application Deadline(s): Summer: May 15.

Tuition and Fees: $1995 (Ayurveda); $645 (Yoga).
Financial Aid: Work study.

Whittier

206. Los Angeles College of Chiropractic
16200 E Amber Valley Dr, Whittier, CA 90609-1166
Phone: (562) 947-8755, (800) 221-5222; *Fax:* (562) 947-5724
E-mail: nathanchurch@lacc.edu
Program Administrator: Reed Phillips, PhD, Pres. *Admissions Contact:* Dr. Nathan Church.
Year Established: 1911.
Staff: Full-time: 54; Part-time: 20.
Avg Enrollment: 250. *Avg Class Size:* 80. *Number of Graduates per Year:* 100.
Wheelchair Access: Yes.
Accreditation/Approval/Licensing: State board: CA Board of Chiropractic; Council on Chiropractic Education; Western Association of Schools and Colleges.
Field of Study: Chiropractic*. *Program Name/Length:* Doctor of Chiropractic, 10 semesters.
Degrees Offered: DC; MS.
License/Certification Preparation: State: CA Board of Chiropractic; National Board of Chiropractic Examiners.
Admission Requirements: Some college (3 yrs), 90 semester hrs.
Application Deadline(s): Fall: Jul 1; Spring: Dec 1.
Tuition and Fees: $5600 per semester.
Financial Aid: Fellowships; Grants; Loans; Scholarships; Work study.
Career Services: Career counseling; Career information; Internships; Interview set up; Resume service.

Windsor

207. Equinology
PO Box 928, Windsor, CA 95492
Phone: (707) 431-8276; *Fax:* (707) 431-7076
E-mail: office@equinology.com *Internet:* http://www.equinology.com
Program Administrator: Debranne Pattillo, Owner. *Admissions Contact:* Debranne Pattillo.
Year Established: 1992.
Staff: Part-time: 12.
Avg Enrollment: 120. *Avg Class Size:* 8. *Number of Graduates per Year:* 60.
Wheelchair Access: No.
Field of Study: Animal Therapy*; Equine Massage*. *Program Name/Length:* Equine Body Worker (EBW) Certification, 100 hrs, 3 levels; Advanced Equine Body Worker (AEBW) Certificate, 400 hrs; Specialized Equine Body Worker (SEBW) Certificate, 400 hrs; Continuing education, independent study.

Degrees Offered: Certificate.
Admission Requirements: Min age: 16; Specific course prerequisites: EBW required for AEBW; AEBW required for SEBW.

Tuition and Fees: $85-$1275 per course.
Financial Aid: Loans.
Career Services: Career counseling.

COLORADO

Aurora

208. Cottonwood School of Massage Therapy
2620 S Parker Rd, Ste 300, Aurora, CO 80014
Phone: (303) 745-7725; *Fax:* (303) 751-1861
Program Administrator: Jackie Otey, Pres. *Admissions Contact:* Jackie Otey.
Year Established: 1993.
Staff: Full-time: 6.
Avg Enrollment: 90. *Avg Class Size:* 15. *Number of Graduates per Year:* 90.
Wheelchair Access: Yes.
Accreditation/Approval/Licensing: State board: CO Dept of Higher Ed.
Field of Study: Aromatherapy; CranioSacral Therapy; Energy Work; Massage Therapy*; Polarity Therapy; Reflexology; Reiki; Shiatsu; Sports Massage. *Program Name/Length:* 1 yr.
Degrees Offered: Certificate.
License/Certification Preparation: National Certification Board for Therapeutic Massage and Bodywork.
Admission Requirements: Min age: 18; High school diploma/GED.
Application Deadline(s): Fall: Sep 1; Winter: Jan 1; Spring: May 1; Summer.
Tuition and Fees: $4000.
Financial Aid: VA approved; Vocational rehabilitation; County government aid; Payment plan.
Career Services: Career information.

Boulder

209. Alexander Technique Institute, Colorado
2545 Vine Pl, Boulder, CO 80304
Phone: (303) 449-4143
E-mail: colinegan@netzero.net
Program Administrator: Colin Egan, Dir. *Admissions Contact:* Colin Egan.
Year Established: 1990.
Staff: Full-time: 2; Part-time: 5.
Accreditation/Approval/Licensing: American Society for the Alexander Technique.
Field of Study: Alexander Technique*. *Program Name/Length:* Teacher Training, 3 yrs.

License/Certification Preparation: American Society for the Alexander Technique.
Admission Requirements: Specific course prerequisites: 30 private lessons in the Alexander Technique, 6 with directors; 3 letters of application; Interview; 3 mo trial term.
Tuition and Fees: $16,000.

210. Artemis Institute of Natural Therapies
875 Alpine Ave, Ste 5, Boulder, CO 80304
Phone: (303) 443-9289; *Fax:* (303) 443-6361
Program Administrator: Peter J. Holmes, MH, Dir. *Admissions Contact:* Janet McKean, Admin.
Year Established: 1988.
Staff: Full-time: 1; Part-time: 3.
Avg Class Size: 14.
Wheelchair Access: No.
Field of Study: Aromatherapy*; Herbal Medicine*. *Program Name/Length:* Professional Certification in Herbal Medicine, 18 mos; Professional Certification in Clinical Aromatherapy, 8 mos.
Degrees Offered: MH; Certificate.
Admission Requirements: Min age: 18; Some college (2 yrs); Interview with director.
Application Deadline(s): Fall: Aug 15; Spring: Mar 15.
Tuition and Fees: $2500 (Herbal Medicine); $1500 (Aromatherapy).

211. Boulder College of Massage Therapy
6255 Longbow, Boulder, CO 80301
Phone: (303) 530-2100, (800) 442-5131; *Fax:* (303) 530-2204
Internet: http://www.bcmt.org
Program Administrator: Christopher Quinn, DC, School Dean. *Admissions Contact:* Carla Stanke, Admissions Coord.
Year Established: 1975.
Staff: Part-time: 35.
Avg Enrollment: 225. *Avg Class Size:* 18. *Number of Graduates per Year:* 225.
Wheelchair Access: Yes.
Accreditation/Approval/Licensing: State board: CO Dept of Higher Ed; National Certification Board for Therapeutic Massage and Bodywork (CEUs).
Field of Study: Chair Massage; Hydrotherapy; Infant Massage; Integrative Massage; Massage Therapy*; Orthopedic Massage; Polarity Therapy; Prenatal Massage; Reflexology; Shiatsu;

Sports Massage; Swedish Massage*. *Program Name/Length:* 1000 hrs, 1 or 2 yrs.
Degrees Offered: Diploma.
License/Certification Preparation: State: IA, ID, ND, NM, NY, WA Licensing/Certification Exams; National Certification Board for Therapeutic Massage and Bodywork.
Admission Requirements: Min age: 21; High school diploma/GED.
Tuition and Fees: $8800 + books, lab fees.
Financial Aid: Federal government aid; Grants; Loans; VA approved; Vocational rehabilitation; Payment plan; Plato loans.
Career Services: Career counseling; Career information; Internships; Referral service; Alumni Association; Career and Field Placement courses.

212. Colorado Institute for Classical Homeopathy

2299 Pearl St, Ste 401, Boulder, CO 80302
Phone: (303) 440-3717
Program Administrator: Barbara Seideneck, CCH, Dir. *Admissions Contact:* Barbara Seideneck.
Year Established: 1991.
Staff: Part-time: 5.
Avg Enrollment: 45. *Avg Class Size:* 20. *Number of Graduates per Year:* 45.
Wheelchair Access: No.
Accreditation/Approval/Licensing: State board: CO Dept of Higher Ed, Div of Private Occupational Schools.
Field of Study: Homeopathy*. *Program Name/Length:* 2 1/2 yrs.
Degrees Offered: CHom.
License/Certification Preparation: State: CO Homeopathic Consultant; Council for Homeopathic Certification; North American Society of Homeopaths.
Admission Requirements: Min age: 21; High school diploma/GED.
Application Deadline(s): Fall: Sep 1; Winter: Jan 15.
Tuition and Fees: $6375.
Financial Aid: State government aid; Vocational rehabilitation; Payment plan.
Career Services: Career counseling.

213. Guild for Structural Integration

3107 28th St, Boulder, CO 80301
Mailing Address: PO Box 1559, Boulder, CO 80306
Phone: (800) 447-0150; *Fax:* (303) 447-0108
E-mail: gsi@rolfguild.org *Internet:* http://www.rolfguild.org
Program Administrator: Susan Melchior, Dir. *Admissions Contact:* Susan Melchior.
Year Established: 1988.
Staff: Full-time: 5.
Avg Enrollment: 100. *Avg Class Size:* 16. *Number of Graduates per Year:* 50.
Wheelchair Access: Yes.

Field of Study: Structural Integration*. *Program Name/Length:* Ida P. Rolf Method of Structural Integration, 1 yr.
Degrees Offered: Certificate.
Admission Requirements: Min age: 21; High school diploma/GED; Specific course prerequisites: anatomy and physiology, massage.
Tuition and Fees: $9000.
Career Services: Career counseling; Career information.

214. Institute of Taoist Education and Acupuncture, Inc

Certificate of Licentiate in Acupuncture
1321 5th St, Boulder, CO 80302
Phone: (303) 440-3492; *Fax:* (303) 440-3492
Program Administrator: Sandra L. Lillie, Pres. *Admissions Contact:* Sandra L. Lillie.
Year Established: 1996.
Staff: Part-time: 25.
Avg Enrollment: 18. *Avg Class Size:* 12.
Wheelchair Access: Yes.
Accreditation/Approval/Licensing: State board: CO Dept of Continuing Ed, Div of Private Occupational Schools.
Field of Study: Acupuncture*. *Program Name/Length:* 3 yrs.
Degrees Offered: Certificate.
License/Certification Preparation: National Certification Commission for Acupuncture and Oriental Medicine.
Admission Requirements: High school diploma/GED; Some college (2 yrs).
Application Deadline(s): Fall: Jun 1.
Tuition and Fees: $6000 per yr.

215. Mandala Institute

Yoga Teacher Training
1800 30th St, Ste 201, Boulder, CO 80301
Phone: (303) 444-7512
Program Administrator: Ravi Dykema, Yoga Master, Owner.
Year Established: 1990.
Staff: Full-time: 1; Part-time: 2.
Avg Enrollment: 15. *Avg Class Size:* 15. *Number of Graduates per Year:* 5.
Wheelchair Access: Yes.
Field of Study: Yoga Teacher Training*. *Program Name/Length:* Advanced Program, 320 hrs (four 2-wk retreats); Masters Program, 800 hrs.
Admission Requirements: Min age: 18.
Career Services: Career counseling; Career information; Internships.

216. Polarity Center of Colorado

1721 Redwood Ave, Boulder, CO 80304-1118
Phone: (303) 443-9847; *Fax:* (303) 415-1839
E-mail: chittyj@aol.com *Internet:* http://www.polaritycolorado.com
Program Administrator: John Chitty, RPP, Dir. *Admissions Contact:* John Chitty. .
Year Established: 1992.

Staff: Part-time: 3.

Avg Enrollment: 50. *Avg Class Size:* 16. *Number of Graduates per Year:* 32.

Wheelchair Access: Yes.

Accreditation/Approval/Licensing: State board: CO Dept of Ed; American Polarity Therapy Association.

Field of Study: CranioSacral Therapy*; Polarity Therapy*. *Program Name/Length:* Polarity Therapy Level I, 16 days; Polarity Therapy Level II, 45 days; CranioSacral Therapy, 2 yrs (10 5-day quarterly modules).

Degrees Offered: Certificate.

License/Certification Preparation: American Polarity Therapy Association; CranioSacral Association of North America.

Admission Requirements: Min age: 21.

Application Deadline(s): Fall: Aug 1; Winter: Dec 1.

Tuition and Fees: $1800 (Polarity Level I); $4800 (Polarity Level II); $4950 (CranioSacral Therapy).

Financial Aid: Payment plan.

Career Services: Career counseling.

217. Rocky Mountain Center for Botanical Studies

2639 Spruce St, Boulder, CO 80302

Mailing Address: PO Box 19254, Boulder, CO 80308-2254

Phone: (303) 442-6861; *Fax:* (303) 442-6294

E-mail: rmcbs@indra.com *Internet:* http://www. herbschool.com

Program Administrator: Feather Jones, Exec Dir. *Admissions Contact:* Becky Haugen, Asst Dir of Academics.

Year Established: 1992.

Staff: Full-time: 5; Part-time: 20.

Avg Enrollment: 125. *Avg Class Size:* 32. *Number of Graduates per Year:* 100.

Wheelchair Access: Yes.

Accreditation/Approval/Licensing: State board: CO Dept of Higher Ed, Div of Private Occupational Schools.

Field of Study: Aromatherapy*; Ayurvedic Medicine; Herbal Medicine*; Traditional Chinese Medicine. *Program Name/Length:* Western Herbalism, 10 mos; Essence of Herbalism, 2 yrs/evenings; Advanced Herbalism, 5 mos; Clinical Internship, 9 mos; Intensive and workshops, 1-3 days.

Degrees Offered: Certificate.

Admission Requirements: Min age: 16; High school diploma/GED preferred.

Application Deadline(s): Fall.

Tuition and Fees: $5200 (Western Herbalism); $4800 (Essence of Herbalism); $3200 (Advanced); $1900 (Clinical).

Financial Aid: Scholarships; Work study; VA approved.

Career Services: Career counseling; Career information; Internships; Interview set up; Job board.

218. Rolf Institute of Structural Integration

205 Canyon Blvd, Boulder, CO 80302

Phone: (303) 449-5903, (800) 530-8875; *Fax:* (303) 449-5978

E-mail: rolfinst@rolf.org *Internet:* http://www. rolf.org

Program Administrator: Rebecca Pembrook, Education Dir. *Admissions Contact:* Holly Hamilton, Student Svcs Coord.

Year Established: 1971.

Staff: Part-time: 35.

Avg Enrollment: 150. *Avg Class Size:* 16. *Number of Graduates per Year:* 70.

Wheelchair Access: No.

Accreditation/Approval/Licensing: State board: CO Dept of Higher Ed, Div of Private Occupational Schools; National Certification Board for Therapeutic Massage and Bodywork (CEUs).

Field of Study: Structural Integration*. *Program Name/Length:* Foundations of Bodywork, 6 wks; Integrated Rolfing Studies, 1 yr; Advanced Rolfing Certification, 6 wks; Rolfing Movement Certification, 1 mo.

Degrees Offered: Certificate.

License/Certification Preparation: National Certification Board for Therapeutic Massage and Bodywork.

Admission Requirements: Min age: 21; High school diploma/GED; Bachelor's degree for Integrated Rolfing; Massage training, exam in anatomy, physiology, and kinesiology required for Integrated Rolfing.

Tuition and Fees: $2500 (Foundations of Bodywork); $11,000 (Integrated Rolfing); $3900 (Advanced Rolfing); $2900 (Rolfing Movement).

Career Services: Career information.

219. Ruseto College of Acupuncture and Chinese Medicine

2900 Valmont Rd, Ste E-1, Boulder, CO 80301

Phone: (303) 449-1686

Program Administrator: Pao-Chin R. Huang, Dir. *Admissions Contact:* Hui-Yu Huang, Pres.

Year Established: 1992.

Staff: Full-time: 2; Part-time: 6.

Avg Enrollment: 7. *Avg Class Size:* 7. *Number of Graduates per Year:* 7.

Wheelchair Access: Yes.

Field of Study: Acupuncture*; Herbal Medicine; Massage Therapy*; Polarity Therapy; Qigong; Reflexology; Shiatsu*; Traditional Chinese Medicine*; Tui Na. *Program Name/Length:* Massage Therapy, 1 yr; Acupuncture and Chinese Medicine, 3 yrs.

Degrees Offered: Certificate.

License/Certification Preparation: National Certification Commission for Acupuncture and Oriental Medicine.

Admission Requirements: Specific course prerequisites: acupuncture, Chinese medicine, medical diagnosis.

Application Deadline(s): Fall: Jul 15; Spring: Dec 15.
Tuition and Fees: $3600 (Massage Therapy); $4800 + $200-$300 books per yr (Acupuncture).
Financial Aid: Payment plan.
Career Services: Career counseling; Internships; Resume service.

220. School of Natural Medicine
PO Box 7369, Boulder, CO 80306-7369
Phone: (303) 443-4882; *Fax:* (303) 443-8276
E-mail: snm@purehealth.com *Internet:* http://www.purehealth.com
Program Administrator: Dr. Farida Sharan, Founder/Dir.
Year Established: 1976.
Staff: Full-time: 2; Part-time: 8.
Avg Enrollment: 100. *Avg Class Size:* 30. *Number of Graduates per Year:* 25.
Wheelchair Access: Yes.
Field of Study: Energy Work; Herbal Medicine*; Iridology*; Naturopathy. *Program Name/Length:* Iridology and Foundations of Natural Medicine; Master Herbalist; Natural Physician; Summer school; Home study/Correspondence.
Degrees Offered: MH; Diploma; Certificate.
Admission Requirements: Min age: 18; High school diploma/GED.
Application Deadline(s): Summer: Aug 9 for Summer school.
Tuition and Fees: $700 (Iridology; Master Herbalist); $3000 (Natural Physician); $1800 (Summer School).
Financial Aid: Work study; Apprentice program.
Career Services: Career counseling; Career information; Internships.

221. SoulWorks Hypnotherapy Training School
Hypnotherapy Certification
1750 30th St, Ste 196, Boulder, CO 80301
Phone: (303) 939-0197
Program Administrator: Lynda Hilburn-Holland, CCH, Dir. *Admissions Contact:* Lynda Hilburn-Holland.
Year Established: 1997.
Staff: Full-time: 1.
Avg Enrollment: 24. *Avg Class Size:* 10. *Number of Graduates per Year:* 24.
Wheelchair Access: Yes.
Accreditation/Approval/Licensing: State board: CO Dept of Ed, Div of Occupational and Private Schools; American Council of Hypnotist Examiners.
Field of Study: Hypnotherapy*. *Program Name/Length:* 250 hrs, 14 weekends.
Degrees Offered: Certificate.
License/Certification Preparation: American Council of Hypnotist Examiners.
Admission Requirements: Min age: 18; High school diploma/GED.

Tuition and Fees: $2600.

222. Southwest Acupuncture School, Boulder
Master of Science in Oriental Medicine
6658 Gunpark Dr, Ste 100, Boulder, CO 80301
Phone: (303) 581-9955; *Fax:* (303) 581-9944
E-mail: swacb@compuserve.com *Internet:* http://www.swacupuncture.com
Program Administrator: Mary Saunders, Dir. *Admissions Contact:* Cindy Wolf, Administrative Dir.
Year Established: 1997.
Staff: Part-time: 20.
Avg Enrollment: 90. *Avg Class Size:* 25. *Number of Graduates per Year:* 20.
Wheelchair Access: Yes.
Accreditation/Approval/Licensing: Accreditation Commission for Acupuncture and Oriental Medicine.
Field of Study: Acupuncture*; Herbal Medicine*; Oriental Medicine*; Qigong; Shiatsu; Traditional Chinese Medicine*. *Program Name/Length:* 3 yrs/accelerated, 4 yrs/full-time or 7 yrs/part-time.
Degrees Offered: MS.
License/Certification Preparation: National Certification Commission for Acupuncture and Oriental Medicine.
Admission Requirements: Min age: 20; Some college (2 yrs, 60 semester credits).
Application Deadline(s): Fall: Mar 15 early, May 15 late.
Tuition and Fees: $30,000 (3 yr program) includes books.
Financial Aid: Federal government aid; Scholarships.

Colorado Springs

223. Collinson School of Therapeutics and Massage
2596 Palmer Park Blvd, Colorado Springs, CO 80909
Phone: (719) 473-0145
Program Administrator: Dr. Torry Collinson, Owner. *Admissions Contact:* Dr. Torry Collinson.
Year Established: 1981.
Staff: Part-time: 3.
Avg Enrollment: 45. *Avg Class Size:* 20. *Number of Graduates per Year:* 30.
Wheelchair Access: Yes.
Field of Study: Acupressure; Aromatherapy; CranioSacral Therapy; Massage Therapy*; Reflexology; Reiki; Shiatsu. *Program Name/Length:* 40 wks.
Degrees Offered: Certificate.
Admission Requirements: Min age: 17.
Application Deadline(s): Fall: Oct; Spring: Apr.
Tuition and Fees: $2800.

224. Colorado Institute of Massage Therapy

2601 E Saint Vrain, Colorado Springs, CO 80909
Phone: (719) 634-7486; *Fax:* (719) 447-9198
E-mail: info@coimt.com *Internet:* http://www. coimt.com
Program Administrator: Togi Kinniman, Director. *Admissions Contact:* Greg Smith, Admissions Advisor.
Year Established: 1985.
Staff: Part-time: 15.
Avg Enrollment: 100. *Avg Class Size:* 25. *Number of Graduates per Year:* 90.
Wheelchair Access: Yes.
Accreditation/Approval/Licensing: National Certification Board for Therapeutic Massage and Bodywork (CEUs).
Field of Study: Acupressure; Fitness Therapy; Massage Therapy*; Neuromuscular Therapy*; Reflexology; Sports Massage. *Program Name/Length:* Massage Therapy, 11 1/5 mos; Fitness Therapy, 3 mos.
Degrees Offered: Certificate.
License/Certification Preparation: National Certification Board for Therapeutic Massage and Bodywork.
Admission Requirements: Min age: 18; High school diploma/GED; Min GPA: 2.0.
Application Deadline(s): Fall: Sep 1; Winter: Dec 15; Spring: Mar 1; Summer: Jun 1.
Tuition and Fees: $6750.
Financial Aid: Loans; Scholarships; State government aid; Work study; VA approved; Vocational rehabilitation.
Career Services: Career counseling; Career information; Internships.

225. Colorado Springs Academy of Therapeutic Massage

3612 Galley, Ste A, Colorado Springs, CO 80909
Phone: (719) 597-0017; *Fax:* (719) 597-6647
Program Administrator: Dr. Daniel A. Sollee, Owner/Dir. *Admissions Contact:* Tina Sollee, Admissions Dir.
Year Established: 1991.
Staff: Full-time: 8; Part-time: 6.
Avg Enrollment: 100. *Avg Class Size:* 33. *Number of Graduates per Year:* 100.
Wheelchair Access: Yes.
Accreditation/Approval/Licensing: State board: CO Dept of Higher Ed.
Field of Study: Deep Tissue Massage; Massage Therapy*; Neuromuscular Therapy; Sports Massage; Swedish Massage*; Trigger Point Therapy. *Program Name/Length:* Certified Massage Therapist, 1100 hrs.
Degrees Offered: Certificate.
License/Certification Preparation: National Certification Board for Therapeutic Massage and Bodywork.

Admission Requirements: Min age: 18; High school diploma/GED; Min GPA: 2.0.
Application Deadline(s): Fall: Aug; Winter: Dec; Spring Apr.
Tuition and Fees: $4950.
Financial Aid: Loans; Scholarships; Work study.
Career Services: Career counseling; Career information.

Crested Butte

226. MountainHeart School of Bodywork and Transformational Therapy

719 5th, Unit A, Crested Butte, CO 81224
Mailing Address: PO Box 575, Crested Butte, CO 81224
Phone: (970) 349-0473, (800) 673-0539; *Fax:* (970) 349-0473
E-mail: cragmc@crestedbutte.net
Program Administrator: Christine McLaughlin, Co-Dir; Craig McLaughlin, Co-Dir. *Admissions Contact:* Christine McLaughlin; Craig McLaughlin.
Year Established: 1997.
Staff: Full-time: 2; Part-time: 2.
Avg Enrollment: 20. *Avg Class Size:* 12. *Number of Graduates per Year:* 18.
Wheelchair Access: No.
Field of Study: Acupressure; Energy Work; Massage Therapy*; Neuromuscular Therapy*; Oriental Medicine; Reflexology. *Program Name/Length:* Massage Therapy, 850 hrs, 6 mos; Transformational Neuromuscular Therapy, 272 hrs.
Degrees Offered: CEUs; Certificate.
License/Certification Preparation: National Certification Board for Therapeutic Massage and Bodywork.
Admission Requirements: Min age: 18.
Application Deadline(s): Winter: Dec 1; Summer: Jun 1.
Tuition and Fees: $6162 (Massage Therapy).
Career Services: Career counseling; Career information.

Crestone

227. Crestone Healing Arts Center

12-Week Massage Certification Intensive
1689 Columbine Overlook, Crestone, CO 81131
Mailing Address: PO Box 156, Crestone, CO 81131
Phone: (719) 256-4036
E-mail: retuta@crestonehac.com *Internet:* http://www.crestonehac.com
Program Administrator: Dan Retuta, Prog Dir.
Year Established: 1995.
Staff: Full-time: 1; Part-time: 2.
Avg Enrollment: 20. *Avg Class Size:* 7. *Number of Graduates per Year:* 7.

Wheelchair Access: No.
Accreditation/Approval/Licensing: State board: CO Dept of Higher Ed, Div of Private Occupational Schools.
Field of Study: Acupressure; Anatomy and Physiology; CPR/First Aid; Herbal Medicine; Integrated Massage; Massage Therapy*; On-Site Massage; Prenatal Massage; Qigong; Reflexology; Shiatsu; Swedish Massage*. *Program Name/Length:* Massage Therapist Certification Intensive, 3 mos.
Degrees Offered: Certificate.
Admission Requirements: Min age: 18; High school diploma/GED; 3-5 letters of recommendation; Interview; On-site visit recommended.
Application Deadline(s): Fall: Sep 15; Winter: Jan 5; Spring: Apr 15.
Tuition and Fees: $4900.
Financial Aid: Payment plan.

Denver

228. Ann Allen and Associates, Biofeedback and Stress Management
Biofeedback Certification Program
1660 S Albion St, Denver, CO 80222
Phone: (303) 757-0508; *Fax:* (303) 758-9203
Program Administrator: Ann Allen, Owner. *Admissions Contact:* Ann Allen.
Year Established: 1993.
Staff: Full-time: 1; Part-time: 2.
Avg Enrollment: 15. *Avg Class Size:* 4. *Number of Graduates per Year:* 15.
Wheelchair Access: Yes.
Accreditation/Approval/Licensing: Biofeedback Certification Institute of America.
Field of Study: Biofeedback*. *Program Name/Length:* Didactic Certification for Biofeedback and Supervision, 60 hrs didactic training + 120 hrs supervised practicum.
Degrees Offered: Certificate.
License/Certification Preparation: Biofeedback Certification Institute of America.
Admission Requirements: Bachelor's degree in health science or psychology.
Tuition and Fees: $1200 didactic training + $800 supervision.

229. Center of Advanced Therapeutics, Inc
1221 S Clarkson St, Ste 412, Denver, CO 80210
Phone: (303) 765-2201
E-mail: center@netsavant.com
Program Administrator: Kins Loree, Pres. *Admissions Contact:* Mary Uhl, Admissions.
Year Established: 1995.
Staff: Part-time: 6.
Avg Class Size: 15. *Number of Graduates per Year:* 80.
Wheelchair Access: Yes.

Accreditation/Approval/Licensing: State board: CO Dept of Higher Ed, Div of Private Occupational Schools.
Field of Study: CranioSacral Therapy; Deep Tissue Massage; Massage Therapy*. *Program Name/Length:* Massage Therapy, 9 mos; Soft Tissue, 1 yr.
Degrees Offered: Certificate.
Admission Requirements: Min age: 18; High school diploma/GED.
Tuition and Fees: $3900-$4400.
Financial Aid: Payment plans.
Career Services: Career information; Internships.

230. Colorado School of Traditional Chinese Medicine
1441 York St, Ste 202, Denver, CO 80210
Phone: (303) 329-6355; *Fax:* (303) 388-8165
Program Administrator: Dr. George H. Kitchie, Pres. *Admissions Contact:* Dr. Steven Juenke, Admin.
Year Established: 1990.
Staff: Part-time: 35.
Avg Enrollment: 125. *Avg Class Size:* 25. *Number of Graduates per Year:* 30.
Wheelchair Access: No.
Accreditation/Approval/Licensing: State board: CO Dept of Higher Ed.
Field of Study: Acupuncture*; Chinese Herbal Medicine*; Qigong*; Traditional Chinese Medicine*. *Program Name/Length:* Traditional Chinese Medicine, 1800 hrs, 3 yrs (program will increase to 2460 hrs).
Degrees Offered: Diploma.
License/Certification Preparation: State: CO Registered Acupuncturist; National Certification Commission for Acupuncture and Oriental Medicine.
Admission Requirements: Min age: 21; Some college (2 yrs); Specific course prerequisites: 90 hrs anatomy and physiology.
Application Deadline(s): Fall: Jul 15; Winter: Dec 15.
Tuition and Fees: $5500 per yr.
Career Services: Career counseling; Career information.

231. Day-Star Method of Yoga
2565 S Meade St, Denver, CO 80219
Phone: (303) 934-6309
E-mail: solsiren@aol.com
Program Administrator: Susan Flanders, Owner/Developer.
Staff: Full-time: 1; Part-time: 2.
Avg Enrollment: 8. *Avg Class Size:* 8. *Number of Graduates per Year:* 8.
Field of Study: Yoga Teacher Training*. *Program Name/Length:* 1 1/2 yrs (1 day per mo); Seminars given in various locations.
Degrees Offered: Certificate.
Admission Requirements: Min age: 18; 1-2 yrs yoga practice preferred.

Tuition and Fees: $1000.
Financial Aid: Payment plan.
Career Services: Internships; Referral service.

232. Just for Health Enterprises, Inc

135 Hour Foot and Hand Reflexology Training
480 S Holly St, Denver, CO 80246
Phone: (303) 341-4384; *Fax:* (303) 360-9118
E-mail: rachel@scicom.alphacdc.com
Program Administrator: Rachel Lord, RN, Dir. *Admissions Contact:* Rachel Lord.
Year Established: 1993.
Staff: Full-time: 1.
Avg Enrollment: 50. *Avg Class Size:* 10. *Number of Graduates per Year:* 40.
Wheelchair Access: Yes.
Field of Study: Acupressure; Anatomy and Physiology; Deep Tissue Massage; Energy Work; Herbal Medicine; Massage Therapy; Reflexology*. *Program Name/Length:* Levels I-V, 135 hrs, 5 weekends (16 hrs each) + 55 hrs out of class.
Degrees Offered: Certificate.
License/Certification Preparation: American Reflexology Certification Board.
Admission Requirements: Min age: 18; Specific course prerequisites: May enter course at Level III with prior training equivalent to Levels I and II.
Tuition and Fees: $1000 + $54 books, charts.
Career Services: Instruction in practice development.

233. Massage Therapy Institute of Colorado

Professional Certified Massage Therapist
1441 York St, Ste 301, Denver, CO 80206
Phone: (303) 329-6345; *Fax:* (303) 388-8165
E-mail: mtickraft@aol.com
Program Administrator: Mark Manton, Dir. *Admissions Contact:* Hilde Kraft, Chief Admin.
Year Established: 1986.
Staff: Full-time: 8; Part-time: 25.
Avg Enrollment: 130. *Avg Class Size:* 18. *Number of Graduates per Year:* 120.
Wheelchair Access: No.
Accreditation/Approval/Licensing: State board: CO Dept of Higher Ed.
Field of Study: Acupressure; Alexander Technique; Aromatherapy; CranioSacral Therapy; Energy Work; Feldenkrais; Herbal Medicine; Homeopathy; Hypnotherapy; Massage Therapy*; Neuromuscular Therapy; Polarity Therapy; Qigong; Reflexology; Reiki; Shiatsu; Sports Massage. *Program Name/Length:* Massage Certification, 1 yr.
Degrees Offered: Certificate.
License/Certification Preparation: National Certification Board for Therapeutic Massage and Bodywork.
Admission Requirements: Min age: 21; High school diploma/GED; Some college preferred;

Life experience accepted in lieu of age and college requirements.
Tuition and Fees: $5135.
Financial Aid: VA approved; Payment plan.
Career Services: Career counseling; Career information; Internships; Referral service.

234. Modern Institute of Reflexology

7043 W Colfax, Denver, CO 80215
Phone: (303) 237-1530; *Fax:* (303) 237-1606
E-mail: footdocs@ix.netcom.com *Internet:* http://www.reflexologyinstitute.com
Program Administrator: Zachary K. Brinkerhoff III, Owner/Pres. *Admissions Contact:* Zachary K. Brinkerhoff III.
Year Established: 1981.
Staff: Full-time: 4; Part-time: 2.
Wheelchair Access: Yes.
Accreditation/Approval/Licensing: State board: CO Dept of Higher Ed.
Field of Study: Reflexology*. *Program Name/Length:* Home Study, 6-12 mos.
Degrees Offered: Certificate.
License/Certification Preparation: State: CO Certification.
Admission Requirements: High school diploma/GED.
Tuition and Fees: $1000.
Financial Aid: Payment plan.

235. University of Colorado, Health Sciences Center

Nurse-Midwifery Option, School of Nursing
4200 E 9th Ave, Box C288-14, Denver, CO 80262
Phone: (303) 315-8654/4324; *Fax:* (303) 315-5666
E-mail: laraine.guyette@uchsc.edu
Program Administrator: Laraine Guyette, PhD, Dir. *Admissions Contact:* Mary Lepley, Dir of Admissions and Student Support.
Staff: Full-time: 3; Part-time: 10.
Avg Enrollment: 30. *Number of Graduates per Year:* 10.
Wheelchair Access: Yes.
Accreditation/Approval/Licensing: State board: CO Board of Nursing; North Central Association of Colleges and Schools; American College of Nurse-Midwives, Division of Accreditation.
Field of Study: Midwifery*.
Degrees Offered: MS.
License/Certification Preparation: Certified Nurse-Midwife, American College of Nurse-Midwives.
Admission Requirements: Bachelor's degree; RN.

Eaton

236. Academy of Natural Therapy

123 Elm Ave, Eaton, CO 80615
Phone: (970) 454-2224; *Fax:* (303) 454-3147
E-mail: mongan@ibm.net

Program Administrator: Dorothy Mongan, Dir. *Admissions Contact:* James Mongan, VP.
Year Established: 1989.
Staff: Full-time: 8; Part-time: 3.
Avg Enrollment: 20. *Avg Class Size:* 10. *Number of Graduates per Year:* 20.
Wheelchair Access: No.
Accreditation/Approval/Licensing: State board: CO Dept of Higher Ed.
Field of Study: Acupressure; Herbal Medicine; Massage Therapy*; Reflexology; Shiatsu. *Program Name/Length:* 1000 hrs, 1 yr.
Degrees Offered: Certificate.
License/Certification Preparation: National Certification Board for Therapeutic Massage and Bodywork.
Admission Requirements: Min age: 18; High school diploma/GED.
Application Deadline(s): Fall: Oct; Spring: Mar.
Tuition and Fees: $5000.
Financial Aid: Scholarships; Payment plan.
Career Services: Career information.

Fort Collins

237. Cooperative Training Systems
Massage Therapist Training
PO Box 1836, Fort Collins, CO 80522
Phone: (970) 416-9956; *Fax:* (970) 472-9522
E-mail: cts@ezlink.com
Program Administrator: Mark F. Beck, Dir. *Admissions Contact:* Mark F. Beck.
Year Established: 1995.
Avg Enrollment: 25. *Avg Class Size:* 4. *Number of Graduates per Year:* 22.
Accreditation/Approval/Licensing: State board: CO Dept of Ed, Div of Private Occupational Schools; ID Dept of Ed; NM Board of Massage Therapy; National Certification Board for Therapeutic Massage and Bodywork (CEUs).
Field of Study: Massage Therapy*. *Program Name/Length:* Correspondence/Mentor Program, 500 hrs.
Degrees Offered: Certificate.
License/Certification Preparation: National Certification Board for Therapeutic Massage and Bodywork.
Admission Requirements: Min age: 18; High school diploma/GED.
Tuition and Fees: $3500-$6000.

Grand Junction

238. BioSomatics
PO Box 206, Grand Junction, CO 81502
Phone: (970) 245-8903; *Fax:* (970) 241-5653
E-mail: biosomatics@gj.net *Internet:* http://www.biosomatics.com
Program Administrator: Carol Welch, Educational Dir. *Admissions Contact:* Carol Welch.

Field of Study: CranioSacral Therapy; Neuromuscular Therapy; Somatic Education*.

Lakewood

239. Colorado School of Healing Arts
7655 W Mississippi, Ste 100, Lakewood, CO 80226
Phone: (303) 986-2320
Program Administrator: Chris Smith, Dir of Ed. *Admissions Contact:* Gina Simpson, Admissions Dir.
Year Established: 1988.
Staff: Part-time: 25.
Avg Enrollment: 260. *Avg Class Size:* 18. *Number of Graduates per Year:* 150.
Wheelchair Access: Yes.
Accreditation/Approval/Licensing: State board: CO Dept of Higher Ed, Div of Private Occupational Schools; Accrediting Commission of Career Schools and Colleges of Technology; International Massage and Somatic Therapies Accreditation Council; National Certification Board for Therapeutic Massage and Bodywork (CEUs).
Field of Study: Aromatherapy; CranioSacral Therapy*; Herbal Medicine; Massage Therapy*; Neuromuscular Therapy*; Reflexology*; Sports Massage*. *Program Name/Length:* Certified Massage Therapy, 670 hrs, 1 yr; Neuromuscular Massage Therapy Certification, 300 hrs; CranioSacral Therapy Certification, 530 hrs; Certificate in Reflexology, 230 hrs, 1 yr; Certificate in Sports Massage, 100 hrs, 1 yr.
Degrees Offered: Certificate.
License/Certification Preparation: National Certification Board for Therapeutic Massage and Bodywork.
Admission Requirements: Min age: 18; High school diploma/GED.
Tuition and Fees: $4120 (CranioSacral); $2295 (Neuromuscular); $1770 (Reflexology); $4850 (Massage); $815 (Sports Massage); $790 (Trauma Touch).
Career Services: Career information; Internships; Job information.

Nederland

240. Qigong Research and Practice Center
Qigong and Indigenous Medicine
PO Box 1727, Nederland, CO 80466
Phone: (303) 258-0971; *Fax:* (303) 258-0971
Program Administrator: Kenneth S. Cohen, Executive Director. *Admissions Contact:* Rebecca D. Cohen, Administrative Director.
Year Established: 1981.
Staff: Full-time: 1; Part-time: 10.
Avg Class Size: 35.
Wheelchair Access: Yes.

Field of Study: Energy Work*; Qigong*; Tai Chi*.
  Program Name/Length: Qigong Teacher
  Training, 3-4 yrs; Tai Chi Teacher Training, 3-4
  yrs; Seminars given in various locations.
Degrees Offered: Certificate.
Admission Requirements: Min age: 17.
Tuition and Fees: $1500 per year.
Financial Aid: Scholarships; Work study; Payment
  plan.
Career Services: Career counseling; Career infor-
  mation; Referral service.
Comments: Courses are offered in Colorado and in
  outreach programs throughout the world.

Pagosa Springs

241. Hahnemann Academy of North America

PO Box 3024, Pagosa Springs, CO 81147
Phone: (970) 731-9681
Admissions Contact: Robin Murphy, ND, Dir.
Field of Study: Homeopathy*.

Telluride

242. Connecting Point School of Massage and Spa Therapies, Inc

104 Society Dr, Telluride, CO 81435
Mailing Address: PO Box 2101, Telluride, CO
  81435
Phone: (870) 728-6424
Program Administrator: Toni Nurnberg, Exec Dir.
  Admissions Contact: Sefra Maples, Administra-
  tive Dir.
Year Established: 1992.
Staff: Full-time: 1; Part-time: 8.
Avg Enrollment: 40. *Avg Class Size:* 15. *Number
  of Graduates per Year:* 40.
Wheelchair Access: Yes.

Field of Study: Acupressure; Aromatherapy; Deep
  Tissue Massage; Massage Therapy*;
  Reflexology; Shiatsu; Spa Therapies*. *Program
  Name/Length:* Massage Therapy, 500 hrs, 8
  mos.
Degrees Offered: Certificate.
License/Certification Preparation: National Certif-
  ication Board for Therapeutic Massage and
  Bodywork.
Admission Requirements: Min age: 18; High
  school diploma/GED.
Application Deadline(s): Fall: Aug; Winter: Apr.

Wheat Ridge

243. Association for Applied Psychophysiology and Biofeedback

10200 W 44th Ave, Ste 304, Wheat Ridge, CO
  80033
Phone: (303) 422-8436; *Fax:* (303) 422-8894
E-mail: aapb@resourcenter.com *Internet:* http://
  www.aapb.org
Program Administrator: Francine Butler, PhD,
  Exec Dir. *Admissions Contact:* Francine Butler.
Year Established: 1969.
Staff: Part-time: 40.
Avg Enrollment: 150. *Avg Class Size:* 30.
Wheelchair Access: Yes.
Accreditation/Approval/Licensing: State board: CA
  Psychological Association; CO Nurses' Associa-
  tion; Biofeedback Certification Institute of
  America; American Psychological Association.
Field of Study: Biofeedback*. *Program
  Name/Length:* AAPB Annual Meeting, 1 1/2-40
  hrs; AAPB Fall Workshops, 25-40 hrs; Seminars
  given in various locations.
Degrees Offered: CEUs.
License/Certification Preparation: Biofeedback
  Certification Institute of America.

CONNECTICUT

Bridgeport

244. University of Bridgeport, College of Chiropractic

75 Linden Ave, Bridgeport, CT 06601
Phone: (203) 576-4279; *Fax:* (203) 576-4351
Internet: http://www.bridgeport.edu/chiro/
Program Administrator: Frank Zolli, DC, Dean.
  Admissions Contact: Laura Hildreth, Admis-
  sions Dir.
Year Established: 1991.
Staff: Full-time: 20; Part-time: 30.

Avg Enrollment: 100. *Avg Class Size:* 50. *Number
  of Graduates per Year:* 75.
Wheelchair Access: Yes.
Accreditation/Approval/Licensing: Council on
  Chiropractic Education; New England Associa-
  tion of Schools and Colleges.
Field of Study: Chiropractic*. *Program
  Name/Length:* Doctor of Chiropractic, 8 semes-
  ters, 4 yrs.
Degrees Offered: DC.

Admission Requirements: Some college (90 credits); Min GPA: 2.5; Specific course prerequisites: 3 semester hrs each: psychology, humanities, social sciences; 6 semester hrs each: communications/language skills, biology, general/inorganic chemistry, organic chemistry, physics; 9 semester hrs humanities or social sciences.
Application Deadline(s): Fall: Mar 1; Spring: Aug 1.
Tuition and Fees: $6200 per semester.
Financial Aid: Loans; Work study.
Career Services: Career information.

245. University of Bridgeport, College of Naturopathic Medicine

60 Lafayette St, Bridgeport, CT 06601
Phone: (203) 576-4109; *Fax:* (203) 576-4107
Internet: http://www.bridgeport.edu/naturopathy/
Program Administrator: Ron Hobbs, ND, Dean.
   Admissions Contact: Miriam Madweb.
Year Established: 1997.
Staff: Full-time: 12; Part-time: 16.
Avg Enrollment: 40. *Avg Class Size:* 30.
Wheelchair Access: Yes.
Accreditation/Approval/Licensing: New England Association of Schools and Colleges.
Field of Study: Acupuncture; Herbal Medicine; Homeopathy; Massage Therapy; Naturopathic Medicine*; Nutrition. *Program Name/Length:* Doctor of Naturopathic Medicine, 4 yrs.
Degrees Offered: ND.
License/Certification Preparation: State: AK, AZ, CT, DC, HI, ME, MT, NH, OR, UT, VT, WA; Naturopathic Physicians Licensing Exam.
Admission Requirements: Bachelor's degree; Min GPA: 2.5.
Application Deadline(s): Fall: Mar 1; Spring: Oct 1.
Tuition and Fees: $6400 per semester.
Financial Aid: Federal government aid.
Career Services: Career counseling; Career information.

New Haven

246. The School of Homeopathy-Devon, England

North American Flexible Learning Program, Administrative Office-U.S.
82 E Pearl St, New Haven, CT 06513
Phone: (203) 624-8783; *Fax:* (203) 624-8783
E-mail: betsy@homeopathyschool.com *Internet:* http://www.homeopathyschool.com
Program Administrator: Misha Norland, Dir; Stuart Gracie, Course Mgr. *Admissions Contact:* Betsy Levine, US Representative.
Year Established: 1981.
Staff: Full-time: 3; Part-time: 12.
Avg Enrollment: 100.
Accreditation/Approval/Licensing: Council on Homeopathic Education.

Field of Study: Anatomy and Physiology; Homeopathy*; Pathology and Disease. *Program Name/Length:* Foundation Certificate, 1 1/2 yrs; Three Year Program + clinical practice and case supervision; Seminars given in various locations; Home study/Correspondence.
Degrees Offered: Diploma; Certificate.
License/Certification Preparation: Council for Homeopathic Certification; North American Society of Homeopaths.
Admission Requirements: Interview.
Tuition and Fees: $2690 (Foundation); $3695 (Three Year Program) or $1595 per yr; $100 registration fee.
Financial Aid: Payment plan.
Career Services: Mentor program.

247. Yale University, School of Nursing

Nurse-Midwifery Program
100 Church St S, Box 9740, New Haven, CT 06536-0740
Phone: (203) 737-2344, 785-2389 (applications); *Fax:* (203) 785-6455
E-mail: lynette.ament@yale.edu *Internet:* http://info.med.yale.edu/nursing/
Program Administrator: Lynette Ament, PhD, Nurse-Midwifery Specialty Dir. *Admissions Contact:* Barbara Reif, Student Affairs Dir.
Year Established: 1956.
Staff: Full-time: 8; Part-time: 1.
Avg Enrollment: 28. *Avg Class Size:* 14. *Number of Graduates per Year:* 14.
Wheelchair Access: Yes.
Accreditation/Approval/Licensing: American College of Nurse-Midwives, Division of Accreditation; National League for Nursing.
Field of Study: Midwifery*. *Program Name/Length:* Program for Nurses, 2 yrs; Program for Non-Nurses, 3 yrs.
Degrees Offered: MSN.
License/Certification Preparation: Certified Nurse-Midwife, American College of Nurse-Midwives.
Admission Requirements: Bachelor's degree; Min GPA: 3.0 preferred; Specific course prerequisites: statistics.
Application Deadline(s): Fall: Nov, for Non-Nurses; Spring: Apr, for Nurses.
Tuition and Fees: $35,200 (Nurses); $24,500/1st yr, then $17,600 per yr (Non-Nurses).
Financial Aid: Federal government aid; Loans; Scholarships; Work study.
Career Services: Career counseling; Career information.

Newington

248. Connecticut Center for Massage Therapy Inc, Newington

75 Kitts Ln, Newington, CT 06111
Phone: (860) 667-1886; *Fax:* (860) 667-2175

E-mail: info@ccmt.com *Internet:* http://www. ccmt.com

Program Administrator: Stephen Kitts, Exec Dir. *Admissions Contact:* Wendy Dorsey, Admissions Dir.

Year Established: 1980.

Staff: Part-time: 30.

Avg Enrollment: 180. *Avg Class Size:* 20. *Number of Graduates per Year:* 180.

Wheelchair Access: Yes.

Accreditation/Approval/Licensing: Commission on Massage Therapy Accreditation; Accrediting Commission of Career Schools and Colleges of Technology; National Certification Board for Therapeutic Massage and Bodywork (CEUs).

Field of Study: Acupressure; Energy Work; Massage Therapy*; Meditation; Neuromuscular Therapy; Reflexology; Reiki; Shiatsu; Sports Massage. *Program Name/Length:* Massage Practitioner Program, 1 yr; Massage Therapist, 16 or 20 mos; Clinical Massage Therapist, 20 mos.

Degrees Offered: Diploma.

License/Certification Preparation: State: CT, NY Licensed Massage Therapist; National Certification Board for Therapeutic Massage and Bodywork.

Admission Requirements: Min age: 18; High school diploma/GED.

Application Deadline(s): Fall: Aug 15; Winter: Dec 15; Summer: Apr 15.

Tuition and Fees: $2000-$2500 per trimester.

Financial Aid: Federal government aid; VA approved; Vocational rehabilitation; Pell grants; Stafford loans.

Career Services: Career counseling; Career information; Internships; Job information.

249. Connecticut Institute for Herbal Studies

87 Market Sq, Newington, CT 06111

Phone: (860) 666-5064; *Fax:* (860) 666-5064

E-mail: laurachina@aol.com *Internet:* http://www. herbworld.com/herbschool

Program Administrator: Laura Mignosa, Owner/Dir. *Admissions Contact:* Laura Mignosa.

Year Established: 1992.

Staff: Part-time: 8.

Avg Class Size: 24.

Wheelchair Access: No.

Field of Study: Herbal Medicine*; Traditional Chinese Medicine*. *Program Name/Length:* Western Herbology, 5 mos; Chinese Herbology, ongoing 5 mo-modules/1 weekend per mo.

Degrees Offered: Certificate.

License/Certification Preparation: National Certification Commission for Acupuncture and Oriental Medicine.

Admission Requirements: Min age: 18; High school diploma/GED.

Tuition and Fees: $795 (Western); $1595 (Chinese).

Westport

250. Connecticut Center for Massage Therapy Inc, Westport

25 Sylvan Rd S, Westport, CT 06880

Phone: (203) 221-7325; *Fax:* (203) 221-0144

E-mail: info@ccmt.com *Internet:* http://www.ccmt .com

Program Administrator: Barry Antoniow, Admin Dir. *Admissions Contact:* Marion Visel, Admissions Rep.

Year Established: 1992.

Staff: Part-time: 20.

Avg Enrollment: 100. *Avg Class Size:* 20. *Number of Graduates per Year:* 100.

Wheelchair Access: Yes.

Accreditation/Approval/Licensing: Commission on Massage Therapy Accreditation; Accrediting Commission of Career Schools and Colleges of Technology; National Certification Board for Therapeutic Massage and Bodywork (CEUs).

Field of Study: Acupressure; Alexander Technique; Aromatherapy; CranioSacral Therapy; Energy Work; Feldenkrais; Massage Therapy*; Neuromuscular Therapy; Polarity Therapy; Reflexology; Reiki; Shiatsu; Sports Massage. *Program Name/Length:* NY Massage Therapist, 20 mos; Clinical Massage Therapist, 20 mos.

Degrees Offered: Diploma.

License/Certification Preparation: State: CT, NY Licensed Massage Therapist; National Certification Board for Therapeutic Massage and Bodywork.

Admission Requirements: Min age: 18; High school diploma/GED.

Application Deadline(s): Fall: Sep; Winter: Jan; Summer: May.

Tuition and Fees: $9750 (NY); $15,000 (Clinical).

Financial Aid: Federal government aid; Pell grants.

Career Services: Career counseling; Career information; Graduate Services Dept.

251. QiGong Institute

361 Post Rd W, Westport, CT 06880

Mailing Address: 121 E 37th St, Ste 4B, New York, NY 10016

Phone: (212) 686-9227; *Fax:* (212) 686-9227

E-mail: akim.070972@aol.com

Program Administrator: Dr. Richard M. Chin, Dir. *Admissions Contact:* Dr. John Patrick, Admissions.

Year Established: 1990.

Staff: Full-time: 2; Part-time: 4.

Avg Enrollment: 10. *Avg Class Size:* 5. *Number of Graduates per Year:* 2.

Wheelchair Access: No.

Field of Study: Acupressure*; CranioSacral Therapy; Energy Work; Herbal Medicine;

Neuromuscular Therapy; Oriental Medicine; Polarity Therapy; Qigong*; Reflexology; Shiatsu*; Traditional Chinese Medicine. *Program Name/Length:* Qigong Therapy, 2 yrs; Acupressure, 2 yrs.
Degrees Offered: Certificate.
License/Certification Preparation: National Certification Commission for Acupuncture and Oriental Medicine; American Oriental Bodywork Therapy Association.
Admission Requirements: Min age: 21; High school diploma/GED; Min GPA: 2.0; Some college (2 yrs); Min GPA 2.0.
Tuition and Fees: $2000 per semester.

252. Rosen Center East, LLC
Rosen Method Practitioner Training
PO Box 5004, Westport, CT 06880
Phone: (203) 319-1090; *Fax:* (203) 319-0032
E-mail: rosenctre@aol.com
Program Administrator: Sue Brenner, Dir. *Admissions Contact:* Asha Stager, Admin.

Year Established: 1988.
Staff: Full-time: 1; Part-time: 2.
Avg Enrollment: 100. *Avg Class Size:* 24. *Number of Graduates per Year:* 4.
Wheelchair Access: Yes.
Accreditation/Approval/Licensing: Accrediting Council for Continuing Education and Training; National Certification Board for Therapeutic Massage and Bodywork (CEUs).
Field of Study: Rosen Method Bodywork*. *Program Name/Length:* 4 yrs or 2 yrs coursework (six 1-wk intensives) with 2 yrs internship.
Degrees Offered: Certificate.
License/Certification Preparation: National Certification Board for Therapeutic Massage and Bodywork.
Admission Requirements: Min age: 25; Specific course prerequisites: health-related disciplines.
Tuition and Fees: $8000 (coursework) + $5100 (internship), additional fees for supervision, private sessions.
Career Services: Internships.

DELAWARE

Greenville

253. Karen Carlson International Academy of Holistic Massage and Science
Twaddell Mill Rd, Greenville, DE 19807
Mailing Address: PO Box 3940, Greenville, DE 19807
Phone: (302) 777-7307
Program Administrator: Karen Carlson, PhD, Dir. *Admissions Contact:* Marilue Hartman, Admin VP.
Year Established: 1977.
Staff: Full-time: 2; Part-time: 12.
Avg Enrollment: 34. *Avg Class Size:* 16. *Number of Graduates per Year:* 34.
Wheelchair Access: Yes.
Accreditation/Approval/Licensing: DE Dept of Ed.
Field of Study: Acupressure; Biofeedback; Energy Work; Feldenkrais; Herbal Medicine; Homeopathy; Massage Therapy*; Reflexology. *Program Name/Length:* Holistic Massage, 960 hrs (26 weekends + home study), 1 yr; Holistic Healing Science, 430 hrs (26 weekends + home study), 1 yr.
Degrees Offered: Diploma; Certificate.
License/Certification Preparation: State: DE Licensed Massage Therapist; National Certification Board for Therapeutic Massage and Bodywork.
Admission Requirements: High school diploma/GED; Specific course prerequisites: Ho-

listic Massage required for Holistic Healing Science.
Application Deadline(s): Fall: Oct 1; Winter: Apr 1.
Tuition and Fees: $6870 (Holistic Massage); $7470 (Holistic Healing Science).
Financial Aid: Work study.
Career Services: Career counseling; Career information.

Wilmington

254. Deep Muscle Therapy School
5317 Limestone Rd, Wilmington, DE 19808
Phone: (302) 239-1613; *Fax:* (302) 239-5195
Program Administrator: Debra Jedlicka, Dir. *Admissions Contact:* Velda Martin, Dir of Admissions.
Year Established: 1986.
Staff: Part-time: 6.
Avg Class Size: 10. *Number of Graduates per Year:* 12.
Wheelchair Access: Yes.
Accreditation/Approval/Licensing: State board: DE Board of Massage and Bodywork.
Field of Study: Deep Tissue Massage*; Massage Therapy*. *Program Name/Length:* Basic, 2 mos; Advanced, 6 mos; 600 hrs, 8 mos.
License/Certification Preparation: State: DE Licensed Massage and Bodywork Therapist; Na-

tional Certification Board for Therapeutic Massage and Bodywork.
Admission Requirements: Min age: 18; High school diploma/GED.

Tuition and Fees: $5500 (600 hrs).
Financial Aid: State government aid; Payment plan.
Career Services: Career counseling.

DISTRICT OF COLUMBIA

Washington

255. Focus on Healing Reflexology Center

2808 Douglas St NE, Washington, DC 20018
Mailing Address: PO Box 26132, Washington, DC 20001
Phone: (301) 779-8005; *Fax:* (301) 779-8006
Program Administrator: Njideka N. Olatunde, Dir. *Admissions Contact:* Phyllis Costley, Admin Asst.
Year Established: 1992.
Staff: Full-time: 1; Part-time: 2.
Avg Enrollment: 48. *Avg Class Size:* 12. *Number of Graduates per Year:* 48.
Wheelchair Access: Yes.
Field of Study: Reflexology*. *Program Name/Length:* Certification, 3 mos.
Degrees Offered: CEUs; Diploma; Certificate.
License/Certification Preparation: State: DC License; American Reflexology Certification Board.
Admission Requirements: Min age: 18; High school diploma/GED; Min GPA: 2.0; Some college; Specific course prerequisites: Introduction to anatomy and physiology.
Application Deadline(s): Fall: Sep; Winter: Jan; Spring: Apr; Summer: Jun.
Tuition and Fees: $1200.
Financial Aid: Work study; Payment plan.
Career Services: Career counseling; Career information; Internships; Referral service.

256. Georgetown University, School of Nursing

Graduate Program in Nurse-Midwifery
3700 Reservoir Rd NW, Washington, DC 20007
Phone: (202) 687-5041; *Fax:* (202) 687-5553
E-mail: midwife@gunet.georgetown.edu *Internet:* http://www.dml.georgetown.edu/schnurs/midwife1.html
Program Administrator: Ann L. Silvonek, MS, Prog Coord. *Admissions Contact:* Michele Havin, Admissions Coord.
Year Established: 1974.
Staff: Full-time: 2-3; Part-time: 2-3.
Avg Enrollment: 37. *Avg Class Size:* 15. *Number of Graduates per Year:* 15.
Wheelchair Access: Yes.

Accreditation/Approval/Licensing: Middle States Association of Colleges and Schools; American College of Nurse-Midwives, Division of Accreditation.
Field of Study: Midwifery*. *Program Name/Length:* 16 mos full-time; 27 mos part-time.
Degrees Offered: MS.
License/Certification Preparation: Certified Nurse-Midwife, American College of Nurse-Midwives.
Admission Requirements: BS in Nursing; Min GPA: 3.0; RN; Specific course prerequisites: statistics (completion of introductory course in statistical methods), GRE or Miller's Analogy Test, TOEFL for non-English speakers.
Application Deadline(s): Fall: Feb 1.
Financial Aid: Federal government aid; Loans; Scholarships; State government aid; Work study.
Career Services: Career information; Internships; Resume service; Job information.

257. Institute for Ethical and Clinical Hypnosis

2510 M St NW, Washington, DC 20037
Mailing Address: PO Box 57374, Washington, DC 20037
Phone: (202) 331-1218; *Fax:* (202) 659-9580
E-mail: payam@netkonnect.net
Program Administrator: Masud Ansari, Pres. *Admissions Contact:* Masud Ansari.
Year Established: 1980.
Staff: Part-time: 2.
Avg Class Size: 12. *Number of Graduates per Year:* 70.
Wheelchair Access: Yes.
Accreditation/Approval/Licensing: Accrediting Council for Continuing Education and Training; Accrediting Commission of Career Schools and Colleges of Technology; American Board of Hypnotherapy.
Field of Study: Hypnotherapy*. *Program Name/Length:* 50 hrs; Seminars given in various locations.
Degrees Offered: Diploma; Certificate.
License/Certification Preparation: American Board of Clinical Hypnosis; American Board of Hypnotherapy.

Admission Requirements: Min age: 18; High school diploma/GED; Some college.
Application Deadline(s): Fall; Winter; Spring; Summer.
Financial Aid: Fellowships.
Career Services: Referral service.

258. Potomac Massage Training Institute

4000 Albemarle St NW, 5th Fl, Washington, DC 20016
Phone: (202) 686-7046; *Fax:* (202) 966-4579
Program Administrator: Rose A. Gowdey, Exec Dir; Daniel Y. Gilham, Dir of Ed. *Admissions Contact:* Philomena Queen, Dir of Admissions.
Year Established: 1976.
Staff: Part-time: 36.
Avg Enrollment: 325. *Avg Class Size:* 18. *Number of Graduates per Year:* 100.
Wheelchair Access: Yes.
Accreditation/Approval/Licensing: Commission on Massage Therapy Accreditation; National Certification Board for Therapeutic Massage and Bodywork (CEUs).
Field of Study: Alexander Technique; Aromatherapy; CranioSacral Therapy; Energy Work; Infant Massage; Massage Therapy*; Myofascial Release; Neuromuscular Therapy; Polarity Therapy; Pregnancy Massage; Qigong; Reflexology; Reiki; Shiatsu; Sports Massage; Traditional Chinese Medicine. *Program Name/Length:* 11 mos/intensive or 18 mos/part-time.
Degrees Offered: Certificate.
License/Certification Preparation: State: DC License, VA Certified Massage Therapist; National Certification Board for Therapeutic Massage and Bodywork.
Admission Requirements: Min age: 18; High school diploma/GED; Basic understanding and experience with massage.
Application Deadline(s): Fall: Jul 15; Winter: Nov 15; Spring: Jan 15.
Tuition and Fees: $5250.
Financial Aid: Scholarships; Vocational rehabilitation; Payment plan.
Career Services: Career counseling; Career information; Job information.

FLORIDA

Altamonte Springs

259. Florida College of Natural Health, Orlando Campus

887 E Altamonte Dr, Altamonte Springs, FL 32701
Phone: (407) 261-0319, (800) 393-7337; *Fax:* (407) 261-0342
E-mail: fcnh@icanect.net *Internet:* http://www. fcnh.com
Program Administrator: Kevin Beaver, Campus Dir. *Admissions Contact:* Thea Depinto, Admissions Coord.
Year Established: 1995.
Staff: Full-time: 3; Part-time: 9.
Avg Enrollment: 400. *Avg Class Size:* 30. *Number of Graduates per Year:* 400.
Wheelchair Access: Yes.
Accreditation/Approval/Licensing: Commission on Massage Therapy Accreditation; Accrediting Commission of Career Schools and Colleges of Technology.
Field of Study: Acupressure; Acupuncture*; Aromatherapy; CranioSacral Therapy; Energy Work; Massage Therapy*; Neuromuscular Therapy*; Reflexology; Shiatsu; Skin Care; Sports Massage; Swedish Massage*. *Program Name/Length:* Massage Therapy, 6-15 mos; Associate of Science in Natural Health, 12-18 mos.
Degrees Offered: Diploma; AS.
License/Certification Preparation: State: FL Licensed Massage Therapist; National Certification Board for Therapeutic Massage and Bodywork.
Admission Requirements: Min age: 18; High school diploma/GED.
Tuition and Fees: $2400-$8500.
Financial Aid: Federal government aid; Grants; Loans; Scholarships; Work study.
Career Services: Career counseling; Career information; Resume service.

Boca Raton

260. Boca Raton Institute

5499 N Federal Hwy, Ste A, Boca Raton, FL 33487
Phone: (561) 241-8105; *Fax:* (561) 241-9789
E-mail: info@bocaschools.com *Internet:* http:// www.bocaschools.com
Program Administrator: Constance M. Gregg, Dir of Ed.
Year Established: 1983.
Staff: Full-time: 4; Part-time: 8.

Avg Enrollment: 200. *Avg Class Size:* 20. *Number of Graduates per Year:* 100.
Wheelchair Access: Yes.
Field of Study: Acupressure; Aromatherapy; CranioSacral Therapy; Massage Therapy*; Neuromuscular Therapy; Polarity Therapy; Reflexology; Shiatsu. *Program Name/Length:* Massage Therapy, 605 hrs.
Degrees Offered: Certificate.
Admission Requirements: Min age: 18; High school diploma/GED.
Tuition and Fees: $4800.
Financial Aid: Federal government aid; Grants; Loans.
Career Services: Career counseling; Career information; Interview set up; Resume service.

Bonita Springs

261. Bonita Springs/Venice School of Massage, Esthetics, Spa/Fitness
10915 Bonita Beach Rd, Ste 2121, Bonita Springs, FL 34135
Mailing Address: 8951 Bonita Beach Rd, Ste 525-222, Bonita Springs, FL 34135
Phone: (941) 495-0714; *Fax:* (941) 498-7164
Program Administrator: Fred Maehr, Owner/Dir. *Admissions Contact:* Fred Maehr; Joy Fiebe, Admin.
Year Established: 1988.
Staff: Full-time: 7; Part-time: 4.
Avg Enrollment: 225. *Avg Class Size:* 18. *Number of Graduates per Year:* 180.
Wheelchair Access: No.
Accreditation/Approval/Licensing: State board: FL Board of Independent Postsecondary Vocational, Technical, Trade and Business Schools.
Field of Study: Aromatherapy; Colon Hydrotherapy*; Herbal Medicine; Massage Therapy*; Neuromuscular Therapy*; Reflexology; Shiatsu*; Spa Therapies*. *Program Name/Length:* Massage Therapy, 500 hrs, 6 mos or 1 yr; Colon Hydrotherapy, 100 hrs; Oriental Shiatsu, 105 hrs; Neuromuscular Therapy, 51 hrs, 6 Sundays; Esthetics/Skin Care, 260 hrs, 18 wks; Spa Therapies, 80 hrs, 10 wks; Nutrition, 100 hrs, 18 wks; Fitness Training, 250 hrs, 12 wks.
Degrees Offered: Diploma; Certificate.
License/Certification Preparation: State: FL Licensed Massage Therapist; National Certification Board for Therapeutic Massage and Bodywork.
Admission Requirements: Min age: 16; High school diploma/GED.
Tuition and Fees: $2750 (Massage); $1550 (Colon Hydrotherapy); $800 (Shiatsu); $570 (Neuromuscular); $1850 (Esthetics); $680 (Spa Therapies); $750 (Nutrition); $2100 (Fitness).
Financial Aid: Grants; Loans; State government aid; Payment plan.

Career Services: Career counseling; Career information; Internships; Interview set up; Resume service; Job information; Referral service; Business management information.

Casselberry

262. Orlando Institute School of Massage Therapy, Inc
3385 S Hwy 17-92, Ste 221, Casselberry, FL 32707
Phone: (407) 331-1101; *Fax:* (407) 331-8331
Program Administrator: Stacee Diehl, Dir. *Admissions Contact:* Stacee Diehl.
Year Established: 1987.
Staff: Full-time: 5.
Avg Enrollment: 50. *Avg Class Size:* 20. *Number of Graduates per Year:* 50.
Wheelchair Access: Yes.
Accreditation/Approval/Licensing: State board: FL Board of Independent Postsecondary Vocational, Technical, Trade and Business Schools.
Field of Study: Aromatherapy; Massage Therapy*; Polarity Therapy; Reflexology; Shiatsu. *Program Name/Length:* 500 hrs.
Degrees Offered: Diploma; Certificate.
License/Certification Preparation: State: FL Licensed Massage Therapist; National Certification Board for Therapeutic Massage and Bodywork.
Admission Requirements: Min age: 18; High school diploma/GED.
Tuition and Fees: $3500.
Financial Aid: Scholarships.
Career Services: Career information; Interview set up.

Clearwater

263. Bhakti Academe School of Intuitive Massage and Healing
25400 US 19 N, Ste 116, Clearwater, FL 33763
Phone: (727) 724-9727
Program Administrator: Dale McNiff, LCSW, Dir. *Admissions Contact:* Dale McNiff.
Year Established: 1993.
Staff: 1.
Avg Enrollment: 120. *Avg Class Size:* 15. *Number of Graduates per Year:* 120.
Wheelchair Access: Yes.
Accreditation/Approval/Licensing: State board: FL Dept of Ed.
Field of Study: Bhakti Bodywork; Energy Work; Massage Therapy*. *Program Name/Length:* Massage, 500 hrs, 6 mos.
Degrees Offered: Diploma.
Admission Requirements: Min age: 18; High school diploma/GED.
Tuition and Fees: $3000.
Career Services: Career counseling; Career information.

Coral Gables

264. University of Miami, School of Nursing
Nurse-Midwifery Program
5801 Red Rd, Coral Gables, FL 33124-3850
Phone: (305) 284-6256
Program Administrator: Virginia Crandall, MSN, Asst Prof.
Avg Enrollment: 25. *Avg Class Size:* 7. *Number of Graduates per Year:* 7.
Wheelchair Access: Yes.
Accreditation/Approval/Licensing: American College of Nurse-Midwives, Division of Accreditation.
Field of Study: Midwifery*. *Program Name/Length:* Master of Science in Nursing, 2 yrs/full-time.
Degrees Offered: MSN.
License/Certification Preparation: Certified Nurse-Midwife, American College of Nurse-Midwives.
Admission Requirements: Bachelor's degree; RN.

DeLand

265. Omni Hypnosis Training Center
830 N Woodland Blvd, DeLand, FL 32720
Mailing Address: 197 Glenwood Rd, DeLand, FL 32720
Phone: (904) 738-9188; *Fax:* (904) 736-7598
E-mail: omni@omnihypnosis.com *Internet:* http://www.omnihypnosis.com
Program Administrator: Gerald F. Kein, Dir. *Admissions Contact:* Jane Arey, Admin Dir.
Year Established: 1979.
Staff: Full-time: 1; Part-time: 1.
Avg Enrollment: 80. *Avg Class Size:* 20. *Number of Graduates per Year:* 80.
Wheelchair Access: Yes.
Accreditation/Approval/Licensing: State board: FL Board of Nursing.
Field of Study: Hypnotherapy*. *Program Name/Length:* Basic/Intermediate and Advanced Hypnosis, 56 hrs; Internship, 50 hrs.
Degrees Offered: Certificate.
License/Certification Preparation: Certification, National Guild of Hypnotists; National Board for Hypnotherapy and Hypnotic Anesthesiology.
Admission Requirements: Min age: 21; High school diploma/GED; Proficiency in English.
Tuition and Fees: $990 (Basic through Advanced); $995 (Internship).

Fort Lauderdale

266. American Institute of Massage Therapy, Fort Lauderdale
Massage Therapy; Colon Therapy
2101 N Federal Hwy, Fort Lauderdale, FL 33301
Phone: (954) 568-6200; *Fax:* (954) 568-6100
E-mail: info@aimt.com *Internet:* http://www.aimt.com
Program Administrator: Lexa Allin Sutherland, Dir. *Admissions Contact:* Gail A. Naas, Dir of Operations.
Year Established: 1987.
Staff: Full-time: 4; Part-time: 20.
Avg Enrollment: 200. *Avg Class Size:* 25. *Number of Graduates per Year:* 200.
Wheelchair Access: Yes.
Accreditation/Approval/Licensing: State board: FL Board of Massage; Accrediting Council for Continuing Education and Training.
Field of Study: Aromatherapy; Colon Hydrotherapy*; CranioSacral Therapy; Massage Therapy*; Neuromuscular Therapy; Reflexology; Sports Massage. *Program Name/Length:* Massage Therapy, 6 mos/full-time or 1 yr/part-time; Colon Therapy, 6 wks.
Degrees Offered: Diploma; Certificate.
License/Certification Preparation: State: FL Licensed Massage Therapist; International Association for Colon Hydrotherapy.
Admission Requirements: Min age: 18; High school diploma/GED.
Application Deadline(s): Fall: Sep 1; Winter: Dec 1; Spring: Mar 1; Summer: Jun 1.
Tuition and Fees: $4500 + $225 books (Massage Therapy); $1750 + $200 books (Colon Therapy).
Financial Aid: Loans; Scholarships; VA approved; Vocational rehabilitation.
Career Services: Career counseling; Career information; Internships.

267. Atlantic Institute of Oriental Medicine
1057 SE 17th St, Fort Lauderdale, FL 33316
Phone: (954) 463-3888, 522-6405 student clinic; *Fax:* (954) 463-3878
E-mail: atom3@ix.netcom.com *Internet:* http://www.khuang.com/atom/
Program Administrator: Terry Goldberg, Admin. *Admissions Contact:* Edith Tonelli, Academic Dean.
Year Established: 1994.
Staff: Full-time: 2; Part-time: 9.
Avg Enrollment: 15. *Avg Class Size:* 12. *Number of Graduates per Year:* 15.
Wheelchair Access: No.
Accreditation/Approval/Licensing: State board: FL Board of Nonpublic Career Education; Candidacy, Accreditation Commission for Acupuncture and Oriental Medicine.
Field of Study: Acupuncture*; Herbal Medicine; Oriental Medicine*; Traditional Chinese Medicine*. *Program Name/Length:* 2718 hrs, 3 yrs.
Degrees Offered: Diploma.
License/Certification Preparation: State: FL Acupuncture Physician; National Certification Commission for Acupuncture and Oriental Medicine.
Application Deadline(s): Fall: Aug; Winter: Sep.

Tuition and Fees: $6000 per yr.
Financial Aid: Vocational rehabilitation.
Career Services: Career counseling.

Fort Myers

268. Florida Academy of Massage
8695 College Pkwy, Ste 110, Fort Myers, FL 33919
Phone: (941) 489-2282, (800) 324-9543; *Fax:* (941)
   489-4065
Internet: http://www.floridaacademymassage.com
Program Administrator: Ronald D. Gray, Pres. *Admissions Contact:* Abby McDonough, Dir of
   Admissions.
Year Established: 1992.
Staff: Full-time: 4; Part-time: 9.
Avg Enrollment: 100. *Avg Class Size:* 20. *Number
   of Graduates per Year:* 80.
Wheelchair Access: Yes.
Accreditation/Approval/Licensing: State board: FL
   Dept of Ed.
Field of Study: Massage Therapy*. *Program
   Name/Length:* 540 hrs, 17 wks/days or 22
   wks/evenings.
Degrees Offered: CEUs; Diploma; Certificate.
License/Certification Preparation: State: FL Licensed Massage Therapist; National Certification Board for Therapeutic Massage and Bodywork.
Admission Requirements: Min age: 17; High
   school diploma/GED.
Tuition and Fees: $3513.
Financial Aid: Loans; Scholarships.
Career Services: Career information; Interview set
   up; Resume service.

Gainesville

269. Florida School of Massage
6421 SW 13th St, Gainesville, FL 32608
Phone: (352) 378-7891; *Fax:* (352) 376-7218
E-mail: info@massageonline.com *Internet:* http://
   www.massageonline.com
Program Administrator: Paul Davenport, BA, Dir.
   Admissions Contact: Dar Mikula, LMT, Admissions.
Year Established: 1973.
Staff: Part-time: 25.
Avg Enrollment: 180. *Avg Class Size:* 60. *Number
   of Graduates per Year:* 180.
Wheelchair Access: Yes.
Accreditation/Approval/Licensing: State board: FL
   Board of Independent Postsecondary Vocational,
   Technical, Trade and Business Schools; Commission on Massage Therapy Accreditation; National Certification Board for Therapeutic Massage and Bodywork (CEUs).
Field of Study: Anatomy and Physiology; Colon
   Hydrotherapy*; Connective Tissue Massage;
   CPR/First Aid; Hydrotherapy; Massage Ther-

apy*; Neuromuscular Therapy; Polarity Therapy*; Reflexology*; Shiatsu; Sports Massage*;
   Structural Integration; Swedish Massage*. *Program Name/Length:* Therapeutic Massage and
   Hydrotherapy, 705-1000 hrs, 6 mos; Colonic Irrigation Therapy Certification, 100 hrs; Polarity
   Therapy Certification, 112 hrs; Sports Massage,
   200 hrs; Therapeutic Hand and Foot
   Reflexology, 205 hrs.
Degrees Offered: Certificate.
License/Certification Preparation: State: FL Licensed Massage Therapist; National Certification Board for Therapeutic Massage and Bodywork.
Admission Requirements: Min age: 19; High
   school diploma/GED; Massage therapist for Polarity Therapy; Massage student or massage
   therapist for Sports Massage and Colonic Irrigation.
Tuition and Fees: $5250 + $250 books, $600 table
   (Therapeutic Massage); $1200 + $75-$100
   books (Colonic); $1425 (Polarity); $1650 +
   $100 books (Sports); $1500 (Reflexology).
Financial Aid: VA approved; Vocational rehabilitation.
Career Services: Instruction in business practices;
   Job information.

270. Florida School of Traditional Midwifery
6501 SW 13 St, Gainesville, FL 32608
Mailing Address: PO Box 5505, Gainesville, FL
   32627
Phone: (352) 338-0766; *Fax:* (352) 338-2013
E-mail: fstm@juno.com
Program Administrator: Jana Borino, AA, Dir. *Admissions Contact:* Glynn Barker, Clinical
   Coord.
Year Established: 1994.
Staff: Part-time: 10.
Avg Enrollment: 10. *Avg Class Size:* 10. *Number
   of Graduates per Year:* 10.
Wheelchair Access: No.
Accreditation/Approval/Licensing: FL Board of Independent Postsecondary Vocational, Technical,
   Trade and Business Schools.
Field of Study: Midwifery*. *Program
   Name/Length:* Midwife Asst, 1 yr; Licensed
   Midwifery, 3 yrs.
Degrees Offered: Certificate; AA.
License/Certification Preparation: State: FL Licensed Midwife; Certified Professional Midwife,
   North American Registry of Midwives.
Admission Requirements: Min age: 18; High
   school diploma/GED; Some college, 3 credits
   math and English.
Application Deadline(s): Winter: Sep 30; Spring:
   Mar 1.
Tuition and Fees: $5400 (Midwife Asst); $18,046
   (Licensed Midwifery) + supplies, equipment, insurance, books for each program.

Hallandale

271. Academy for Five Element Acupuncture

Licentiate in Acupuncture
1170-A E Hallandale Beach Blvd, Hallandale, FL 33009
Phone: (954) 456-6336; *Fax:* (954) 456-3944
E-mail: afea@compuserve.com
Program Administrator: Dorit Reznek, Exec Dir.
   Admissions Contact: Isaac Goren, Bus Affairs.
Year Established: 1989.
Staff: Part-time: 38.
Avg Enrollment: 20. *Avg Class Size:* 20. *Number of Graduates per Year:* 20.
Wheelchair Access: Yes.
Accreditation/Approval/Licensing: State board: FL Board of Independent Postsecondary Vocational, Technical, Trade and Business Schools; Accreditation Commission for Acupuncture and Oriental Medicine.
Field of Study: Acupuncture*; Herbal Medicine*.
Program Name/Length: Five Element Acupuncture, 27 mos (Years 1 and 2: two 3-wk sessions; Year 3: residential).
Degrees Offered: Diploma.
License/Certification Preparation: National Certification Commission for Acupuncture and Oriental Medicine.
Admission Requirements: High school diploma/GED; Some college (60 semester credits); Specific course prerequisites: 60 hrs basic science; before graduation: 120 hrs anatomy and physiology, 30 hrs western medical terminology.
Application Deadline(s): Summer: Aug.
Tuition and Fees: $24,950.
Financial Aid: Loans.
Career Services: Career counseling; Career information.

Jacksonville

272. Alpha School of Massage, Inc

Massage Therapy
4642 San Juan Ave, Jacksonville, FL 32210
Phone: (904) 389-9117; *Fax:* (904) 389-6496
Program Administrator: Edward L. Driggers, LMT, Admin. *Admissions Contact:* Angela R. Warren, LMT, Admin Asst.
Year Established: 1993.
Staff: Full-time: 2; Part-time: 2.
Avg Enrollment: 100. *Avg Class Size:* 12. *Number of Graduates per Year:* 100.
Wheelchair Access: Yes.
Accreditation/Approval/Licensing: State board: FL Board of Massage; FL Dept of Ed.
Field of Study: Acupressure; Aromatherapy; Energy Work; Herbal Medicine; Homeopathy; Massage Therapy*; Neuromuscular Therapy; Reflexology; Reiki; Shiatsu; Sports Massage.

Program Name/Length: Massage Therapy, 501 hrs, 6 mos or 1 yr.
Degrees Offered: Certificate.
License/Certification Preparation: State: FL Licensed Massage Therapist; National Certification Board for Therapeutic Massage and Bodywork.
Admission Requirements: Min age: 18; High school diploma/GED.
Application Deadline(s): Fall: Sep; Winter: Jan; Spring: Mar; Summer: Jun.
Tuition and Fees: $3100.
Financial Aid: Work study; VA approved; Vocational rehabilitation; Payment plan.
Career Services: Career counseling; Career information; Job information.

273. Biofeedback Therapist Training Institute

1826 University Blvd W, Jacksonville, FL 32217
Phone: (904) 737-5821; *Fax:* (904) 730-3821
E-mail: hartje@aol.com *Internet:* http://www.hartje.com
Program Administrator: Jack C. Hartje, PhD, Dir.
   Admissions Contact: Susan Farrar, Prog Mgr; Catherine Navarre, Prog Mgr.
Year Established: 1988.
Accreditation/Approval/Licensing: Biofeedback Certification Institute of America; American Psychological Association.
Field of Study: Biofeedback*. *Program Name/Length:* Fundamentals of Biofeedback, 60 hrs; Home study/Correspondence; Personalized Workshops, 20 hrs, 3 days.
License/Certification Preparation: Biofeedback Certification Institute of America.
Admission Requirements: Min age: 18.
Tuition and Fees: $695-$780.

274. Birth Buddies

Doula Training
5329 Buggy Whip Dr N, Jacksonville, FL 32257
Phone: (904) 268-5629; *Fax:* (904) 363-6356
E-mail: doulasue@aol.com
Program Administrator: Susan Toffolon, Dir. *Admissions Contact:* Susan Toffolon.
Year Established: 1995.
Staff: Full-time: 1; Part-time: 1.
Avg Enrollment: 27. *Avg Class Size:* 9. *Number of Graduates per Year:* 25.
Wheelchair Access: Yes.
Accreditation/Approval/Licensing: Doulas of North America.
Field of Study: Doula*. *Program Name/Length:* Professional Labor Support, 18 hrs; Seminars given in various locations.
Degrees Offered: Certificate.
License/Certification Preparation: Doulas of North America.
Admission Requirements: Min age: 18; Specific course prerequisites: Extensive knowledge and/or work experience in the birth field.

Tuition and Fees: $195 per course.
Career Services: Career information; Internships; Referral service.

275. Classical Acupuncture Institute
4237 Salisbury Rd, Ste 108, Jacksonville, FL 32216
Phone: (904) 296-0906
Program Administrator: Michael Kowalski, AP, Dir of Acupuncture. *Admissions Contact:* Debbie Rewis, Office Mgr.
Year Established: 1986.
Avg Enrollment: 35. *Avg Class Size:* 8. *Number of Graduates per Year:* 22.
Wheelchair Access: Yes.
Accreditation/Approval/Licensing: State board: FL Board of Independent Postsecondary Vocational, Technical, Trade and Business Schools.
Field of Study: Acupuncture*. *Program Name/Length:* 3 yrs.
Degrees Offered: Diploma.
License/Certification Preparation: State: FL Acupuncture Physician; National Certification Commission for Acupuncture and Oriental Medicine.
Admission Requirements: Min age: 21; High school diploma/GED; Some college (2 yrs).
Application Deadline(s): Fall: Aug 15.
Tuition and Fees: $21,500.

276. Jacksonville School of Massage Therapy
5305 San Juan Ave, Jacksonville, FL 32210
Phone: (904) 389-3878
Program Administrator: Earl F. Kennedy, LMT, Dir. *Admissions Contact:* Earl F. Kennedy, Dir.
Year Established: 1980.
Staff: Full-time: 1; Part-time: 3.
Avg Enrollment: 30. *Number of Graduates per Year:* 30.
Wheelchair Access: Yes.
Accreditation/Approval/Licensing: State board: FL Board of Independent Postsecondary Vocational, Technical, Trade and Business Schools.
Field of Study: Acupressure; Aromatherapy; Ayurvedic Medicine; Biofeedback; Colon Hydrotherapy; Massage Therapy*; Polarity Therapy; Reflexology; Reiki; Shiatsu; Traditional Chinese Medicine. *Program Name/Length:* 500 hrs, 6 mos.
Degrees Offered: Certificate.
License/Certification Preparation: State: FL Licensed Massage Therapist; National Certification Board for Therapeutic Massage and Bodywork.
Admission Requirements: Min age: 18; High school diploma/GED.
Tuition and Fees: $2800.
Financial Aid: Scholarships; State government aid; Payment plan.
Career Services: Career counseling; Career information; Job information; Referral service.

277. Southeastern School of Neuromuscular and Massage Therapy Inc, Jacksonville
9088 Golfside Dr, Jacksonville, FL 32256
Phone: (904) 448-9499; *Fax:* (904) 448-9270
E-mail: ses-jax@btitelecom.net *Internet:* http://www.se-massage.com
Program Administrator: Kyle C. Wright, LMT, Owner/Founder. *Admissions Contact:* David W. Dolan, LMT, Dir.
Year Established: 1992.
Staff: Full-time: 6; Part-time: 4.
Avg Enrollment: 100. *Avg Class Size:* 25. *Number of Graduates per Year:* 100.
Wheelchair Access: Yes.
Accreditation/Approval/Licensing: State board: FL Board of Independent Postsecondary Vocational, Technical, Trade and Business Schools; National Certification Board for Therapeutic Massage and Bodywork (CEUs).
Field of Study: Acupressure; CranioSacral Therapy; Feldenkrais; Herbal Medicine; Homeopathy; Massage Therapy*; Neuromuscular Therapy*; Polarity Therapy; Reflexology; Reiki; Shiatsu. *Program Name/Length:* 500 hrs, 6 mos.
Degrees Offered: Diploma.
License/Certification Preparation: State: FL Licensed Massage Therapist; National Certification Board for Therapeutic Massage and Bodywork.
Admission Requirements: Min age: 18; High school diploma/GED.
Application Deadline(s): Fall: Aug; Winter: Nov; Spring: Feb; Summer: May.
Tuition and Fees: $5300.
Financial Aid: Loans; Vocational rehabilitation; Payment plan.
Career Services: Placement assistance.

278. University of Florida, Health Science Center
Nurse-Midwifery Program, College of Nursing
653 W 8th St, Bldg 1, 2nd Fl, Jacksonville, FL 32209-6561
Phone: (904) 549-3245
E-mail: bixenpm.ufcon@shands.ufl.edu *Internet:* http://con.ufl.edu
Program Administrator: Alice H. Poe, CNM, Dir.
Accreditation/Approval/Licensing: American College of Nurse-Midwives, Division of Accreditation.
Field of Study: Midwifery*.
Degrees Offered: MSN; MN.
License/Certification Preparation: Certified Nurse-Midwife, American College of Nurse-Midwives.
Admission Requirements: Bachelor's degree; RN.

Jacksonville Beach

279. Holistic Health Services

Reiki Training Level I

1551 S 1st St, Ste 701, Jacksonville Beach, FL
32250

Phone: (904) 246-6064; *Fax:* (904) 247-1266

E-mail: powerprogm@aol.com

Program Administrator: Gail Greenfield, RN. *Admissions Contact:* Gail Greenfield.

Year Established: 1998.

Staff: Part-time: 1.

Wheelchair Access: Yes.

Accreditation/Approval/Licensing: American Holistic Nurses Association.

Field of Study: Reiki*. *Program Name/Length:*
Reiki Level I; Seminars given in various locations.

Degrees Offered: Certificate.

Admission Requirements: RN.

Tuition and Fees: $150.

Key Largo

280. Reiki Plus Institute

707 Barcelona Rd, Key Largo, FL 33037

Phone: (305) 451-9881

E-mail: reikiplus@bellsouth.net *Internet:* http://
www.reikiplus.com

Program Administrator: David G. Jarrell, Reiki
Plus Master, Founder/Dir. *Admissions Contact:*
David G. Jarrell.

Year Established: 1983.

Staff: Full-time: 2; Part-time: 7.

Avg Enrollment: 175. *Avg Class Size:* 12. *Number
of Graduates per Year:* 25.

Wheelchair Access: No.

Accreditation/Approval/Licensing: National Certification Board for Therapeutic Massage and
Bodywork (CEUs).

Field of Study: Energy Work*; Reiki*. *Program
Name/Length:* Reiki Plus First Degree, 20 hrs;
Reiki Plus Second Degree, 20 hrs; Reiki Plus
Practitioner, 100 hrs, 1-2 yrs; Reiki Plus Master,
45 hrs + tutorial; Seminars given in various locations.

Degrees Offered: Certificate.

Tuition and Fees: $200 (First Degree); $300 (Second Degree); $1300 (Practitioner).

Kissimmee

281. Wood Hygienic Institute

2220 E Irlo Bronson Hwy, Kissimmee, FL 34744

Phone: (407) 933-0009

Accreditation/Approval/Licensing: State board: FL
Board of Independent Postsecondary Vocational,
Technical, Trade and Business Schools.

Field of Study: Colon Hydrotherapy*; Massage
Therapy*. *Program Name/Length:* Massage
Therapy, 500 hrs; Colonic Irrigation, 100 hrs.

License/Certification Preparation: State: FL Licensed Massage Therapist; National Certification Board for Therapeutic Massage and Bodywork.

Lake Park

282. Alpha Institute of South Florida, Inc

Massage Therapy; Facial Specialist

904 Park Ave, Lake Park, FL 33403

Phone: (561) 845-1400; *Fax:* (561) 845-1360

Program Administrator: Douglas C. Espie, Admin.
Admissions Contact: Douglas C. Espie.

Year Established: 1992.

Staff: Part-time: 6.

Avg Enrollment: 110. *Avg Class Size:* 15. *Number
of Graduates per Year:* 75.

Wheelchair Access: Yes.

Accreditation/Approval/Licensing: State board: FL
Board of Massage; FL Dept of Ed; Accrediting
Commission of Career Schools and Colleges of
Technology.

Field of Study: Aromatherapy; CranioSacral Therapy; Deep Tissue Massage; Energy Work;
Hypnotherapy; Massage Therapy*; Oriental
Medicine; Polarity Therapy; Reflexology; Reiki;
Shiatsu; Skin Care. *Program Name/Length:*
Massage Therapy, 500 hrs, 6 mos; Facial Specialist, 240 hrs, 4 mos.

Degrees Offered: Certificate.

License/Certification Preparation: State: FL Licensed Massage Therapist; FL Board of Cosmetology Specialty Registration; National Certification Board for Therapeutic Massage and
Bodywork.

Admission Requirements: Min age: 18 or high
school diploma/GED.

Tuition and Fees: $3250 (Massage Therapy);
$1925 (Facial Specialist).

Financial Aid: Loans.

Career Services: Career information.

Lake Worth

283. Academy of Healing Arts, Massage and Facial Skin Care, Inc

3141 S Military Trail, Lake Worth, FL 33463

Phone: (561) 965-5550; *Fax:* (561) 641-2603

Program Administrator: Angela K. Artemik, Dir of
Training. *Admissions Contact:* Mary Wright,
Admin Asst.

Year Established: 1983.

Staff: Full-time: 3; Part-time: 5.

Avg Class Size: 50.

Accreditation/Approval/Licensing: Accrediting
Commission of Career Schools and Colleges of

Technology; National Certification Board for Therapeutic Massage and Bodywork (CEUs).

Field of Study: Acupressure; Aromatherapy; Massage Therapy*; Reflexology; Shiatsu. *Program Name/Length:* Massage Therapy, 500 hrs, 6 mos; 600 hrs, 7 mo.

Degrees Offered: Diploma; Certificate.

License/Certification Preparation: State: FL Licensed Massage Therapist; National Certification Board for Therapeutic Massage and Bodywork.

Admission Requirements: Min age: 18; High school diploma/GED.

Tuition and Fees: $2850-$4100.

Financial Aid: Federal government aid; Grants; Loans; VA approved.

Career Services: Career counseling; Career information.

284. Seminar Network International, Inc d/b/a SNI School of Massage and Allied Therapies

518 N Federal Hwy, Lake Worth, FL 33460

Phone: (561) 582-5349, (800) 882-0903; *Fax:* (561) 582-0807

E-mail: snimassage@mindspring.com

Program Administrator: Larry E. Loving, Admin. *Admissions Contact:* Nancy Putzan, Admissions Rep.

Year Established: 1987.

Staff: Full-time: 3; Part-time: 10.

Avg Enrollment: 125. *Avg Class Size:* 25. *Number of Graduates per Year:* 125.

Wheelchair Access: Yes.

Accreditation/Approval/Licensing: State board: FL Board of Independent Postsecondary Vocational, Technical, Trade, and Business Schools; National Certification Board for Therapeutic Massage and Bodywork (CEUs).

Field of Study: Colon Hydrotherapy*; Massage Therapy*. *Program Name/Length:* Massage Therapy, 600 hrs; Colon Therapy, 100 hrs.

Degrees Offered: CEUs; Diploma.

License/Certification Preparation: State: FL Licensed Massage Therapist; National Certification Board for Therapeutic Massage and Bodywork.

Admission Requirements: Min age: 18; High school diploma/GED.

Application Deadline(s): Fall; Winter; Spring; Summer.

Tuition and Fees: $5000 (Massage Therapy).

Financial Aid: Grants; Loans; VA approved; Vocational rehabilitation.

Career Services: Career information; Interview set up.

Leesburg

285. Central Florida Hypnosis Institute

9737 Fairway Circle, Leesburg, FL 34788

Phone: (352) 315-0555; *Fax:* (352) 315-0383

E-mail: ejyawman@aol.com

Program Administrator: Earl J. Yawman, Exec Dir. *Admissions Contact:* Earl J. Yawman.

Year Established: 1990.

Staff: Full-time: 1; Part-time: 2.

Avg Enrollment: 50. *Avg Class Size:* 12. *Number of Graduates per Year:* 50.

Wheelchair Access: Yes.

Accreditation/Approval/Licensing: National Guild of Hypnotists.

Field of Study: Hypnotherapy*. *Program Name/Length:* Introduction to Hypnosis, 16 hrs; Basic Hypnotherapy, 50 hrs; Advanced Hypnotherapy, 100 hrs.

Degrees Offered: CEUs; Certificate.

License/Certification Preparation: National Guild of Hypnotists.

Admission Requirements: Min age: 18; High school diploma/GED; Min GPA: 2.5.

Tuition and Fees: $295-$950 per course.

Miami

286. Acupressure-Acupuncture Institute

Oriental Medicine; Massage Therapy

10506 N Kendall Dr, Miami, FL 33176

Phone: (305) 595-9500; *Fax:* (305) 595-2622

E-mail: aai@acupuncture.pair.com *Internet:* http://www.acupuncture.pair.com

Program Administrator: Nancy Browne, Admin Dir. *Admissions Contact:* Nancy Browne.

Staff: Full-time: 2; Part-time: 15.

Avg Enrollment: 100. *Avg Class Size:* 30. *Number of Graduates per Year:* 40.

Wheelchair Access: Yes.

Accreditation/Approval/Licensing: FL Board of Independent Postsecondary Vocational, Technical, Trade and Business Schools; Candidate, Accreditation Commission for Acupuncture and Oriental Medicine.

Field of Study: Acupressure*; Acupuncture*; Herbal Medicine; Homeopathy*; Massage Therapy*; Oriental Medicine*; Qigong; Reiki; Shiatsu*; Traditional Chinese Medicine*. *Program Name/Length:* Massage Therapy, 6 mos; Oriental Medicine, 36 mos, 4 academic yrs.

Degrees Offered: Diploma; Certificate.

License/Certification Preparation: State: FL Acupuncture Physician, FL Massage Therapist; American Oriental Bodywork Therapy Association; National Board of Homeopathic Examiners; National Certification Board for Therapeutic Massage and Bodywork; National Certification Commission for Acupuncture and Oriental Medicine.

Admission Requirements: Min age: 18; High school diploma/GED for Massage; Some college (2 yrs) for Oriental Medicine.

Application Deadline(s): Fall: Aug 15; Winter: Feb 1.

Tuition and Fees: $3500 (Massage); $18,125 (Oriental Medicine).

Financial Aid: VA approved; Vocational rehabilitation; Payment plan.

Career Services: Career counseling; Career information; Job information.

287. Educating Hands School of Massage

Therapeutic Massage Training Program
120 SW 8th St, Miami, FL 33130
Phone: (305) 285-6991; *Fax:* (305) 857-0298
E-mail: eduhands@aol.com *Internet:* http://massagetherapynetwork.com/edhand1.html
Program Administrator: Iris Burman, Dir; Ray Infante, Admin. *Admissions Contact:* Kathy Ozzard, Admissions Dir.
Year Established: 1981.
Staff: Part-time: 15.
Avg Enrollment: 120. *Avg Class Size:* 20. *Number of Graduates per Year:* 120.
Wheelchair Access: Yes.
Accreditation/Approval/Licensing: State board: FL Board of Independent Postsecondary Vocational, Technical, Trade and Business Schools; National Certification Board for Therapeutic Massage and Bodywork (CEUs).
Field of Study: Massage Therapy*. *Program Name/Length:* Therapeutic Massage and Bodywork Professional Training, 624 hrs (6, 8, or 11 mos); Continuing Education, 6-100 hrs.
Degrees Offered: Diploma.
License/Certification Preparation: State: FL Licensed Massage Therapist; National Certification Board for Therapeutic Massage and Bodywork.
Admission Requirements: Min age: 18; High school diploma/GED; English comprehension exam.
Application Deadline(s): Fall; Winter; Spring; Summer.
Tuition and Fees: $4900.
Financial Aid: Loans; State government aid; VA approved; Vocational rehabilitation; Private tuition financing.
Career Services: Career counseling; Career information; Job information.

288. Florida College of Natural Health, Miami

7925 NW 12th St, Ste 201, Miami, FL 33126
Phone: (305) 597-9599, (800) 599-9599; *Fax:* (305) 597-9110
E-mail: fcnh@icanect.net *Internet:* http://www.fcnh.com
Program Administrator: Lourdes Kamadia, Dir. *Admissions Contact:* Lucy Bonilla; Wanda Ramos; Jessica Soto.
Year Established: 1986.
Staff: Full-time: 4; Part-time: 11.
Avg Class Size: 25.
Wheelchair Access: Yes.

Accreditation/Approval/Licensing: State board: FL Board of Independent Postsecondary Vocational, Technical, Trade and Business Schools; Commission on Massage Therapy Accreditation; Accrediting Commission of Career Schools and Colleges of Technology.
Field of Study: Acupressure; Acupuncture*; Aromatherapy; CranioSacral Therapy; Massage Therapy*; Myofascial Release; Neuromuscular Therapy; Polarity Therapy; Reflexology; Shiatsu; Sports Massage. *Program Name/Length:* Therapeutic Massage, 5-6 mos; Advanced Therapeutic Massage, 9-12 mos; Associate of Science, 13-17 mos; Acupuncture, 3 yrs.
Degrees Offered: AS.
License/Certification Preparation: State: FL Licensed Massage Therapist, FL Acupuncture Physician; National Certification Commission for Acupuncture and Oriental Medicine; National Certification Board for Therapeutic Massage and Bodywork.
Admission Requirements: Min age: 18; High school diploma/GED or entrance exam.
Tuition and Fees: $5500 (Therapeutic Massage); $180 per credit (Associate of Science); $21,000 (Acupuncture).
Financial Aid: Federal government aid; Grants; Loans; Payment plan; Work study.
Career Services: Career information; Interview set up; Resume service.

289. Yoga Institute of Miami

9350 S Dadeland Blvd, Ste 207, Miami, FL 33156
Phone: (305) 670-0558; *Fax:* (305) 661-9943
Program Administrator: Bobbi Goldin, Dir. *Admissions Contact:* Bobbi Goldin.
Year Established: 1979.
Staff: Full-time: 3; Part-time: 6.
Avg Enrollment: 15. *Avg Class Size:* 15. *Number of Graduates per Year:* 15.
Wheelchair Access: Yes.
Field of Study: Yoga Teacher Training*. *Program Name/Length:* 1 wk.
License/Certification Preparation: Certification, Iyengar Yoga National Association.
Admission Requirements: Yoga practitioner or teacher.
Career Services: Career counseling; Career information; Internships.

Naples

290. Florida Health Academy, Naples

261 Ninth St S, Naples, FL 34102
Phone: (941) 263-9391; *Fax:* (941) 263-8680
Internet: http://www.ceuonline.org
Program Administrator: Clara E. McElroy, Dir. *Admissions Contact:* Clara E. McElroy, Dir.
Year Established: 1994.
Staff: Full-time: 10; Part-time: 5.

Avg Enrollment: 30. *Avg Class Size:* 12. *Number of Graduates per Year:* 20.
Wheelchair Access: Yes.
Accreditation/Approval/Licensing: State board: FL Dept of Ed.
Field of Study: Acupuncture*; Aromatherapy; Herbal Medicine; Massage Therapy*; Skin Care; Traditional Chinese Medicine. *Program Name/Length:* Massage Therapy, 6 mos; Acupuncture, 3 yrs; Facials and Skin Care, 13 wks.
Degrees Offered: Diploma; Certificate.
License/Certification Preparation: State: FL Licensed Massage Therapist, FL Acupuncture Physician; National Certification Commission for Acupuncture and Oriental Medicine; National Certification Board for Therapeutic Massage and Bodywork.
Admission Requirements: Min age: 18; High school diploma/GED.
Application Deadline(s): Fall: Sep 1; Winter: Jan 2; Spring: Apr 1; Summer: Jun 1.
Tuition and Fees: $2500 (Massage); $15,000 (Acupuncture); $1200 (Facials).
Financial Aid: Loans; VA approved.
Career Services: Career counseling; Career information.

North Palm Beach

291. East-West Therapy Institute
745 US Hwy 1, Ste 103, North Palm Beach, FL 33408
Phone: (561) 881-1228
E-mail: bie@flinet.com *Internet:* http://www.east-westtherapy.com
Program Administrator: Thomas Herakovich, Owner. *Admissions Contact:* Thomas Herakovich.
Year Established: 1998.
Staff: Full-time: 1.
Avg Class Size: 10.
Wheelchair Access: Yes.
Accreditation/Approval/Licensing: State board: FL Board of Massage (CEUs); National Certification Board for Therapeutic Massage and Bodywork (CEUs).
Field of Study: Meditation; Reiki*. *Program Name/Length:* Reiki I, 12 hrs; Reiki II, 12 hrs; Reiki III, 12 hrs; Meditation, individual hourly sessions.
Degrees Offered: CEUs; Certificate.
Admission Requirements: Specific course prerequisites: Reiki I required for Reiki II; Must be licensed or nationally certified massage therapist for CEUs.

Orlando

292. National College of Oriental Medicine
7100 Lake Ellenor Dr, Orlando, FL 32809

Phone: (407) 888-8689; *Fax:* (407) 888-8211
E-mail: info@acupunctureschool.com *Internet:* http://www.acupunctureschool.com
Program Administrator: Marvin D. Kelly, PhD, Admin. *Admissions Contact:* Lloyd Buss, Admissions Officer.
Year Established: 1991.
Staff: Full-time: 5; Part-time: 4.
Avg Enrollment: 24. *Avg Class Size:* 10. *Number of Graduates per Year:* 18.
Wheelchair Access: Yes.
Accreditation/Approval/Licensing: Accreditation Commission for Acupuncture and Oriental Medicine.
Field of Study: Acupuncture*; Herbal Medicine*; Oriental Medicine*; Traditional Chinese Medicine*. *Program Name/Length:* Diploma in Oriental Medicine, 3 yrs.
Degrees Offered: Diploma.
License/Certification Preparation: State: FL Acupuncture Physician; National Certification Commission for Acupuncture and Oriental Medicine.
Admission Requirements: Min age: 18; Some college (2 yrs); Min GPA: 2.0.
Application Deadline(s): Fall: Aug; Winter: Jan.
Tuition and Fees: $25,200.
Financial Aid: Federal government aid; State government aid; VA approved.
Career Services: Career counseling; Career information; Internships.

Palm Beach Gardens

293. The Upledger Institute
11211 Prosperity Farms Rd, D-325, Palm Beach Gardens, FL 33410
Phone: (561) 622-4334, (800) 233-5880; *Fax:* (561) 622-4771
E-mail: upledger@upledger.com *Internet:* http://www.upledger. com
Program Administrator: Kathy Lewis, Curriculum Dir. *Admissions Contact:* Kevin Roberts, Educational Svcs Dir.
Year Established: 1985.
Staff: Full-time: 80.
Avg Class Size: 35. *Number of Graduates per Year:* 2500.
Wheelchair Access: Yes.
Accreditation/Approval/Licensing: National Certification Board for Therapeutic Massage and Bodywork (CEUs).
Field of Study: CranioSacral Therapy*; Mechanical Link; Visceral Manipulation; Zero Balancing*. *Program Name/Length:* 4 day seminars.
Degrees Offered: Certificate.
License/Certification Preparation: CranioSacral Therapy Certification.
Admission Requirements: Specific course prerequisites: anatomy; Licensed health care professional.
Tuition and Fees: $495-$750 per course.

Pensacola

294. Florida's Therapeutic Massage School

1300 E Gadsden St, Pensacola, FL 32501
Phone: (850) 433-8212
Program Administrator: Geraldine Vaurigaud, LMT, Owner/Dir. *Admissions Contact:* Kat Miller, Admin.
Year Established: 1992.
Staff: Part-time: 12.
Avg Enrollment: 88. *Avg Class Size:* 22. *Number of Graduates per Year:* 80.
Wheelchair Access: Yes.
Accreditation/Approval/Licensing: State board: FL Board of Massage.
Field of Study: Acupressure; Aromatherapy; Herbal Medicine; Hydrotherapy*; Massage Therapy*; Neuromuscular Therapy*; Oriental Medicine; Polarity Therapy; Reflexology; Shiatsu; Sports Massage. *Program Name/Length:* Therapeutic Massage and Hydrotherapy, 6 mos.
Degrees Offered: Diploma.
License/Certification Preparation: State: FL Licensed Massage Therapist.
Admission Requirements: Min age: 18; High school diploma/GED.
Tuition and Fees: $3150.
Financial Aid: VA approved; Vocational rehabilitation.
Career Services: Career counseling; Career information; Internships; Referral service.

Pinellas Park

295. The Humanities Center Institute of Allied Health/School of Massage

Therapeutic Massage
4045 Park Blvd, Pinellas Park, FL 33781
Phone: (727) 541-5200; *Fax:* (727) 545-0053
E-mail: info@2touch.com *Internet:* http://www. 2touch.com
Program Administrator: Sherry L. Fears, Dir. *Admissions Contact:* Sherry L. Fears, Dir.
Year Established: 1981.
Staff: Full-time: 5; Part-time: 5.
Avg Enrollment: 250. *Avg Class Size:* 16. *Number of Graduates per Year:* 150.
Wheelchair Access: Yes.
Accreditation/Approval/Licensing: State board: FL Board of Independent Postsecondary Vocational, Technical, Trade and Business Schools; Accrediting Commission of Career Schools and Colleges of Technology.
Field of Study: Massage Therapy*; Neuromuscular Therapy. *Program Name/Length:* 7 mos.
Degrees Offered: Certificate.
License/Certification Preparation: State: FL Licensed Massage Therapist; National Certification Board for Therapeutic Massage and Bodywork.

Admission Requirements: Min age: 20; High school diploma/GED; Min GPA: 2.5.
Tuition and Fees: $5820.
Financial Aid: Grants; Loans; Vocational rehabilitation.
Career Services: Career information.

Pompano Beach

296. Florida College of Natural Health, Fort Lauderdale Campus

2001 W Sample, Ste 100, Pompano Beach, FL 33064
Phone: (954) 975-6400; *Fax:* (954) 975-9633
E-mail: fcnh@icanect.net *Internet:* http://www. fcnh.com
Program Administrator: Dorothy Artioli, Campus Dir. *Admissions Contact:* Kristi Mollis, VP of Admissions and Mktg.
Year Established: 1986.
Staff: Full-time: 6; Part-time: 12.
Avg Enrollment: 500. *Avg Class Size:* 35. *Number of Graduates per Year:* 225.
Wheelchair Access: Yes.
Accreditation/Approval/Licensing: Commission on Massage Therapy Accreditation; Accrediting Commission of Career Schools and Colleges of Technology; National Certification Board for Therapeutic Massage and Bodywork (CEUs).
Field of Study: Acupuncture*; Massage Therapy*; Skin Care. *Program Name/Length:* Therapeutic Massage Training, 5 mos; Associate of Science in Natural Health, 18 mos; Acupuncture, 3 yrs.
Degrees Offered: Diploma; AS.
License/Certification Preparation: State: FL Licensed Massage Therapist; FL Skin Care Specialist; National Certification Commission for Acupuncture and Oriental Medicine; National Certification Board for Therapeutic Massage and Bodywork.
Admission Requirements: Min age: 18; High school diploma/GED; Entrance exam.
Tuition and Fees: $5500 (Therapeutic Massage); $180 per credit (Associate of Science).
Financial Aid: Federal government aid; Grants; Loans; Scholarships; State government aid; Work study; VA approved; Vocational rehabilitation.
Career Services: Career counseling; Career information; Interview set up; Resume service.

Saint Augustine

297. HealthBuilders School of Therapeutic Massage, Inc

2180 State Rd A1A, Saint Augustine, FL 32084
Phone: (904) 471-8828; *Fax:* (904) 471-8838
E-mail: law@aug.com *Internet:* http://www. oldcity.com/hb

Program Administrator: Lydia Williams, Owner/Dir. *Admissions Contact:* Karen Peters, Admin Asst.
Year Established: 1994.
Staff: Full-time: 8; Part-time: 4.
Avg Enrollment: 25. *Avg Class Size:* 10. *Number of Graduates per Year:* 25.
Wheelchair Access: Yes.
Accreditation/Approval/Licensing: State board: FL Board of Massage; FL Dept of Ed.
Field of Study: Aromatherapy*; Deep Tissue Massage*; Energy Work*; Massage Therapy*; Polarity Therapy*; Reflexology*; Reiki*. *Program Name/Length:* 500 hrs, 6 mos.
Degrees Offered: Diploma.
License/Certification Preparation: State: FL Licensed Massage Therapist; National Certification Board for Therapeutic Massage and Bodywork.
Admission Requirements: Min age: 19; High school diploma/GED.
Tuition and Fees: $3600.
Financial Aid: Payment plan.
Career Services: Career counseling.

Saint Petersburg

298. Florida Institute of Traditional Chinese Medicine

Acupuncture and Traditional Chinese Medicine
5335 66th St N, Saint Petersburg, FL 33709
Phone: (813) 546-6565; *Fax:* (813) 547-0703
E-mail: fitcm@gte.net *Internet:* http://www.fitcm.com
Program Administrator: Dr. Su Liang Ku, Dir. *Admissions Contact:* Dr. W. Adams, Dir of Academic Admin.
Year Established: 1986.
Staff: Full-time: 11.
Avg Enrollment: 80. *Avg Class Size:* 40.
Wheelchair Access: Yes.
Accreditation/Approval/Licensing: Candidacy, Accreditation Commission for Acupuncture and Oriental Medicine.
Field of Study: Acupuncture*; Herbal Medicine; Traditional Chinese Medicine*; Tui Na. *Program Name/Length:* 6 semesters, 3 yrs.
Degrees Offered: Diploma.
License/Certification Preparation: State: FL Acupuncture Physician; National Certification Commission for Acupuncture and Oriental Medicine.
Admission Requirements: Some college (2 yrs).
Tuition and Fees: $3750 per semester.
Financial Aid: Federal government aid; Grants; Loans; VA approved; Vocational rehabilitation.
Career Services: Career information; Internships.

299. Integrated Health Care Systems

Complementary and Integrative Health Care
PO Box 67153, Saint Petersburg, FL 33736
Phone: (813) 367-3063; *Fax:* (813) 367-3170

E-mail: ssbegley@aol.com
Program Administrator: Shirley Spear Begley, RN, Exec Dir. *Admissions Contact:* Shirley Spear Begley.
Year Established: 1982.
Staff: Full-time: 1; Part-time: 3.
Avg Enrollment: 200. *Avg Class Size:* 20. *Number of Graduates per Year:* 200.
Wheelchair Access: Yes.
Accreditation/Approval/Licensing: State board: FL Board of Registered Nurses; FL Board of Clinical Social Work, Marriage and Family Therapy, and Mental Health Counseling; FL Board of Massage; National Certification Board for Therapeutic Massage and Bodywork (CEUs); Nurse Healers Professional Associates; International Therapeutic Touch Teacher's Cooperative.
Field of Study: Energy Work*; Guided Imagery*; Holistic Nursing*; Hypnotherapy; Therapeutic Touch*. *Program Name/Length:* Beginning Therapeutic Touch, 14 hrs, 2 days; Intermediate Therapeutic Touch, 14 hrs, 2 days; Advanced Therapeutic Touch, 16 hrs, 2 1/2 days; On-going Therapeutic Touch Mentorship, 4-12 mos; Guided Imagery, 14 hrs, 2 days; Mentorship Program in Holistic Nursing and Health Care, 48 hrs, 1 yr.
Degrees Offered: CEUs; Certificate.
License/Certification Preparation: State: FL Re-Licensure; Certified Holistic Nurse; International Therapeutic Touch Teacher's Cooperative; Nurse Healers Professional Associates.
Admission Requirements: Interview.
Tuition and Fees: $225-$1250.
Financial Aid: Payment plan.
Career Services: Career counseling; Career information; Internships.

300. International Institute of Reflexology

5650 1st Ave N, Saint Petersburg, FL 33710
Mailing Address: PO Box 12642, Saint Petersburg, FL 33733-2642
Phone: (727) 343-4811/1722; *Fax:* (727) 381-2807
E-mail: ftreflex@concentric.net
Program Administrator: Dwight C. Byers, Pres. *Admissions Contact:* Dwight C. Byers; Nancy Byers, VP.
Year Established: 1973.
Staff: Full-time: 25; Part-time: 30.
Avg Enrollment: 800. *Avg Class Size:* 40. *Number of Graduates per Year:* 350.
Wheelchair Access: Yes.
Accreditation/Approval/Licensing: State board: FL Board of Independent Postsecondary Vocational, Technical, Trade and Business Schools; National Certification Board for Therapeutic Massage and Bodywork (CEUs).
Field of Study: Reflexology*. *Program Name/Length:* Original Ingham Method of Reflexology Certification, 1 yr.
Degrees Offered: Diploma; Certificate.

License/Certification Preparation: State: FL;
American Reflexology Certification Board; National Certification Board for Therapeutic Massage and Bodywork.
Tuition and Fees: $740 + books, materials.

Sarasota

301. Academy of Chinese Healing Arts, Inc
Oriental Medicine
505 S Orange Ave, Sarasota, FL 34236
Phone: (941) 955-4456; *Fax:* (941) 330-1951
E-mail: acha@gte.net *Internet:* http://www.acha.
net
Program Administrator: Cynthia O'Donnell, AP,
CEO. *Admissions Contact:* Meredith Slaughter.
Year Established: 1994.
Staff: Full-time: 3; Part-time: 19.
Avg Enrollment: 30. *Avg Class Size:* 12. *Number
of Graduates per Year:* 7.
Wheelchair Access: Yes.
Accreditation/Approval/Licensing: State board: FL
Board of Independent Postsecondary Vocational,
Technical, Trade and Business Schools; Candidate, Accreditation Commission for Acupuncture and Oriental Medicine.
Field of Study: Acupressure; Acupuncture*; Herbal
Medicine; Homeopathy; Oriental Medicine*;
Qigong; Shiatsu; Traditional Chinese Medicine*.
Program Name/Length: Master's level diploma
in Oriental Medicine, 2700 hrs, 3 yrs.
Degrees Offered: CEUs; Diploma.
License/Certification Preparation: State: FL Acupuncture Physician; National Certification Commission for Acupuncture and Oriental Medicine.
Admission Requirements: Min age: 18; Some college (2 yrs in BA or RN program); Min GPA:
2.0.
Application Deadline(s): Fall: Aug 1; Winter: Dec
1; Spring: Apr 1.
Tuition and Fees: $20,000.
Financial Aid: VA approved; Payment plan.
Career Services: Career counseling; Career information; Internships; Job information.

302. American Yoga Association
Easy Does It Yoga
PO Box 19986, Sarasota, FL 34276
Phone: (941) 927-4977; *Fax:* (941) 921-9844
E-mail: yogamerica@aol.com *Internet:* http://
www.users.aol.com/amyogaassn
Program Administrator: Alice Christensen, Exec
Dir. *Admissions Contact:* Patricia Rockwood.
Year Established: 1975.
Field of Study: Yoga Teacher Training*. *Program
Name/Length:* Easy Does It Yoga Trainer Program, 1 day to 10 wks (weekly classes); Seminars given in various locations.

303. Florida College of Natural Health, Sarasota
8216 S Tamiami Trail, Sarasota, FL 34238
Phone: (941) 966-7117, (800) 966-7117
E-mail: fcnh@icanect.net *Internet:* http://www.
fcnh.com
Program Administrator: Prudence Sterling, Campus Dir. *Admissions Contact:* Prudence Sterling.
Year Established: 1978.
Staff: Full-time: 10; Part-time: 10.
Avg Enrollment: 100-250. *Avg Class Size:* 30-35.
Number of Graduates per Year: 100-200.
Wheelchair Access: Yes.
Accreditation/Approval/Licensing: Accrediting
Commission of Career Schools and Colleges of
Technology; State board: FL Board of Independent Postsecondary Vocational, Technical, Trade
and Business Schools.
Field of Study: Acupressure; Acupuncture*;
Aromatherapy; CranioSacral Therapy; Herbal
Medicine; Homeopathy; Massage Therapy*;
Neuromuscular Therapy; Polarity Therapy;
Reflexology; Reiki; Shiatsu; Skin Care; Sports
Massage; Traditional Chinese Medicine*. *Program Name/Length:* Therapeutic Massage
Training Program, 6 mos; Acupuncture/Traditional Chinese Medicine, 3 yrs; Skin Care
Training Program, 4-5 mos.
Degrees Offered: Diploma.
License/Certification Preparation: State: FL Licensed Massage Therapist, FL Acupuncture
Physician; National Certification Board for
Therapeutic Massage and Bodywork.
Admission Requirements: Min age: 18; High
school diploma/GED; Some college (60 credits
for Acupuncture Program only).
Tuition and Fees: $5500 (Massage); $21,000 (Acupuncture); $2850 (Skin Care).
Financial Aid: Federal government aid; Grants;
Loans; Work study; Payment plan.
Career Services: Career counseling.

304. Sarasota School of Massage Therapy
1970 Main St, 3rd Fl, Sarasota, FL 34236
Phone: (941) 957-0577; *Fax:* (941) 957-1049
Internet: http://www.sarasota.com/ssmt
Program Administrator: Michael Rosen-Pyros,
DC, Dir. *Admissions Contact:* Donald Brechner,
Dir of Finance and Admissions.
Year Established: 1979.
Staff: Full-time: 2; Part-time: 8.
Avg Enrollment: 120. *Avg Class Size:* 20. *Number
of Graduates per Year:* 100.
Wheelchair Access: Yes.
Accreditation/Approval/Licensing: State board: FL
Board of Independent Postsecondary Vocational, Technical, Trade and Business Schools;
Council on Occupational Education.
Field of Study: Aromatherapy; CranioSacral Therapy; Massage Therapy*; Neuromuscular Ther-

apy; Polarity Therapy; Reflexology. *Program Name/Length:* Massage Therapy, 540 hrs, 6 mos.
Degrees Offered: Diploma.
License/Certification Preparation: State: FL Licensed Massage Therapist; National Certification Board for Therapeutic Massage and Bodywork.
Admission Requirements: Min age: 18; High school diploma/GED.
Application Deadline(s): Fall: Sep; Winter: Jan; Spring: Mar; Summer: Jul.
Tuition and Fees: $3895.
Financial Aid: Payment plan.
Career Services: Career information; Job information.

Seminole

305. Saint John Neuromuscular Pain Relief Institute
10710 Seminole Blvd, Ste 1, Seminole, FL 33778
Phone: (727) 397-5525, (888) 668-4325; *Fax:* (727) 397-5808
E-mail: info@stjohnnmtseminars.com *Internet:* http://www.stjohnnmtseminars.com
Program Administrator: Paul St. John, LMT, Dir.
Year Established: 1978.
Accreditation/Approval/Licensing: National Certification Board for Therapeutic Massage and Bodywork (CEUs).
Field of Study: Neuromuscular Therapy*. *Program Name/Length:* St. John Neuromuscular Therapy, Seminars 1-7; Seminars given in various locations.
Degrees Offered: Certificate.
Admission Requirements: Licensed health care professional.

Sunrise

306. Academy of Lymphatic Studies
12651 W Sunrise Blvd, Sunrise, FL 33323
Mailing Address: 102 Redgrave Dr, Sebastian, FL 32958
Phone: (954) 846-7855, (800) 863-5935; *Fax:* (954) 845-9207
E-mail: joezuther@aol.com *Internet:* http://www.zutheracademy.com
Program Administrator: Joachim E. Zuther, Dir.
Admissions Contact: Joachim E. Zuther.
Year Established: 1994.
Staff: Full-time: 2; Part-time: 3.
Avg Enrollment: 100. *Avg Class Size:* 22. *Number of Graduates per Year:* 100.
Wheelchair Access: No.
Accreditation/Approval/Licensing: American Polarity Therapy Association; FL Physical Therapy Association; FL Occupational Therapy Association.

Field of Study: Complete Decongestive Physiotherapy; Manual Lymph Drainage*. *Program Name/Length:* Manual Lymph Drainage/Complete Decongestive Physiotherapy, 135 hrs; Seminars given in various locations.
Degrees Offered: Certificate.
Admission Requirements: Massage therapist (minimum 500 hrs), physical or occupational therapist, nurse or MD.
Tuition and Fees: $2500.
Career Services: Career information.

Tallahassee

307. CORE Institute School of Massage Therapy and Structural Bodywork
223 W Carolina St, Tallahassee, FL 32301
Phone: (850) 222-8673; *Fax:* (850) 561-6160
E-mail: core@nettally.com *Internet:* http://www.coreinstitute.com
Program Administrator: George Kousaleos, Dir.
Admissions Contact: Philip Arcuri, Assoc Dir.
Year Established: 1990.
Staff: Part-time: 16.
Avg Enrollment: 100. *Avg Class Size:* 20. *Number of Graduates per Year:* 100.
Wheelchair Access: Yes.
Accreditation/Approval/Licensing: State board: FL Board of Independent Postsecondary Vocational, Technical, Trade and Business Schools; FL Board of Massage; Commission on Massage Therapy Accreditation; National Certification Board for Therapeutic Massage and Bodywork (CEUs).
Field of Study: Massage Therapy*; Myofascial Release. *Program Name/Length:* Professional Massage Therapy Training, 650 hrs, 8 mos/full-time or 1 yr/part-time.
Degrees Offered: Diploma.
License/Certification Preparation: State: FL Licensed Massage Therapist; National Certification Board for Therapeutic Massage and Bodywork.
Admission Requirements: Min age: 20; High school diploma/GED; Some college (2 yrs); Min GPA: 2.0; Biographical essay; Medical history; 2 letters of reference.
Application Deadline(s): Fall: Aug; Winter: Jan; Spring: Apr.
Tuition and Fees: $5200.
Financial Aid: Work study.
Career Services: Career counseling; Career information; Internships; Job information.

Tampa

308. Atlantic Institute of Aromatherapy
2514 W Kennedy Blvd, Tampa, FL 33609
Phone: (813) 265-2222; *Fax:* (813) 265-2222
Internet: http://www.atlanticinstitute.com

Program Administrator: Sylla Sheppard-Hanger, Founder/Dir. *Admissions Contact:* Sylla Sheppard-Hanger.
Year Established: 1989.
Staff: Part-time: 5.
Avg Enrollment: 375. *Avg Class Size:* 5.
Accreditation/Approval/Licensing: State board: FL Board of Massage.
Field of Study: Aromatherapy*. *Program Name/Length:* Correspondence; Basic, 2 days; Advanced, 3 days; Medical/Nursing, 3 days; Chemistry/Perfume, 3 days.
Degrees Offered: Diploma; Certificate.
Admission Requirements: Health care professional.
Tuition and Fees: $275 per course.

309. Delphi Center for Midwifery Studies

3102 W Cypress St, Ste B, Tampa, FL 33607-5108
Phone: (813) 873-7135; *Fax:* (813) 873-0274
E-mail: delphicntr@aol.com
Program Administrator: Karin Kearns, LM, Exec Dir. *Admissions Contact:* Lisa McColl, Registrar.
Year Established: 1996.
Staff: Full-time: 1; Part-time: 12.
Avg Enrollment: 4. *Avg Class Size:* 4. *Number of Graduates per Year:* 1.
Wheelchair Access: Yes.
Accreditation/Approval/Licensing: Candidate, Midwifery Education Accreditation Council.
Field of Study: Midwifery*. *Program Name/Length:* Midwifery Asst, 1 yr; Midwifery Direct Entry, 3 yrs; Clinical Review and Assessment for FL Licensing, 6 mos; Childbirth Education, 31 classroom hrs and self-paced modules, 1 yr.
Degrees Offered: Diploma; Certificate; Associate's degree.
License/Certification Preparation: State: FL Licensed Midwife; Certified Professional Midwife, North American Registry of Midwives.
Admission Requirements: Min age: 18; High school diploma/GED; Min GPA: 3.0; Some college; Min GPA: 3.0; Specific course prerequisites: anatomy and physiology, chemistry, health sciences, medical terminology, microbiology; Out-of-state licensed midwife for Clinical Review and Assessment.
Tuition and Fees: $4150 + $400 books (Midwifery Asst); $14,150 + $1100 books, insurance, supplies, equipment (Midwifery); $1950 (Clinical Review); $950 (Childbirth Ed).
Financial Aid: Work exchange.
Career Services: Career counseling; Career information; Referral service.

310. Florida Institute of Postural Integration

5837 Mariner Dr, Tampa, FL 33609
Phone: (813) 286-2273; *Fax:* (813) 287-2870
E-mail: drjoy@johnsonmail.com *Internet:* http://www.quantumbalance.com
Program Administrator: Dr. Joy K. Johnson, PhD, Dir. *Admissions Contact:* Dr. Joy K. Johnson.
Year Established: 1988.
Staff: Full-time: 1; Part-time: 1.
Avg Enrollment: 4. *Avg Class Size:* 4. *Number of Graduates per Year:* 4.
Wheelchair Access: No.
Field of Study: Acupressure*; Deep Tissue Massage*. *Program Name/Length:* 2 1/2 wks.
Degrees Offered: Diploma; Certificate.
License/Certification Preparation: International Center for Release and Integration.
Admission Requirements: Background in health field.
Tuition and Fees: $3100.

311. ReNew Life and Dotolo Institute School of Colon Hydrotherapy

1007 N MacDill, Tampa, FL 33607
Phone: (813) 871-3200; *Fax:* (813) 877-2640
E-mail: rdotolo@dotoloresearch.com *Internet:* http://www.dotoloresearch.com
Program Administrator: Suzanne M. Gray, Owner/Admin; Brenda Gray, Owner/Admin. *Admissions Contact:* Suzanne M. Gray.
Year Established: 1996.
Staff: Full-time: 2.
Avg Enrollment: 30. *Avg Class Size:* 8.
Wheelchair Access: Yes.
Accreditation/Approval/Licensing: State board: FL Board of Independent Postsecondary Vocational, Technical, Trade and Business Schools; Accrediting Council for Continuing Education and Training.
Field of Study: Colon Hydrotherapy*. *Program Name/Length:* 100 hrs.
Degrees Offered: Certificate.
License/Certification Preparation: State: FL Licensed Colon Hydrotherapist.
Admission Requirements: High school diploma/GED; Some college; Specific course prerequisites: anatomy and physiology; Massage therapy license required for FL residents.
Application Deadline(s): Fall: Sep; Winter: Jan; Spring: Mar; Summer Jul.
Tuition and Fees: $1550.
Career Services: Career information.

312. Suncoast Center for Natural Health, Inc

4910 W Cypress St, Tampa, FL 33607
Phone: (813) 287-1099; *Fax:* (813) 287-1914
Program Administrator: Kathy Reid, Dir.
Year Established: 1982.
Staff: Part-time: 14.
Accreditation/Approval/Licensing: State board: FL Board of Independent Postsecondary Vocational, Technical, Trade and Business Schools; Accrediting Commission of Career Schools and Colleges of Technology.
Field of Study: Anatomy and Physiology; Hydrotherapy*; Massage Therapy*;

Neuromuscular Therapy; Sports Massage. *Program Name/Length:* Basic Massage and Hydrotherapy, 500-600 hrs, 6 mos.
Degrees Offered: Diploma.
License/Certification Preparation: State: FL Licensed Massage Therapist; National Certification Board for Therapeutic Massage and Bodywork.
Admission Requirements: Min age: 18; High school diploma/GED; Interview.
Tuition and Fees: $4275-$5275 + $400 books.
Financial Aid: Federal government aid; Grants; Loans; VA approved; Vocational rehabilitation.
Career Services: Job information.

West Palm Beach

313. The Bramham Institute
1014 N Olive Ave, West Palm Beach, FL 33401
Phone: (800) 575-0518; *Fax:* (561) 832-6642
E-mail: bramhami@aol.com *Internet:* http://www.spamastery.com
Program Administrator: Anne Bramham, Dir of Ed. *Admissions Contact:* Sara Eavenson, Exec Admin.
Year Established: 1996.
Staff: Full-time: 1; Part-time: 7.
Avg Enrollment: 200. *Avg Class Size:* 10.
Wheelchair Access: Yes.
Accreditation/Approval/Licensing: National Certification Board for Therapeutic Massage and Bodywork (CEUs); State board: FL Board of Massage; FL Physical Therapy Association; Accrediting Council for Continuing Education and Training.
Field of Study: Aromatherapy; Connective Tissue Massage; Hydrotherapy; Manual Lymph Drainage*; Reflexology; Spa Therapies*. *Program Name/Length:* Dr. Vodder Manual Lymph Drainage, 1 mo; The Spa Certification Program, 200 hrs, 5 wks; Spa Management Certification, 8 days.
Degrees Offered: CEUs; Certificate.
License/Certification Preparation: American Spa Therapy Education and Certification Council.

Admission Requirements: Min age: 18; High school diploma/GED; Health care professional.
Tuition and Fees: $2400 (Manual Lymph Drainage); $2700 (Spa certification); $1200 (Spa management).
Financial Aid: Loans.
Career Services: Career counseling; Career information; Internships; Job placement.

Winter Haven

314. Ridge Technical Center
Massage Therapy
7700 State Rd 544, Winter Haven, FL 33881
Phone: (941) 299-2512, ext 247; 419-3062, ext 247; *Fax:* (941) 419-3060
Program Administrator: Eileen Harriman, Instr. *Admissions Contact:* Steve Strodman, Adult Guidance Counselor.
Year Established: 1993.
Staff: Full-time: 1; Part-time: 1.
Avg Enrollment: 36. *Avg Class Size:* 24 day, 12 evening. *Number of Graduates per Year:* 36.
Wheelchair Access: Yes.
Accreditation/Approval/Licensing: State board: FL Board of Massage; Southern Association of Colleges and Schools; Accrediting Commission of the Council on Occupational Ed.
Field of Study: Massage Therapy*. *Program Name/Length:* 850 hrs.
Degrees Offered: Certificate.
License/Certification Preparation: State: FL Licensed Massage Therapist; National Certification Board for Therapeutic Massage and Bodywork.
Admission Requirements: Min age: 18; High school diploma/GED.
Application Deadline(s): Spring: Jan; Summer: Aug.
Tuition and Fees: $1700 includes books, supplies, and national certification exam and state licensing fees.
Financial Aid: Federal government aid; Grants; Scholarships; Vocational rehabilitation.
Career Services: Resume service; Career Assessment.

GEORGIA

Atlanta

315. The Academy of Somatic Healing Arts
1924 Cliff Valley Way, Atlanta, GA 30329
Phone: (404) 315-0394; *Fax:* (404) 633-1270

Program Administrator: Jim Gabriel, Dir. *Admissions Contact:* Rebecca Noll, Admissions Coord.
Year Established: 1991.
Staff: Full-time: 10; Part-time: 3.

Avg Enrollment: 80. *Avg Class Size:* 20. *Number of Graduates per Year:* 56.
Wheelchair Access: Yes.
Accreditation/Approval/Licensing: State board: GA Nonpublic Postsecondary Ed.
Field of Study: Massage Therapy*; Neuromuscular Therapy; Sports Massage. *Program Name/Length:* 9 mos/days or 1 yr/evenings and weekends.
Degrees Offered: Certificate.
License/Certification Preparation: State: FL Licensed Massage Therapist; National Certification Board for Therapeutic Massage and Bodywork.
Admission Requirements: Min age: 18; High school diploma/GED.
Tuition and Fees: $6000.
Financial Aid: Federal government aid; Loans; State government aid; VA approved; Vocational rehabilitation; Payment plan.
Career Services: Career counseling; Career information.

316. Alexander Technique of Atlanta

4246 Peachtree Rd, Ste 6, Atlanta, GA 30319
Phone: (770) 454-1177
Program Administrator: Ron Dennis, EdD, Dir.
Year Established: 1994.
Accreditation/Approval/Licensing: American Society for the Alexander Technique.
Field of Study: Alexander Technique. *Program Name/Length:* Teacher Training, 1600 hrs, 3 yrs.
License/Certification Preparation: American Society for the Alexander Technique.
Admission Requirements: Min age: 21; Bachelor's degree or equivalent life experience; Specific course prerequisites: 10 private lessons with certified teacher; Letter of reference from teacher; 3 lesson/interviews with director.
Tuition and Fees: $3900 per yr.

317. Atlanta School of Massage

2300 Peachford Rd, Ste 3200, Atlanta, GA 30338
Phone: (770) 454-7167, (888) 276-6277; *Fax:* (770) 454-7367
Year Established: 1980.
Staff: Full-time: 6; Part-time: 38.
Avg Enrollment: 225. *Avg Class Size:* 24. *Number of Graduates per Year:* 150.
Wheelchair Access: No.
Accreditation/Approval/Licensing: Commission on Massage Therapy Accreditation; National Certification Board for Therapeutic Massage and Bodywork (CEUs); Accrediting Commission of Career Schools and Colleges of Technology.
Field of Study: Acupressure; Aromatherapy; Deep Tissue Massage; Integrative Massage; Massage Therapy*; Polarity Therapy; Reflexology; Shiatsu; Spa Therapies*. *Program Name/Length:* Integrative Massage and Deep Tissue Therapy, 620 hrs; Clinical Massage, 620

hrs; Wellness Massage and Spa Therapies, 620 hrs.
Degrees Offered: Certificate.
License/Certification Preparation: State: FL Licensed Massage Therapist; National Certification Board for Therapeutic Massage and Bodywork.
Admission Requirements: Min age: 18; High school diploma/GED.
Financial Aid: Grants; Loans.
Career Services: Career information.

318. Capelli Learning Center

Massage Therapy
2581 Piedmont Rd, Ste C-1000, Atlanta, GA 30324
Phone: (404) 261-5261; *Fax:* (404) 261-5069
Program Administrator: Deb Elkin, LMT, Dir. *Admissions Contact:* Deb Elkin.
Year Established: 1994.
Staff: Part-time: 11.
Avg Enrollment: 40. *Avg Class Size:* 10. *Number of Graduates per Year:* 35.
Wheelchair Access: Yes.
Accreditation/Approval/Licensing: State board: FL Board of Massage; GA Non-Public Postsecondary Ed Commission.
Field of Study: Deep Tissue Massage; Massage Therapy*; Qigong; Reflexology; Thai Massage*; Traditional Chinese Medicine. *Program Name/Length:* Massage Therapy, 618 hrs, 6 mos.
Degrees Offered: Certificate.
License/Certification Preparation: State: FL Licensed Massage Therapist; National Certification Board for Therapeutic Massage and Bodywork.
Admission Requirements: Min age: 18; High school diploma/GED; Awareness of oriental philosophies preferred; Interview.
Tuition and Fees: $5400 + $800 additional expenses.
Financial Aid: Grants; Loans; Institutional financing.
Career Services: Career information; Job board.

319. Emory University, Nell Hodgson Woodruff School of Nursing

Nurse-Midwifery Program
Atlanta, GA 30322
Phone: (404) 727-6961; *Fax:* (404) 727-0536
E-mail: makelle@nurse.emory.edu *Internet:* http://www.nurse.emory.edu
Program Administrator: Maureen Kelley, PhD, Dir. *Admissions Contact:* L. Leusch.
Year Established: 1978.
Staff: Full-time: 4.
Avg Class Size: 16. *Number of Graduates per Year:* 16.
Wheelchair Access: Yes.
Accreditation/Approval/Licensing: American College of Nurse-Midwives, Division of Accreditation.

Field of Study: Midwifery*. *Program Name/Length:* Master of Science in Nursing, 4 semesters, 16 mos.
Degrees Offered: MSN.
License/Certification Preparation: Certified Nurse-Midwife, American College of Nurse-Midwives.
Admission Requirements: Bachelor's degree; Min GPA: 3.0.
Financial Aid: Fellowships; Loans; Scholarships.

320. New Life Institute, Inc, School of Massage Excellence
4330 Georgetown Sq, Ste 500, Atlanta, GA 30338
Phone: (770) 457-2021; *Fax:* (770) 457-5614
Internet: http://www.yp.bellsouth.com/newlifemassage
Program Administrator: Dr. Bruce Costello, Exec Dir. *Admissions Contact:* Sandy Jones, Admissions Dir.
Year Established: 1994.
Staff: Part-time: 88.
Avg Enrollment: 100. *Avg Class Size:* 12. *Number of Graduates per Year:* 93.
Wheelchair Access: No.
Accreditation/Approval/Licensing: State board: GA Nonpublic Postsecondary Education Commission.
Field of Study: Massage Therapy*. *Program Name/Length:* 630 hrs, 6 mos, 9 mos or 12 mos.
Degrees Offered: Certificate.
License/Certification Preparation: National Certification Board for Therapeutic Massage and Bodywork.
Admission Requirements: Min age: 18; High school diploma/GED.
Application Deadline(s): Fall: Sep 15; Winter: Dec 15; Spring: Mar 15; Summer: Jun 15.
Tuition and Fees: $5975 + $400 books.
Financial Aid: Loans; VA approved; Vocational rehabilitation; Payment plan.
Career Services: Career counseling.

321. The Polarity Training Institute
566 Pharr Rd, Atlanta, GA 30305
Phone: (770) 704-5170
E-mail: will65928@aol.com
Program Administrator: Will Leichnitz, RPP, Dir. *Admissions Contact:* Will Leichnitz.
Accreditation/Approval/Licensing: American Polarity Therapy Association.
Field of Study: Polarity Therapy*. *Program Name/Length:* Associate Polarity Practitioner, 155 hrs; Seminars given in various locations.
License/Certification Preparation: APP; American Polarity Therapy Association.

Augusta

322. Georgia Institute of Therapeutic Massage LLC
Certificate in Massage Therapy
2160 Centra Ave, Augusta, GA 30904
Mailing Address: PO Box 3657, Augusta, GA 30914-3657
Phone: (706) 738-7695; *Fax:* (706) 738-6232
E-mail: vnp@massageone.com *Internet:* http://www.massageone.com
Program Administrator: Vicki N. Platt, Exec Dir. *Admissions Contact:* Daniel H. Platt.
Year Established: 1995.
Staff: Full-time: 1; Part-time: 7.
Avg Enrollment: 25. *Avg Class Size:* 15. *Number of Graduates per Year:* 25.
Wheelchair Access: Yes.
Field of Study: Acupressure; Massage Therapy*; Neuromuscular Therapy*; Polarity Therapy; Reflexology; Shiatsu; Sports Massage; Swedish Massage*. *Program Name/Length:* Massage Certification, 10 mos/days or nights.
Degrees Offered: Certificate.
License/Certification Preparation: State: FL and SC Licensed Massage Therapist; National Certification Board for Therapeutic Massage and Bodywork.
Admission Requirements: Min age: 18; High school diploma/GED; Min GPA: 2.0; Health release; 2 letters of recommendation.
Application Deadline(s): Fall: Sep (night class); Winter: Feb (day class).
Tuition and Fees: $5100 + $700-$1000 books and table.
Financial Aid: VA approved; Vocational rehabilitation; Payment plan.
Career Services: Career information; Job information; Referral service.

Gainesville

323. Lake Lanier School of Massage
Professional Massage Therapy Training
400 Brenau Ave, Gainesville, GA 30501
Phone: (770) 287-0377; *Fax:* (770) 536-7350
Internet: http://www.massageschool.net
Program Administrator: Sandra Easterbrooks, Dir. *Admissions Contact:* Sandra Easterbrooks.
Year Established: 1994.
Staff: Full-time: 1; Part-time: 4.
Avg Enrollment: 35. *Avg Class Size:* 10. *Number of Graduates per Year:* 33.
Wheelchair Access: No.
Accreditation/Approval/Licensing: State board: GA Nonpublic Postsecondary Ed; FL Dept of Business and Professional Regulation; International Massage and Somatic Therapies Accreditation Council; National Certification Board for Therapeutic Massage and Bodywork (CEUs).

Field of Study: Massage Therapy*. *Program Name/Length:* Professional Massage Therapy, 550 hrs, 6 mos.
Degrees Offered: Certificate.
License/Certification Preparation: State: FL Licensed Massage Therapist; National Certification Board for Therapeutic Massage and Bodywork.
Admission Requirements: Min age: 16; High school diploma/GED.
Tuition and Fees: $5500.
Financial Aid: VA approved; Payment plan.
Career Services: Career counseling; Career information; Resume service.

Marietta

324. Life University, School of Chiropractic
1269 Barclay Cir, Marietta, GA 30060
Phone: (770) 426-2884, (800) 543-3345; *Fax:* (770) 428-9886
E-mail: admission@life.edu *Internet:* http://www.life.edu
Program Administrator: Dr. Ron Kirk, Dean. *Admissions Contact:* Dr. Harry Harrison, Dir.
Year Established: 1974.

Staff: Full-time: 100; Part-time: 20.
Avg Enrollment: 3000. *Number of Graduates per Year:* 900.
Wheelchair Access: Yes.
Accreditation/Approval/Licensing: State board: GA Board of Chiropractic; Accrediting Council for Continuing Education and Training; Council on Chiropractic Education; Southern Association of Colleges and Schools.
Field of Study: Chiropractic*. *Program Name/Length:* Doctor of Chiropractic, 4400 hrs.
Degrees Offered: DC.
License/Certification Preparation: State: GA Board of Chiropractic; National Board of Chiropractic Examiners.
Admission Requirements: High school diploma/GED; Some college (2 yrs); Min GPA 2.25.
Application Deadline(s): Fall: Sep; Winter: Dec; Spring: Mar; Summer: Jun.
Tuition and Fees: $3400 per qtr + $200 fees.
Financial Aid: Federal government aid; Grants; Loans; Scholarships; Work study; VA approved; Payment plan.
Career Services: Career counseling; Career information; Internships; Job information.

HAWAII

Hanalei

325. Aloha Kaui Massage Workshop
PO Box 622, Hanalei, HI 96714
Phone: (808) 826-9990; *Fax:* (808) 826-6180
Program Administrator: Devaki Holman, Owner/Instr. *Admissions Contact:* Devaki Holman.
Year Established: 1985.
Staff: Full-time: 2.
Avg Enrollment: 28. *Avg Class Size:* 14. *Number of Graduates per Year:* 28.
Wheelchair Access: Yes.
Accreditation/Approval/Licensing: State board: HI Board of Massage Therapy.
Field of Study: Massage Therapy*. *Program Name/Length:* Pre-Licensing Massage, 150 hrs, 3 mos; Apprenticeship Massage, 420 hrs, 6 mos.
License/Certification Preparation: State: HI Licensed Massage Therapist.
Admission Requirements: Min age: 18.
Tuition and Fees: $1950 (Pre-Licensing); $1600 (Apprenticeship).
Financial Aid: Discount for early payment.

Hilo

326. Big Island Academy of Massage, Inc
211 Kinoole St, Hilo, HI 96720
Phone: (808) 935-1405
E-mail: nasisu@bigisland.com
Program Administrator: Nancy Kahalewai, LMT. *Admissions Contact:* Paul Rambo, Admin Asst.
Year Established: 1992.
Staff: Full-time: 2; Part-time: 3.
Avg Enrollment: 32. *Avg Class Size:* 16. *Number of Graduates per Year:* 30.
Wheelchair Access: Yes.
Accreditation/Approval/Licensing: State board: HI Dept of Commerce and Consumer Affairs.
Field of Study: Acupressure; Aromatherapy; Deep Tissue Massage; Energy Work; LomiLomi*; Massage Therapy*; Polarity Therapy; Reflexology; Reiki; Shiatsu; Sports Massage. *Program Name/Length:* Basic Massage Therapy, 100-150 hrs, 1-2 semesters; Seminars given in various locations; Professional Pre-Licensing, 600 hrs, 3-5 semesters; Seminars given in various locations.
Degrees Offered: Certificate.

License/Certification Preparation: State: HI Licensed Massage Therapist; National Certification Board for Therapeutic Massage and Bodywork.
Admission Requirements: Min age: 18; Interview.
Application Deadline(s): Fall: Sep 1; Spring: Jan 15.
Tuition and Fees: $900 (100 hrs); $1350 (150 hrs); $3200 (600 hrs).
Financial Aid: Loans; Payment plans.
Career Services: Career counseling; Career information; Internships; Referral service.

Honolulu

327. Aisen Shiatsu School

1314 S King St, Ste 601, Honolulu, HI 96814
Phone: (808) 596-7354; *Fax:* (808) 593-8282
Internet: http://www.gtesupersite.com/aisenshiatsu
Program Administrator: Fumihiko Indei, LMT, Dir. *Admissions Contact:* Fumihiko Indei.
Year Established: 1977.
Staff: Full-time: 3; Part-time: 5.
Avg Class Size: 15.
Accreditation/Approval/Licensing: State board: HI Dept of Ed.
Field of Study: Shiatsu*. *Program Name/Length:* 200 hrs, 4 mos.
Degrees Offered: Certificate.
License/Certification Preparation: State: HI Board of Massage Therapy.
Admission Requirements: High school diploma/GED; Health release including negative TB; 3 letters of reference; Narrative personal history; Interview.
Tuition and Fees: $4800.

328. Hawaii College of Health Sciences, Inc

1750 Kalakaua Ave, Ste 2404, Honolulu, HI 96826
Phone: (808) 941-8223; *Fax:* (808) 944-8343
Program Administrator: Dr. Randall H. James, Principal. *Admissions Contact:* Evelyn James, Office Mgr.
Year Established: 1989.
Staff: Part-time: 18.
Avg Enrollment: 60. *Avg Class Size:* 18. *Number of Graduates per Year:* 48.
Wheelchair Access: Yes.
Accreditation/Approval/Licensing: State board: HI Board of Massage.
Field of Study: Acupressure; CranioSacral Therapy; Deep Tissue Massage; Herbal Medicine; Massage Therapy*; Reflexology; Shiatsu; Traditional Chinese Medicine. *Program Name/Length:* Phase I and Phase II, 570 hrs, 12-18 mos.
Degrees Offered: Diploma; Certificate.
License/Certification Preparation: State: HI Licensed Massage Therapist.
Admission Requirements: Min age: 16.

Tuition and Fees: $3075-$4275.
Financial Aid: State government aid; Vocational rehabilitation.
Career Services: Career counseling; Career information; Internships.

329. Honolulu School of Massage, Inc

1136 12th Ave, Ste 240, Honolulu, HI 96816
Phone: (808) 733-0000; *Fax:* (808) 733-0045
E-mail: hsminc@msn.com
Program Administrator: Gayle E. Volger, Dir of Ed. *Admissions Contact:* Gayle E. Volger.
Year Established: 1982.
Staff: Part-time: 10.
Avg Enrollment: 160. *Avg Class Size:* 12. *Number of Graduates per Year:* 90.
Wheelchair Access: No.
Accreditation/Approval/Licensing: State board: HI Dept of Ed; HI Nursing Association.
Field of Study: Applied Kinesiology; CranioSacral Therapy; Deep Tissue Massage; Hydrotherapy*; LomiLomi Massage*; Massage Therapy*; Neuromuscular Therapy; Reflexology; Shiatsu; Sports Massage. *Program Name/Length:* Basic Massage Therapy Training, 3 1/2 mos part-time; AMTA Professional Massage Therapy Training, 7 mos part-time.
Degrees Offered: CEUs; Diploma; Certificate.
License/Certification Preparation: State: HI Licensed Massage Therapist; National Certification Board for Therapeutic Massage and Bodywork.
Admission Requirements: Min age: 18; High school diploma/GED; Specific course prerequisites: Basic Massage required for Professional level courses; Statement of intention; 2 letters of reference; TB release.
Application Deadline(s): Fall: Aug; Winter: Dec; Spring: Apr.
Tuition and Fees: $1950 (Basic Massage); $6550 (AMTA Professional).
Financial Aid: State government aid; VA approved; Vocational rehabilitation.
Career Services: Career information; Work opportunity at school clinic.

330. Institute of Clinical Acupuncture and Oriental Medicine

1270 Queen Emma St, Ste 107, Honolulu, HI 96813
Phone: (808) 521-2288; *Fax:* (808) 521-2288
E-mail: icaomhi@msn.com
Program Administrator: Wai Hoa Low, Pres. *Admissions Contact:* Catherine Low, Clinic Dir.
Year Established: 1997.
Staff: Full-time: 1; Part-time: 7.
Avg Enrollment: 8. *Avg Class Size:* 8.
Wheelchair Access: Yes.
Accreditation/Approval/Licensing: State board: HI Dept of Ed.
Field of Study: Acupuncture*; Herbal Medicine*; Oriental Medicine*; Traditional Chinese Medi-

cine*. *Program Name/Length:* Master Level Oriental Medicine Diploma, 4 yrs.
Degrees Offered: Diploma.
License/Certification Preparation: State: HI Licensed Acupuncturist; National Certification Commission for Acupuncture and Oriental Medicine.
Admission Requirements: Some college (2 yrs, 60 semester credits).
Application Deadline(s): Fall: Jul 31; Spring: Dec 31.
Financial Aid: Payment plan.
Career Services: Career information; Internships.

331. Tai Hsuan Foundation: College of Acupuncture and Herbal Medicine

Master of Acupuncture and Oriental Medicine
2600 S King St, Rm 206, Honolulu, HI 96826
Mailing Address: PO Box 11130, Honolulu, HI 96828
Phone: (800) 942-4788; *Fax:* (808) 949-1005
E-mail: taihsuan@acupuncture-hi.com *Internet:* http://www.acupuncture-hi.com
Program Administrator: Dr. Gayle Todoki, Pres. *Admissions Contact:* Phyllis Ono, Lily Chen, Admissions.
Year Established: 1970.
Staff: Part-time: 12.
Avg Enrollment: 32. *Avg Class Size:* 35. *Number of Graduates per Year:* 8.
Wheelchair Access: Yes.
Accreditation/Approval/Licensing: Accreditation Commission for Acupuncture and Oriental Medicine.
Field of Study: Acupressure; Acupuncture*; Herbal Medicine*; Oriental Medicine*; Qigong; Traditional Chinese Medicine*. *Program Name/Length:* 4 yrs.
Degrees Offered: MAcOM.
License/Certification Preparation: State: HI Acupuncture License; National Certification Commission for Acupuncture and Oriental Medicine.
Admission Requirements: Min age: 18; Some college (2 yrs); Min GPA: 2.0.
Tuition and Fees: $3450 per semester.
Financial Aid: Federal government aid; Loans; State government aid; VA approved; Vocational rehabilitation.
Career Services: Career counseling; Career information; Internships.

332. University of Health Science

1778 Ala Moana Blvd, Ste 1307, Honolulu, HI 96815
Phone: (808) 951-8242; *Fax:* (808) 951-8242
Program Administrator: Lucy Han Lee, Pres. *Admissions Contact:* David Ai-He Zhu, VP.
Year Established: 1986.
Staff: Full-time: 4; Part-time: 7.
Avg Enrollment: 10. *Avg Class Size:* 5. *Number of Graduates per Year:* 3.
Wheelchair Access: No.

Field of Study: Acupressure*; Acupuncture*; Herbal Medicine*; Homeopathy; Iridology; Qigong; Reflexology; Shiatsu*; Traditional Chinese Medicine*. *Program Name/Length:* Acupuncture, 3 yrs; Herbal Medicine/Traditional Chinese Medicine, 1 yr; Acupressure/Shiatsu, 1 yr.
Degrees Offered: MS; OMD; Certificate.
License/Certification Preparation: State: HI Licensed Acupuncturist; National Certification Commission for Acupuncture and Oriental Medicine.
Admission Requirements: Min age: 18; High school diploma/GED; Some college (2 yrs).
Application Deadline(s): Fall: Sep; Spring: Feb.
Tuition and Fees: $16,000-$17,000 (Acupuncture); $6000 (Herbal); $5000-$6000 (Acupressure).
Financial Aid: Scholarships; Work study.

Kailua

333. American Institute of Massage Therapy, Kailua

State Licensed Massage Therapy Training
407 Uluniu St, Ste 204A, Kailua, HI 96734
Phone: (808) 266-2468; *Fax:* (808) 266-2460
E-mail: ereveley@compuserve.com *Internet:* http://www.aimt-hi@l-netmall/shops/massage
Program Administrator: Elizabeth Reveley, Dir. *Admissions Contact:* Elizabeth Reveley.
Year Established: 1984.
Staff: Part-time: 4.
Avg Enrollment: 30. *Avg Class Size:* 10. *Number of Graduates per Year:* 30.
Wheelchair Access: Yes.
Accreditation/Approval/Licensing: State board: HI Board of Massage.
Field of Study: Acupressure; Aromatherapy; CranioSacral Therapy; Deep Tissue Massage; Energy Work*; Healing Touch; Hypnotherapy; Massage Therapy*; Reflexology.
Degrees Offered: Diploma.
License/Certification Preparation: State: HI Licensed Massage Therapist; National Certification Board for Therapeutic Massage and Bodywork.
Admission Requirements: Min age: 18; High school diploma/GED.
Application Deadline(s): Fall: Sep 10; Winter: Jan 10; Summer: May 10.
Tuition and Fees: $3000 includes books, supplies.
Career Services: Career counseling; Career information.

Kailua-Kona

334. The Hawaiian Islands School of Body Therapies

Professional Massage Therapy Program
78-6739 Alii Dr, Kailua-Kona, HI 96740

Mailing Address: PO Box 390188, Kailua-Kona, HI 96739
Phone: (808) 322-0048; *Fax:* (808) 322-4971
E-mail: massages@gte.net
Program Administrator: Peter Wind, Principal; Lynn Wind, Dir. *Admissions Contact:* Lynn Wind; Gretchen Markley, Admin Asst.
Year Established: 1984.
Staff: Full-time: 2; Part-time: 3.
Avg Enrollment: 26. *Avg Class Size:* 16. *Number of Graduates per Year:* 16.
Wheelchair Access: Yes.
Accreditation/Approval/Licensing: State board: HI Dept of Ed.
Field of Study: Aromatherapy; CranioSacral Therapy; Massage Therapy*; Polarity Therapy; Reflexology; Restorative Treatment Therapy; Shiatsu. *Program Name/Length:* Basic Massage Therapy Training, 645 hrs, 1 yr; Professional Massage Therapy Training, 1000 hrs, 15 mos.
Degrees Offered: Diploma.
License/Certification Preparation: State: HI Licensed Massage Therapist; National Certification Board for Therapeutic Massage and Bodywork.
Admission Requirements: Min age: 18; High school diploma/GED.
Application Deadline(s): Fall: Aug; Winter: Dec; Spring: Mar; Summer: Mar.
Tuition and Fees: $5700 (Basic); $7600 (Professional).
Financial Aid: Payment plan.
Career Services: Career counseling; Career information.

Kamuela

335. Traditional Chinese Medical College of Hawaii
Diploma in Oriental Medicine
PO Box 2288, Kamuela, HI 96743
Phone: (808) 885-9226; *Fax:* (808) 885-9226
E-mail: chinese@ilhawaii.com *Internet:* http://www.ilhawaii.net/~chinese
Accreditation/Approval/Licensing: Candidate, Accreditation Commission for Acupuncture and Oriental Medicine.
Field of Study: Acupuncture*; Oriental Medicine*; Traditional Chinese Medicine*.
Degrees Offered: Diploma.

Kihei

336. Maui Academy of the Healing Arts
1993 S Kihei Rd, Ste 210, Kihei, HI 96753
Phone: (808) 879-4266; *Fax:* (808) 879-4484
E-mail: sancorp@maui.net *Internet:* http://maui.net/~sancorp/

Program Administrator: John Sanderson, Dir. *Admissions Contact:* John Sanderson; Sora Rose, Admin Asst.
Year Established: 1988.
Staff: Part-time: 12.
Avg Enrollment: 24. *Avg Class Size:* 12. *Number of Graduates per Year:* 20.
Wheelchair Access: Yes.
Accreditation/Approval/Licensing: State board: HI Dept of Ed.
Field of Study: Acupressure; Esalen Massage*; LomiLomi Massage*; Lymphatic Massage; Massage Therapy*; Reflexology; Shiatsu; Sports Massage; Swedish Massage*; Thai Massage. *Program Name/Length:* Prelicensure Massage Therapy, 450 classroom hrs and 150 practice hrs.
Degrees Offered: Certificate.
License/Certification Preparation: State: HI Licensed Massage Therapist.
Admission Requirements: Min age: 18; High school diploma/GED.
Application Deadline(s): Winter: Feb 15; Summer: Aug 15.
Tuition and Fees: $3900.
Financial Aid: State government aid; Vocational rehabilitation; Payment plan.
Career Services: Career counseling; Career information; Interview set up.

Kilauea

337. Pacific Center for Awareness and Bodywork
Connective Bodywork; Present Centered Hypnotherapy
7703 Koolau Rd, Kilauea, HI 96754
Mailing Address: PO Box 672, Kilauea, HI 96754
Phone: (808) 828-6797; *Fax:* (808) 828-6797
E-mail: presence@gte.net *Internet:* http://www.home1.gte.net/presence/index.htm
Program Administrator: Lee Joseph, Co-Dir; Carole Madsen, Co-Dir. *Admissions Contact:* Lee Joseph; Carole Madsen.
Year Established: 1990.
Staff: Full-time: 2; Part-time: 5.
Avg Enrollment: 24. *Avg Class Size:* 12. *Number of Graduates per Year:* 24.
Wheelchair Access: Yes.
Accreditation/Approval/Licensing: State board: HI Board of Ed; National Certification Board for Therapeutic Massage and Bodywork (CEUs); American Council of Hypnotist Examiners.
Field of Study: Acupressure; Awareness Practices; Connective Bodywork; Hypnotherapy*; Massage Therapy*; Neuromuscular Therapy; Polarity Therapy; Reflexology; Structural Integration*. *Program Name/Length:* Massage Therapy, 2 1/2 mos; Structural Bodywork and Awareness, 2-6 mos; Hypnotherapy, 1-3 mos; Weekend workshops.

Degrees Offered: Certificate.
License/Certification Preparation: State: HI Certification; American Council of Hypnotist Examiners; National Certification Board for Therapeutic Massage and Bodywork.
Admission Requirements: Min age: 18.
Application Deadline(s): Fall: Sep 15; Spring: Feb 15.
Tuition and Fees: $675-$2000.
Financial Aid: State government aid; Work study; Vocational rehabilitation.
Career Services: Career counseling; Career information; Internships.

Kula

338. Hawaii College of Traditional Oriental Medicine
PO Box 457, Kula, HI 96790
Phone: (808) 573-0899; *Fax:* (808) 573-2450
E-mail: info@hawaiicollege.com *Internet:* http://www.hawaiicollege.com
Year Established: 1994.
Staff: Full-time: 9; Part-time: 5.
Avg Enrollment: 12. *Avg Class Size:* 12.
Wheelchair Access: Yes.
Accreditation/Approval/Licensing: Candidate, Accreditation Commission for Acupuncture and Oriental Medicine.
Field of Study: Acupressure; Acupuncture*; Herbal Medicine*; Oriental Medicine*; Qigong; Shiatsu; Traditional Chinese Medicine*. *Program Name/Length:* Master of Traditional Oriental Medicine, 3 yrs.
Degrees Offered: MTOM.

License/Certification Preparation: State: HI Licensed Acupuncturist; National Certification Commission for Acupuncture and Oriental Medicine.
Admission Requirements: High school diploma/GED; Some college (2 yrs).
Financial Aid: Scholarships.

Makawao

339. American Viniyoga Institute
Viniyoga Teacher and Therapist Training
PO Box 88, Makawao, HI 96768
Phone: (808) 572-1414
E-mail: info@viniyoga.com
Program Administrator: Gary Kraftsow, Dir. *Admissions Contact:* Mary Lou Mellinger, Mgmt Asst.
Year Established: 1983.
Staff: Full-time: 2; Part-time: 2.
Avg Class Size: 50.
Accreditation/Approval/Licensing: International Association of Yoga Therapists; Krishnamacharya Yoga Mandiram.
Field of Study: Yoga Teacher Training*; Yoga Therapy*. *Program Name/Length:* Viniyoga Teacher Training, 3 yrs; Viniyoga Therapist Training, 2-3 yrs.
Degrees Offered: Certificate.
Admission Requirements: Participation in open workshops and foundation trainings.
Financial Aid: Payment plan.
Career Services: Career counseling; Job information.

IDAHO

Boise

340. Idaho Institute of Wholistic Studies
Massage Practitioner Certification
1412 W Washington, Boise, ID 83702
Phone: (208) 345-2704; *Fax:* (208) 367-9242
Program Administrator: Barbera Bashan, Co-Dir; Karen Mangan, Co-Dir; Brandie Reanger, Co-Dir. *Admissions Contact:* Martha Scism, Admissions Counselor.
Year Established: 1993.
Staff: Full-time: 3; Part-time: 3.
Avg Class Size: 15.
Wheelchair Access: Yes.
Accreditation/Approval/Licensing: State board: ID Board of Ed.

Field of Study: Acupressure; Massage Therapy*; Shiatsu; Sports Massage; Traditional Chinese Medicine. *Program Name/Length:* 1-3 yrs.
Degrees Offered: Certificate.
Tuition and Fees: $3770.
Financial Aid: Vocational rehabilitation.

341. Idaho School of Massage Therapy
5353 Franklin Rd, Boise, ID 83705
Phone: (208) 343-1847
Program Administrator: Cindy J. Langston, Admin. *Admissions Contact:* Ruth R. Haefer, Dir.
Year Established: 1983.
Staff: Part-time: 8.
Avg Enrollment: 110. *Avg Class Size:* 14. *Number of Graduates per Year:* 20.

Wheelchair Access: Yes.
Field of Study: Connective Tissue Massage; Deep Tissue Massage; Massage Therapy*; Reflexology; Shiatsu; Sports Massage; Swedish Massage*. *Program Name/Length:* Basic Swedish Technician, 155 hrs, 4 mos; Massage Practitioner, 350 hrs, 6-9 mos; Massage Therapist, 1 yr.
Degrees Offered: Certificate.
License/Certification Preparation: National Certification Board for Therapeutic Massage and Bodywork.
Admission Requirements: Min age: 18.
Application Deadline(s): Fall: Sep 4; Winter: Jan 4; Spring: April 30.
Tuition and Fees: $1400 (Basic); $4000 (Massage Practitioner); $5500 (Massage Therapist).
Financial Aid: Payment plan.
Career Services: Career counseling; Career information; Referral service.

Moscow

342. Moscow School of Massage
S 600 Main, Moscow, ID 83843

Phone: (208) 882-7867
Program Administrator: Lisa O'Leary, Co-Dir; Jan Roberts, Co-Dir.
Year Established: 1994.
Staff: Full-time: 2; Part-time: 5.
Avg Enrollment: 16. *Avg Class Size:* 16. *Number of Graduates per Year:* 16.
Wheelchair Access: Yes.
Accreditation/Approval/Licensing: State board: ID Registered Vocational School; WA Board of Massage.
Field of Study: Deep Tissue Massage*; Massage Therapy*; Oriental Medicine; Qigong. *Program Name/Length:* 9 mos (Sep-Jun).
Degrees Offered: Diploma.
License/Certification Preparation: State: WA Licensed Massage Practitioner; National Certification Board for Therapeutic Massage and Bodywork.
Admission Requirements: Min age: 18; High school diploma/GED; Interview.
Application Deadline(s): Spring: Mar 30.
Tuition and Fees: $4550 + $320 books.
Financial Aid: Payment plan.
Career Services: Career information; Job information.

ILLINOIS

Chicago

343. Chicago National College of Naprapathy
Doctor of Naprapathy Program
3330 N Milwaukee Ave, Chicago, IL 60641
Phone: (773) 282-2686; *Fax:* (773) 282-2688
E-mail: naprapath@aol.com *Internet:* http://www.naprapathy.edu
Program Administrator: Dr. Paul Maguire, DN, CEO; Dr. Alexanne Osinski, DN, Admin. *Admissions Contact:* Dr. Joanne Reisner, DN, Admissions Dir.
Year Established: 1907.
Staff: Part-time: 23.
Avg Enrollment: 70. *Avg Class Size:* 30. *Number of Graduates per Year:* 30.
Wheelchair Access: No.
Accreditation/Approval/Licensing: State board: IL Board of Higher Ed; Council of the American Naprapathic Association.
Field of Study: Naprapathy*; Neuromuscular Therapy*. *Program Name/Length:* Doctor of Naprapathy, 3 yrs full-time.
Degrees Offered: Diploma; DN.
License/Certification Preparation: State: IL Licensed Naprapath.

Admission Requirements: Some college (2 yrs); Min GPA: 2.0; Specific course prerequisites: biology; general ed.
Application Deadline(s): Fall: Oct; Winter: Jan; Spring: Apr; Summer: Jul.
Tuition and Fees: $7800 per yr.
Financial Aid: VA approved; Vocational rehabilitation.
Career Services: Internships.

344. The Chicago School of Massage Therapy
Massage Therapy Diploma Program
2918 N Lincoln Ave, Chicago, IL 60657
Phone: (773) 477-9444; *Fax:* (773) 477-7256
E-mail: csmtinfo@csmt.com *Internet:* http://www.csmt.com
Program Administrator: Robert K. King, Pres. *Admissions Contact:* Jeff Marzano, Admissions Dir.
Year Established: 1981.
Staff: Part-time: 25.
Avg Enrollment: 280. *Avg Class Size:* 60. *Number of Graduates per Year:* 250.
Wheelchair Access: Yes.
Accreditation/Approval/Licensing: State board: IL Board of Ed; Commission on Massage Therapy

Accreditation; National Certification Board for Therapeutic Massage and Bodywork (CEUs).
Field of Study: Acupressure; Anatomy and Physiology; CranioSacral Therapy; Energy Work; Massage Therapy*; Myofascial Release; Reflexology; Reiki; Shiatsu; Sports Massage. *Program Name/Length:* Massage Therapy Diploma Program, 16 mos.
Degrees Offered: Diploma.
License/Certification Preparation: National Certification Board for Therapeutic Massage and Bodywork.
Admission Requirements: Min age: 18; High school diploma/GED; Specific course prerequisites: introductory massage class.
Application Deadline(s): Fall: Aug; Winter: Jan; Spring: May.
Tuition and Fees: $7300.
Financial Aid: Payment plan.
Career Services: Job information.

345. International Thai Therapists Association, Inc

Thai Massage; Nuat Thai; Nuad Boran
47 W Polk St, Ste 100-329, Chicago, IL 60605
Phone: (773) 792-4121; *Fax:* (773) 326-6442
E-mail: itta@ix.netcom.com *Internet:* http://www.thaimassage.com
Program Administrator: Anthony B. James, PhD, Dir of Ed. *Admissions Contact:* Kat Bartel, Pres, Admissions Dir.
Year Established: 1986.
Staff: Full-time: 2; Part-time: 10.
Avg Enrollment: 700. *Avg Class Size:* 20. *Number of Graduates per Year:* 700.
Wheelchair Access: Yes.
Field of Study: Acupressure; Aromatherapy; Ayurvedic Medicine; CranioSacral Therapy; Energy Work; Herbal Medicine; Massage Therapy; Neuromuscular Therapy; Oriental Medicine; Qigong; Reflexology; Reiki; Shiatsu; Thai Massage*; Traditional Chinese Medicine. *Program Name/Length:* Nuat Thai Basic Practitioner Certification, 5 levels.
Degrees Offered: Diploma; Certificate; Facilitator; Instructor; Master Instructor.
Admission Requirements: High school diploma/GED.
Application Deadline(s): Fall; Winter; Spring; Summer.
Tuition and Fees: $200-$3195.
Financial Aid: Grants; Scholarships; Work study.
Career Services: Career counseling; Career information; Internships; Resume service; Referral service; Online Directory of Practitioners.

346. Midwest Center for the Study of Oriental Medicine, Chicago

4334 N Hazel, Ste 206, Chicago, IL 60613
Phone: (773) 975-1295
E-mail: dunbrdoc@aol.com *Internet:* http://www.acupuncture.edu

Program Administrator: Dr. William Dunbar, Pres.
Avg Class Size: 30.
Accreditation/Approval/Licensing: Accreditation Commission for Acupuncture and Oriental Medicine.
Field of Study: Acupressure; Acupuncture*; Herbal Medicine; Oriental Medicine*; Traditional Chinese Medicine*. *Program Name/Length:* Acupuncture Therapist, 27 mos; Master of Science in Oriental Medicine, 3 yrs.
Degrees Offered: MS.
License/Certification Preparation: National Certification Commission for Acupuncture and Oriental Medicine.
Admission Requirements: Some college (2 yrs), Min GPA: 2.0.
Tuition and Fees: $2790 per qtr.
Financial Aid: Grants; Loans.

347. University of Illinois at Chicago, College of Nursing

Nurse-Midwifery Program
845 S Damen Ave, Chicago, IL 60612
Phone: (312) 996-7937
Internet: http://www.uic.edu/nursing/mcn.htm
Program Administrator: Janet Engstrom, PhD, Dir.
Accreditation/Approval/Licensing: American College of Nurse-Midwives, Division of Accreditation.
Field of Study: Midwifery*.
Degrees Offered: MS; PhD.
License/Certification Preparation: Certified Nurse-Midwife, American College of Nurse-Midwives.
Admission Requirements: Bachelor's degree; RN.

Crystal Lake

348. Pamela Arwine

Reiki Training; Hypnotherapy Intensive
1701 Marguerite St, Crystal Lake, IL 60014
Phone: (815) 455-4502
Program Administrator: Pamela Arwine, CHt, Reiki Master, Certified Rubenfeld Synergist. *Admissions Contact:* Pamela Arwine.
Year Established: 1996.
Staff: Full-time: 1.
Avg Enrollment: 65 Reiki, 18 Hypnotherapy. *Avg Class Size:* 8. *Number of Graduates per Year:* 50 Reiki, 15 Hypnotherapy.
Wheelchair Access: No.
Accreditation/Approval/Licensing: National Certification Board for Therapeutic Massage and Bodywork (CEUs); American Board of Hypnotherapy.
Field of Study: Hypnotherapy*; Reiki*. *Program Name/Length:* Reiki, Levels 1-4, 42 hrs; Seminars given in various locations; Reiki Advanced Training; Hypnotherapy, Units 1-4, 72 hrs; Seminars given in various locations.
Degrees Offered: CEUs; Certificate.

Admission Requirements: Min age: 21.
Tuition and Fees: $150 per course (Reiki 1 and 2); $200 per course (Reiki 3 and 4; Advanced Training); $300 per unit (Hypnotherapy).
Financial Aid: Payment plan.
Career Services: Career information; Marketing class.

East Moline

349. Best Institute of Hypnosis
832 16th Ave, East Moline, IL 61244-2124
Phone: (309) 755-2378; *Fax:* (309) 755-1669
Program Administrator: Kenn Geiger, CHt, Dir. *Admissions Contact:* Kenn Geiger.
Year Established: 1988.
Staff: Full-time: 1.
Avg Enrollment: 10. *Avg Class Size:* 5. *Number of Graduates per Year:* 9.
Accreditation/Approval/Licensing: International Medical and Dental Hypnotherapy Association.
Field of Study: Hypnotherapy*. *Program Name/Length:* Three 40-hr courses.
Degrees Offered: Certificate.
License/Certification Preparation: International Medical and Dental Hypnotherapy Association.
Admission Requirements: Min age: 18; High school diploma/GED.
Tuition and Fees: $550 per course.
Financial Aid: Payment plan.
Career Services: Mentor program.

Evanston

350. Ohashiatsu Chicago
825 Chicago Ave, Evanston, IL 60202
Phone: (847) 864-1130; *Fax:* (847) 733-9473
Program Administrator: Matthew Sweigart, Dir. *Admissions Contact:* Linda Gonnerman, Admin Asst.
Year Established: 1988.
Staff: Full-time: 1; Part-time: 20.
Avg Enrollment: 200. *Avg Class Size:* 15. *Number of Graduates per Year:* 10.
Wheelchair Access: No.
Field of Study: Acupressure*; Shiatsu*. *Program Name/Length:* Ohashiatsu, 1 1/2-3 yrs.
Degrees Offered: Certificate.
Tuition and Fees: $4500.
Financial Aid: Work study; Discount for advance registration.
Career Services: Internships.

Galena

351. Integrative Yoga Therapy
1207 Lincoln Ave, Galena, IL 61036
Phone: (815) 777-6068, (800) 750-9642; *Fax:* (815) 777-6629

E-mail: iyt@cruzio.com
Program Administrator: Joseph LePage, Dir. *Admissions Contact:* Joseph LePage.
Year Established: 1991.
Staff: Full-time: 2; Part-time: 8.
Avg Enrollment: 150. *Avg Class Size:* 40. *Number of Graduates per Year:* 125.
Field of Study: Yoga Teacher Training*. *Program Name/Length:* Yoga and Mind Body Health, 6-12 mos; Seminars given in various locations.
Degrees Offered: Certificate.
Admission Requirements: Min age: 18.
Tuition and Fees: $1675.
Financial Aid: Work study.
Career Services: Career counseling; Career information; Internships.

Herrin

352. Edens Institute of Alternative Therapy
212 N Park, Herrin, IL 62948
Mailing Address: 550 Packentack Rd, Ozark, IL 62972
Phone: (618) 942-8825
E-mail: lorim@midwest.net
Program Administrator: Lori McCraw, ND, Dir. *Admissions Contact:* E. J. Engram, ND.
Year Established: 1996.
Staff: Full-time: 2.
Avg Class Size: 8. *Number of Graduates per Year:* 8.
Wheelchair Access: Yes.
Accreditation/Approval/Licensing: State board: IL Board of Ed.
Field of Study: Massage Therapy*. *Program Name/Length:* 100 hrs; 500 hrs.
Application Deadline(s): Fall: Aug 1; Winter: Jan 1.
Tuition and Fees: $600 (100 hrs); $3000 (500 hrs).
Financial Aid: Loans; Job Training Partnership Act.

Lombard

353. The National College of Chiropractic
200 E Roosevelt Rd, Lombard, IL 60148
Phone: (630) 629-2000, (800) 826-6285; *Fax:* (630) 889-6554
Internet: http://www.national.chiropractic.edu
Program Administrator: James F. Winterstein, DC, Pres. *Admissions Contact:* Julia Talarico, Admissions Dir.
Year Established: 1906.
Staff: Full-time: 73; Part-time: 20.
Avg Enrollment: 850. *Number of Graduates per Year:* 270.
Wheelchair Access: Yes.
Accreditation/Approval/Licensing: State board: IL State Board of Chiropractic; Council on

Chiropractic Education; North Central Association of Colleges and Schools.

Field of Study: Acupuncture; Chiropractic*. *Program Name/Length:* Doctor of Chiropractic, 10 trimesters.

Degrees Offered: BS; DC.

License/Certification Preparation: State: IL Doctor of Chiropractic.

Admission Requirements: Min age: 20; High school diploma/GED; Min GPA: 2.5; Bachelor's degree.

Tuition and Fees: $6200 per trimester.

Financial Aid: Fellowships; Federal government aid; Grants; Loans; Scholarships; State government aid; Work study.

Career Services: Career counseling; Career information; Internships; Preceptorship program.

Peoria

354. LifePath School of Massage Therapy

7820 N University, Ste 110, Peoria, IL 61614

Phone: (888) 2-LifePath (254-3372); *Fax:* (309) 693-7293

E-mail: rwasher@flink.com

Program Administrator: Rhonda Washer, MS, Dir.

Year Established: 1991.

Staff: Full-time: 2; Part-time: 9.

Avg Enrollment: 22. *Avg Class Size:* 22. *Number of Graduates per Year:* 22.

Wheelchair Access: Yes.

Accreditation/Approval/Licensing: State board: IL Board of Ed; International Massage and Somatic Therapies Accreditation Council; National Certification Board for Therapeutic Massage and Bodywork (CEUs).

Field of Study: CranioSacral Therapy; Massage Therapy*; Neuromuscular Therapy; Polarity Therapy; Reflexology; Shiatsu; Sports Massage; Swedish Massage*. *Program Name/Length:* Therapeutic Massage and Bodywork Training, 10 mos.

Degrees Offered: Diploma.

License/Certification Preparation: National Certification Board for Therapeutic Massage and Bodywork.

Admission Requirements: Min age: 18; High school diploma/GED; Min GPA: 2.0.

Application Deadline(s): Fall: Aug.

Tuition and Fees: $7000.

Financial Aid: Loans.

Rock Island

355. Kurashova Institute, Inc

Russian Neuro-Muscular Re-Education

PO Box 6246, Rock Island, IL 61201

Phone: (309) 786-4888; *Fax:* (309) 786-8687

Program Administrator: Zhenya K. Wine, Pres. *Admissions Contact:* Dir of Ed.

Year Established: 1986.

Staff: Full-time: 2; Part-time: 2.

Avg Enrollment: 600. *Avg Class Size:* 20. *Number of Graduates per Year:* 100.

Wheelchair Access: Yes.

Accreditation/Approval/Licensing: National Certification Board for Therapeutic Massage and Bodywork (CEUs).

Field of Study: Massage Therapy*; Neuromuscular Therapy*; Russian Massage*. *Program Name/Length:* 8-100 hrs; Seminars given in various locations.

Degrees Offered: Diploma.

License/Certification Preparation: Saskatchewan, Canada; National Certification Board for Therapeutic Massage and Bodywork.

Admission Requirements: Massage therapy course; RN recommended.

Tuition and Fees: $150-$1300.

Financial Aid: Payment plan.

Career Services: Internships.

Schaumburg

356. The Leidecker Institute

Hypnotherapy

1901 N Roselle Rd, Ste 800, Schaumburg, IL 60195

Phone: (847) 844-1933

E-mail: nghschool@aol.com *Internet:* http://www.brightfuture.org

Program Administrator: Arthur A. Leidecker, CH, Dir. *Admissions Contact:* Lynsi Brule, Admissions.

Year Established: 1970.

Staff: Full-time: 1; Part-time: 4.

Avg Class Size: 20.

Wheelchair Access: Yes.

Field of Study: Acupressure; Aromatherapy; Hypnotherapy*; Reflexology; Reiki*. *Program Name/Length:* Hypnotherapy, 100 hrs; Seminars given in various locations; Reiki, 100 hrs.

Degrees Offered: Certificate.

License/Certification Preparation: National Guild of Hypnotists.

Admission Requirements: Min age: 18; High school diploma/GED.

Application Deadline(s): Fall; Winter; Spring; Summer.

Financial Aid: Payment plan.

Career Services: Career counseling; Career information; Internships; Marketing classes.

Sycamore

357. Northern Prairie School of Therapeutic Massage and Bodywork, Inc

Massage Therapy; Therapeutic Herbalism

138 N Fair St, Sycamore, IL 60178

Phone: (815) 899-3382; *Fax:* (815) 899-3381

Program Administrator: Jeannette Vaupel, RN,
Dir. *Admissions Contact:* Jeannette Vaupel.
Year Established: 1993.
Staff: Part-time: 20.
Avg Enrollment: 50. *Avg Class Size:* 18. *Number
of Graduates per Year:* 45.
Wheelchair Access: Yes.
Accreditation/Approval/Licensing: State board: IL
Board of Ed; International Massage and Somatic
Therapies Accreditation Council; National Cer-
tification Board for Therapeutic Massage and
Bodywork (CEUs).
Field of Study: Acupressure; Aromatherapy;
Ayurvedic Medicine; Biofeedback; CranioSacral
Therapy; Energy Work; Herbal Medicine*; Ho-
meopathy; Hypnotherapy; Massage Therapy*;
Oriental Medicine; Polarity Therapy; Qigong;
Reflexology; Reiki; Shiatsu; Traditional Chinese
Medicine. *Program Name/Length:* Massage
Therapy, 600 hrs, 11 mos; Therapeutic
Herbalism, 200 hrs, 9 mos; Seminars given in
various locations.
Degrees Offered: Diploma.
License/Certification Preparation: National Certif-
ication Board for Therapeutic Massage and
Bodywork.
Admission Requirements: Min age: 18; High
school diploma/GED.
Application Deadline(s): Fall: Dec 1; Summer:
Aug 1.
Tuition and Fees: $8800 (Massage Therapy);
$3000 (Herbalism).

Urbana

358. Urbana Center for the Alexander Technique

508 W Washington St, Urbana, IL 61801
Phone: (217) 367-3172
Program Administrator: Joan Murray, Co-Dir; Al-
exander Murray, Co-Dir; Rose Bronec, Co-Dir;
Richard Carbaugh, Co-Dir.
Year Established: 1977.
Accreditation/Approval/Licensing: American Soci-
ety for the Alexander Technique.
Field of Study: Alexander Technique*. *Program
Name/Length:* Teacher Training, 3 yrs.
License/Certification Preparation: American Soci-
ety for the Alexander Technique.
Admission Requirements: Specific course prerequi-
sites: prior lessons in the Alexander Technique.
Tuition and Fees: $4200 per yr.

Woodridge

359. Center for Therapeutic Massage and Wellness

2704 Woodridge Dr, Woodridge, IL 60517

Phone: (708) 960-9053
Program Administrator: Bea Stanton, Dir. *Admis-
sions Contact:* Bea Stanton.
Year Established: 1987.
Staff: Full-time: 1; Part-time: 6.
Avg Enrollment: 30. *Avg Class Size:* 10. *Number
of Graduates per Year:* 28.
Wheelchair Access: No.
Accreditation/Approval/Licensing: State board: IL
Board of Ed.
Field of Study: CranioSacral Therapy; Energy
Work; Massage Therapy*; Qigong; Reflexology;
Reiki; Sports Massage; Therapeutic Touch. *Pro-
gram Name/Length:* Basic Therapeutic Mas-
sage, 9 mos.
Degrees Offered: CEUs; Certificate.
Admission Requirements: Min age: 18; High
school diploma/GED.
Application Deadline(s): Fall: Sep.
Tuition and Fees: $2550.
Financial Aid: Payment plan.

360. Wellness and Massage Training Institute

Massage Therapy; Oriental Studies
1051 Internationale Pkwy, Woodridge, IL 60517
Phone: (630) 325-3773
E-mail: info@wmti.com *Internet:* http://www.
wmti.com
Program Administrator: Raymond Miller, Dir. *Ad-
missions Contact:* Sandy Kessel, Admissions
Dir.
Year Established: 1989.
Staff: Part-time: 40.
Avg Enrollment: 750. *Avg Class Size:* 20. *Number
of Graduates per Year:* 75.
Wheelchair Access: Yes.
Accreditation/Approval/Licensing: State board: IL
Board of Ed; Commission on Massage Therapy
Accreditation; National Certification Board for
Therapeutic Massage and Bodywork (CEUs).
Field of Study: Aromatherapy; CranioSacral Ther-
apy; Massage Therapy*; Oriental Medicine;
Ortho-Bionomy*; Qigong; Reflexology*;
Shiatsu; Sports Massage; Traditional Chinese
Medicine*. *Program Name/Length:* Profes-
sional Massage Therapy Training, 2-3 yrs; Ori-
ental Studies, 2-3 yrs.
Degrees Offered: Diploma.
License/Certification Preparation: National Certif-
ication Board for Therapeutic Massage and
Bodywork.
Admission Requirements: Min age: 18; High
school diploma/GED; Comprehensive reading
test.
Application Deadline(s): Fall: Jul; Winter: Nov;
Spring: Mar.
Tuition and Fees: $7500 per program.
Career Services: Job information.

INDIANA

Alexandria

361. Alexandria School of Scientific Therapeutics, Inc
Swedish Massage Therapy and Pfrimmer Deep Muscle Therapy
809 S Harrison St, Alexandria, IN 46001
Mailing Address: PO Box 287, Alexandria, IN 46001
Phone: (765) 724-9152; *Fax:* (765) 724-9156
E-mail: alexssi@netusa1.net *Internet:* http://www.assti.com
Program Administrator: Herbert L. Hobbs, Admin. *Admissions Contact:* Herbert L. Hobbs.
Year Established: 1982.
Staff: Full-time: 3; Part-time: 10.
Avg Enrollment: 96. *Avg Class Size:* 34. *Number of Graduates per Year:* 96.
Wheelchair Access: Yes.
Accreditation/Approval/Licensing: State board: IN Commission on Proprietary Ed.
Field of Study: Acupressure; Aromatherapy; Ayurvedic Medicine; Deep Muscle Massage; Energy Work; Feldenkrais; Herbal Medicine; Homeopathy; Massage Therapy*; Neuromuscular Therapy; Oriental Medicine; Polarity Therapy; Reflexology; Shiatsu; Sports Massage; Swedish Massage*. *Program Name/Length:* 10 1/2 mos.
Degrees Offered: Diploma.
License/Certification Preparation: National Certification Board for Therapeutic Massage and Bodywork.
Admission Requirements: Min age: 18; High school diploma/GED; 2 letters of recommendation; Interview with administrator.
Application Deadline(s): Summer: Jul 15.
Tuition and Fees: $5800.
Financial Aid: Loans; Vocational rehabilitation.
Career Services: Referral service.

Crown Point

362. American Certified Massage School
Massage Therapist Course
109 1/2 W Joliet St, Crown Point, IN 46307
Phone: (219) 661-9099; *Fax:* (219) 661-8978
Internet: http://www.hhgi.net/gale.miller.htm
Program Administrator: Gale Miller, Dir. *Admissions Contact:* Gale Miller.
Year Established: 1998.
Staff: Part-time: 4.
Avg Enrollment: 32. *Avg Class Size:* 8. *Number of Graduates per Year:* 32.

Wheelchair Access: No.
Accreditation/Approval/Licensing: State board: IN Commission on Proprietary Ed.
Field of Study: Aromatherapy; Deep Tissue Massage; Massage Therapy*; Reflexology; Sports Massage. *Program Name/Length:* Massage Therapist, 662 hrs; Reflexology and Sports Massage, 24 hrs.
Degrees Offered: Certificate.
Admission Requirements: Min age: 18.
Application Deadline(s): Fall: Sep 21; Winter: Jan 31; Spring: May 31.
Career Services: Career counseling.

Fort Wayne

363. Ivy Tech State College
Massage Therapy
3800 N Anthony Blvd, Fort Wayne, IN 46805
Phone: (219) 482-9171; *Fax:* (219) 480-4149
E-mail: drogers@ivy.tec.in.us *Internet:* http://www.ivy.tec.in.us/fortwayne
Program Administrator: Dee Rogers, MS, Health and Human Svcs Division Chair. *Admissions Contact:* Neal Davis, Admissions.
Year Established: 1996.
Staff: Part-time: 6.
Avg Class Size: 14.
Wheelchair Access: Yes.
Accreditation/Approval/Licensing: North Central Association of Colleges and Schools.
Field of Study: Massage Therapy*. *Program Name/Length:* Associate of Applied Science in Massage Therapy, 5-6 semesters.
Degrees Offered: AAS.
License/Certification Preparation: National Certification Board for Therapeutic Massage and Bodywork.
Admission Requirements: Min age: 18; High school diploma/GED.
Application Deadline(s): Fall; Winter; Spring; Summer.
Tuition and Fees: $66.50 per credit hr.
Financial Aid: Federal government aid; Loans; Scholarships; Work study; VA approved; Vocational rehabilitation.
Career Services: Career counseling; Career information; Resume service.

364. Midwest Training Institute of Hypnosis
Hypnosis and Regression Therapy
2121 Engle Rd, Ste 3A, Fort Wayne, IN 46809
Phone: (219) 747-6774; *Fax:* (219) 747-6774

Program Administrator: Gisella Zukausky, CHt, Dir. *Admissions Contact:* Gisella Zukausky.
Year Established: 1987.
Staff: Full-time: 1.
Wheelchair Access: Yes.
Accreditation/Approval/Licensing: State board: IN Commission on Proprietary Ed; International Medical and Dental Hypnotherapy Association.
Field of Study: Hypnotherapy*. *Program Name/Length:* Hypnosis and Regression Therapy, 120 hrs; Nonverbal Technique, 30 hrs; Seminars given in various locations; Home study/Correspondence.
Degrees Offered: Certificate.
License/Certification Preparation: International Medical and Dental Hypnotherapy Association.
Admission Requirements: Min age: 18; High school diploma/GED.
Tuition and Fees: $789 (120 hrs); $365 (30 hrs).

Indianapolis

365. Academy of Reflexology and Health Therapy International
8397 E 10th St, Indianapolis, IN 46219-5330
Phone: (317) 897-5111; *Fax:* (317) 897-5115
Program Administrator: E. James O'Donnell, Admin Dir; Dr. Christina J. Brown, Exec Dir. *Admissions Contact:* E. James O'Donnell, Admin Dir.
Year Established: 1990.
Staff: Full-time: 2; Part-time: 4.
Avg Enrollment: 40. *Avg Class Size:* 15. *Number of Graduates per Year:* 30.
Wheelchair Access: Yes.
Accreditation/Approval/Licensing: State board: IN Commission on Proprietary Ed.
Field of Study: Acupressure; Alexander Technique; Energy Work; Feldenkrais; Homeopathy*; Massage Therapy*; Polarity Therapy; Reflexology*; Sports Massage. *Program Name/Length:* Reflexology, 175 hrs, 10 weekends; Healing Massage Techniques, 200 hrs, 12 weekends.
Degrees Offered: Certificate.
Admission Requirements: Min age: 18; High school diploma/GED.
Tuition and Fees: $1400 (Reflexology); $1600 (Massage).
Financial Aid: Payment plan.
Career Services: Training and counseling in business promotion.

366. Indiana University, Purdue University at Indianapolis
Massage Therapy Program
620 N Union Dr, Rm 142, Indianapolis, IN 46202

Phone: (317) 274-2887; *Fax:* (317) 274-2638
Program Administrator: Tom McCarthy, Prog Admin. *Admissions Contact:* Janis Legendre, Prog Coord.
Year Established: 1994.
Staff: Full-time: 4; Part-time: 12.
Avg Enrollment: 75. *Avg Class Size:* 22. *Number of Graduates per Year:* 70.
Wheelchair Access: Yes.
Accreditation/Approval/Licensing: State board: IN Board of Postsecondary Ed; Accrediting Council for Continuing Education and Training; North Central Association of Colleges and Schools.
Field of Study: Massage Therapy*. *Program Name/Length:* 500 hrs and 100 log sessions, 3 semesters, 11 mos.
Degrees Offered: Certificate.
License/Certification Preparation: National Certification Board for Therapeutic Massage and Bodywork.
Admission Requirements: Min age: 18; High school diploma/GED.
Application Deadline(s): Fall: Jul 1; Spring: Feb 15.
Tuition and Fees: $3750.
Financial Aid: Federal government aid; VA approved.

Long Beach

367. Dancing Feet Yoga Center, Inc
YogaKids Facilitator Certification
2501 Oriole Trail, Long Beach, IN 46360
Phone: (219) 872-9611, (800) 968-0694; *Fax:* (219) 873-7612
E-mail: innerwrk@niia.net *Internet:* http://www.yogakids.com
Program Administrator: Marsha Wenig, Creative Dir. *Admissions Contact:* Marsha Wenig.
Year Established: 1997.
Staff: Full-time: 1.
Avg Enrollment: 100. *Avg Class Size:* 15. *Number of Graduates per Year:* 10.
Wheelchair Access: Yes.
Field of Study: Yoga Teacher Training*. *Program Name/Length:* 8-14 mos.
Degrees Offered: Certificate; Certified YogaKids Facilitator.
Admission Requirements: Min age: 18; Bachelor's degree.
Application Deadline(s): Fall; Winter; Spring; Summer.
Tuition and Fees: $1550 + yearly licensing fees.
Financial Aid: Payment plan.
Career Services: Career counseling; Job information; Referral service.

IOWA

Anamosa

368. Carlson College of Massage Therapy
11809 County Rd X 28, Anamosa, IA 52205
Phone: (319) 462-3402; *Fax:* (319) 462-5990
E-mail: carlc@inab.net
Program Administrator: Ruth A. Carlson, Dir. *Admissions Contact:* Wayne Anthony Pakulis, Admin.
Year Established: 1984.
Staff: Full-time: 3; Part-time: 5.
Avg Enrollment: 60. *Avg Class Size:* 30. *Number of Graduates per Year:* 58.
Wheelchair Access: No.
Accreditation/Approval/Licensing: State board: IA Dept of Health Massage Therapy Advisory Board; Commission on Massage Therapy Accreditation.
Field of Study: Aromatherapy; Energy Work; Herbal Medicine; Massage Therapy*; Polarity Therapy; Reflexology; Shiatsu; Sports Massage. *Program Name/Length:* 5 1/2 mos.
Degrees Offered: CEUs; Diploma.
License/Certification Preparation: State: IA Licensed Massage Therapist; National Certification Board for Therapeutic Massage and Bodywork.
Admission Requirements: Min age: 18; High school diploma/GED.
Application Deadline(s): Fall: Sep 1; Spring: Mar 1.
Tuition and Fees: $5000.
Financial Aid: VA approved; Vocational rehabilitation.
Career Services: Internships; Job listings board.

Cedar Rapids

369. Capri College of Massage Therapy, Cedar Rapids
315 2nd Ave SE, Cedar Rapids, IA 52401
Mailing Address: PO Box 74912, Cedar Rapids, IA 52407-4912
Phone: (319) 364-1541
E-mail: cradm@mwci.net *Internet:* http://www.capricollege.com
Program Administrator: Melissa Strouf, LMT, Prog Dir. *Admissions Contact:* Joni Westphall, Admissions Dir.
Year Established: 1994.
Staff: Full-time: 2; Part-time: 1.
Avg Enrollment: 36. *Avg Class Size:* 12. *Number of Graduates per Year:* 35.
Wheelchair Access: No.

Accreditation/Approval/Licensing: State board: IA Board of Massage; Accrediting Commission of Career Schools and Colleges of Technology.
Field of Study: Acupressure; Aromatherapy*; Deep Tissue Massage*; Massage Therapy*; Reflexology*. *Program Name/Length:* Massage Therapy, 650 hrs.
Degrees Offered: Diploma.
License/Certification Preparation: State: IA Licensed Massage Therapist; National Certification Board for Therapeutic Massage and Bodywork.
Admission Requirements: Min age: 18; High school diploma/GED; Min GPA: 2.0.
Application Deadline(s): Fall: Sep 1; Winter: Jan 1; Spring: May 1.
Tuition and Fees: $5600-$6000.
Financial Aid: Federal government aid; Scholarships; State government aid; VA approved; Vocational rehabilitation.
Career Services: Career information.

Davenport

370. Capri College, Davenport
Massage Therapy
425 E 59th St, Davenport, IA 52807
Phone: (319) 388-6642
Internet: http://www.capricollege.com
Program Administrator: Bob Cox, Massage Therapy Dir. *Admissions Contact:* Heather McClanahan, Admissions Representative.
Year Established: 1994.
Staff: Full-time: 2; Part-time: 4.
Avg Enrollment: 40. *Avg Class Size:* 14. *Number of Graduates per Year:* 40.
Wheelchair Access: Yes.
Accreditation/Approval/Licensing: State board: IA Board of Massage Therapy; Accrediting Commission of Career Schools and Colleges of Technology.
Field of Study: Acupressure; Aromatherapy; Massage Therapy*; Neuromuscular Therapy; Polarity Therapy; Reflexology; Reiki; Shiatsu; Sports Massage. *Program Name/Length:* 650 hrs, 28 wks.
Degrees Offered: Diploma.
License/Certification Preparation: State: IA Licensed Massage Therapist; National Certification Board for Therapeutic Massage and Bodywork.
Admission Requirements: High school diploma/GED; Min GPA: 2.0; 2 reference letters; high school and any college transcripts.
Tuition and Fees: $6200.

Financial Aid: Federal government aid; Grants; Loans; VA approved; Vocational rehabilitation; Payment plan.

Career Services: Career counseling; Career information; Internships; Resume service; Job information.

371. Institute of Therapeutic Massage and Wellness

516 W 35th St, Davenport, IA 52806
Phone: (319) 445-1055; *Fax:* (319) 285-5201
Program Administrator: Dan Howes, DC, Dir of Admin. *Admissions Contact:* Bonita Howes, LMT.
Year Established: 1997.
Staff: Full-time: 8; Part-time: 20.
Avg Enrollment: 60. *Avg Class Size:* 20. *Number of Graduates per Year:* 60.
Wheelchair Access: Yes.
Accreditation/Approval/Licensing: State board: IA Dept of Health; IA Massage Therapy Board.
Field of Study: Acupressure; Aromatherapy; CranioSacral Therapy; Energy Work; Massage Therapy*; Neuromuscular Therapy; Polarity Therapy; Reflexology; Reiki; Shiatsu; Sports Massage; Yoga Teacher Training. *Program Name/Length:* Massage Therapy, 650 hrs, 9 mos/days or 1 yr/evenings.
Degrees Offered: Diploma; Certificate.
License/Certification Preparation: State: IA Licensed Massage Therapist; National Certification Board for Therapeutic Massage and Bodywork.
Admission Requirements: Min age: 18; High school diploma/GED.
Application Deadline(s): Fall: Aug, days; Winter: Jan, evenings; Summer: Jul, evenings.
Tuition and Fees: $4500 + $300 books, fees.
Financial Aid: Loans; Work study; Vocational rehabilitation; Payment plan.
Career Services: Career information; Internships; Interview set up; Job information; Referral service.

372. Palmer College of Chiropractic

1000 Brady St, Davenport, IA 52803
Phone: (319) 884-5000; *Fax:* (319) 884-5897
E-mail: pcadmit@palmer.edu
Program Administrator: Guy F. Riekeman, DC, Pres. *Admissions Contact:* David B. Anderson, DC, Dir of Admissions.
Year Established: 1897.
Staff: Full-time: 124; Part-time: 7.
Avg Enrollment: 1800. *Avg Class Size:* 185. *Number of Graduates per Year:* 550.
Wheelchair Access: Yes.
Accreditation/Approval/Licensing: Council on Chiropractic Education; North Central Association of Colleges and Schools.
Field of Study: Chiropractic*. *Program Name/Length:* Chiropractic Technology, 4 trimesters, 1 1/2 yrs; Bachelor of Science, 10 trimesters, 3 1/3 yrs; Doctor of Chiropractic, 10 trimesters, 3 1/3 yrs.
Degrees Offered: BS; DC; MS; Chiropractic Technology.
License/Certification Preparation: National Board of Chiropractic Examiners.
Admission Requirements: High school diploma/GED; Some college (2 yrs); Specific course prerequisites: 6 semester hrs each (with lab): biology, organic chemistry, inorganic chemistry, physics; 3 semester hrs psychology; 6 semester hrs English/communication skills; 15 semester hrs social science/humanities; Min GPA: 2.0.
Application Deadline(s): Fall: Oct; Spring: Feb; Summer: Jun.
Tuition and Fees: $4990 per trimester.
Financial Aid: Federal government aid; Grants; Loans; Scholarships; State government aid; Work study.
Career Services: Professional Opportunities Office.

Fairfield

373. Maharishi University of Management

College of Maharishi Vedic Medicine
Fairfield, IA 52557
Phone: (515) 472-1110; *Fax:* (515) 472-1179
E-mail: admissions@mum.edu *Internet:* http://www.mum.edu/CMVM
Program Administrator: Robert Schneider, MD, Dean. *Admissions Contact:* John Revolinski, Assoc Dir of Admissions.
Year Established: 1997.
Staff: Full-time: 8; Part-time: 2.
Avg Enrollment: 40. *Avg Class Size:* 40.
Wheelchair Access: Yes.
Accreditation/Approval/Licensing: North Central Association of Colleges and Schools.
Field of Study: Ayurvedic Medicine*; Herbal Medicine; Maharishi Vedic Medicine*. *Program Name/Length:* BA/BS, 4 yrs (major is 2 yrs with fieldwork each yr); PhD, 4 yrs + 2 yr foundation program (undergraduate major).
Degrees Offered: BS; PhD.
Admission Requirements: Min age: 17; High school diploma/GED; Bachelor's degree for PhD.
Application Deadline(s): Fall: prefer by Apr 30.
Tuition and Fees: $20,230 per yr.
Financial Aid: Federal government aid; Grants; Loans; Scholarships; State government aid; Work study.
Career Services: Career counseling; Career information; Internships; Interview set up.

Fort Dodge

374. Millenium College of Massage and Reflexology
934 S 17th St, Fort Dodge, IA 50501
Phone: (515) 955-2296; *Fax:* (515) 955-7709
E-mail: dreamer2@frontiernet.net
Program Administrator: Angie Eldridge, Owner.
   Admissions Contact: Angie Eldridge.
Year Established: 1984.
Staff: Full-time: 1; Part-time: 2.
Avg Enrollment: 15. *Avg Class Size:* 8. *Number of
   Graduates per Year:* 15.
Wheelchair Access: Yes.
Accreditation/Approval/Licensing: State board: IA
   Dept of Health Massage Therapy Advisory
   Board.
Field of Study: Acupressure; Aromatherapy;
   CranioSacral Therapy; Massage Therapy*;
   Reflexology*. *Program Name/Length:* 576 hrs,
   8 mos; 1000 hrs, 6 mos.
Degrees Offered: Diploma; Certificate.
License/Certification Preparation: State: IA Li-
   censed Massage Therapist; National Certifica-
   tion Board for Therapeutic Massage and Body-
   work.
Admission Requirements: Min age: 18; High
   school diploma/GED; Min GPA: 2.5.
Tuition and Fees: $5000 (576 hrs); $7500 (1000
   hrs).

Financial Aid: Loans.
Career Services: Internships.

West Union

375. MotherCare Doula Training
244 S Walnut, West Union, IA 52175
Phone: (319) 422-8833, (800) 648-3662
E-mail: theyoungs@trxinc.com
Program Administrator: Debbie Young, CD, Dir.
   Admissions Contact: Debbie Young.
Year Established: 1993.
Staff: Full-time: 1; Part-time: 1.
Avg Enrollment: 70. *Avg Class Size:* 20. *Number
   of Graduates per Year:* 70.
Accreditation/Approval/Licensing: Doulas of
   North America.
Field of Study: Doula*. *Program Name/Length:*
   Doula Training, 16 hrs; Seminars given in vari-
   ous locations.
Degrees Offered: Certificate.
License/Certification Preparation: Fulfills one step
   toward DONA certification.
Admission Requirements: Childbirth education
   course or knowledge of labor as RN.
Tuition and Fees: $300.
Financial Aid: Scholarships; Payment plan.
Career Services: Job information.

KANSAS

Overland Park

376. BMSI Institute, LLC
Massage Therapy
8665 W 96th St, Ste 300, Overland Park, KS 66212
Phone: (913) 649-3322; *Fax:* (913) 649-1010
E-mail: psmith3027@aol.com *Internet:* http://
   www.bmsi-institute.com
Program Administrator: Peggy Smith, Dir of Ed.
   Admissions Contact: Peggy Smith.
Year Established: 1994.
Staff: Full-time: 3; Part-time: 14.
Avg Enrollment: 46. *Avg Class Size:* 16 (Tech-
   niques), 36 (Theory). *Number of Graduates per
   Year:* 30.
Wheelchair Access: Yes.
Accreditation/Approval/Licensing: State board: KS
   Board of Ed; National Certification Board for
   Therapeutic Massage and Bodywork (CEUs).
Field of Study: Acupressure; Aromatherapy;
   CranioSacral Therapy; Energy Work; Massage
   Therapy*; Polarity Therapy; Qigong;
   Reflexology; Reiki; Sports Massage; Traditional

Chinese Medicine. *Program Name/Length:* 500
   hrs, 2 yrs, self-paced.
Degrees Offered: Diploma.
License/Certification Preparation: State: IA Li-
   censed Massage Therapist; Kansas City license.
Admission Requirements: Min age: 18; High
   school diploma/GED.
Application Deadline(s): Fall: Aug 5; Spring: Dec
   5; Summer: May 5.
Tuition and Fees: $4750.
Financial Aid: Work study; VA approved; Voca-
   tional rehabilitation; Job Training Partnership
   Act; Payment plan.
Career Services: Career counseling; Career infor-
   mation.

377. Johnson County Community College
Therapeutic Massage Certification/Center for Pro-
fessional Education
9780 W 87th St, Overland Park, KS 66212
Mailing Address: 12345 College Blvd, Box 67,
   Overland Park, KS 66210
Phone: (913) 469-4422; *Fax:* (913) 649-1050

E-mail: mcdaniel@jccc.net *Internet:* http://www.jccc.net/conted/cpc

Program Administrator: Karen McDaniel, Prog Dir.

Year Established: 1995.

Staff: Part-time: 10.

Avg Enrollment: 42. *Avg Class Size:* 16. *Number of Graduates per Year:* 30.

Wheelchair Access: Yes.

Accreditation/Approval/Licensing: North Central Association of Colleges and Schools.

Field of Study: Aromatherapy; CranioSacral Therapy; Hydrotherapy; Massage Therapy*; Reflexology. *Program Name/Length:* Certificate, 3 semesters; CEUs, 8-30 hrs.

Degrees Offered: CEUs; Certificate.

License/Certification Preparation: National Certification Board for Therapeutic Massage and Bodywork.

Admission Requirements: High school diploma/GED; Specific course prerequisites: human anatomy and physiology; 3 one-hr massages.

Application Deadline(s): Fall: Apr 30; Winter: Oct 30.

Tuition and Fees: $4200.

Financial Aid: Payment plan; Pending, VA approval.

Career Services: Career counseling; Job information.

Wichita

378. Kansas College of Chinese Medicine
9235 E Harry St, Bldg 100, Ste 1A, Wichita, KS 67207

Phone: (316) 691-8822; *Fax:* (316) 691-8868

E-mail: kccm@southwind.net

Program Administrator: Dr. Qizhi Gao, Pres. *Admissions Contact:* Lawrence Scott, Exec Dir.

Year Established: 1997.

Staff: Full-time: 3; Part-time: 7.

Avg Enrollment: 18. *Avg Class Size:* 6.

Wheelchair Access: Yes.

Accreditation/Approval/Licensing: State board: KS Board of Ed.

Field of Study: Acupressure; Acupuncture*; CranioSacral Therapy; Deep Tissue Massage; Energy Work; Herbal Medicine*; Massage Therapy*; Oriental Medicine; Qigong; Shiatsu; Sports Massage; Traditional Chinese Medicine*. *Program Name/Length:* Massage, 525 contact hrs (35 credit hrs), 1 yr; Acupuncture, 2002 contact hrs (121 credit hrs), 3 yrs; Herbal Medicine, 2370 contact hrs (158 credit hrs), 4 yrs.

Degrees Offered: Diploma; Certificate.

License/Certification Preparation: National Certification Commission for Acupuncture and Oriental Medicine; National Certification Board for Therapeutic Massage and Bodywork.

Admission Requirements: Min age: 21; Some college (AA or 60 hrs); Min GPA: 3.0; Specific course prerequisites: biology, chemistry, and physics may be taken concurrently.

Application Deadline(s): Fall: Jul 5; Spring: Nov 5.

Tuition and Fees: $125 per credit hr/full-time; $150 per credit hr/part-time.

Financial Aid: Payment plan.

Career Services: Career counseling; Career information; Internships.

KENTUCKY

Hyden

379. Frontier School of Midwifery and Family Nursing
Community-Based Nurse-Midwifery Education Program (CNEP)

Hospital Hill, Hyden, KY 41749

Mailing Address: PO Box 528, Hyden, KY 41749

Phone: (606) 672-2312

E-mail: cnep@midwives.org *Internet:* http://www.midwives.org

Program Administrator: Susan E. Stone, CNM, Prog Dir. *Admissions Contact:* Jeanette Woods, Registrar.

Year Established: 1939.

Staff: Full-time: 10; Part-time: 30.

Avg Enrollment: 100. *Avg Class Size:* 40. *Number of Graduates per Year:* 120.

Wheelchair Access: Yes.

Accreditation/Approval/Licensing: American College of Nurse-Midwives, Division of Accreditation.

Field of Study: Midwifery*. *Program Name/Length:* 2 yrs.

Degrees Offered: MS; Certificate.

License/Certification Preparation: Certified Nurse-Midwife, American College of Nurse-Midwives.

Admission Requirements: Bachelor's degree; Min GPA: 3.0; RN.

Application Deadline(s): Fall: Oct 31; Spring: Mar 31.

Tuition and Fees: $16,200.
Financial Aid: Fellowships; Federal government aid; Grants; Loans; Scholarships; State government aid.
Career Services: Career counseling; Career information.

LaGrange

380. Infinite Light Healing Studies Center, Inc

3509 W Dogwood Cir, LaGrange, KY 40031
Phone: (502) 454-0430; *Fax:* (502) 241-8732
E-mail: lauramaya@aol.com
Program Administrator: Laurelle Gaia, Dir. *Admissions Contact:* Laurelle Gaia.
Year Established: 1991.
Staff: Full-time: 1.
Avg Enrollment: 350. *Avg Class Size:* 10. *Number of Graduates per Year:* 350.
Accreditation/Approval/Licensing: National Certification Board for Therapeutic Massage and Bodywork (CEUs); American Holistic Nurses Association.
Field of Study: Energy Work*; Reiki*. *Program Name/Length:* Reiki Training; Seminars given in various locations.
Degrees Offered: Certificate.
Admission Requirements: Min age: 18.

Lexington

381. Bluegrass Professional School of Massage Therapy

Theory and Practice of Therapeutic Massage
501 Darby Creek, Ste 14, Lexington, KY 40509
Phone: (606) 264-1450; *Fax:* (606) 264-1450
E-mail: bpsmass@aol.com *Internet:* http://www.bpmassage.com
Program Administrator: James R. Sloan, Pres. *Admissions Contact:* Terri Sloan, Co-Dir.
Year Established: 1989.
Staff: Full-time: 2.
Avg Enrollment: 24. *Avg Class Size:* 6. *Number of Graduates per Year:* 24.
Wheelchair Access: No.
Field of Study: Acupressure; Aromatherapy; Deep Tissue Massage; Massage Therapy*; Reflexology; Sports Massage. *Program Name/Length:* Theory and Practice of Therapeutic Massage, 500 hrs.
Degrees Offered: Certificate.
License/Certification Preparation: National Certification Board for Therapeutic Massage and Bodywork.
Admission Requirements: Min age: 18; High school diploma/GED; CPR certification completed by end of course.
Application Deadline(s): Fall: May; Winter: Dec.
Tuition and Fees: $3000.

Financial Aid: Payment plan.
Career Services: Job board.

Louisville

382. Louisville School of Massage

7410 New LaGrange Rd, Louisville, KY 40222
Phone: (502) 429-5765; *Fax:* (502) 429-8581
E-mail: bcwilliams@kih.net
Program Administrator: Brent C. Williams, Dir.
Year Established: 1994.
Staff: Full-time: 4.
Avg Enrollment: 100. *Avg Class Size:* 18. *Number of Graduates per Year:* 75.
Wheelchair Access: Yes.
Accreditation/Approval/Licensing: State board: KY Board of Proprietary Ed.
Field of Study: Massage Therapy*. *Program Name/Length:* 600 hrs.
Degrees Offered: Diploma; Certificate.
License/Certification Preparation: National Certification Board for Therapeutic Massage and Bodywork.
Admission Requirements: Min age: 18; High school diploma/GED.
Financial Aid: Payment plan.

Mayfield

383. Sun Touch Massage School

914 W Broadway, Mayfield, KY 42066
Phone: (502) 247-8923; *Fax:* (502) 247-6110
E-mail: yzba67a@prodigy.com *Internet:* http://www.festivalusa.com/suntouch-enterprises
Program Administrator: Marilyn Gossett, Admin. *Admissions Contact:* Marilyn Gossett.
Year Established: 1998.
Staff: Full-time: 2; Part-time: 3.
Avg Enrollment: 25. *Avg Class Size:* 10. *Number of Graduates per Year:* 20.
Wheelchair Access: Yes.
Accreditation/Approval/Licensing: State board: KY Board of Proprietary Ed.
Field of Study: Aromatherapy; Deep Tissue Massage; Massage Therapy*; Polarity Therapy; Qigong; Reflexology; Swedish Massage*. *Program Name/Length:* 100 hrs; 500 hrs.
Degrees Offered: Certificate.
License/Certification Preparation: National Certification Board for Therapeutic Massage and Bodywork.
Admission Requirements: Min age: 18; High school diploma/GED.
Application Deadline(s): Winter: Jan 15; Summer: Jul 15.
Tuition and Fees: $950 (100 hrs); $4750 (500 hrs).
Financial Aid: Loans; Work study.
Career Services: Career counseling; Career information.

LOUISIANA

Kenner

384. Blue Cliff School of Therapeutic Massage, Kenner

1919 Veterans Blvd, Ste 310, Kenner, LA 70062
Phone: (504) 471-0294; *Fax:* (504) 466-8514
E-mail: massage@ametro.net *Internet:* http://
www.bluecliffschool.com
Program Administrator: J. Vernon Smith, PhD,
Pres. *Admissions Contact:* Richard Denny, Dir.
Year Established: 1987.
Staff: Full-time: 5; Part-time: 15.
Avg Enrollment: 150. *Avg Class Size:* 28. *Number
of Graduates per Year:* 120.
Wheelchair Access: Yes.
Accreditation/Approval/Licensing: State board: LA
Dept of Ed; Commission on Massage Therapy
Accreditation; Accrediting Commission of Ca-
reer Schools and Colleges of Technology; Na-
tional Certification Board for Therapeutic Mas-
sage and Bodywork (CEUs); American Oriental
Bodywork Therapy Association.
Field of Study: Acupressure; CranioSacral Ther-
apy; Energy Work; Healing Touch; Massage
Therapy*; Neuromuscular Therapy; Oriental
Medicine; Qigong; Reflexology; Shiatsu*;
Sports Massage*; Traditional Chinese Medicine.
Program Name/Length: Massage Therapy and
Oriental Bodywork, 600 hrs; Advanced Oriental
Studies, 300 hrs; Sports Massage, 750 hrs.
Degrees Offered: Diploma.
License/Certification Preparation: State: LA Li-
censed Massage Therapist; American Oriental
Bodywork Therapy Association; National Certif-
ication Board for Therapeutic Massage and
Bodywork.
Admission Requirements: Min age: 18; High
school diploma/GED; Min GPA: 2.0.
Tuition and Fees: $4900 + $550 books, insurance
(Massage Therapy); $2500 (Advanced Oriental
Studies); $6000 + $600 books, insurance (Sports
Massage).
Financial Aid: Grants; Loans; State government
aid; VA approved; Vocational rehabilitation.
Career Services: Career counseling; Career infor-
mation; Referral registry.

Lafayette

385. Blue Cliff School of Therapeutic Massage, Lafayette

103 Calco Blvd, Lafayette, LA 70503
Phone: (318) 269-0620; *Fax:* (318) 269-0688
E-mail: blueclif@bellsouth.net *Internet:*

http://www.bluecliffschool.com
Program Administrator: Claudette Hymel, Admin.
Admissions Contact: Claudette Hymel.
Year Established: 1993.
Staff: Full-time: 2; Part-time: 15.
Avg Enrollment: 60. *Avg Class Size:* 15. *Number
of Graduates per Year:* 15.
Wheelchair Access: Yes.
Accreditation/Approval/Licensing: State board: LA
Proprietary Schools.
Field of Study: CranioSacral Therapy; Massage
Therapy*; Neuromuscular Therapy; Shiatsu;
Sports Massage. *Program Name/Length:* Mas-
sage Therapy, 600 hrs.
Degrees Offered: Diploma.
License/Certification Preparation: State: LA Li-
censed Massage Therapist; National Certifica-
tion Board for Therapeutic Massage and Body-
work.
Admission Requirements: Min age: 18; High
school diploma/GED.
Tuition and Fees: $4900 + $550 registration,
books.
Financial Aid: VA approved; Vocational rehabili-
tation; Payment plan; Job Training Partnership
Act.
Career Services: Job information; Referral service.

Lake Charles

386. Louisiana Institute of Massage Therapy

1108 Lafitte St, Lake Charles, LA 70601
Phone: (318) 474-9435; *Fax:* (318) 474-9432
E-mail: salvo.breaux@usaunwired.net
Program Administrator: Susan Salvo, Dir. *Admis-
sions Contact:* Michael Breaux, Admissions.
Year Established: 1987.
Staff: Full-time: 3; Part-time: 3.
Avg Enrollment: 50. *Avg Class Size:* 25.
Wheelchair Access: BY.
Accreditation/Approval/Licensing: State board: LA
Dept of Ed; TX Dept of Ed.
Field of Study: Hydrotherapy; Infant Massage;
Massage Therapy*; Pregnancy Massage;
Reflexology; Sports Massage. *Program
Name/Length:* 500 hrs, 1 yr (every other week-
end).
License/Certification Preparation: State: LA Li-
censed Massage Therapist; National Certifica-
tion Board for Therapeutic Massage and Body-
work.
Admission Requirements: High school di-
ploma/GED.

Tuition and Fees: $3700.
Financial Aid: Payment plan; State government aid.
Career Services: Internships.

Monroe

387. Career Training Specialists
Massage Therapy
Mid-City Plaza, 1611 Louisville Ave, Monroe, LA 71201
Phone: (318) 323-2889; *Fax:* (318) 324-9883
E-mail: whiteros@bayou.com
Program Administrator: Dr. Lloydelle Hopkins, School Dir. *Admissions Contact:* Keith Hopkins, Admissions Dir.
Year Established: 1996.
Staff: Full-time: 1; Part-time: 6.
Avg Enrollment: 48. *Avg Class Size:* 24. *Number of Graduates per Year:* 44.
Wheelchair Access: Yes.
Accreditation/Approval/Licensing: State board: LA Board of Massage; Bureau on Occupational Ed.
Field of Study: Aromatherapy; Deep Tissue Massage*; Massage Therapy*; Reflexology; Shiatsu. *Program Name/Length:* Therapeutic Massage, 660 hrs, 30 wks; Massage Therapy, 780 hrs, 35 wks.
Degrees Offered: Certificate.
License/Certification Preparation: State: LA Licensed Massage Therapist; National Certification Board for Therapeutic Massage and Bodywork.
Admission Requirements: Min age: 18; High school diploma/GED.
Application Deadline(s): Winter: Jan; Summer: Jun.
Tuition and Fees: $6000 (Therapeutic Massage); $7100 (Massage Therapy).
Financial Aid: Federal government aid; Grants; Loans.
Career Services: Career counseling; Career information; Interview set up.

Pineville

388. Central Louisiana School of Therapeutic Massage, Inc
2901 Hwy 28 E, Stes C and D, Pineville, LA 71360
Phone: (318) 449-1111; *Fax:* (318) 445-5498
Program Administrator: Andrea R. Martin, Dir. *Admissions Contact:* Andrea R. Martin.
Year Established: 1995.
Staff: 1; Part-time: 6.
Avg Class Size: 15.
Wheelchair Access: Yes.

Accreditation/Approval/Licensing: LA Board of Massage Therapy; LA Licensed Proprietary School.
Field of Study: Acupressure; Deep Tissue Massage; Massage Therapy*; Reflexology; Shiatsu. *Program Name/Length:* 500 hrs, 7 mos/evenings and weekends.
Degrees Offered: Diploma.
License/Certification Preparation: State: FL and LA Licensed Massage Therapist; TX Registered Massage Therapist; National Certification Board for Therapeutic Massage and Bodywork.
Admission Requirements: Min age: 18; High school diploma/GED.
Tuition and Fees: $3830 + $300 supplies.
Financial Aid: Vocational rehabilitation; Job Training Partnership Act.
Career Services: Career information; Internships.

Shreveport

389. Blue Cliff School of Therapeutic Massage, Shreveport
3823 Gilbert Dr, Ste 103, Shreveport, LA 71104
Phone: (318) 861-5959; *Fax:* (318) 861-5957
E-mail: bluecliff@shreve.net *Internet:* http://www.bluecliffschool.com
Program Administrator: Brenda Chadwick, Admin. *Admissions Contact:* Brenda Chadwick.
Year Established: 1987.
Staff: Part-time: 15.
Avg Enrollment: 60. *Avg Class Size:* 20. *Number of Graduates per Year:* 35.
Wheelchair Access: Yes.
Accreditation/Approval/Licensing: State board: LA Board of Massage Therapy; Pending, Accrediting Commission of Career Schools and Colleges of Technology.
Field of Study: Acupressure; CranioSacral Therapy; Deep Tissue Massage; Energy Work; Massage Therapy*; Reflexology; Shiatsu. *Program Name/Length:* 600 hrs, 6-7 mos/days or 1 yr/evenings; Seminars given in various locations.
Degrees Offered: Diploma.
License/Certification Preparation: State: LA Licensed Massage Therapist; National Certification Board for Therapeutic Massage and Bodywork.
Admission Requirements: Min age: 18; High school diploma/GED.
Application Deadline(s): Fall: Aug 1; Spring: Mar 1.
Tuition and Fees: $4950.
Financial Aid: Loans; VA approved; Vocational rehabilitation.

MAINE

Alna

390. Footloose, Inc, Professional Reflexology Training
Egypt Rd, Box 112, Alna, ME 04535
Phone: (207) 586-6751; *Fax:* (207) 586-6702
E-mail: footloos@gwi.net *Internet:* http://www.
  portlandwebsmith.com/footloose/
Program Administrator: Janet E. Stetser, DSc, Dir.
  Admissions Contact: Janet E. Stetser.
Year Established: 1983.
Staff: Full-time: 1; Part-time: 2.
Avg Enrollment: 8. *Avg Class Size:* 8. *Number of
  Graduates per Year:* 6.
Wheelchair Access: Yes.
Field of Study: Hypnotherapy; Reflexology*. *Pro-
  gram Name/Length:* 300 hrs, 8-9 mos.
Degrees Offered: Certificate.
License/Certification Preparation: American
  Reflexology Certification Board.
Admission Requirements: Min age: 18; High
  school diploma/GED.
Application Deadline(s): Fall: Aug; Winter: Jan.
Tuition and Fees: $3200.
Financial Aid: Payment plan.
Career Services: Career information.

Bangor

391. Childbirth Support Consultants of Northern New England
Doula Training
28 Merrimac St, Bangor, ME 04401
Phone: (207) 945-9804, (603) 626-3933; *Fax:* (603)
  666-5937
E-mail: ybcdoula@aol.com, dbdoula@cmss.com
Program Administrator: Evelyn Conrad, Co-Dir;
  Donna Basiliou, Co-Dir. *Admissions Contact:*
  Evelyn Conrad.
Year Established: 1998.
Staff: Part-time: 2.
Avg Enrollment: 60. *Avg Class Size:* 22.
Wheelchair Access: Yes.
Accreditation/Approval/Licensing: Doulas of
  North America.
Field of Study: Doula*. *Program Name/Length:*
  Childbirth Support, 2 1/2 days; Seminars given
  in various locations.
Degrees Offered: Certificate.
License/Certification Preparation: Doulas of North
  America.
Admission Requirements: High school di-
  ploma/GED.
Tuition and Fees: $250.

Career Services: Referral service.

Bridgton

392. New Hampshire Institute for Therapeutic Arts School of Massage Therapy, Bridgton
39 Main St, Bridgton, ME 04009
Phone: (207) 647-3794; *Fax:* (603) 598-9101
Program Administrator: Patrick Cowan, PhD, Ad-
  ministrative Dir. *Admissions Contact:* Patrick
  Cowan.
Year Established: 1983.
Avg Enrollment: 24. *Avg Class Size:* 24. *Number
  of Graduates per Year:* 24.
Accreditation/Approval/Licensing: National Certif-
  ication Board for Therapeutic Massage and
  Bodywork (CEUs).
Field of Study: Acupressure*; Lymphatic Massage;
  Massage Therapy*; Neuromuscular Therapy;
  Polarity Therapy*; Reflexology*; Sports Mas-
  sage*; Swedish Massage*. *Program
  Name/Length:* 9 mos (Sep-Jun, 2 terms).
Degrees Offered: Certificate.
License/Certification Preparation: ME Licensed
  Massage Therapist; NH Licensed Massage Prac-
  titioner; NY Licensed Massage Therapist; Na-
  tional Certification Board for Therapeutic Mas-
  sage and Bodywork.
Admission Requirements: Min age: 18; High
  school diploma/GED.
Application Deadline(s): Fall: Aug 1.
Tuition and Fees: $5635 + $300 books, $500 table,
  $200 supplies.
Financial Aid: State government aid; Payment
  plan; Canadian government loans.
Career Services: Career counseling; Career information; Job information; Referral service.

Portland

393. Polarity Realization Institute, Inc, Portland
222 St John St, Ste 300, Portland, ME 04101
Phone: (978) 356-0980; *Fax:* (978) 356-9818
E-mail: admissions@ryse.com *Internet:* http://
  www.holistic-massage.com
Program Administrator: Nancy Risley, RPP, Dir.
Year Established: 1980.
Staff: Part-time: 14.
Avg Enrollment: 300. *Avg Class Size:* 24. *Number
  of Graduates per Year:* 60.
Wheelchair Access: Yes.

Accreditation/Approval/Licensing: Accrediting Council for Continuing Education and Training; International Massage and Somatic Therapies Accreditation Council; American Polarity Therapy Association; National Certification Board for Therapeutic Massage and Bodywork (CEUs).

Field of Study: Aromatherapy; CranioSacral Therapy; Deep Tissue Massage; Energy Work*; Massage Therapy*; Polarity Therapy*; Reflexology; Yoga Teacher Training. *Program Name/Length:* Holistic Massage Therapy, 600 hrs, 9-24 mos; Polarity Realization Therapy, 650 hrs, 14-18 mos; Seminars given in various locations.

Degrees Offered: Certificate.

License/Certification Preparation: National Certification Board for Therapeutic Massage and Bodywork; American Polarity Therapy Association.

Admission Requirements: High school diploma/GED.

Tuition and Fees: $1500-$8000.

Financial Aid: Loans.

Waldoboro

394. Downeast School of Massage
99 Moose Meadow Ln, Waldoboro, ME 04572
Mailing Address: PO Box 24, Waldoboro, ME 04572
Phone: (207) 832-5531; *Fax:* (207) 832-0504

E-mail: dsm@midcoast.com *Internet:* http://www.midcoast.com/~dsm

Program Administrator: Nancy Dail, Dir. *Admissions Contact:* Christa Gerrish, Admissions Dir.

Year Established: 1981.

Staff: Part-time: 20.

Avg Enrollment: 70. *Avg Class Size:* 20. *Number of Graduates per Year:* 70.

Wheelchair Access: Yes.

Accreditation/Approval/Licensing: State board: ME State board; Commission on Massage Therapy Accreditation; National Certification Board for Therapeutic Massage and Bodywork (CEUs).

Field of Study: Massage Therapy*; Shiatsu*; Sports Massage*. *Program Name/Length:* Swedish Massage and Sports Massage, 11 mos; Swedish Massage and Body-Mind, 11 mos; Swedish Massage and Shiatsu, 11 mos.

Degrees Offered: Diploma.

License/Certification Preparation: State: ME Licensed Massage Therapist.

Admission Requirements: Min age: 18; High school diploma/GED.

Application Deadline(s): Fall: Aug; Winter: Nov.

Tuition and Fees: $5625 (Swedish and Sports); $5500 (Swedish and Body-Mind); $6200 (Swedish and Shiatsu).

Financial Aid: Scholarships; Payment plan.

Career Services: Career counseling; Career information; Interview set up; Job information.

MARYLAND

Baltimore

395. Baltimore School of Massage
Basic Massage; Professional Massage; Professional Program in Comprehensive Massage Therapy for a Medical or Clinical Setting
6401 Dogwood Rd, Baltimore, MD 21207
Phone: (410) 944-8855; *Fax:* (410) 944-8859
E-mail: registrar@bhhc.com *Internet:* http://www.bsom.com

Program Administrator: Cindi Pridgen, Admin. *Admissions Contact:* Carol Burke, Dir of Ed.

Year Established: 1981.

Staff: Part-time: 14.

Avg Enrollment: 650. *Avg Class Size:* 22. *Number of Graduates per Year:* 250.

Wheelchair Access: Yes.

Accreditation/Approval/Licensing: State board: MD Higher Ed Commission; Accrediting Commission of Career Schools and Colleges of Technology; National Certification Board for Therapeutic Massage and Bodywork (CEUs).

Field of Study: Massage Therapy*. *Program Name/Length:* Basic Massage Training Program, 5 mos; Professional Massage Training Program, 510 hrs, 18 mos; Professional Program in Comprehensive Massage Therapy, 610 hrs, 21 mos.

Degrees Offered: CEUs; Certificate.

License/Certification Preparation: National Certification Board for Therapeutic Massage and Bodywork.

Admission Requirements: Min age: 18; High school diploma/GED.

Application Deadline(s): Fall: Aug; Spring: Feb.

Tuition and Fees: $775 (Basic); $4750 (Professional); $5850 (Comprehensive).

Financial Aid: Federal government aid; Loans.

Career Services: Career information.

396. The Maryland Institute for Ericksonian Hypnosis and Psychotherapy
6118 Park Heights Ave, Baltimore, MD 21215
Phone: (410) 358-1381; *Fax:* (410) 358-5815
E-mail: mehyp@aol.com
Admissions Contact: Hillel Zeitlin, LCSW, Dir.
Year Established: 1987.
Staff: Part-time: 4.
Avg Class Size: 12.
Wheelchair Access: No.
Accreditation/Approval/Licensing: State board: MD Board of Psychologists and Social Workers; American Society of Clinical Hypnosis.
Field of Study: Hypnotherapy*. *Program Name/Length:* Trance Forms: Foundation Skills in Clinical Hypnosis, 10 mos.
Degrees Offered: Certificate.
License/Certification Preparation: American Board of Clinical Hypnosis.
Admission Requirements: Master's degree.
Tuition and Fees: $600.
Financial Aid: Scholarships.

Bethesda

397. Maryland Institute of Traditional Chinese Medicine
3-Year Professional Acupuncture Diploma Program
4641 Montgomery Ave, Ste 400, Bethesda, MD 20814
Phone: (301) 718-7373; *Fax:* (301) 718-0735
E-mail: martindell@aol.com *Internet:* http://www.mitcm.org
Program Administrator: Jay Martindell, CEO. *Admissions Contact:* Hee Junj Sunj; Dir of Admin.
Year Established: 1987.
Staff: Full-time: 2; Part-time: 15.
Avg Enrollment: 50. *Avg Class Size:* 25. *Number of Graduates per Year:* 25.
Wheelchair Access: Yes.
Accreditation/Approval/Licensing: State board: MD Higher Ed Commission; Accreditation Commission for Acupuncture and Oriental Medicine.
Field of Study: Acupuncture*; Herbal Medicine*; Qigong; Traditional Chinese Medicine*. *Program Name/Length:* Professional Diploma in Acupuncture, 3 yrs.
Degrees Offered: Diploma.
License/Certification Preparation: National Certification Commission for Acupuncture and Oriental Medicine.
Admission Requirements: Some college (2 yrs); Specific course prerequisites: 6 semester hrs anatomy and physiology.
Application Deadline(s): Fall: Aug 1; Spring: Dec 1.
Tuition and Fees: $3565 per semester.
Financial Aid: Federal government aid; Loans; VA approved.

Career Services: Career counseling; Career information.

398. Unity Woods Yoga Center
4853 Cordell Ave, Ste PH9, Bethesda, MD 20814
Phone: (301) 656-8992; *Fax:* (301) 656-7792
Program Administrator: John Schumacher, Dir.
   Admissions Contact: Esther Geiger, Admin.
Year Established: 1979.
Staff: Full-time: 1.
Avg Enrollment: 26. *Avg Class Size:* 26.
Wheelchair Access: Yes.
Field of Study: Yoga Teacher Training*.
License/Certification Preparation: Certification, Iyengar Yoga National Association.
Admission Requirements: Specific course prerequisites: 3 yrs Iyengar yoga study and practice; 1 yr apprentice or training with certified Iyengar teacher.
Financial Aid: Scholarships; Work study.
Career Services: Career counseling; Interview set up.

Columbia

399. Traditional Acupuncture Institute
American City Bldg, 10227 Wincopin Cir, Ste 100, Columbia, MD 21044-3422
Phone: (301) 596-6006; *Fax:* (410) 964-3544
Internet: http://www.acupuncture.com/TCMSchools/TAI1.htm
Accreditation/Approval/Licensing: State board: CA Acupuncture Board; Accreditation Commission for Acupuncture and Oriental Medicine.
Field of Study: Acupuncture*; Traditional Chinese Medicine*. *Program Name/Length:* Track A, 7 trimesters, 2 yrs + 5 mos; Track B, 10 trimesters, 3 yrs + 4 mos.
Degrees Offered: Master of Acupuncture.
License/Certification Preparation: National Certification Commission for Acupuncture and Oriental Medicine.
Admission Requirements: Bachelor's degree; Specific course prerequisites: 15 semester credits in biosciences (including anatomy, physiology, nutrition) and social sciences (including introductory-level psychology, sociology); Min GPA: 2.0; 200 hrs clinical work experience in medical setting; Letter from practitioner documenting Five Element treatment; 3 letters of reference; Current CPR certification, tuberculosis skin test (PPD), and hepatitis B vaccination.
Tuition and Fees: $27,865.
Financial Aid: Federal government aid; VA approved.

400. The Yoga Center
8950 Rte 108, Ste 114, Columbia, MD 21045
Phone: (410) 720-4340; *Fax:* (410) 461-4799
E-mail: yoga@samadhiyoga.com *Internet:* http://www.samadhiyoga.com

Program Administrator: Bob Glickstein,
Owner/Dir. *Admissions Contact:* Bob Glickstein.
Year Established: 1990.
Staff: Full-time: 5.
Avg Class Size: 15.
Wheelchair Access: Yes.
Field of Study: Yoga Teacher Training*. *Program
Name/Length:* 6 mos.
Degrees Offered: Certificate.
License/Certification Preparation: Certification,
Iyengar Yoga National Association.
Admission Requirements: Specific course prerequi-
sites: Level I yoga class.
Tuition and Fees: $995.

Ellicott

401. Ohashiatsu Maryland

8659 Baltimore Nat'l Pike, Ellicott, MD 21043
Phone: (410) 313-8501; *Fax:* (410) 313-8500
E-mail: om.chung@mindspring.com *Internet:*
http://www.ohashiatsu.com
Program Administrator: Hazel Chung, Dir. *Admis-
sions Contact:* Hazel Chung.
Year Established: 1985.
Staff: Full-time: 3; Part-time: 3.
Avg Enrollment: 150. *Avg Class Size:* 8. *Number
of Graduates per Year:* 6.
Wheelchair Access: Yes.
Accreditation/Approval/Licensing: Accrediting
Council for Continuing Education and Training.
Field of Study: Shiatsu*. *Program Name/Length:*
Ohashiatsu Curriculum, 6 levels, 2 yrs;
Ohashiatsu Instructor Training, 12-18 mos.
Degrees Offered: Certificate.
License/Certification Preparation: American Ori-
ental Bodywork Therapy Association.
Tuition and Fees: $425-$825 per level.
Financial Aid: Work study.
Career Services: Career counseling; Career infor-
mation; Internships; Interview set up.

McHenry

402. Garrett Community College

Continuing Education and Training, Massage Ther-
apy Program
687 Mosser Rd, McHenry, MD 21541
Mailing Address: PO Box 151, McHenry, MD 21541
Phone: (301) 387-3084; *Fax:* (301) 387-3096
E-mail: tstead@gcnet.net *Internet:* http://garrett.
gcc.cc.md.us/
Program Administrator: Thomas H. Kierstead, As-
sociate Prog Dir. *Admissions Contact:* Carol
Newman, Sec.
Year Established: 1993.
Staff: Part-time: 15.
Avg Enrollment: 10. *Avg Class Size:* 10. *Number
of Graduates per Year:* 10.
Wheelchair Access: Yes.

Accreditation/Approval/Licensing: State board:
MD Higher Ed Commission; Middle States As-
sociation of Colleges and Schools.
Field of Study: Deep Tissue Massage; Massage
Therapy*. *Program Name/Length:* Massage
Therapy, 5 semesters.
License/Certification Preparation: National Certif-
ication Board for Therapeutic Massage and
Bodywork.
Admission Requirements: High school diploma/GED.
Tuition and Fees: $5000.
Career Services: College placement office.

Silver Spring

403. American Hypnosis Training Academy, Inc

8750 Georgia Ave, Ste 125E, Silver Spring, MD 20910
Phone: (301) 565-0103, (800) 343-9915
Program Administrator: Ron Klein, Certified Mas-
ter Hypnotherapist, Dir. *Admissions Contact:*
Ron Klein.
Staff: Part-time: 3.
Accreditation/Approval/Licensing: State board:
MD Board of Examiners of Psychologists; NJ
Academy of Psychology; American Psychologi-
cal Association; National Association.
Field of Study: Hypnotherapy*. *Program
Name/Length:* Ericksonian Approaches to Hyp-
nosis, 60 hrs, 8 days; Seminars given in various
locations.
Degrees Offered: CEUs; Certificate.
License/Certification Preparation: National Board
for Certified Clinical Hypnotherapists.
Admission Requirements: Mental health profes-
sional.
Tuition and Fees: $850-$950.

Takoma Park

404.The Polarity Center and Shamanic Studies

9 Philadelphia, Takoma Park, MD 10912
E-mail: bkhalsa@aol.com *Internet:* http://www.
erols.com/bkhalsa
Program Administrator: Rose Diana Khalsa, Dir.
Admissions Contact: Rose Diana Khalsa.
Year Established: 1986.
Staff: Full-time: 1; Part-time: 5.
Avg Enrollment: 35. *Avg Class Size:* 12. *Number
of Graduates per Year:* 20 APP, 10 RPP.
Wheelchair Access: No.
Accreditation/Approval/Licensing: Accrediting
Council for Continuing Education and Training;
American Polarity Therapy Association.
Field of Study: CranioSacral Therapy; Energy
Work*; Polarity Therapy*; Qigong;
Reflexology; Yoga. *Program Name/Length:*
Associate Polarity Practitioner, 155 hrs, 8 mos;
Registered Polarity Practitioner, 2 yrs.
Degrees Offered: Certificate.

License/Certification Preparation: APP and RPP; American Polarity Therapy Association.
Admission Requirements: Min age: 18; Background in healing preferred.

Application Deadline(s): Fall: Sep 1 RPP.
Tuition and Fees: $1650 (APP); $4900 (RPP).

MASSACHUSETTS

Amherst

405. Alexander Technique School of New England
94 Lessey St, Amherst, MA 01002
Phone: (413) 253-2595
E-mail: mvine@netscape.com
Program Administrator: Missy Vineyard, Dir. *Admissions Contact:* Missy Vineyard.
Year Established: 1987.
Staff: Full-time: 1; Part-time: 5.
Avg Enrollment: 8. *Avg Class Size:* 3. *Number of Graduates per Year:* 3.
Wheelchair Access: No.
Accreditation/Approval/Licensing: American Society for the Alexander Technique.
Field of Study: Alexander Technique*. *Program Name/Length:* Teacher Training, 1600 hrs, 3 yrs.
Degrees Offered: Certificate.
License/Certification Preparation: American Society for the Alexander Technique.
Admission Requirements: Min age: 21; Bachelor's degree; Private lesson and interview with director; Specific course prerequisites: 25 private lessons in the Alexander Technique.
Tuition and Fees: $4300 per yr.
Career Services: Career counseling; Career information; Internships.

406. Ellen Evert Hopman Introduction to Botanical Medicine and Self Care
PO Box 219, Amherst, MA 01004
Phone: (413) 323-4494
E-mail: saille333@aol.com
Program Administrator: Ellen Evert Hopman, MEd, Master Herbalist, Teacher. *Admissions Contact:* Ellen Evert Hopman.
Year Established: 1983.
Staff: Full-time: 1; Part-time: 1.
Avg Enrollment: 20. *Avg Class Size:* 20. *Number of Graduates per Year:* 15.
Wheelchair Access: No.
Field of Study: Aromatherapy*; Herbal Medicine*; Homeopathy*. *Program Name/Length:* Amherst area program, 6 mos.
Degrees Offered: Certificate.
Admission Requirements: Min age: 18 or parental consent; High school diploma/GED.

Application Deadline(s): Fall: Oct 1.
Tuition and Fees: $800.

407. New England School of Homeopathy
356 Middle St, Amherst, MA 01002
Phone: (413) 256-5949; *Fax:* (413) 256-6223
E-mail: nesh@nesh.com *Internet:* http://www.nesh.com
Program Administrator: Dr. Amy Rothenberg, Coord; Dr. Paul Herscu, Coord. *Admissions Contact:* Dr. Amy Rothenberg.
Year Established: 1987.
Staff: Part-time: 3.
Avg Enrollment: 100. *Avg Class Size:* 25. *Number of Graduates per Year:* 40.
Wheelchair Access: Yes.
Accreditation/Approval/Licensing: Council on Homeopathic Education; Homeopathic Academy of Naturopathic Physicians; World Health Organization.
Field of Study: Homeopathy*. *Program Name/Length:* Professional Course, 3 yrs; Postgraduate for Medically Licensed, 2 yrs; Weekend Seminars.
Degrees Offered: Certificate.
License/Certification Preparation: Council for Homeopathic Certification; Homeopathic Academy of Naturopathic Physicians.
Tuition and Fees: $2600 per yr (Professional); $3800 per yr (Postgraduate); $525+ (Seminars).

408. The School for Body-Mind Centering
Practitioner Certification Program
189 Pondview Dr, Amherst, MA 01002-3230
Phone: (413) 256-8615; *Fax:* (413) 256-8239
E-mail: bmcschool@aol.com
Program Administrator: Myra Avedon, Programs Dir. *Admissions Contact:* Dawn G. Chamberlin, Admin.
Year Established: 1982.
Avg Enrollment: 50.
Wheelchair Access: Yes.
Field of Study: Body-Mind Centering*. *Program Name/Length:* 2 phase program, 4 yrs (Berkeley, CA, or Amherst, MA).
Degrees Offered: Certificate.
License/Certification Preparation: National Certification Board for Therapeutic Massage and Bodywork.

Admission Requirements: Specific course prerequisites: anatomy and physiology, kinesiology; Movement or bodywork experience.
Tuition and Fees: $4090.

Andover

409. Greater New England Academy of Hypnosis, Inc
Clinical Hypnosis
PO Box 975, Andover, MA 01810
Phone: (978) 474-4601; *Fax:* (978) 474-4601
E-mail: gneah@greennet.net *Internet:* http://www.gneah.com
Program Administrator: Alphonse M. Tatarunis, EdD, Pres. *Admissions Contact:* Alphonse M. Tatarunis.
Year Established: 1979.
Staff: Full-time: 2.
Avg Enrollment: 100. *Avg Class Size:* 10.
Accreditation/Approval/Licensing: State board: MA Nurses Association; American Association of Nurse Anesthetists.
Field of Study: Hypnotherapy*. *Program Name/Length:* 2 days; Seminars given in various locations.
Degrees Offered: CEUs; Certificate.
Admission Requirements: RN.
Tuition and Fees: $350.

Boston

410. Boston University, School of Public Health
Nurse-Midwifery Education Program, Department of Maternal and Child Health
715 Albany St, Rm A-207, Boston, MA 02118
Phone: (617) 638-5012
Internet: http://www.bumc.bu.edu
Program Administrator: Mary Barger, CNM, Dir.
Accreditation/Approval/Licensing: American College of Nurse-Midwives, Division of Accreditation.
Field of Study: Midwifery*.
Degrees Offered: MPH.
License/Certification Preparation: Certified Nurse-Midwife, American College of Nurse-Midwives.
Admission Requirements: Bachelor's degree; RN.

411. New England School of Whole Health Education, Boston
581 Boylston St, Ste 506, Boston, MA 02216
Phone: (617) 267-0516; *Fax:* (617) 247-0896
E-mail: healthed@tiac.net *Internet:* http://www.wholehealtheducation.com
Program Administrator: Dr. Georgianna Donadio-McCormack, Dir. *Admissions Contact:* Nancy Steeves, Registrar.
Year Established: 1977.

Staff: Part-time: 10.
Avg Enrollment: 50. *Avg Class Size:* 22. *Number of Graduates per Year:* 35.
Wheelchair Access: Yes.
Accreditation/Approval/Licensing: State board: MA Dept of Ed; MA Association of Private Career Schools.
Field of Study: Holistic Health*. *Program Name/Length:* Whole Health Educator, 2 yrs/part-time (every other Sat).
Degrees Offered: Certificate.
Admission Requirements: High school diploma/GED.
Application Deadline(s): Fall; Winter.
Tuition and Fees: $3800 (1st yr); $4400 (2nd yr).
Career Services: Career counseling; Career information; Internships; Interview set up; Referral service.

Brookline

412. Yoga Therapy Center
120-A Westbourne Terrace, Brookline, MA 02446
Phone: (617) 739-1146
E-mail: yogimuk@banet.net
Program Administrator: Mukunda Stiles, Dir.
Year Established: 1978.
Staff: Full-time: 1; Part-time: 2.
Avg Enrollment: 8. *Avg Class Size:* 6-12. *Number of Graduates per Year:* 6.
Wheelchair Access: Yes.
Accreditation/Approval/Licensing: World Union of Yoga.
Field of Study: Yoga Teacher Training*. *Program Name/Length:* Structural Yoga Therapy, 500 hrs; Ayurveda Yoga Therapy, 300 hrs; Seminars given in various locations.
Degrees Offered: Certificate.
Admission Requirements: 2 yrs yoga experience.
Application Deadline(s): Fall: Sep 1; Spring: Apr 1.
Financial Aid: Payment plan.
Career Services: Referral service.

Cambridge

413. Association of Labor Assistants and Childbirth Educators
Labor Assistant Certification; Childbirth Educator Certification
552 Massachusetts Ave, Cambridge, MA 02139
Mailing Address: PO Box 382724, Cambridge, MA 02238-2724
Phone: (888) 222-5223; *Fax:* (617) 441-3167
Program Administrator: Jessica Porter, Pres.
Year Established: 1994.
Staff: Part-time: 5.
Avg Enrollment: 300. *Avg Class Size:* 15. *Number of Graduates per Year:* 275.
Wheelchair Access: Yes.

Field of Study: Childbirth Education*; Doula*.
Program Name/Length: Labor Assistant (Birth Doula) Certification, 6-12 mos; Childbirth Educator Certification, 6-12 mos; Seminars given in various locations; Home study/Correspondence.
Degrees Offered: Certificate.
Tuition and Fees: $395 (Labor Assistant); $575-$695 (Childbirth Educator).
Career Services: Referral service.

414. Center for Traditional Medicine

1770 Mass Ave, Ste 624, Cambridge, MA 02140
Phone: (781) 643-1918
E-mail: lekorn@wco.com *Internet:* http://www.halcyon.com/fwdp/medicine/tmp.html
Program Administrator: Leslie Korn, PhD, Dir. *Admissions Contact:* Dr. Rudolph Ryser.
Year Established: 1976.
Staff: Full-time: 3; Part-time: 25.
Avg Enrollment: 30. *Avg Class Size:* 20.
Field of Study: CranioSacral Therapy*; Energy Work*; Herbal Medicine*; Massage Therapy*; Naturopathic Medicine*; Polarity Therapy*.
Program Name/Length: 1 wk seminars-1 yr clinical internships; 2 yr certificate; BA and MA programs.
Degrees Offered: BS; Certificate; BA, MA.
Admission Requirements: Min age: 18.
Tuition and Fees: $1500 per wk-$9000 per yr.
Financial Aid: Fellowships; Grants; Loans; Scholarships.
Career Services: Career counseling; Internships.
Comments: Additional address: 1001 Cooper Point Rd SW, Ste 140-214, Olympia, WA 98502.

415. The Dimon School for the Alexander Technique

15 Day St, Cambridge, MA 02140
Phone: (617) 876-3434
Program Administrator: Ted Dimon, Dir. *Admissions Contact:* Ted Dimon.
Year Established: 1996.
Accreditation/Approval/Licensing: American Society for the Alexander Technique.
Field of Study: Alexander Technique*. *Program Name/Length:* Teacher Training, 3 yrs.
License/Certification Preparation: American Society for the Alexander Technique.
Admission Requirements: Bachelor's degree; Specific course prerequisites: 20-30 private lessons in the Alexander Technique; Interview and lessons with director.
Tuition and Fees: $6500 per yr.

416. East/West Institute of Alternative Medicine

Shiatsu Certification; Integrative Ayurvedic Health Care Practitioner Certification
1972 Massachusetts Ave, Cambridge, MA 02140
Phone: (617) 876-4048; *Fax:* (617) 497-4892
E-mail: eastwestinst@mindspring.com *Internet:* http://www.eastwestinstitute.com

Program Administrator: Kikuko Zutrau Miyazaki, Dir. *Admissions Contact:* Erik Zutrau, Admin.
Year Established: 1985.
Staff: Full-time: 2; Part-time: 7.
Avg Enrollment: 100. *Avg Class Size:* 15. *Number of Graduates per Year:* 30.
Wheelchair Access: Yes.
Accreditation/Approval/Licensing: American Oriental Bodywork Therapy Association.
Field of Study: Acupressure*; Ayurvedic Medicine*; Shiatsu*; Traditional Chinese Medicine. *Program Name/Length:* Zen Shiatsu, 720 hrs, 18 mos; Ayurvedic Practitioner, 300 hrs.
Degrees Offered: Diploma; Certificate.
License/Certification Preparation: American Oriental Bodywork Therapy Association.
Admission Requirements: Min age: 18; High school diploma/GED.
Application Deadline(s): Fall: Sep 1; Winter: Nov 15; Spring: Mar 1; Summer: May 15.
Tuition and Fees: $7200 (Shiatsu).
Financial Aid: Loans.
Career Services: Career information; Internships; Job listings.

417. Muscular Therapy Institute

122 Rindge Ave, Cambridge, MA 02140
Phone: (617) 576-1300; *Fax:* (617) 864-8283
Internet: http://www.mtti.com
Program Administrator: Joelle Andre, Education Dir. *Admissions Contact:* Elizabeth M. Harvey, Admissions Dir.
Year Established: 1974.
Staff: Full-time: 20; Part-time: 30.
Avg Enrollment: 170. *Avg Class Size:* 30. *Number of Graduates per Year:* 122.
Wheelchair Access: No.
Accreditation/Approval/Licensing: Accrediting Council for Continuing Education and Training; National Certification Board for Therapeutic Massage and Bodywork (CEUs).
Field of Study: Massage Therapy*. *Program Name/Length:* 900 hrs, 3-4 semesters.
Degrees Offered: Diploma.
Admission Requirements: Min age: 20; High school diploma/GED.
Application Deadline(s): Fall: Sep; Winter: Feb.
Tuition and Fees: $12,890.
Financial Aid: Federal government aid; Grants; Loans; VA approved; Vocational rehabilitation.
Career Services: Career counseling; Career information; Job information; Outreach opportunities.

Chestnut Hill

418. Alexander Technique Training Center

803 Boylston St, Chestnut Hill, MA 02167
Phone: (617) 734-6898
E-mail: kilroyr@tiac.net
Program Administrator: Ruth Kilroy, Dir. *Admissions Contact:* Ruth Kilroy.

Year Established: 1993.
Staff: Full-time: 1; Part-time: 4.
Avg Class Size: 6-8.
Wheelchair Access: No.
Accreditation/Approval/Licensing: American Society for the Alexander Technique.
Field of Study: Alexander Technique*. *Program Name/Length:* Teacher Training, 3 yrs.
Degrees Offered: Certificate.
License/Certification Preparation: American Society for the Alexander Technique.
Admission Requirements: Specific course prerequisites: 25 private lessons in the Alexander Technique, 6 with faculty; Interview with director.
Tuition and Fees: $5575 per yr.
Career Services: Internships.

Dover

419. New England School of Whole Health Education, Dover

60 Farm St, Dover, MA 02030
Phone: (508) 785-0309; *Fax:* (508) 785-9743
E-mail: healthed@tiac.net *Internet:* http://www.wholehealtheducation.com
Program Administrator: Dr. Georgianna Donadio-McCormack, Dir. *Admissions Contact:* Nancy Steeves, Registrar.
Year Established: 1977.
Staff: Part-time: 10.
Avg Enrollment: 50. *Number of Graduates per Year:* 35.
Wheelchair Access: Yes.
Accreditation/Approval/Licensing: State board: MA Dept of Ed; MA Association of Private Career Schools.
Field of Study: Holistic Health*. *Program Name/Length:* Whole Health Educator, 2 yrs/part-time (every other Sat).
Degrees Offered: Certificate.
Admission Requirements: High school diploma/GED.
Application Deadline(s): Fall; Winter.
Tuition and Fees: $3800 (1st yr); $4400 (2nd yr).
Career Services: Career counseling; Career information; Internships; Interview set up; Referral service.

Greenfield

420. Greenfield Community College

Massage Therapy Program
270 Main St, Greenfield, MA 01301
Mailing Address: PO Box 15, Hatfield, MA 01038
Phone: (413) 775-1620; *Fax:* (413) 774-2285
E-mail: nursing@gcc.mass.edu *Internet:* http://www.gcc.mass.edu
Program Administrator: Patricia Wachter, Prog Dir. *Admissions Contact:* Laura Earl.
Year Established: 1980.

Staff: Part-time: 12.
Avg Enrollment: 30. *Avg Class Size:* 30. *Number of Graduates per Year:* 30.
Wheelchair Access: Yes.
Accreditation/Approval/Licensing: State board: MA Dept of Ed; National Certification Board for Therapeutic Massage and Bodywork (CEUs).
Field of Study: Massage Therapy*; Polarity Therapy; Reflexology; Shiatsu. *Program Name/Length:* 10 mos.
Degrees Offered: Diploma.
License/Certification Preparation: State: NY Licensed Massage Therapist, NH Licensed Massage Practitioner.
Admission Requirements: Min age: 21; High school diploma/GED.
Application Deadline(s): Fall: Jul 31; Winter: Jan 1.
Tuition and Fees: $4300 (in state); $9500 (out of state).
Career Services: Career information.

Housatonic

421. Phoenix Rising Yoga Therapy

Professional Certification Training
402 Park St, Housatonic, MA 02136
Mailing Address: PO Box 819, Housatonic, MA 01236
Phone: (413) 274-3515; *Fax:* (413) 274-6166
E-mail: moreinfo@pryt.com *Internet:* http://www.pryt.com
Program Administrator: Becky McFarland, Bus Mgr. *Admissions Contact:* Becky McFarland.
Year Established: 1986.
Staff: Full-time: 3; Part-time: 44.
Avg Enrollment: 200. *Avg Class Size:* 25. *Number of Graduates per Year:* 150.
Wheelchair Access: Yes.
Accreditation/Approval/Licensing: International Association of Yoga Therapists; National Board of Certified Counselors.
Field of Study: Yoga Therapy*. *Program Name/Length:* Level 1 Professional Training, 4 days; Level 2, 6 days; Level 3, 6 mos/part-time (includes residential and home study).
Degrees Offered: Certificate.
License/Certification Preparation: Phoenix Rising Yoga Therapy Practitioner.
Admission Requirements: Min age: 21; High school diploma/GED; 3 mos yoga practice.
Application Deadline(s): Winter: Nov 15 for Level 3; Summer: May 15 for Level 3.
Tuition and Fees: $545 (Level 1); $680 (Level 2); $2850 (Level 3).
Financial Aid: Work study; Payment plan.
Career Services: Career counseling; Marketing kit.

Ipswich

422. Polarity Realization Institute, Inc, Ipswich
Holistic and Therapeutic Massage; Polarity Realization Therapy
126 High St, Ipswich, MA 01938
Phone: (508) 356-0980; *Fax:* (508) 356-9818
E-mail: polaritytherapy@msn.com *Internet:* http://www.ryse.com
Program Administrator: Nancy Risley, RPP, Dir.
 Admissions Contact: Nicole Romano, Dir of Admissions.
Year Established: 1980.
Staff: Part-time: 15-20.
Avg Enrollment: 350. *Avg Class Size:* 20. *Number of Graduates per Year:* 90.
Wheelchair Access: No.
Accreditation/Approval/Licensing: State board: MA Dept of Ed; ME Dept of Ed; International Massage and Somatic Therapies Accreditation Council; American Polarity Therapy Association; National Certification Board for Therapeutic Massage and Bodywork (CEUs).
Field of Study: Energy Work*; Massage Therapy*; Polarity Therapy*. *Program Name/Length:* Polarity Realization Certification: Level I, 160 hrs, 7 mos; Polarity Realization Certification: Advanced, 650 hrs, 6 mos or 11 mos; Holistic Massage and Bodywork: Module I, 180 hrs, 6 mos; Holistic Massage and Bodywork, 600 hrs, 6 mos or 11 mos.
Degrees Offered: CEUs; Certificate.
License/Certification Preparation: APP and RPP; American Polarity Therapy Association.
Admission Requirements: Min age: 18; High school diploma/GED.
Application Deadline(s): Fall: Oct; Spring: Apr; Winter: Jan; Summer: Jul.
Tuition and Fees: $1900 (160 hr Polarity); $7000 (650 hr Polarity); $2100 (180 hr Massage); $6500 (600 hr Massage).
Financial Aid: Payment plan.
Career Services: Career information.

Plymouth

423. Dovestar Institute, Plymouth
120 Court St, Plymouth, MA 02360
Phone: (508) 830-0068, (888) 222-5603; *Fax:* (508) 830-0288
Internet: http://www.dovestar.edu
Program Administrator: Kamala Renner, Dir.
Year Established: 1973.
Staff: Full-time: 3; Part-time: 12.
Avg Class Size: 12.
Wheelchair Access: Yes.
Accreditation/Approval/Licensing: State board: MA Dept of Ed.

Field of Study: Acupressure; Breathwork; Colon Hydrotherapy; Energy Work*; Hypnotherapy*; Kriya Massage*; Massage Therapy*; Qigong; Reflexology; Reiki*; Shiatsu; Yoga Teacher Training*. *Program Name/Length:* Colon Hydrotherapy, 2 mos; Reiki-Alchemia, 3 mos; Alchemical Synergy/Hypnotherapy, 6 mos; Kriya Massage, 9 mos; Alchemia Yoga Teacher Training, 1 yr.
Degrees Offered: Certificate.
License/Certification Preparation: American Council of Hypnotist Examiners; American Oriental Bodywork Therapy Association; National Certification Board for Therapeutic Massage and Bodywork.
Tuition and Fees: $2000-$6000.
Financial Aid: State government aid; Work study; Vocational rehabilitation.
Career Services: Career counseling; Career information; Internships.

424. Polarity Realization Institute, Inc, Plymouth
59 Industrial Park Rd, Plymouth, MA 02360
Phone: (978) 356-0980; *Fax:* (978) 356-9818
E-mail: admissions@ryse.com *Internet:* http://www.holistic-massage.com
Program Administrator: Nancy Risley, RPP, Dir.
Year Established: 1980.
Staff: Part-time: 14.
Avg Enrollment: 300. *Avg Class Size:* 24. *Number of Graduates per Year:* 60.
Wheelchair Access: Yes.
Accreditation/Approval/Licensing: Accrediting Council for Continuing Education and Training; International Massage and Somatic Therapies Accreditation Council; American Polarity Therapy Association; National Certification Board for Therapeutic Massage and Bodywork (CEUs).
Field of Study: Aromatherapy; CranioSacral Therapy; Deep Tissue Massage; Energy Work*; Massage Therapy*; Polarity Therapy*; Reflexology; Yoga Teacher Training. *Program Name/Length:* Holistic Massage Therapy, 600 hrs, 9-24 mos; Seminars given in various locations; Polarity Realization Therapy, 650 hrs, 14-18 mos; Seminars given in various locations.
Degrees Offered: Certificate.
License/Certification Preparation: National Certification Board for Therapeutic Massage and Bodywork; American Polarity Therapy Association.
Admission Requirements: High school diploma/GED.
Tuition and Fees: $1500-$8000.
Financial Aid: Loans.

Shelburne Falls

425. Blazing Star Herbal School
119 Pfersick Rd, Shelburne Falls, MA 01370

Mailing Address: PO Box 6, Shelburne Falls, MA 01370
Phone: (413) 625-6875; *Fax:* (413) 625-6972
E-mail: blazingstarherbs@hotmail.com
Program Administrator: Gail Ulrich, Dir. *Admissions Contact:* Gail Ulrich.
Year Established: 1984.
Staff: Full-time: 1; Part-time: 2.
Avg Enrollment: 20. *Avg Class Size:* 15. *Number of Graduates per Year:* 15.
Wheelchair Access: No.
Field of Study: Herbal Medicine*; Plant Spirit Medicine. *Program Name/Length:* Therapeutic Herbalism, 7 mos; Herbal Apprenticeship, 10 mos.
Degrees Offered: Certificate.
Admission Requirements: High school diploma/GED.
Application Deadline(s): Winter: for Apprenticeship; Summer: for Therapeutic Herbalism.
Tuition and Fees: $1000 (Therapeutic Herbalism); $1400 (Apprenticeship).
Financial Aid: Work study; Vocational rehabilitation; VT Student's Assistance Fund.

Shutesbury

426. The Certificate Program in Holistic Nursing

c/o Seeds and Bridges, Inc
PO Box 307, Shutesbury, MA 01072
Phone: (413) 253-0443; *Fax:* (413) 259-1034
E-mail: cphn@seedsandbridges.com *Internet:* http://www.seedsandbridges.com
Program Administrator: Veda Andrus, EdD, Prog Dir. *Admissions Contact:* Beth Dichter, Admin.
Year Established: 1987.
Staff: Full-time: 2; Part-time: 11.
Avg Enrollment: 600. *Avg Class Size:* 35. *Number of Graduates per Year:* 120.
Wheelchair Access: No.
Field of Study: Holistic Nursing*. *Program Name/Length:* Phase I: Introduction to Holistic Nursing, 3 1/2 days; Phase II: Core Concepts in Holistic Nursing, 4 1/2 days; Phase III: Independent Practicum in Holistic Nursing, 8-12 mos; Phase IV: Advancing Concepts in Holistic Nursing, 3 1/2 days.
Degrees Offered: Certificate.
License/Certification Preparation: Board Certified Certification in Holistic Nursing (HNC).
Admission Requirements: RN or LPN.
Tuition and Fees: $375-$450 (Phase I); $575-$625 (Phase II); $750 (Phase III); $400 (Phase IV) + materials fee for each seminar.
Financial Aid: Scholarships; Discount for AHNA members, full-time nursing students and senior citizens.

Somerville

427. BKS Iyengar Yoga Center of Greater Boston

Yoga Teacher Training
240A Elm St, Ste 23, Somerville, MA 02144
Phone: (617) 666-9551; *Fax:* (617) 296-6194
E-mail: yogactr@world.std.com
Program Administrator: Patricia Walden, Dir. *Admissions Contact:* Elizabeth Shields.
Year Established: 1993.
Staff: Full-time: 3.
Avg Enrollment: 20. *Avg Class Size:* 20. *Number of Graduates per Year:* 20.
Wheelchair Access: Yes.
Accreditation/Approval/Licensing: BKS Iyengar Yoga National Association (IYNAUS).
Field of Study: Yoga Teacher Training*. *Program Name/Length:* 2 years, 40 hrs/yr.
License/Certification Preparation: Preparation for certification with IYNAUS.
Admission Requirements: Minimum 2 years Iyengar yoga experience.
Application Deadline(s): Fall.
Tuition and Fees: $1200 per yr.
Financial Aid: Work study.
Career Services: Job placement assistance.

428. Massage Institute of New England

Massage Therapist Certification
22 McGrath Hwy, Ste 11, Somerville, MA 02143
Phone: (617) 666-3700; *Fax:* (617) 666-0109
E-mail: mineinc@aol.com
Program Administrator: Henry Corley, Admin Dir. *Admissions Contact:* Monique Illona, Registrar.
Year Established: 1982.
Staff: Full-time: 2; Part-time: 18.
Avg Enrollment: 150. *Avg Class Size:* 26. *Number of Graduates per Year:* 120.
Wheelchair Access: No.
Accreditation/Approval/Licensing: State board: MA Dept of Ed.
Field of Study: Energy Work; Massage Therapy*; Neuromuscular Therapy; Sports Massage; Swedish Massage*. *Program Name/Length:* 9 mos/days or 18 mos/evenings.
Degrees Offered: Certificate.
License/Certification Preparation: National Certification Board for Therapeutic Massage and Bodywork.
Admission Requirements: Min age: 18; High school diploma/GED.
Tuition and Fees: $7500.
Financial Aid: Loans.
Career Services: Career information.

Spencer

429. The Central Mass School of Massage and Therapy

200 Main St, Spencer, MA 01562

Phone: (508) 885-0306, (800) 766-6572
Program Administrator: Gregory St. Jacques, Dir
of Ed. *Admissions Contact:* Gregory St.
Jacques.
Year Established: 1970.
Staff: Part-time: 8.
Avg Enrollment: 52. *Avg Class Size:* 13. *Number
of Graduates per Year:* 52.
Wheelchair Access: Yes.
Accreditation/Approval/Licensing: State board:
MA Dept of Ed.
Field of Study: Acupressure*; Aromatherapy*;
Deep Tissue Massage*; Energy Work*; Herbal
Medicine; Massage Therapy*; Meditation*; Po-
larity Therapy*; Reflexology*; Reiki*. *Program
Name/Length:* Diploma in Massage and Ther-
apy, 500 hrs, 1 yr.
Degrees Offered: Diploma.
License/Certification Preparation: National Certif-
ication Board for Therapeutic Massage and
Bodywork.
Admission Requirements: High school di-
ploma/GED; Some college preferred.
Application Deadline(s): Fall: Sep; Spring: Apr.
Tuition and Fees: $8395.
Financial Aid: Work study; Payment plan.
Career Services: Career counseling; Career infor-
mation; Interview set up; Resume service.

Springfield

430. Baystate Medical Center
Nurse-Midwifery Education Program
759 Chestnut St, Springfield, MA 01199
Phone: (413) 794-4448; *Fax:* (413) 794-8770
Internet: http://www.baystatehealth.com
Program Administrator: Susan DeJoy, CNM, Dir.
Admissions Contact: Susan DeJoy.
Year Established: 1991.
Staff: Full-time: 6; Part-time: 2.
Avg Enrollment: 8. *Avg Class Size:* 8. *Number of
Graduates per Year:* 8.
Wheelchair Access: No.
Accreditation/Approval/Licensing: American Col-
lege of Nurse-Midwives, Division of Accredita-
tion.
Field of Study: Midwifery*. *Program
Name/Length:* Nurse-Midwifery, 1 yr/full-time
or 2 yrs/part-time.
Degrees Offered: Certificate.
License/Certification Preparation: State: MA Li-
censed, Certified Nurse-Midwife; Certified
Nurse-Midwife, American College of
Nurse-Midwives.
Admission Requirements: Bachelor's degree; Min
GPA: 2.5; RN; Specific course prerequisites:
physical assessment; 2 yrs nursing experience, 1
in labor and delivery, or other maternal child
health experience.
Application Deadline(s): Winter: Jun 1 for Jan 2
admission.

Tuition and Fees: $12,100 (full-time) or $7100 per
yr (part-time).
Financial Aid: Loans; Scholarships.

Stockbridge

431. Kripalu Center for Yoga and Health
West St, Stockbridge, MA 01262
Mailing Address: PO Box 793, Lenox, MA 01240
Phone: (800) 741-7353; *Fax:* (413) 448-3384
Internet: http://www.kripalu.org
Program Administrator: John Willey, Dir of Yoga
Teacher Development. *Admissions Contact:*
Reservations Dept.
Year Established: 1972.
Staff: Part-time: 10.
Avg Enrollment: 220. *Avg Class Size:* 55. *Number
of Graduates per Year:* 215.
Wheelchair Access: Yes.
Field of Study: Holistic Health*; Massage Ther-
apy*; Yoga Teacher Training*. *Program
Name/Length:* Kripalu Yoga Teacher Training
Basic Certification, 210 hrs, 1 mo or three 9-day
components; Kripalu Bodywork Certification,
200 hrs, 1 mo; Holistic Health Teacher Training,
1 mo.
Degrees Offered: Certificate.
Admission Requirements: 6 mos Hatha Yoga prac-
tice, 1 hr daily; familiarity with Kripalu Yoga
through a Kripalu Certified Teacher.
Tuition and Fees: $2492-$5124.
Financial Aid: Scholarships.
Career Services: Career information; Kripalu Yoga
Teachers Association membership.

Watertown

432. American School for Energy Therapies
17 Spring St, Watertown, MA 02172
Phone: (617) 924-9150, (800) 875-6347; *Fax:* (617)
924-2828
Program Administrator: Douglas Janssen, RPP,
Dir.
Year Established: 1990.
Staff: Full-time: 5; Part-time: 2.
Avg Enrollment: 50. *Avg Class Size:* 12. *Number
of Graduates per Year:* 20.
Wheelchair Access: No.
Accreditation/Approval/Licensing: State board:
MA Dept of Ed; American Polarity Therapy As-
sociation.
Field of Study: CranioSacral Therapy*; Polarity
Therapy*. *Program Name/Length:* Level 1:
Registered Polarity Practitioner Training (APP),
170 hrs, 10 mos; Level 2: Registered Polarity
Practitioner Training, 530 hrs, 3 yrs (six 5-mo
semesters).
Degrees Offered: Certificate.
License/Certification Preparation: APP and RPP;
American Polarity Therapy Association.

Admission Requirements: Min age: 18; High school diploma/GED.

Application Deadline(s): Fall: Sep; Spring: Mar; Summer: May.

Financial Aid: Work study.

Career Services: Career information.

433. New England School of Acupuncture

30 Common St, Watertown, MA 02172

Phone: (617) 926-1788; *Fax:* (617) 924-4167

E-mail: info@nesa.edu *Internet:* http://www.nesa.edu

Program Administrator: Daniel Seitz, Pres. *Admissions Contact:* Cindy Rosenbaum, Dean of Admissions.

Year Established: 1975.

Staff: Part-time: 60.

Avg Enrollment: 90. *Avg Class Size:* 45. *Number of Graduates per Year:* 90.

Wheelchair Access: No.

Accreditation/Approval/Licensing: State board: MA Dept of Ed; Accreditation Commission for Acupuncture and Oriental Medicine.

Field of Study: Acupuncture*; Herbal Medicine*; Oriental Medicine*; Qigong; Traditional Chinese Medicine*. *Program Name/Length:* Master of Acupuncture, 3 yrs.

Degrees Offered: MAc.

License/Certification Preparation: State: MA Licensed Acupuncturist; National Certification Commission for Acupuncture and Oriental Medicine.

Admission Requirements: Min age: 21; Bachelor's degree; Min GPA: 2.5; (exemption possible for RN).

Application Deadline(s): Fall: May 1.

Tuition and Fees: $9225 per yr.

Financial Aid: Federal government aid; Loans.

Career Services: Career information.

Wilmington

434. Bach International Education Program

Nelson Bach USA, Ltd.

100 Research Dr, Wilmington, MA 01887

Phone: (978) 988-3833, (800) 334-0843; *Fax:* (978) 988-0233

E-mail: education@nelsonbach.com *Internet:* http://www.nelsonbach.com

Program Administrator: Karen Zilinek, Training Mgr; Lucille Arcouet, National Education Mgr. *Admissions Contact:* Education Dept.

Year Established: 1995.

Staff: Full-time: 2; Part-time: 4.

Avg Enrollment: 1000. *Avg Class Size:* 30 Level 2, 20 Level 3.

Accreditation/Approval/Licensing: State board: MA Nurses Association (CEUs for Level 1); Recognized by Bach Centre, Mount Vernon, England.

Field of Study: Flower Essences*. *Program Name/Length:* Level 1: Introduction, 2 days; Level 2: Advanced, 2 days; Level 3: Practitioner, 4 days + 6 mos home study; Seminars given in various locations.

Degrees Offered: CEUs; Certificate.

Admission Requirements: Specific course prerequisites: Level 1 required for Level 2; Level 2 required for Level 3.

Tuition and Fees: $199 per course (Levels 1 and 2); $695 (Level 3).

Financial Aid: Work study.

Career Services: Career information; Referral service; International Register of Bach Centre.

Worcester

435. Bancroft School of Massage Therapy

333 Shrewsbury St, Worcester, MA 01604

Phone: (508) 757-7923; *Fax:* (508) 791-5930

E-mail: bsmttank@aol.com *Internet:* http://www.bancroftsmt.com

Program Administrator: Steven Tankanow, Dir/Pres. *Admissions Contact:* Judie Morin, Admissions Rep.

Year Established: 1950.

Staff: Part-time: 17.

Avg Enrollment: 180. *Avg Class Size:* 24. *Number of Graduates per Year:* 120.

Wheelchair Access: Yes.

Accreditation/Approval/Licensing: State board: MA Dept of Ed; Accrediting Commission of Career Schools and Colleges of Technology; National Certification Board for Therapeutic Massage and Bodywork (CEUs).

Field of Study: Massage Therapy*. *Program Name/Length:* 18 mos/days or 23 mos/evenings.

Degrees Offered: CEUs; Certificate.

License/Certification Preparation: National Certification Board for Therapeutic Massage and Bodywork.

Admission Requirements: Min age: 20; High school diploma/GED.

Application Deadline(s): Fall: Aug 20; Winter: Dec 20; Spring: Mar 20.

Tuition and Fees: $10,950.

Financial Aid: Federal government aid; State government aid; Stafford and PLUS loans.

Career Services: Career counseling; Career information; Internships; Resume service.

436. The Center for Universal and Holistic Studies, Worcester

Reflexology Certification Program

3 Ruthven Ave, Worcester, MA 01606

Mailing Address: PO Box 569, Clinton, MA 01510-1812

Phone: (978) 365-6104

Program Administrator: Janice L. Lucht, Dir/Principal Instr. *Admissions Contact:* Janice L. Lucht.

Year Established: 1993.
Staff: Part-time: 1.
Avg Enrollment: 36. *Avg Class Size:* 6. *Number of Graduates per Year:* 36.
Wheelchair Access: No.
Field of Study: Aromatherapy; Reflexology*; Reiki. *Program Name/Length:* Reflexology, 7 wks (1 day per wk).
Degrees Offered: Diploma.
License/Certification Preparation: American Reflexology Certification Board.
Admission Requirements: Min age: 18; High school diploma/GED.
Application Deadline(s): Fall; Winter; Spring; Summer.
Tuition and Fees: $1200.
Financial Aid: Payment plan.
Career Services: Career information.

437. International Ayurvedic Institute, Inc
Advanced Ayurveda
111 Elm St, Stes 103-105, Worcester, MA 01609

Phone: (508) 755-3744; *Fax:* (508) 770-0618
E-mail: ayurveda@hotmail.com *Internet:* http://www.gis.net/~AYURVEDA
Program Administrator: Abbas Qutab, MD, DC, PhD, Dir. *Admissions Contact:* Dorothy Ciak, Admissions Mgr.
Year Established: 1991.
Staff: Full-time: 6; Part-time: 11.
Avg Enrollment: 65. *Avg Class Size:* 60. *Number of Graduates per Year:* 60.
Wheelchair Access: Yes.
Field of Study: Ayurvedic Medicine*. *Program Name/Length:* 10 weekends/1 yr.
Degrees Offered: Diploma.
Admission Requirements: High school diploma/GED; Min GPA: 3.0.
Application Deadline(s): Spring: Apr 5.
Tuition and Fees: $4200.
Career Services: Career counseling; Career information.

MICHIGAN

Ann Arbor

438. Ann Arbor Institute of Massage Therapy
2835 Carpenter Rd, Ann Arbor, MI 48108
Phone: (734) 677-4430; *Fax:* (734) 677-4520
Program Administrator: Jocelyn Granger, Co-Dir; Jane Anderson, Co-Dir. *Admissions Contact:* Barbara McComb, School Admin.
Year Established: 1993.
Staff: Full-time: 6; 6 assistants.
Avg Enrollment: 80. *Avg Class Size:* 35. *Number of Graduates per Year:* 80.
Wheelchair Access: Yes.
Field of Study: Massage Therapy*; Neuromuscular Therapy; Shiatsu; Sports Massage. *Program Name/Length:* 11 mos.
Degrees Offered: Diploma.
License/Certification Preparation: National Certification Board for Therapeutic Massage and Bodywork.
Admission Requirements: High school diploma/GED.
Application Deadline(s): Fall: Sep 10; Winter: Feb 1.
Tuition and Fees: $6000.
Career Services: Career information.

439. Ann Arbor School of Massage and Bodywork
1530 Northwood, Ann Arbor, MI 48103-4667

Phone: (734) 662-1572; *Fax:* (734) 662-2246
E-mail: luisa@umich.edu
Program Administrator: Barry Ryder, Dir. *Admissions Contact:* Deborah Salerno, Admin.
Year Established: 1992.
Staff: Part-time: 2.
Avg Enrollment: 20. *Avg Class Size:* 20. *Number of Graduates per Year:* 18.
Wheelchair Access: Yes.
Field of Study: Massage Therapy*. *Program Name/Length:* 500 hrs, 2 yrs; 700 hrs, 2 yrs; 900 hrs, 2 yrs.
Degrees Offered: Diploma.
License/Certification Preparation: National Certification Board for Therapeutic Massage and Bodywork.
Admission Requirements: Min age: 18.
Tuition and Fees: $3500-$6300.

440. University of Michigan, School of Nursing
Nurse-Midwifery Program
400 N Ingalls, Rm 3320, Ann Arbor, MI 48109-0482
Phone: (734) 763-3710; *Fax:* (734) 647-0351
E-mail: dswalker@umich.edu *Internet:* http://www-personal.umich.edu/~dswalker/umhome.html
Program Administrator: Deborah S. Walker, FNP, Asst Professor. *Admissions Contact:* Gloria Crothers, Nurse-Midwifery Sec.

Year Established: 1990.
Staff: Full-time: 2; Part-time: 4.
Avg Enrollment: 42. *Avg Class Size:* 14. *Number of Graduates per Year:* 14.
Wheelchair Access: Yes.
Accreditation/Approval/Licensing: North Central Association of Colleges and Schools; American College of Nurse-Midwives, Division of Accreditation.
Field of Study: Midwifery*. *Program Name/Length:* 2 yrs/full-time or 3-4 yrs/part-time.
Degrees Offered: MS.
License/Certification Preparation: State: MI Nurse-Midwifery Certificate; Certified Nurse-Midwife, American College of Nurse-Midwives.
Admission Requirements: High school diploma/GED; Min GPA: 3.0; Bachelor's degree; Min GPA: 3.0A; RN; Specific course prerequisites: statistics, physical assessment, nursing research.
Application Deadline(s): Winter: Feb 1.
Tuition and Fees: $5000/resident, $10,000/nonresident per semester.
Financial Aid: Fellowships; Federal government aid; Grants; Loans; Scholarships; State government aid; Work study.
Career Services: Career information.

Berkley

441. Michigan School of Myomassology
3270 Greenfield Rd, Berkley, MI 48072
Phone: (248) 542-7228; *Fax:* (248) 542-5830
E-mail: touch@concentric.net *Internet:* http://www.therapeutic-touch.com
Program Administrator: Marilyn A. Rotko, CMT, Dir. *Admissions Contact:* Karrie Sladewski, Admin.
Year Established: 1992.
Staff: Full-time: 4; Part-time: 16.
Avg Enrollment: 95. *Avg Class Size:* 18.
Wheelchair Access: Yes.
Accreditation/Approval/Licensing: State board: MI Dept of Ed.
Field of Study: Acupressure; Aromatherapy; CranioSacral Therapy; Energy Work; Massage Therapy*; Myomassology; Neuromuscular Therapy; Polarity Therapy; Reflexology; Reiki; Shiatsu; Sports Massage. *Program Name/Length:* 11 mos.
Degrees Offered: Diploma; Certificate.
License/Certification Preparation: National Certification Board for Therapeutic Massage and Bodywork.
Admission Requirements: Min age: 17; High school diploma/GED.
Application Deadline(s): Fall: Sep; Winter: Jan; Spring: May.

Financial Aid: State government aid; Payment plan.
Career Services: Job information; Referral service.

Dearborn

442. Polarity Center of Dearborn
5824 Chase, Dearborn, MI 48126
Phone: (313) 582-5034
Program Administrator: John Bodary, Dir. *Admissions Contact:* John Bodary.
Year Established: 1986.
Staff: Full-time: 1; Part-time: 2.
Avg Enrollment: 30. *Avg Class Size:* 16. *Number of Graduates per Year:* 12.
Wheelchair Access: No.
Accreditation/Approval/Licensing: American Polarity Therapy Association.
Field of Study: CranioSacral Therapy; Polarity Therapy*. *Program Name/Length:* Associate Polarity Practitioner, 230 hrs, 16 mos.
Degrees Offered: Certificate.
License/Certification Preparation: APP; American Polarity Therapy Association.
Admission Requirements: Min age: 18; Specific course prerequisites: anatomy and physiology.
Application Deadline(s): Fall: Sep 1; Spring: Mar 1.
Tuition and Fees: $1850.

East Lansing

443. Institute of Transformational Hypnotherapy
PO Box 1293, East Lansing, MI 48826
Phone: (517) 374-6156
Program Administrator: Robert Ranger, Dir. *Admissions Contact:* Robert Ranger.
Year Established: 1992.
Staff: Full-time: 2; Part-time: 2.
Avg Enrollment: 18. *Avg Class Size:* 18. *Number of Graduates per Year:* 16.
Wheelchair Access: No.
Accreditation/Approval/Licensing: International Medical and Dental Hypnotherapy Association.
Field of Study: Hypnotherapy*. *Program Name/Length:* Hypnotherapy Training, 7 mos; Seminars given in various locations.
Degrees Offered: Certificate.
License/Certification Preparation: International Medical and Dental Hypnotherapy Association; National Board for Hypnotherapy and Hypnotic Anesthesiology.
Admission Requirements: High school diploma/GED; Experience in a helping profession; Interview.
Application Deadline(s): Fall: Sep.
Tuition and Fees: $595.

444. Yogic Sciences Research Foundation
1228 Daisy Ln, East Lansing, MI 48823
Phone: (517) 351-3056
E-mail: reschbach@yahoo.com
Program Administrator: Robert Eschbach, Dir. *Admissions Contact:* Robert Eschbach.
Year Established: 1991.
Staff: Part-time: 7.
Avg Class Size: 12. *Number of Graduates per Year:* 5.
Wheelchair Access: Yes.
Field of Study: Yoga Teacher Training*. *Program Name/Length:* 10-wk intensive; Seminars given in various locations; Home study/Correspondence.
Degrees Offered: Certificate.
Tuition and Fees: Free.

Fenwick

445. Discovery Institute of Hypnotherapy
6451 Belding Ave, Fenwick, MI 48834
Phone: (616) 761-3453; *Fax:* (616) 761-3710
E-mail: discovery@ud/ager.net
Program Administrator: Charles Kinney, Dir.
Year Established: 1994.
Staff: Full-time: 2; Part-time: 2.
Avg Enrollment: 30. *Avg Class Size:* 12. *Number of Graduates per Year:* 30.
Wheelchair Access: Yes.
Accreditation/Approval/Licensing: International Medical and Dental Hypnotherapy Association.
Field of Study: Hypnotherapy*. *Program Name/Length:* Basic/Self-Hypnosis, Advanced Therapy, Clinical Hypnoanalysis (3 mos).
Degrees Offered: Certificate.
License/Certification Preparation: International Medical and Dental Hypnotherapy Association.
Admission Requirements: Min age: 18; High school diploma/GED.

Grand Rapids

446. Blue Heron Academy of the Healing Arts and Sciences
2020 Raybrook SE, Ste 203, Grand Rapids, MI 49546
Phone: (616) 285-9999; *Fax:* (616) 956-7777
Internet: http://www.imagroup.com
Program Administrator: Gregory T. Lawton, DC, Dir.
Year Established: 1980.
Staff: Full-time: 10; Part-time: 10.
Avg Enrollment: 300. *Avg Class Size:* 15. *Number of Graduates per Year:* 300.
Wheelchair Access: Yes.
Accreditation/Approval/Licensing: State board: MI Board of Higher Ed.

Field of Study: Acupressure*; CranioSacral Therapy; Herbal Medicine*; Homeopathy; Massage Therapy*; Naturopathic Medicine; Neuromuscular Therapy; Oriental Medicine; Qigong; Sports Massage*; Tai Chi; Traditional Chinese Medicine. *Program Name/Length:* Clinical Massage Therapy, 6 mos; Medical Herbalism for the Professional Therapist, 10 mos; Acupressure for the Professional Therapist, 10 mos; Continuing Education Seminars; Seminars given in various locations.
Degrees Offered: MH; Certificate.
Admission Requirements: High school diploma/GED; Some college.
Tuition and Fees: $2800 (Clinical Massage); $200 per mo + $100 workbook (Medical Herbalism; Acupressure); $100 per seminar + $25 workbook (Continuing Education).
Financial Aid: Federal government aid; State government aid; Payment plan.
Career Services: Career counseling; Career information; Internships; Resume service; Job information; Referral service.

Hancock

447. Institute of Natural Therapies
PO Box 222, Hancock, MI 49930
Phone: (906) 482-2222
Admissions Contact: Hal Rudnianin, Dir.
Year Established: 1994.
Staff: Full-time: 1; Part-time: 3.
Avg Enrollment: 10. *Avg Class Size:* 10. *Number of Graduates per Year:* 10.
Wheelchair Access: Yes.
Field of Study: Acupressure; CranioSacral Therapy; Massage Therapy*; Qigong; Traditional Chinese Medicine. *Program Name/Length:* Massage Professional Therapist, 1 yr.
Degrees Offered: Certificate.
License/Certification Preparation: National Certification Board for Therapeutic Massage and Bodywork.
Admission Requirements: Min age: 18; High school diploma/GED.
Application Deadline(s): Fall: Sep 1.
Tuition and Fees: $4000.
Financial Aid: State government aid.
Career Services: Career counseling; Career information; Interview set up.

Kalamazoo

448. Kalamazoo Center for the Healing Arts
3715 W Main, Ste 3, Kalamazoo, MI 49006-2842
Phone: (616) 373-0910; *Fax:* (616) 373-0271
E-mail: kchands@aol.com *Internet:* http://www.kcha.com

Program Administrator: Jim Herweg, Co-Dir; Su Bibik, Co-Dir. *Admissions Contact:* Cathy Esman, Registrar.
Year Established: 1993.
Staff: Full-time: 2; Part-time: 3.
Avg Enrollment: 60. *Avg Class Size:* 22. *Number of Graduates per Year:* 25.
Wheelchair Access: Yes.
Accreditation/Approval/Licensing: International Massage and Somatic Therapies Accreditation Council.
Field of Study: Acupressure; CranioSacral Therapy; Massage Therapy*; Polarity Therapy; Reflexology. *Program Name/Length:* Professional Massage Training, 4 semesters.
Degrees Offered: Certificate.
License/Certification Preparation: National Certification Board for Therapeutic Massage and Bodywork.
Admission Requirements: Min age: 18.
Application Deadline(s): Fall: Oct 1; Spring: Feb 1; Summer: Jun 1.
Tuition and Fees: $4720.
Financial Aid: Loans; State government aid; Work study.
Career Services: Career information; Apprenticeships.

Lansing

449. Lansing Community College
Polarity Therapy Program
PO Box 40010, Lansing, MI 48901-7210
Phone: (517) 887-1670
Program Administrator: Sheila Cook, RPP, Dir.
Accreditation/Approval/Licensing: American Polarity Therapy Association.
Field of Study: Polarity Therapy*. *Program Name/Length:* Polarity Therapy I, 32 hrs; Polarity Therapy II, 32 hrs.

Lapeer

450. Health Enrichment Center, Inc
1820 N Lapeer Rd, Lapeer, MI 48446
Phone: (810) 667-9453; *Fax:* (810) 667-4095
E-mail: hec@tir.com *Internet:* http://www. healthenrichment.com
Program Administrator: Sandy Fritz, Owner/Dir.
Year Established: 1985.
Staff: Part-time: 22.
Avg Enrollment: 350. *Avg Class Size:* 24. *Number of Graduates per Year:* 300.
Wheelchair Access: Yes.
Accreditation/Approval/Licensing: Accrediting Council for Continuing Education and Training; National Certification Board for Therapeutic Massage and Bodywork (CEUs).
Field of Study: Acupressure; CranioSacral Therapy; Massage Therapy*; Polarity Therapy;

Reflexology; Shiatsu. *Program Name/Length:* Level I: Therapeutic Massage, 1000 hrs, 6-10 mos; Level II: Advanced Practitioner, 1500 hrs, 2-4 yrs; Level III: Master Bodywork Therapist, 2500 hrs, 3-6 yrs.
Degrees Offered: Diploma; Certificate.
License/Certification Preparation: National Certification Board for Therapeutic Massage and Bodywork.
Admission Requirements: Min age: 18; High school diploma/GED.
Tuition and Fees: $4500 (Level I); $6000-7000 (Level II); $15,000-$20,000 (Level III).
Financial Aid: Scholarships.
Career Services: Career information; Internships.

Mikado

451. The Michigan School of Traditional Midwifery and Herbology
PO Box 162, Mikado, MI 48745
Phone: (517) 736-6583
E-mail: mstm@i-star.com *Internet:* http://www. oscoda.net/mstm
Program Administrator: Casey Makela, Dir. *Admissions Contact:* Casey Makela.
Year Established: 1994.
Accreditation/Approval/Licensing: North American Guild of Traditional Midwives.
Field of Study: Herbal Medicine*; Midwifery*. *Program Name/Length:* Traditional Midwifery Program, 2 yrs (distance learning with workshops); Well-woman Herbology, 1 yr; Seminars given in various locations; Home study/Correspondence.
Degrees Offered: Certificate.
License/Certification Preparation: Certified Professional Midwife, North American Registry of Midwives.
Admission Requirements: Min age: 18; High school diploma/GED.
Tuition and Fees: $575 per yr.
Financial Aid: Scholarships; Payment plan.
Career Services: Career counseling; Career information; Job information; Referral service.

Mount Pleasant

452. Naturopathic Institute of Therapies and Education
1410 S Mission, Mount Pleasant, MI 48848
Phone: (517) 773-1714; *Fax:* (517) 775-7319
Program Administrator: Bessheen Baker, ND, Dir. *Admissions Contact:* Beth Flaugher, Asst Dir.
Year Established: 1997.
Staff: Full-time: 2; Part-time: 7.
Avg Enrollment: 84. *Avg Class Size:* 20. *Number of Graduates per Year:* 60.
Wheelchair Access: Yes.

Accreditation/Approval/Licensing: State board: MI Board of Ed.

Field of Study: Aromatherapy; CranioSacral Therapy; Energy Work; Flower Essences; Herbal Medicine; Homeopathy; Iridology; Massage Therapy*; Naturopathic Medicine*; Neuromuscular Therapy; Nutrition*; Reflexology; Sports Massage; Traditional Chinese Medicine. *Program Name/Length:* Therapeutic Bodywork Practitioner, 11 courses, 600 hrs; Naturopathic Therapist and Educator, 11 courses, 600 hrs; Advanced Naturopathic Practitioner, 11 courses, 600 hrs; Nutritional Therapist, 5 courses, 600 hrs.

Degrees Offered: Diploma.

Admission Requirements: Min age: 18; High school diploma/GED.

Tuition and Fees: $225 per course.

Financial Aid: Payment plan.

Career Services: Resume service; Job information; Referral service.

Novi

453. Institute of Natural Health Sciences

Homeotherapeutics and the Natural Health Sciences
43000 Nine Mile Rd, Novi, MI 48375
Mailing Address: 20270 Middlebelt Rd, Livonia, MI 48152
Phone: (248) 473-8522; *Fax:* (248) 473-8141
Program Administrator: Kenneth S. Pittaway, PhD, Pres. *Admissions Contact:* C. Lois Grice, DHom, Sec.
Year Established: 1988.
Staff: Full-time: 4; Part-time: 5.
Avg Enrollment: 15. *Avg Class Size:* 15. *Number of Graduates per Year:* 9.
Wheelchair Access: Yes.
Accreditation/Approval/Licensing: State board: MI Dept of Ed; Candidate, Council on Homeopathic Education.
Field of Study: Herbal Medicine; Homeopathy*.
  Program Name/Length: Homeotherapeutics and the Natural Health Sciences, 18 mos; Seminars given in various locations; Bio-Energetics and the Natural Health Sciences, 18 mos; Seminars given in various locations.
Degrees Offered: Diploma.
Admission Requirements: Some college (2 yrs); Specific course prerequisites: anatomy, biology, chemistry, physiology.
Application Deadline(s): Fall.
Tuition and Fees: $4705.

Royal Oak

454. Infinity International Institute of Hypnotherapy

4110 Edgeland, Ste 800, Royal Oak, MI 48073-2285

Phone: (248) 549-5594; *Fax:* (248) 549-5421
E-mail: aspencer@infinityinst.com *Internet:* http://www.infinityinst.com
Program Administrator: Anne H. Spencer, PhD, Exec Dir. *Admissions Contact:* Christina Manson, Dir.
Year Established: 1980.
Staff: Full-time: 2; Part-time: 2.
Avg Enrollment: 150. *Avg Class Size:* 22. *Number of Graduates per Year:* 100.
Wheelchair Access: Yes.
Accreditation/Approval/Licensing: State board: MI Certified Addiction Counselors; MI Dept of Higher Ed; MI Nurses Association; International Medical and Dental Hypnotherapy Association; National Association of Alcohol and Drug Abuse; Westbrook University.
Field of Study: Hypnotherapy*; Reiki; Therapeutic Touch. *Program Name/Length:* Basic Hypnosis, 1 mo; Advanced Hypnotherapy, 1 mo; Hypnoanalysis, 1 mo; Reiki, Therapeutic Touch, weekend workshops.
Degrees Offered: CEUs; Diploma; Certificate.
License/Certification Preparation: International Medical and Dental Hypnotherapy Association.
Admission Requirements: Min age: 18; High school diploma/GED.
Application Deadline(s): Fall: Sep 10; Winter: Jan 10; Spring: Apr 1.
Tuition and Fees: $575 per course.
Financial Aid: Scholarships.
Career Services: Career information; Mentor program.

Saint Clair Shores

455. Wellspring Institute School of Therapeutic Bodywork

20312 Chalon St, Saint Clair Shores, MI 48080
Phone: (810) 772-8520
Program Administrator: Sandra J. Todt, Dir. *Admissions Contact:* Sandra J. Todt.
Year Established: 1981.
Staff: Full-time: 2; Part-time: 3.
Avg Enrollment: 75. *Avg Class Size:* 15.
Wheelchair Access: No.
Field of Study: Acupressure; CranioSacral Therapy; Energy Work; Hypnotherapy; Massage Therapy*; Polarity Therapy; Qigong; Reflexology; Shiatsu; Sports Massage; Therapeutic Touch. *Program Name/Length:* Massage Therapy, 300 hrs, 6-12 mos; Therapeutic Bodywork, 500 hrs, 1-2 yrs.
Degrees Offered: Diploma.
Admission Requirements: Min age: 18.
Tuition and Fees: $3085 (Massage Therapy); $4455 (Therapeutic Bodywork).
Financial Aid: Payment plan.
Career Services: Career counseling; Career information; Referral service.

Southfield

456. The International Center for Reiki Training

21421 Hilltop, Ste 28, Southfield, MI 48034
Phone: (800) 332-8112; *Fax:* (248) 948-8112
E-mail: reikicen@aol.com *Internet:* http://www.
reiki.org
Program Administrator: William Lee Rand, Pres.
Admissions Contact: William Lee Rand.
Year Established: 1988.
Staff: Full-time: 20.
Avg Enrollment: 1200. *Avg Class Size:* 20. *Number of Graduates per Year:* 1200.
Accreditation/Approval/Licensing: National Athletic Trainers Association Board of Certification.
Field of Study: Reiki*. *Program Name/Length:*
Reiki I/II, 2 days; Art/III Master, 3 days;
Karuna, 3 days.
Degrees Offered: CEUs; Certificate.
Admission Requirements: Min age: 18.
Career Services: Career counseling; Career information.

457. Irene's Myomassology Institute, Inc

18911 Ten Mile, Southfield, MI 48075
Phone: (248) 569-4263; *Fax:* (248) 569-4261
Internet: http://www.myomassology.com

Program Administrator: Kathleen Gauthier Grogan, Admin. *Admissions Contact:* Danielle Osborn, Public Relations.
Year Established: 1993.
Staff: Part-time: 15.
Avg Enrollment: 300. *Avg Class Size:* 22. *Number of Graduates per Year:* 150.
Wheelchair Access: No.
Accreditation/Approval/Licensing: State board: MI Board of Higher Ed; International Myomassethics Federation.
Field of Study: Aromatherapy; CranioSacral Therapy; Herbal Medicine; Massage Therapy*; Myomassology*; Polarity Therapy; Prenatal Massage; Qigong; Reflexology; Shiatsu; Sports Massage; Thai Massage. *Program Name/Length:* Myomassology, 1 yr.
Degrees Offered: Diploma.
License/Certification Preparation: National Certification Board for Therapeutic Massage and Bodywork; Certification, International Myomassethics Federation.
Admission Requirements: High school diploma/GED.
Application Deadline(s): Fall: Aug; Winter: Dec; Spring: Apr.
Tuition and Fees: $3990.
Financial Aid: Scholarships.
Career Services: Career information; Job information.

MINNESOTA

Bloomington

458. Northwestern College of Chiropractic

2501 W 84th St, Bloomington, MN 55431
Phone: (612) 888-4777; *Fax:* (612) 888-6713
E-mail: admit@nwchiro.edu *Internet:* http://www.
nwchiro.edu
Program Administrator: John F. Allenburg, DC,
Pres. *Admissions Contact:* Henry Kaynes, PhD,
Admissions Dir.
Year Established: 1941.
Staff: Full-time: 55; Part-time: 20.
Avg Enrollment: 700. *Avg Class Size:* 70. *Number of Graduates per Year:* 170.
Wheelchair Access: Yes.
Accreditation/Approval/Licensing: State board:
MN Higher Ed Services Office; Council on Chiropractic Education; North Central Association of Colleges and Schools.
Field of Study: Acupressure; Acupuncture*;
Chiropractic*. *Program Name/Length:* Doctor of Chiropractic, 10 semesters.
Degrees Offered: BS; DC.

Admission Requirements: High school diploma/GED; Some college (3 yrs); Min GPA: 2.5.
Tuition and Fees: $5000 per semester.
Financial Aid: Grants; Loans; Scholarships; Work study; VA approved.
Career Services: Career counseling; Career information; Internships.

Duluth

459. Lake Superior College

Massage Therapy Program
2101 Trinity Rd, Duluth, MN 55811
Phone: (218) 733-5921, (800) 432-2884
E-mail: daveburson@lsc.edu
Program Administrator: Dave Burson, Prog Dir.
Admissions Contact: Dave Burson.
Year Established: 1998.
Field of Study: Massage Therapy*. *Program Name/Length:* 5 1/2 mos.
Tuition and Fees: $5600.

Eagan

460. Hypnosis Research and Training Center

Hypnotherapy Certification
1960 Cliff Lake Rd, Stes 112-200, Eagan, MN 55122
Phone: (612) 707-1898; *Fax:* (612) 707-1898
E-mail: meta@ix.netcom.com *Internet:* http://www.hollys.com/success-dynamics
Program Administrator: Kevin Hogan, PhD, Dir. *Admissions Contact:* Kevin Hogan.
Year Established: 1998.
Staff: Full-time: 1; Part-time: 3.
Avg Enrollment: 60. *Avg Class Size:* 15. *Number of Graduates per Year:* 58.
Wheelchair Access: Yes.
Accreditation/Approval/Licensing: International Medical and Dental Hypnotherapy Association.
Field of Study: Hypnotherapy*; Neuro-Linguistic Programming*. *Program Name/Length:* Hypnotherapy Certification, 130 hrs; NLP Certification, 130 hrs; Seminars given in various locations; Home study/Correspondence.
Degrees Offered: Certificate.
License/Certification Preparation: International Medical and Dental Hypnotherapy Association.
Admission Requirements: Min age: 18.
Application Deadline(s): Fall: Aug 31; Winter: Feb 28; Spring: Apr 30.

Edina

461. Biofeedback Training and Treatment Center, Inc

7300 France Ave S, Ste 200, Edina, MN 55435
Phone: (612) 893-9400; *Fax:* (612) 893-0615
E-mail: pills@aol.com
Program Administrator: Lilli Ann Jeffrey-Smith, PhD, Dir. *Admissions Contact:* Lilli Ann Jeffrey-Smith.
Year Established: 1983.
Staff: Part-time: 1.
Avg Enrollment: 10. *Avg Class Size:* 5. *Number of Graduates per Year:* 10.
Wheelchair Access: Yes.
Accreditation/Approval/Licensing: Accrediting Council for Continuing Education and Training; Biofeedback Certification Institute of America.
Field of Study: Biofeedback*. *Program Name/Length:* 60 hrs; 200 hrs.
Degrees Offered: Certificate.
License/Certification Preparation: Biofeedback Certification Institute of America.
Admission Requirements: Bachelor's degree in health care field; Specific course prerequisites: anatomy, counseling.
Tuition and Fees: $950 (60 hrs); $2000 (200 hrs).
Career Services: Internships.

Mankato

462. Sister Rosalind Gefre School of Professional Massage, Mankato

165 W Lind Ct, Mankato, MN 56001
Phone: (507) 344-0220
Staff: Part-time: 80 over 4 campuses.
Accreditation/Approval/Licensing: International Massage and Somatic Therapies Accreditation Council; National Certification Board for Therapeutic Massage and Bodywork (CEUs).
Field of Study: Deep Tissue Massage; Massage Therapy*; Reflexology. *Program Name/Length:* Intro class; Professional Massage Therapy, 650 hrs.
Degrees Offered: CEUs; Certificate.
License/Certification Preparation: National Certification Board for Therapeutic Massage and Bodywork.
Admission Requirements: Min age: 18; High school diploma/GED.
Application Deadline(s): Fall: Aug; Winter: Feb.
Tuition and Fees: $495 (Intro); $5554 (Professional).
Financial Aid: VA approved; Vocational rehabilitation; Payment plan.
Career Services: Career information.

Minneapolis

463. BKS Iyengar Yoga Center

2736 Lyndale Ave S, Minneapolis, MN 55408
Phone: (612) 872-8708; *Fax:* (612) 872-1893
E-mail: chirh001@tc.umn.edu
Program Administrator: Lee Sverkerson, Co-Dir; Kristin Chirhart, Co-Dir. *Admissions Contact:* Lee Sverkerson; Kristin Chirhart.
Year Established: 1982.
Staff: Full-time: 2.
Avg Enrollment: 12. *Avg Class Size:* 12. *Number of Graduates per Year:* 12.
Wheelchair Access: Yes.
Field of Study: Yoga Teacher Training*. *Program Name/Length:* Iyengar Yoga Teacher Training, 3 yrs; In-depth Studies, 3 yrs.
License/Certification Preparation: Certification, Iyengar Yoga National Association.
Admission Requirements: Specific course prerequisites: 2 yrs of Iyengar yoga study required for Teacher Training, 1 yr for In-depth Studies.
Application Deadline(s): Fall: Sep 1.
Tuition and Fees: $700 per yr.

464. Minneapolis School of Massage and Bodywork, Inc

85 22nd Ave NE, Minneapolis, MN 55418
Phone: (612) 788-8907; *Fax:* (612) 788-8907
E-mail: msmb@mplsschoolofmassage.org
Internet: http://www.mplsschoolofmassage.org
Program Administrator: Joan Crawford-Dietsch, Dir of Ed.

Year Established: 1975.

Staff: Full-time: 3; Part-time: 11.

Avg Enrollment: 300. *Avg Class Size:* 14. *Number of Graduates per Year:* 300.

Wheelchair Access: Yes.

Accreditation/Approval/Licensing: International Massage and Somatic Therapies Accreditation Council; Accrediting Commission of Career Schools and Colleges of Technology.

Field of Study: Deep Tissue Massage*; Massage Therapy*; Sports Massage*. *Program Name/Length:* Massage Practitioner, 6 mos; Deep Tissue/Sports Massage, 1 yr; Comprehensive Massage Therapy, 18 mos.

Degrees Offered: Certificate.

Admission Requirements: Min age: 18; High school diploma/GED.

Financial Aid: State government aid.

Career Services: Career information; Job information.

465. Minnesota Center for Shiatsu Study

Professional Shiatsu Training Program
1313 5th St SE, Ste 336, Minneapolis, MN 55414
Phone: (612) 379-3565; *Fax:* (612) 379-3568
E-mail: shiatsumn@aol.com
Program Administrator: Cari Johnson Pelava, Dir. *Admissions Contact:* Contact admissions for more information.

Year Established: 1992.

Staff: Full-time: 2; Part-time: 14.

Avg Enrollment: 75. *Avg Class Size:* 15. *Number of Graduates per Year:* 35.

Wheelchair Access: Yes.

Accreditation/Approval/Licensing: American Oriental Bodywork Therapy Association.

Field of Study: Shiatsu*; Traditional Chinese Medicine. *Program Name/Length:* Professional Shiatsu Training, 560 hrs, 1 yr/full-time or 2 yrs/evenings.

Degrees Offered: Certificate.

License/Certification Preparation: American Oriental Bodywork Therapy Association.

Admission Requirements: Min age: 18; High school diploma/GED.

Application Deadline(s): Fall: Aug 15; Winter: Jan 15.

Tuition and Fees: $5875-$6125.

Financial Aid: Loans; State government aid; VA approved; Payment plan.

466. Northern Lights School of Massage Therapy

Massage Therapy Training Program
1313 SE 5th St, Ste 209, Minneapolis, MN 55414
Phone: (612) 379-3822; *Fax:* (612) 379-5971
Program Administrator: Jackson Petersburg, Exec Dir. *Admissions Contact:* Deni Dantis, Admissions Dir.

Year Established: 1985.

Staff: Part-time: 9.

Avg Enrollment: 70. *Avg Class Size:* 12 full-time, 25 part-time. *Number of Graduates per Year:* 70.

Wheelchair Access: Yes.

Field of Study: Massage Therapy*. *Program Name/Length:* 600 hrs, 1 yr/full-time or 2 yrs/part-time.

Degrees Offered: Certificate.

License/Certification Preparation: National Certification Board for Therapeutic Massage and Bodywork.

Admission Requirements: Min age: 18; High school diploma/GED.

Application Deadline(s): Fall: Jul; Winter: Nov.

Tuition and Fees: $5000.

Financial Aid: Loans.

Career Services: Job information.

467. University of Minnesota, Academic Health Program

Center for Spirituality and Healing
308 Harvard St SE, 6-101 WDH, Minneapolis, MN 55455
Phone: (612) 624-9459; *Fax:* (612) 624-3174
Internet: http://www.nursing.umn.edu
Program Administrator: Mary Jo Kreitzer, PhD, Dir.

Staff: Full-time: 2; Part-time: 3.

Wheelchair Access: Yes.

Accreditation/Approval/Licensing: North Central Association of Colleges and Schools; American College of Nurse-Midwives, Division of Accreditation.

Field of Study: Midwifery*. *Program Name/Length:* Nurse-Midwifery, 6 qtrs, 2 yrs.

Degrees Offered: MS.

License/Certification Preparation: Certified Nurse-Midwife, American College of Nurse-Midwives.

Admission Requirements: Bachelor's degree; Min GPA: 3.0; RN; 1 yr RN experience, OB preferred.

Application Deadline(s): Fall: Dec 15.

Tuition and Fees: $1560/resident, $3130/nonresident per qtr.

Financial Aid: Federal government aid; Federal traineeships; Scholarships.

Career Services: Job information.

Plymouth

468. Northwestern School of Homeopathy

10700 Old County Rd 15, Ste 300, Plymouth, MN 55441
Phone: (612) 794-6445; *Fax:* (612) 525-9518
E-mail: info@homeopathicschool.org *Internet:* http://www.homeopathicschool.org
Program Administrator: Eric Sommermann, Dean. *Admissions Contact:* Jan Forsberg, Admin.

Year Established: 1994.

Staff: Full-time: 2; Part-time: 5.

Avg Enrollment: 25. *Avg Class Size:* 25. *Number of Graduates per Year:* 22.
Wheelchair Access: Yes.
Accreditation/Approval/Licensing: State board: MN Board of Higher Ed; Candidate, Council on Homeopathic Education.
Field of Study: Homeopathy*. *Program Name/Length:* Classical Homeopathy: Academic and Clinical Training, 6 semesters, 3 yrs.
Degrees Offered: Certificate.
License/Certification Preparation: Council for Homeopathic Certification; Homeopathic Academy of Naturopathic Physicians; North American Society of Homeopaths.
Admission Requirements: Min age: 18; Some college; Specific course prerequisites: psychology, biology, chemistry, anatomy and physiology, scientific and medical terminology, microbiology, human pathology, emergency training.
Tuition and Fees: $2450 per semester.
Career Services: Career counseling; Career information; Mentorship.

Rochester

469. Sister Rosalind Gefre School of Professional Massage, Rochester

300 Elton Hills Dr NW, Rochester, MN 55901
Phone: (507) 286-8608; *Fax:* (507) 282-2893
Program Administrator: Rolf Bollingberg, Admin. *Admissions Contact:* Rolf Bollingberg.
Year Established: 1995.
Staff: Part-time: 20.
Avg Enrollment: 60. *Avg Class Size:* 10. *Number of Graduates per Year:* 15.
Wheelchair Access: Yes.
Accreditation/Approval/Licensing: International Massage and Somatic Therapies Accreditation Council; National Certification Board for Therapeutic Massage and Bodywork (CEUs).
Field of Study: Deep Tissue Massage; Massage Therapy*; Reflexology. *Program Name/Length:* Intro class; Professional Massage Therapy, 650 hrs.
Degrees Offered: CEUs; Certificate.
License/Certification Preparation: National Certification Board for Therapeutic Massage and Bodywork.
Admission Requirements: Min age: 18; High school diploma/GED.
Application Deadline(s): Fall: Aug; Winter: Feb.
Tuition and Fees: $495 (Intro); $5554 (Professional).
Financial Aid: VA approved; Vocational rehabilitation; Payment plan.
Career Services: Career information.

Saint Paul

470. Sister Rosalind Gefre School of Professional Massage, Saint Paul

400 Selby Ave, Ste G, Saint Paul, MN 55102
Phone: (651) 228-0960; *Fax:* (651) 698-7436
Program Administrator: Page Dunn-Albertie, School Admin. *Admissions Contact:* Audry Handland, Student Advisor.
Year Established: 1973.
Staff: Part-time: 80 over 4 campuses.
Avg Enrollment: 200. *Avg Class Size:* 16. *Number of Graduates per Year:* 20.
Wheelchair Access: Yes.
Accreditation/Approval/Licensing: International Massage and Somatic Therapies Accreditation Council.
Field of Study: Acupressure; Chair Massage*; CranioSacral Therapy; Massage Therapy*; Neuromuscular Therapy; On-Site Massage; Reflexology*; Sports Massage. *Program Name/Length:* Intro to Swedish; Massage Certification, 650 hrs, 15 mos; Reflexology Certificate, 6 mos; On-Site Chair Certification, 6-8 mos.
Degrees Offered: Certificate.
License/Certification Preparation: American Oriental Bodywork Therapy Association; American Reflexology Certification Board; National Certification Board for Therapeutic Massage and Bodywork.
Admission Requirements: Min age: 18; High school diploma/GED; Min GPA: 2.5; Specific course prerequisites: Intro to Swedish required for Massage and On-Site Certification.
Tuition and Fees: $495 (Intro to Swedish); $5554 (Massage Certification); $2158 (Reflexology); $1247 (On-Site).
Financial Aid: Loans; Work study; VA approved.
Career Services: Career counseling; Career information; Internships; Job information; Sister Rosalind Gefre Professional Massage Centers.

471. Minnesota Institute of Acupuncture and Herbal Studies

1821 University Ave W, Ste 278-S, Saint Paul, MN 55104
Phone: (612) 603-0994; *Fax:* (612) 603-0995
E-mail: miahs@millcomm.com *Internet:* http://www.millcomm.com/~miahs/miahs.htm
Program Administrator: Isaac Rodman, Pres. *Admissions Contact:* Page Purdy, Registrar.
Year Established: 1990.
Staff: Part-time: 20.
Avg Enrollment: 80. *Avg Class Size:* 25. *Number of Graduates per Year:* 12.
Wheelchair Access: Yes.
Accreditation/Approval/Licensing: Candidacy, Accreditation Commission for Acupuncture and Oriental Medicine.

Field of Study: Acupuncture*; Herbal Medicine*; Oriental Medicine*; Traditional Chinese Medicine*. *Program Name/Length:* Professional Acupuncture, 3 1/4 yrs; Oriental Medicine (Acupuncture and Herbs), 4 yrs.
Degrees Offered: Diploma.
License/Certification Preparation: State: MN Licensed Acupuncturist; National Certification Commission for Acupuncture and Oriental Medicine.
Admission Requirements: Min age: 18; Some college (2 yrs); Personal statement; Professional references; Interview.
Application Deadline(s): Fall: Sep.
Tuition and Fees: $8000 per yr.
Financial Aid: Loans; State government aid; VA approved.
Career Services: Career counseling; Career information.

West Saint Paul

472. Center for A Balanced Life, Inc
Massage Practitioner Program
1535 Livingston, Ave, Ste 105, West Saint Paul, MN 55118-3411

Phone: (612) 455-0473
Internet: http://www.saintpaul.com/bodywork.htm
Program Administrator: Sister M. Janine Rajkowski, Exec Dir. *Admissions Contact:* Sister M. Janine Rajkowski.
Year Established: 1994.
Staff: Full-time: 1; Part-time: 3.
Avg Enrollment: 10. *Avg Class Size:* 5. *Number of Graduates per Year:* 5.
Wheelchair Access: Yes.
Accreditation/Approval/Licensing: State board: MN Private Postsecondary Ed.
Field of Study: Acupressure; Massage Therapy*; Polarity Therapy; Reflexology. *Program Name/Length:* Massage Practitioner, 15-20 mos.
Degrees Offered: Certificate.
License/Certification Preparation: National Certification Board for Therapeutic Massage and Bodywork.
Admission Requirements: Min age: 18; High school diploma/GED.
Tuition and Fees: $6700-$7000.
Career Services: Internship required; Work opportunities at Center.

MISSISSIPPI

Gulfport

473. Blue Cliff School of Therapeutic Massage, Gulf Coast Campus
942 E Beach Blvd, Gulfport, MS 39507
Phone: (228) 896-9727; *Fax:* (228) 896-8659
E-mail: bluecliff@datasync.com *Internet:* http://www.bluecliffschool.com
Program Administrator: Richard Lee Berry, Admin. *Admissions Contact:* Richard Lee Berry.
Year Established: 1997.
Staff: Part-time: 15.
Avg Enrollment: 100. *Avg Class Size:* 18.
Wheelchair Access: Yes.
Accreditation/Approval/Licensing: State board: MS Commission on Proprietary School and College Registration.
Field of Study: Acupressure; CranioSacral Therapy; Healing Touch; Massage Therapy*; Neuromuscular Therapy; Reflexology; Shiatsu; Sports Massage. *Program Name/Length:* Massage Therapist, 7 mos/days or 13 mos/nights.
Degrees Offered: Diploma.

License/Certification Preparation: National Certification Board for Therapeutic Massage and Bodywork.
Admission Requirements: Min age: 18; High school diploma/GED.
Tuition and Fees: $4950 includes books.
Financial Aid: Loans; Payment plan.
Career Services: Career counseling; Career information; Referral service.

Jackson

474. Blue Cliff School of Therapeutic Massage, Jackson
600 Hour Massage Therapist Program
5120 Galaxie Dr, Jackson, MS 39206
Phone: (601) 362-3624; *Fax:* (601) 362-3694
Program Administrator: Cheryl Sproles, Dir/Admin. *Admissions Contact:* Dee A. Meux, Admissions Counselor.
Year Established: 1996.
Staff: Full-time: 4; Part-time: 6.
Avg Class Size: 12. *Number of Graduates per Year:* 40.

Accreditation/Approval/Licensing: State board: MS Commission on Proprietary School and College Registration.
Field of Study: Aromatherapy; CranioSacral Therapy; Deep Tissue Massage*; Energy Work; Massage Therapy*; Neuromuscular Therapy*; Reflexology; Reiki; Shiatsu*. *Program Name/Length:* 600 hrs, 6 1/2 mos/days or 13 1/2 mos/evenings.

Degrees Offered: Diploma.
License/Certification Preparation: National Certification Board for Therapeutic Massage and Bodywork.
Admission Requirements: Min age: 18; High school diploma/GED.
Tuition and Fees: $4400 + $550 books, fees.
Financial Aid: Loans; VA approved.
Career Services: Career information; Job board.

MISSOURI

Chesterfield

475. Logan College of Chiropractic
1851 Schoettler Rd, Chesterfield, MO 63017
Mailing Address: PO Box 1065, Chesterfield, MO 63006-1065
Phone: (314) 227-2100, (800) 533-9210; *Fax:* (314) 207-2424
E-mail: loganadm@logan.edu *Internet:* http://www.logan.edu
Program Administrator: George A. Goodman, DC, Pres.
Accreditation/Approval/Licensing: Council on Chiropractic Education.
Field of Study: Chiropractic*.
Degrees Offered: DC.
Admission Requirements: Some college.

Columbia

476. Massage Therapy Institute of Missouri (MTIM)
5 S 9th St, Ste 202, Columbia, MO 65201
Phone: (573) 875-7905; *Fax:* (573) 443-7933
E-mail: eruvalca@digmo.org
Program Administrator: Mirra Greenway, Esteban Ruvalcaba, co-owners. *Admissions Contact:* Mirra Greenway, NCTMB, Admissions Dir.
Year Established: 1994.
Staff: Full-time: 2; Part-time: 10.
Avg Enrollment: 20. *Avg Class Size:* 6-8. *Number of Graduates per Year:* 3-6.
Wheelchair Access: No.
Field of Study: Deep Tissue Massage; Energy Work*; Massage Therapy*; Sports Massage*; Swedish Massage*. *Program Name/Length:* Deep Tissue Massage: 500 hrs; Sports (Clinical) Massage: 500 hrs; Swedish/Integrative Massage: 500 hrs; Energetic Studies: 500 hrs.
Degrees Offered: Certificate.
License/Certification Preparation: National Certification Board for Therapeutic Massage and Bodywork.

Admission Requirements: Min age: 16; High school diploma/GED.
Financial Aid: Payment plan; Scholarships; Work study.
Career Services: Career counseling; Career information; Internships; Interview set up; Regional networking.

477. University of Missouri, Columbia, Sinclair School of Nursing
Nurse-Midwifery Program
Columbia, MO 65211
Phone: (573) 882-0235; *Fax:* (573) 884-4544
E-mail: nurssche@showme.missouri.edu
Program Administrator: Donna Scheideberg, PhD, Coord. *Admissions Contact:* Nancy Johnson, Student Admissions.
Year Established: 1995.
Staff: Full-time: 3; Part-time: 12.
Avg Enrollment: 8. *Avg Class Size:* 8. *Number of Graduates per Year:* 7.
Wheelchair Access: Yes.
Accreditation/Approval/Licensing: State board: MO Board of Nursing; Southern Association of Colleges and Schools; American College of Nurse-Midwives, Division of Accreditation.
Field of Study: Midwifery*. *Program Name/Length:* Nurse-Midwifery, 5 semesters/full-time or 8-10 semesters/part-time.
Degrees Offered: MS; Certificate.
License/Certification Preparation: Certified Nurse-Midwife, American College of Nurse-Midwives.
Admission Requirements: Bachelor's degree; Min GPA: 3.0; RN; Min GRE: 1500.
Application Deadline(s): Fall: Jun 1.
Tuition and Fees: $1700/resident, $3600/nonresident per semester.
Financial Aid: Fellowships; Loans; Scholarships; State government aid.
Career Services: Career counseling; Career information; Resume service.

Kansas City

478. Cleveland Chiropractic College, Kansas City

6401 Rockhill Rd, Kansas City, MO 64131
Phone: (816) 501-0100; *Fax:* (816) 361-0272
E-mail: admis@clevelandchiropractic.edu *Internet:* http://www.clevelandchiropractic.edu
Program Administrator: Carl S. Cleveland III, DC, Pres. *Admissions Contact:* Brenda Holland, Dir of Admissions.
Year Established: 1922.
Wheelchair Access: Yes.
Accreditation/Approval/Licensing: Council on Chiropractic Education; North Central Association of Colleges and Schools.
Field of Study: Chiropractic*. *Program Name/Length:* 9 semesters, 4 academic yrs; 12 semesters, 5 1/2 academic yrs.
Degrees Offered: BS; DC.
License/Certification Preparation: State: All 50 states; National Board of Chiropractic Examiners.
Admission Requirements: Some college.

479. Massage Therapy Training Institute, LLC

9140 Ward Pkwy, Ste 100, Kansas City, MO 64114
Phone: (816) 523-9140
Program Administrator: Terri Oglesby, Admin. *Admissions Contact:* Connie Orman, School Manager.
Year Established: 1988.
Staff: Part-time: 21.
Avg Enrollment: 450. *Avg Class Size:* 16. *Number of Graduates per Year:* 20.
Wheelchair Access: Yes.
Accreditation/Approval/Licensing: State board: MO Coordinating Board for Higher Ed; Accrediting Council for Continuing Education and Training; International Massage and Somatic Therapies Accreditation Council; National Certification Board for Therapeutic Massage and Bodywork (CEUs).
Field of Study: Aromatherapy; CranioSacral Therapy; Energy Work*; Herbal Medicine; Massage Therapy*; Myofascial Release; Neuromuscular Therapy; Polarity Therapy; Qigong; Reflexology; Shiatsu; Sports Massage; Therapeutic Touch; Trigger Point Therapy. *Program Name/Length:* Massage Therapy Practitioner, 500 hrs, 18-24 mos; Personal Trainer/Wellness Consultant, 300 hrs, 18-24 mos; Energy Therapy, 200 hrs, 1 yr.
Degrees Offered: CEUs; Diploma; Certificate.
License/Certification Preparation: Kansas City License; National Certification Board for Therapeutic Massage and Bodywork.
Admission Requirements: Min age: 18; High school diploma/GED.

Tuition and Fees: $5800 (Massage Therapy); $3500 (Personal Trainer); $2300 (Energy Trainer).
Career Services: Job postings.

Saint Charles

480. Saint Charles School of Massage Therapy

2440 Executive Dr, Saint Charles, MO 63301
Phone: (314) 498-0777; *Fax:* (314) 498-0708
E-mail: oasis@anet-stl.com *Internet:* http://www.britestar.net/oasis
Program Administrator: Kathleen Crawford, Dir. *Admissions Contact:* Kathleen Crawford.
Year Established: 1987.
Staff: Full-time: 2; Part-time: 6.
Avg Enrollment: 75. *Avg Class Size:* 10. *Number of Graduates per Year:* 75.
Wheelchair Access: Yes.
Accreditation/Approval/Licensing: State board: MO Coordinating Board for Higher Ed.
Field of Study: Aromatherapy; CranioSacral Therapy; Massage Therapy*; Polarity Therapy; Reflexology; Reiki; Shiatsu. *Program Name/Length:* Professional Massage Therapy Training, 500 hrs, 6 mos.
Degrees Offered: Certificate.
Admission Requirements: Min age: 18; High school diploma/GED.
Tuition and Fees: $4900.
Financial Aid: Loans.

Saint Louis

481. Inochi Institute, Inc.

Master of Acupuncture and Oriental Bodywork
70-D Grasso Plaza, Saint Louis, MO 63123
Mailing Address: PO Box 28803, Saint Louis, MO 63123
Phone: (314) 544-9600; *Fax:* (314) 631-0223
E-mail: inochi_institute@hotmail.com
Program Administrator: Dr. Thomas Duckworth, Admin. *Admissions Contact:* Dr. Thomas Duckworth, Admin.
Year Established: 1998.
Staff: Full-time: 2-3; Part-time: 3-4.
Avg Class Size: 10-12.
Wheelchair Access: Yes.
Accreditation/Approval/Licensing: State board: Missouri; Accrediting Council for Continuing Education and Training; Accreditation Commission for Acupuncture and Oriental Medicine.
Field of Study: Acupressure; Acupuncture*; Energy Work; Herbal Medicine; Homeopathy; Kototama Medicine; Massage Therapy; Naturopathic Medicine; Neuromuscular Therapy; Oriental Medicine*; Shiatsu*; Traditional Japanese Medicine*. *Program Name/Length:* Shiatsu-Oriental bodywork therapist, 1 yr.

Degrees Offered: CEUs; MS; Diploma.
License/Certification Preparation: State: Missouri; National Certification Commission for Acupuncture and Oriental Medicine.
Admission Requirements: Min age: 19; High school diploma/GED (for bodywork); Some college (Min 2 yrs for acupuncture).
Application Deadline(s): Fall.
Tuition and Fees: pay per course.

Springfield

482. Professional Massage Training Center
200 E Commercial, Springfield, MO 65803
Phone: (417) 863-7682; *Fax:* (417) 863-7652
E-mail: juliet@cland.net
Program Administrator: Juliet Mee, Dir. *Admissions Contact:* Debbie Jolley, Supervisor.
Year Established: 1994.
Staff: Part-time: 5.
Avg Enrollment: 15. *Avg Class Size:* 15. *Number of Graduates per Year:* 15.
Wheelchair Access: Yes.
Accreditation/Approval/Licensing: State board: MO Coordinating Board for Higher Ed.
Field of Study: Massage Therapy*. *Program Name/Length:* 600 hrs.
Degrees Offered: Certificate.
License/Certification Preparation: National Certification Board for Therapeutic Massage and Bodywork.
Admission Requirements: Min age: 18; High school diploma/GED; 2 professional massages.
Tuition and Fees: $5025 + $500 books, supplies.
Financial Aid: Loans; Work study; VA approved; Vocational rehabilitation; Payment plan.
Career Services: Career counseling; Career information; Internships; Resume service; Job information.

MONTANA

Helena

483. Big Sky Somatic Institute
1802 11th Ave, Ste A, Helena, MT 59601
Phone: (406) 442-8998
Program Administrator: Ron Floyd, Co-Dir; Jennifer Hicks, Co-Dir. *Admissions Contact:* Linus Carleton, Admin.
Year Established: 1996.
Staff: Part-time: 10.
Avg Enrollment: 30. *Avg Class Size:* 16.
Wheelchair Access: No.
Accreditation/Approval/Licensing: State board: MT Dept of Commerce, Div of Postsecondary Ed.
Field of Study: Acupressure; Energy Work; Herbal Medicine; Massage Therapy*; Neuromuscular Therapy; Qigong*; Shiatsu*; Thai Massage*; Traditional Chinese Medicine. *Program Name/Length:* Introduction to Massage and Bodywork, 130 hrs, 6-12 mos; Intermediate Massage and Bodywork, 520 hrs, 1-2 yrs; Oriental Healing Arts, 550 hrs.
Degrees Offered: Certificate.
License/Certification Preparation: National Certification Board for Therapeutic Massage and Bodywork.
Admission Requirements: High school diploma/GED.
Application Deadline(s): Fall: Aug; Spring: Jan.
Tuition and Fees: $977 (Introduction); $4547 (Intermediate); $4675 (Oriental).

Hot Springs

484. Rocky Mountain Herbal Institute
Traditional Chinese Herbal Sciences
305 2nd Ave S, Hot Springs, MT 59845
Mailing Address: PO Box 579, Hot Springs, MT 59845
Phone: (406) 741-3811
E-mail: rmhi@rmhiherbal.org *Internet:* http://www.rmhiherbal.org
Program Administrator: Roger W. Wicke, PhD, Dir. *Admissions Contact:* Roger W. Wicke, PhD.
Year Established: 1991.
Staff: Full-time: 1; Part-time: 2.
Avg Enrollment: 6. *Avg Class Size:* 6. *Number of Graduates per Year:* 4.
Wheelchair Access: No.
Accreditation/Approval/Licensing: American Association of Drugless Practitioners.
Field of Study: Herbal Medicine*; Traditional Chinese Medicine*. *Program Name/Length:* 2 yrs.
Degrees Offered: Certificate.
Admission Requirements: Some college; Specific course prerequisites: B in anatomy and physiology or graduate degree in clinical health field; Achieve 70 percent on sample homework assignment.
Application Deadline(s): Fall: Sep.
Tuition and Fees: $4100.
Career Services: Career counseling; Career information; Referral service.

Missoula

485. Starfire Massage School and Healing Center
9819 Waldo Rd, Missoula, MT 59808
Phone: (406) 721-7519; *Fax:* (406) 721-7519
E-mail: starfiremassageschool@yahoo.com
Internet: http://www.montana.com/massage
Program Administrator: Victoria Noble, Co-Dir.
   Admissions Contact: Mary Marron, Co-Dir.
Year Established: 1995.
Staff: Part-time: 12.
Avg Enrollment: 22. *Avg Class Size:* 11. *Number of Graduates per Year:* 20.
Wheelchair Access: Yes.
Accreditation/Approval/Licensing: National Certification Board for Therapeutic Massage and Bodywork (CEUs).

Field of Study: Acupressure*; Energy Work; Hydrotherapy; Massage Therapy*; Reiki*; Shamanic Healing; Shiatsu*; Sound Healing. *Program Name/Length:* Certified Massage Practitioner, 165 hrs; Certified Massage Therapist, 500 hrs or 600 hrs.
Degrees Offered: CEUs; Certificate.
License/Certification Preparation: National Certification Board for Therapeutic Massage and Bodywork.
Admission Requirements: Min age: 18; High school diploma/GED.
Application Deadline(s): Fall: Aug 15; Spring: Jan 15.
Tuition and Fees: $1500 (165 hrs); $4400 (500 hrs); $4900 (600 hrs).
Career Services: Job information; Referral service.

NEBRASKA

Lincoln

486. Myotherapy Institute
6020 S 58th St, Lincoln, NE 68516
Phone: (402) 421-7410; *Fax:* (402) 421-6736
Accreditation/Approval/Licensing: State board: NE Depts of Health and Ed.
Field of Study: Hydrotherapy; Massage Therapy*; Medical Massage; Spa Therapies. *Program Name/Length:* 1000 hrs, 10 mos (days or evenings).
License/Certification Preparation: State: NE Licensed Massage Therapist; National Certification Board for Therapeutic Massage and Bodywork.
Application Deadline(s): Fall: Aug; Spring: Jan.

Omaha

487. Omaha School of Massage Therapy
9748 Park Dr, Omaha, NE 68127
Phone: (402) 331-3694; *Fax:* (402) 331-0280
E-mail: osmtschool@aol.com *Internet:* http://www.osmt.com
Admissions Contact: Ann Reuck, Dir.
Year Established: 1991.
Staff: Part-time: 8.
Avg Enrollment: 75. *Avg Class Size:* 12. *Number of Graduates per Year:* 55.
Wheelchair Access: Yes.
Accreditation/Approval/Licensing: State board: NE Depts of Health and Ed; Accrediting Commission of Career Schools and Colleges of Technology.

Field of Study: Acupressure; Aromatherapy; Energy Work; Massage Therapy*; Reflexology; Sports Massage; Swedish Massage*. *Program Name/Length:* Massage Therapy, 9 mos (prelicensing).
Degrees Offered: Diploma.
License/Certification Preparation: State: NE Licensed Massage Therapist; National Certification Board for Therapeutic Massage and Bodywork.
Admission Requirements: Min age: 18; High school diploma/GED.
Tuition and Fees: $7580.
Financial Aid: Federal government aid; Grants; Loans; VA approved; Vocational rehabilitation.

488. Universal Center of Healing Arts
School of Massage Therapy
109 N 50th St, Omaha, NE 68132
Phone: (402) 556-4456; *Fax:* (402) 561-0635
Program Administrator: Paulette Genthon, Exec Dir. *Admissions Contact:* Patrick Davis, Asst Dir.
Year Established: 1994.
Staff: Full-time: 3; Part-time: 6.
Avg Enrollment: 60. *Number of Graduates per Year:* 50.
Accreditation/Approval/Licensing: State board: NE and IA Depts of Health.
Field of Study: Acupressure; Aromatherapy; Ayurvedic Medicine; CranioSacral Therapy; Energy Work; Herbal Medicine; Massage Therapy*; Neuromuscular Therapy; Oriental Medicine; Polarity Therapy; Qigong; Reflexology;

Reiki; Shiatsu; Sports Massage; Tai Chi; Traditional Chinese Medicine; Yoga. *Program Name/Length:* Seminars given in various locations 500 hrs; Home study/Correspondence 1000 hrs, 9-11 mos.
Degrees Offered: Diploma; Certificate.
License/Certification Preparation: State: NE and IA Licensed Massage Therapist; National Certification Board for Therapeutic Massage and Bodywork.
Admission Requirements: Min age: 18; High school diploma/GED.
Tuition and Fees: $6561.
Financial Aid: Loans; Scholarships; VA approved; Vocational rehabilitation; Payment plan.
Career Services: Career information; Internships; Job information.

South Sioux City

489. Gateway College of Massage Therapy
2607 Dakota Ave, South Sioux City, NE 68776
Phone: (402) 494-8390; *Fax:* (402) 494-4561
E-mail: gcmass@pionet.net *Internet:* http://www.busdir.com/gatewaycol/index.html
Program Administrator: Darrell J. Peck, PhD, Exec Dir/Co-Owner; Joan E. Knott, Co-Owner. *Admissions Contact:* Darrell J. Peck.
Year Established: 1995.
Staff: Full-time: 1; Part-time: 5.
Avg Enrollment: 50. *Avg Class Size:* 8. *Number of Graduates per Year:* 40.
Wheelchair Access: Yes.
Accreditation/Approval/Licensing: State board: IA Dept of Health and Ed; NE Depts of Health and Ed.
Field of Study: Acupressure; CranioSacral Therapy; Massage Therapy*; Neuromuscular Therapy; Reflexology; Sports Massage; Swedish Massage*. *Program Name/Length:* Iowa, 9 mos; Nebraska, 1000 hrs, 1 yr.
Degrees Offered: Diploma.
License/Certification Preparation: National Certification Board for Therapeutic Massage and Bodywork.
Admission Requirements: Min age: 18; High school diploma/GED.
Application Deadline(s): Fall: Oct 15; Winter: Jan 15; Spring: Apr 15; Summer: Jul 15.
Tuition and Fees: $4950 (Iowa); $5950 (Nebraska).
Financial Aid: VA approved.
Career Services: Career counseling; Career information; Internships; Job information.

NEVADA

Incline Village

490. Aston-Patterning Training Center/A Continuing Education Service
PO Box 3568, Incline Village, NV 89450
Phone: (702) 831-8228
Program Administrator: Judith Aston, Dir/Pres. *Admissions Contact:* Judith Aston.
Year Established: 1971.
Staff: Full-time: 1; Part-time: 10.
Avg Class Size: 15. *Number of Graduates per Year:* 20.
Accreditation/Approval/Licensing: National Certification Board for Therapeutic Massage and Bodywork (CEUs).
Field of Study: Aston-Patterning Bodywork and Movement*. *Program Name/Length:* Basic Aston-Patterning Certification, 20 wks; Movement Certification, 13 wks; Electives-Arthrokinetics, 7 wks; Fitness, 5 wks; Facial Fitness, 2 wks.
Degrees Offered: Certificate.
Admission Requirements: Min age: 21; Bachelor's degree; Licensed health care professional; State-ment of purpose; Recommendation from Aston-Patterning Practitioner; 6 private Aston-Patterning sessions with certified practitioner; Specific course prerequisites: anatomy, kinesiology.
Tuition and Fees: $110-$125 per day.

Las Vegas

491. Dahan Institute of Massage Studies
3430 E Tropicana, Ste 62, Las Vegas, NV 89121
Phone: (702) 434-1338; *Fax:* (702) 434-3449
Internet: http://www.dahanmassage.com
Program Administrator: Serge Dahan, School Dir.
Year Established: 1993.
Staff: Full-time: 6; Part-time: 6.
Avg Enrollment: 150. *Avg Class Size:* 20. *Number of Graduates per Year:* 135.
Wheelchair Access: Yes.
Accreditation/Approval/Licensing: State board: NV Commission on Postsecondary Ed.
Field of Study: Acupressure; Aromatherapy; Massage Therapy*; Polarity Therapy; Reflexology;

Shiatsu; Sports Massage. *Program Name/Length:* Massage Therapist, 650 hrs.
Degrees Offered: Certificate.
License/Certification Preparation: National Certification Board for Therapeutic Massage and Bodywork.
Admission Requirements: Min age: 18; High school diploma/GED.
Tuition and Fees: $5900.
Financial Aid: Loans; VA approved; Vocational rehabilitation.
Career Services: Career counseling; Career information.

Reno

492. International BioMedical Research Institute

Homeopathic and Integrative Medicine
6490 S McCarran Blvd, C-24, Reno, NV 89509
Phone: (702) 827-1444; *Fax:* (702) 827-2424
E-mail: cora@bioregen.reno.nv.us
Program Administrator: Corazon I. Ibarra, MD, Research Dir. *Admissions Contact:* Edna Edsig, Sec.
Year Established: 1993.
Staff: Full-time: 2; Part-time: 2.

Avg Enrollment: 3. *Avg Class Size:* 3. *Number of Graduates per Year:* 3.
Field of Study: Herbal Medicine; Homeopathy*. *Program Name/Length:* 2 yrs; Home study/Correspondence.
License/Certification Preparation: State: NV Board of Homeopathic Medical Examiners.
Admission Requirements: Medical degree.
Application Deadline(s): Fall.
Tuition and Fees: $4000.

493. Ralston School of Massage

Washoe Med Ctr, 77 Pringle Way, Reno, NV 89520-0109
Phone: (775) 982-5450; *Fax:* (775) 982-5452
E-mail: 2relax@intercomm.com
Program Administrator: Robert H. Oliver, Dir. *Admissions Contact:* Debra Rilea.
Year Established: 1988.
Staff: Full-time: 1; Part-time: 3.
Avg Class Size: 20.
Wheelchair Access: Yes.
Field of Study: Massage Therapy*. *Program Name/Length:* 560 hrs, 10 mos-2 yrs (day, afternoon, or evening classes).
Admission Requirements: Min age: 18; High school diploma/GED.
Tuition and Fees: $3495 + $500 books, insurance.

NEW HAMPSHIRE

Hooksett

494. Dovestar Institute, Hooksett

50 Whitehall Rd, Hooksett, NH 03106
Phone: (603) 669-5104, (888) 222-5603; *Fax:* (603) 625-1919
Internet: http://www.dovestar.edu
Program Administrator: Kamala Renner, CEO. *Admissions Contact:* Heather Horton, Dir.
Year Established: 1973.
Staff: Full-time: 3; Part-time: 12.
Avg Enrollment: 60. *Avg Class Size:* 12. *Number of Graduates per Year:* 50.
Wheelchair Access: Yes.
Accreditation/Approval/Licensing: State board: NH Postsecondary Ed Commission.
Field of Study: Acupressure; Colon Hydrotherapy*; CranioSacral Therapy; Hypnotherapy*; Kriya Massage*; Neuromuscular Therapy; Qigong; Reflexology; Reiki*; Shiatsu; Yoga Teacher Training*. *Program Name/Length:* Colon Hydrotherapy, 2 mos; Reiki-Alchemia, 3 mos; Alchemical Synergy/Hypnotherapy, 6 mos; Kriya Massage, 9 mos; Alchemia Yoga Teacher Training, 1 yr.

Degrees Offered: CEUs; Certificate.
License/Certification Preparation: State: NH Licensed Massage Practitioner; National Certification Board for Therapeutic Massage and Bodywork.
Tuition and Fees: $2000-$6000.
Financial Aid: State government aid; Work study; Vocational rehabilitation.
Career Services: Career counseling; Career information; Internships.

Hudson

495. New Hampshire Institute for Therapeutic Arts School of Massage Therapy, Hudson

153 Lowell Rd, Hudson, NH 03051
Phone: (603) 882-3022; *Fax:* (603) 598-9101
Program Administrator: Patrick Cowan, MA, PhD, Administrative Dir. *Admissions Contact:* Patrick Cowan.
Year Established: 1983.
Staff: Full-time: 6; Part-time: 6.
Avg Enrollment: 36. *Avg Class Size:* 36.

Wheelchair Access: 36.
Accreditation/Approval/Licensing: National Certification Board for Therapeutic Massage and Bodywork (CEUs).
Field of Study: Acupressure*; Lymphatic Massage; Massage Therapy*; Neuromuscular Therapy; Polarity Therapy*; Reflexology*; Sports Massage*; Swedish Massage*. *Program Name/Length:* 9 mos (Sep-Jun, 2 terms).
Degrees Offered: Certificate.
License/Certification Preparation: ME Licensed Massage Therapist; NH Licensed Massage Practitioner; NY Licensed Massage Therapist; National Certification Board for Therapeutic Massage and Bodywork.
Admission Requirements: Min age: 18; High school diploma/GED.
Application Deadline(s): Fall: Aug 1.
Tuition and Fees: $5635 + $300 books, $500 table, $200 supplies.
Financial Aid: State government aid; Payment plan; Canadian government loans.
Career Services: Career counseling; Career information; Job information; Referral service.

Manchester

496. North Eastern Institute of Whole Health, Inc

22 Bridge St, Manchester, NH 03101-1655
Phone: (603) 623-5018; *Fax:* (603) 641-5928
Program Administrator: Dr. Gabrielle M. Grigore, Institute Dir. *Admissions Contact:* Douglas DuVerger, Academic Dir.
Year Established: 1993.
Staff: Full-time: 20; Part-time: 10.
Avg Enrollment: 100. *Avg Class Size:* 30. *Number of Graduates per Year:* 100.
Wheelchair Access: No.
Accreditation/Approval/Licensing: State board: NH Dept of Postsecondary Ed; National Certification Board for Therapeutic Massage and Bodywork (CEUs).
Field of Study: Acupressure; Anatomy and Physiology; Aromatherapy; Chair Massage; CPR/First Aid; CranioSacral Therapy; Esalen Massage; Herbal Medicine; Hydrotherapy; Hypnotherapy; LomiLomi Massage; Lymphatic Massage; Massage Therapy*; Neuromuscular Therapy; Oriental Medicine; Polarity Therapy; Pregnancy Massage; Qigong; Reflexology; Reiki; Shiatsu; Sports Massage; Traditional Chinese Medicine; Trigger Point Therapy. *Program Name/Length:* Diploma of Massage Therapy, 750 hrs, 1 yr.
Degrees Offered: Diploma; Certificate.

License/Certification Preparation: State: NH Licensed Massage Practitioner; National Certification Board for Therapeutic Massage and Bodywork.
Admission Requirements: Min age: 18; High school diploma/GED.
Application Deadline(s): Fall: Sep; Spring: Mar.
Tuition and Fees: $6000.
Financial Aid: Loans; Scholarships; State government aid; VA approved; Vocational rehabilitation; Payment plan; NH Charitable Foundation; NH Job Training Council.
Career Services: Career information; Internships; Job information.

Nashua

497. New England Academy of Therapeutic Sciences

402 Amherst St, Nashua, NH 03063
Phone: (603) 886-8433; *Fax:* (603) 880-8654
E-mail: maureen@neats.com *Internet:* http://www.neats.com
Program Administrator: Maureen J. Healy, Dir. *Admissions Contact:* Maureen J. Healy.
Year Established: 1993.
Staff: Full-time: 4; Part-time: 4.
Avg Enrollment: 55. *Avg Class Size:* 12. *Number of Graduates per Year:* 55.
Wheelchair Access: Yes.
Accreditation/Approval/Licensing: State board: NH Postsecondary Ed Approving Agency; National Certification Board for Therapeutic Massage and Bodywork (CEUs).
Field of Study: Acupressure; Animal Therapy*; CranioSacral Therapy; Equine Massage*; Herbal Medicine; Homeopathy; Hypnotherapy; Massage Therapy*; Neuromuscular Therapy; Polarity Therapy; Reflexology; Shiatsu; Swedish Massage*; Traditional Chinese Medicine. *Program Name/Length:* Massage Therapy, 830 hrs, 9 mos; Equine Massage, 3 levels, 3 wks per level.
Degrees Offered: Certificate.
License/Certification Preparation: State: NH Licensed Massage Practitioner; National Certification Board for Therapeutic Massage and Bodywork.
Admission Requirements: Min age: 18; High school diploma/GED.
Tuition and Fees: $9000 (Massage Therapy); $1500 per wk (Equine Massage).
Financial Aid: Payment plan; Work study.
Career Services: Career counseling; Career information; Externships; Internships.

NEW JERSEY

Belle Mead

498. Health Choices Center for the Healing Arts

170 Township Line Rd, Bldg B, Belle Mead, NJ
08502
Phone: (908) 359-3995; *Fax:* (908) 359-3902
E-mail: hc@health-choices.com *Internet:* http://
www.health-choices.com
Program Administrator: Renate M. Novak,
Owner/Co-Dir. *Admissions Contact:* Neil
Campbell Tucker, Dir of Operations.
Year Established: 1976.
Staff: Full-time: 3; Part-time: 10.
Avg Enrollment: 80. *Avg Class Size:* 20. *Number
of Graduates per Year:* 56.
Wheelchair Access: Yes.
Accreditation/Approval/Licensing: State board: NJ
Dept of Ed; Accrediting Council for Continuing
Education and Training; National Certification
Board for Therapeutic Massage and Bodywork
(CEUs).
Field of Study: Acupressure; Aromatherapy; Mas-
sage Therapy*; Neuromuscular Therapy; Polar-
ity Therapy; Qigong; Reflexology; Reiki;
Shiatsu. *Program Name/Length:* Massage Ther-
apy Training, 600 hrs, 1 yr; Continuing Educa-
tion, weekend workshops.
Degrees Offered: CEUs; Certificate; CMT.
License/Certification Preparation: National Certif-
ication Board for Therapeutic Massage and
Bodywork.
Application Deadline(s): Fall: Sep; Winter: Mar.
Tuition and Fees: $5885 (Massage Therapy).
Financial Aid: Federal government aid; State gov-
ernment aid.
Career Services: Career counseling; Career infor-
mation; Resume service.

Broadway

499. Herbal Therapeutics School of Botanical Medicine

PO Box 553, Broadway, NJ 08808
Phone: (908) 835-0822; *Fax:* (908) 835-0824
E-mail: dwherbal@nac.net
Program Administrator: David Winston, Herbalist,
Primary Instr/Dean. *Admissions Contact:* David
Winston.
Year Established: 1980.
Staff: Full-time: 1; Part-time: 3.
Avg Enrollment: 50. *Avg Class Size:* 25. *Number
of Graduates per Year:* 25.
Wheelchair Access: No.

Field of Study: Herbal Medicine*. *Program
Name/Length:* Herbalist training (includes Chinese Herbal Medicine, Field Botany, Herbal
Pharmacy, Materia Medica and Therapeutics),
450 hrs, 2 yrs (1 eve/wk); Graduate program, 75
hrs (1 weekend/mo).
Degrees Offered: Certificate.
Admission Requirements: Min age: 18; Licensed
health care professional or extensive study of
herbal medicine; Specific course prerequisites:
college-level anatomy and physiology.
Tuition and Fees: $1600-$1800.
Financial Aid: Work study.
Career Services: Career counseling; Career information.

Cherry Hill

500. School of Asian Healing Arts

Executive Mews G-38, 1930 E Marlton Pk, Cherry
Hill, NJ 08003
Phone: (609) 424-7501; *Fax:* (609) 424-7379
E-mail: acwsaha@bellatlantic.net *Internet:* http://
www.members.bellatlantic.net/~acwsaha
Program Administrator: Ruth Dalphin, Dir. *Ad-
missions Contact:* Maureen Esterland.
Year Established: 1989.
Staff: Part-time: 5.
Avg Enrollment: 25. *Avg Class Size:* 10. *Number
of Graduates per Year:* 4.
Wheelchair Access: Yes.
Accreditation/Approval/Licensing: State board: NJ
Dept of Ed; American Oriental Bodywork Ther-
apy Association.
Field of Study: Acupressure; Qigong; Reflexology;
Reiki; Shiatsu*; Thai Massage*; Traditional
Chinese Medicine; Yoga Teacher Training*.
Program Name/Length: Shiatsu, 150 hrs, 6
mos-1 yr; Shiatsu, 500 hrs, 18 mos-3 yrs; Yoga
Teacher Training, 200 hrs, 1 yr; Thai Massage,
100 hrs.
Degrees Offered: Certificate.
License/Certification Preparation: State: NJ; Na-
tional Certification Commission for Acupunc-
ture and Oriental Medicine; American Oriental
Bodywork Therapy Association.
Admission Requirements: Min age: 18; High
school diploma/GED.
Tuition and Fees: $1500-$1750 (150 hr Shiatsu);
$5000-$6000 (500 hr Shiatsu); $2000 (Yoga);
$1000 (Thai Massage).
Financial Aid: Payment plan.
Career Services: Career counseling; Career infor-
mation.

Collingswood

501. Our Lady of Lourdes Institute of Wholistic Studies

900 Haddon Ave, Ste 118, Collingswood, NJ 08108
Phone: (609) 869-3134; *Fax:* (609) 869-3129
Internet: http://www.loudesnet.org
Program Administrator: Erika MacWilliams, Institute Coord. *Admissions Contact:* Erika MacWilliams.
Year Established: 1993.
Staff: Part-time: 10.
Avg Enrollment: 35. *Avg Class Size:* 20. *Number of Graduates per Year:* 35.
Wheelchair Access: Yes.
Field of Study: Aromatherapy; Ayurvedic Medicine; Feldenkrais; Guided Imagery; Massage Therapy*; Reflexology; Reiki; Shiatsu*; Sports Massage; Therapeutic Touch; Traditional Chinese Medicine; Yoga Teacher Training*. *Program Name/Length:* Wholistic Massage Certification, 550 hrs; Shiatsu Certification, 3 mos; Wholistic Yoga Teacher Training, 2 mos.
Degrees Offered: Certificate.
License/Certification Preparation: National Certification Board for Therapeutic Massage and Bodywork.
Admission Requirements: Min age: 18; High school diploma/GED.
Application Deadline(s): Fall: Sep; Winter: Feb; Summer: Jul.
Tuition and Fees: $4190 (Massage).
Financial Aid: Loans; Work study.
Career Services: Career information; Job information.

Denville

502. Classic Center for Health and Healing

Therapeutic Touch
25 Orchard St, Ste 101, Denville, NJ 07834-2160
Phone: (973) 627-4833
Program Administrator: Zoe Elva Putnam, MA, Dir. *Admissions Contact:* Zoe Elva Putnam.
Year Established: 1991.
Staff: Full-time: 1.
Avg Enrollment: 60. *Avg Class Size:* 20. *Number of Graduates per Year:* 60.
Wheelchair Access: Yes.
Accreditation/Approval/Licensing: American Nurses Association.
Field of Study: Therapeutic Touch*. *Program Name/Length:* Basic, Intermediate, and Advanced Workshops, 35 hrs; Seminars given in various locations.
Degrees Offered: Certificate.
Tuition and Fees: $245 (Basic); $245 (Intermediate); $265 (Advanced).
Financial Aid: Payment plan.

503. Morris Institute of Natural Therapeutics

3108 Rte 10 W, Denville, NJ 07834
Phone: (201) 989-8939; *Fax:* (201) 989-5554
Program Administrator: Vincent R. Iuppo, Dir.
Admissions Contact: Elizabeth Iuppo, Registrar.
Year Established: 1963.
Staff: Full-time: 4; Part-time: 8.
Avg Enrollment: 200. *Avg Class Size:* 10.
Wheelchair Access: No.
Field of Study: Acupressure; Applied Kinesiology; Aromatherapy; Chair Massage; CranioSacral Therapy; Manual Lymph Drainage; Massage Therapy*; Neuromuscular Therapy; Reflexology; Shiatsu; Sports Massage. *Program Name/Length:* 3-day to 3-yr programs.
Degrees Offered: Certificate.
License/Certification Preparation: American Oriental Bodywork Therapy Association; National Certification Board for Therapeutic Massage and Bodywork.
Admission Requirements: Min age: 18; High school diploma/GED.
Application Deadline(s): Fall: Sep; Winter: Dec; Spring: Apr.
Tuition and Fees: $325-$3000.
Career Services: Career information.

Englewood

504. Academy of Massage Therapy

401 S Van Brunt St, Englewood, NJ 07631
Phone: (201) 568-3220; *Fax:* (201) 568-5181
Program Administrator: Joanna Sechuk, Exec Dir.
Admissions Contact: Young Lee, Admissions Representative.
Year Established: 1992.
Staff: Full-time: 3; Part-time: 6.
Avg Enrollment: 70. *Avg Class Size:* 16. *Number of Graduates per Year:* 65.
Wheelchair Access: Yes.
Accreditation/Approval/Licensing: Accrediting Commission of Career Schools and Colleges of Technology; National Certification Board for Therapeutic Massage and Bodywork (CEUs).
Field of Study: Aromatherapy; Massage Therapy*; Medical Massage; Qigong; Reflexology*; Reiki; Shiatsu*; Sports Massage; Thai Massage. *Program Name/Length:* NY Licensed Massage Therapist.
Degrees Offered: Certificate.
License/Certification Preparation: State: NY Licensed Massage Therapist; National Certification Board for Therapeutic Massage and Bodywork.
Admission Requirements: Min age: 18; High school diploma/GED.
Application Deadline(s): Fall: Sep; Winter: Jan; Spring: Apr; Summer: Jul.

Tuition and Fees: $4200 (Massage); $1100 (Shiatsu); $4200 (Oriental Bodywork).

Financial Aid: Federal government aid; Loans; State government aid; VA approved; Vocational rehabilitation; Payment plan.

Career Services: Career counseling; Career information; Internships; Interview set up; Job information; Referral service.

Flanders

505. Massage Therapy Center for Healing and Learning

4 Deerfield Pl, Flanders, NJ 07836

Phone: (973) 927-3151

Program Administrator: Jack Hicks, Dir. *Admissions Contact:* Jack Hicks.

Year Established: 1996.

Staff: Full-time: 4; Part-time: 1.

Avg Enrollment: 16. *Avg Class Size:* 8. *Number of Graduates per Year:* 16.

Wheelchair Access: No.

Accreditation/Approval/Licensing: Accrediting Commission of Career Schools and Colleges of Technology.

Field of Study: CranioSacral Therapy; Deep Tissue Massage; Massage Therapy*; Reflexology*; Reiki. *Program Name/Length:* 526 hrs, 6 mos.

Degrees Offered: Certificate.

License/Certification Preparation: National Certification Board for Therapeutic Massage and Bodywork.

Admission Requirements: Min age: 18; High school diploma/GED.

Application Deadline(s): Fall; Spring.

Tuition and Fees: $3800 includes books.

Financial Aid: State government aid.

Haddon Heights

506. Healing Hands School of Massage

515 Whitehorse Pike, Haddon Heights, NJ 08035

Phone: (215) 676-9891 am, (609) 546-7471 pm; *Fax:* (609) 546-7491

E-mail: edheisco@aol.com *Internet:* http://www.healingartsinstituteinc.baweb.com

Program Administrator: Kristina Shaw, Dir. *Admissions Contact:* Kristina Shaw.

Year Established: 1982.

Staff: Full-time: 2; Part-time: 5.

Avg Enrollment: 22. *Avg Class Size:* 11. *Number of Graduates per Year:* 20.

Wheelchair Access: Yes.

Accreditation/Approval/Licensing: State board: NJ Dept of Ed.

Field of Study: Acupressure; CranioSacral Therapy; Deep Tissue Massage*; Herbal Medicine; Hydrotherapy; Massage Therapy*; Myofascial Release; Neuromuscular Therapy; Polarity Therapy; Reflexology; Shiatsu*; Swedish Massage*;

Traditional Chinese Medicine*. *Program Name/Length:* Introduction to Massage, 65 hrs, 3 mos; Therapeutic and Deep Tissue Bodywork (includes Chinese and Western anatomy), 200 hrs; Professional Massage and Holistic Studies/Nutrition, 550 hrs, 1 yr (2 mornings or evenings per wk + 1 weekend per mo); Chinese Five Elements Nutrition and Shiatsu, 65 hrs.

Degrees Offered: Diploma; Certificate.

License/Certification Preparation: State: NJ Certified Massage Therapist; National Certification Board for Therapeutic Massage and Bodywork.

Admission Requirements: Min age: 21; High school diploma/GED; Specific course prerequisites: Introduction to Massage required for 200 hr and 550 hr programs.

Application Deadline(s): Fall: Intro class; Nov, for Professional Massage; Spring: Intro class; Summer: Intro class.

Tuition and Fees: $750 (65 hrs); $5600 (550 hrs).

Financial Aid: Loans; Payment plan; Work study.

Career Services: Career counseling; Career information; Internships; National exam tutoring.

Comments: South Jersey location, 10 minutes from Philadelphia.

Lakewood

507. Garden State Center for Holistic Health Care

1203 Rte 70 W and Airport Rd, Lakewood, NJ 08701

Phone: (732) 364-0882; *Fax:* (732) 364-7096

Internet: http://www.bodywork4u.com

Program Administrator: Gloria Coppola, Dir. *Admissions Contact:* Gloria Coppola.

Year Established: 1993.

Staff: Full-time: 2; Part-time: 4.

Avg Enrollment: 30. *Avg Class Size:* 14. *Number of Graduates per Year:* 28.

Wheelchair Access: Yes.

Accreditation/Approval/Licensing: State board: NJ Dept of Ed; National Certification Board for Therapeutic Massage and Bodywork (CEUs).

Field of Study: Acupressure; Aromatherapy; CranioSacral Therapy; Energy Work; Massage Therapy*; Neuromuscular Therapy; Reiki; Swedish Massage*; Thai Massage. *Program Name/Length:* Certified Massage Therapist, 675 hrs, 1 yr.

Degrees Offered: CMT.

License/Certification Preparation: National Certification Board for Therapeutic Massage and Bodywork.

Admission Requirements: High school diploma/GED.

Application Deadline(s): Fall: Aug 15; Winter: Dec 30.

Financial Aid: Vocational rehabilitation.

Career Services: Career counseling; Career information; Internships.

Long Branch

508. New Jersey Institute of Reflexology
Practitioner Certification Program
155 Franklin Ave, Long Branch, NJ 07740-6616
Phone: (888) 722-NJIR (6547)
Internet: http://www.njir.com
Program Administrator: Mary Alice Arre,
Founder/Dir. *Admissions Contact:* Mary Alice
Arre.
Year Established: 1994.
Staff: Full-time: 1; Part-time: 4.
Avg Enrollment: 100. *Avg Class Size:* 12. *Number
of Graduates per Year:* 75.
Wheelchair Access: No.
Field of Study: Reflexology*. *Program
Name/Length:* 150-200 hrs, 3-6 mos; Seminars
given in various locations.
Degrees Offered: Certificate.
License/Certification Preparation: American
Reflexology Certification Board.
Admission Requirements: Min age: 18.
Tuition and Fees: $1450-$2000.
Financial Aid: Payment plan.
Career Services: Career information; Referral ser-
vice.

Madison

509. Studio Yoga
2 Green Village Rd, Rm 301, Madison, NJ 07940
Mailing Address: PO Box 99, Chatham, NJ 07928
Phone: (973) 966-5311; *Fax:* (973) 966-1477
E-mail: studioyoga@yoga.com
Program Administrator: Theresa Rowland, Dir.
Admissions Contact: Theresa Rowland.
Year Established: 1989.
Staff: Full-time: 1; Part-time: 14.
Avg Enrollment: 20. *Avg Class Size:* 10.
Wheelchair Access: No.
Field of Study: Yoga Teacher Training*. *Program
Name/Length:* Yoga Instructor Certification
Program for YMCA and Health Club Instruc-
tors, 1 yr; First Degree Iyengar Yoga Teacher
Certification, 2 yrs; Advanced Degree Yoga
Teacher Certification.
Degrees Offered: Certificate.
License/Certification Preparation: Certification,
Iyengar Yoga National Association.
Admission Requirements: Specific course prerequi-
sites: 1 yr of study with certified Iyengar yoga
instructor or equivalent.
Financial Aid: Scholarships; Work study.
Career Services: Career counseling; Career infor-
mation; Internships; Interview set up.

Manalapan

510. The Institute of Hypnotherapy
10 Darby Ct, Manalapan, NJ 07726

Phone: (732) 446-5995
E-mail: drjaimef@aol.com *Internet:* http://www.
members.aol.com/insthypno
Program Administrator: Dr. Jaime Feldman, Dir.
Admissions Contact: Dr. Jaime Feldman.
Year Established: 1994.
Staff: Full-time: 1; Part-time: 3.
Avg Enrollment: 75. *Avg Class Size:* 10. *Number
of Graduates per Year:* 75.
Wheelchair Access: Yes.
Accreditation/Approval/Licensing: State board: NJ
Board of Social Workers; American Board of
Hypnotherapy; International Association of
Counselors and Therapists; International Medi-
cal and Dental Hypnotherapy Association.
Field of Study: Hypnotherapy*; Neuro-Linguistic
Programming. *Program Name/Length:*
Hypnotherapy and NLP, 40 hrs or 80 hrs; Holis-
tic Philosophy, 20 hrs or 40 hrs; Seminars given
in various locations.
Degrees Offered: Certificate.
License/Certification Preparation: State: NJ Board
of Social Workers; American Board of
Hypnotherapy; International Association of
Counselors and Therapists; International Medi-
cal and Dental Hypnotherapy Association.
Admission Requirements: Min age: 18; Proficiency
in English.

Metuchen

511. The Center for Transpersonal BodyMind Studies
51 Upland Ave, Metuchen, NJ 08840
Phone: (732) 548-8579
Program Administrator: Joanne Rossi, Dir. *Admis-
sions Contact:* Joanne Rossi.
Year Established: 1990.
Staff: Full-time: 5; Part-time: 2.
Avg Enrollment: 40. *Avg Class Size:* 14. *Number
of Graduates per Year:* 37.
Wheelchair Access: Yes.
Field of Study: Aromatherapy; Energy Work*;
Massage Therapy; Polarity Therapy; Somatic
Psychology*. *Program Name/Length:* 9 mos;
Seminars given in various locations.
Degrees Offered: Certificate; independent college
credits.
License/Certification Preparation: National Certif-
ication Board for Therapeutic Massage and
Bodywork.
Admission Requirements: Min age: 18; High
school diploma/GED.
Application Deadline(s): Fall: Sep; Winter: Jan;
Spring: May.
Tuition and Fees: $2150.
Financial Aid: Scholarships.
Career Services: Career counseling; Career infor-
mation; Internships; Resume service.

Mount Lakes

512. Five Elements School of Classical Homeopathy

115 Rte 46, Bldg D-29, Mount Lakes, NJ 07046
Phone: (201) 402-8510; *Fax:* (201) 402-9753
Program Administrator: Jane Cicchetti, RS Hom (NA), Dir. *Admissions Contact:* Jane Cicchetti.
Year Established: 1991.
Staff: Full-time: 1; Part-time: 2.
Avg Enrollment: 60. *Avg Class Size:* 20. *Number of Graduates per Year:* 11.
Wheelchair Access: Yes.
Field of Study: Homeopathy*. *Program Name/Length:* 3 yrs (8 weekends/yr).
Degrees Offered: Certificate.
License/Certification Preparation: Council for Homeopathic Certification; North American Society of Homeopaths.
Admission Requirements: Specific course prerequisites: introductory course or self-study in homeopathy.
Application Deadline(s): Fall: Sep 15.
Tuition and Fees: $1700 per yr.
Financial Aid: Work study.

Newark

513. University of Medicine and Dentistry of New Jersey, School of Health Related Professions

Nurse-Midwifery Program
65 Bergen St, Newark, NJ 07107-3001
Phone: (973) 972-4298
E-mail: diegmaek@umdnj.edu *Internet:* http://www.umdnj.edu.shrp.eb.home.htm
Program Administrator: Elaine Diegmann, CNM, Dir.
Accreditation/Approval/Licensing: American College of Nurse-Midwives, Division of Accreditation.
Field of Study: Midwifery*. *Program Name/Length:* Nurse-Midwifery Certificate.
Degrees Offered: Certificate.
License/Certification Preparation: Certified Nurse-Midwife, American College of Nurse-Midwives.
Admission Requirements: RN.

Paramus

514. The Center for Universal and Holistic Studies, Paramus

Reflexology Therapist Trainings
PO Box 1306, Paramus, NJ 07653
Phone: (973) 686-9700
E-mail: feeteze@aol.com
Program Administrator: Elaine Gordon, Principal/Founder.
Year Established: 1997.

Staff: Full-time: 7.
Avg Enrollment: 55. *Avg Class Size:* 8. *Number of Graduates per Year:* 55.
Field of Study: Energy Work*; Reflexology*. *Program Name/Length:* 230 hrs, 7 wk intensive with 100 hrs home study; Seminars given in various locations.
Degrees Offered: Diploma.
License/Certification Preparation: American Reflexology Certification Board.
Admission Requirements: Min age: 18.
Application Deadline(s): Fall; Winter; Spring; Summer.
Tuition and Fees: $1500 + $50 books.
Financial Aid: Payment plan.
Career Services: Internships.

Parsippany

515. North Jersey Massage Training Center

3699 Rt 46 E, Parsippany, NJ 07054
Phone: (973) 263-2229; *Fax:* (973) 402-1222
Internet: http://www.n.j.massage.com
Program Administrator: Larry Heisler, Dir.
Year Established: 1980.
Staff: Full-time: 2; Part-time: 3.
Avg Enrollment: 24. *Avg Class Size:* 8. *Number of Graduates per Year:* 24.
Wheelchair Access: Yes.
Accreditation/Approval/Licensing: State board: NJ Dept of Ed.
Field of Study: Acupressure; Massage Therapy*; Neuromuscular Therapy; Qigong; Reflexology; Shiatsu*; Sports Massage; Swedish Massage*; Yoga Teacher Training*. *Program Name/Length:* 500 hrs, 6 mos.
Degrees Offered: Certificate.
License/Certification Preparation: State: NJ Certification; National Certification Board for Therapeutic Massage and Bodywork.
Admission Requirements: Min age: 18; High school diploma/GED.
Tuition and Fees: $5200.
Financial Aid: Loans; Work study; Vocational rehabilitation; Workforce development.
Career Services: Career counseling; Career information; Practice management program.

Pompton Lakes

516. Institute for Therapeutic Massage, Inc

Therapeutic Massage and Bodywork Program
125 Wanaque Ave, Pompton Lakes, NJ 07442
Phone: (201) 839-6131; *Fax:* (201) 839-9878
E-mail: itminc@erols.com *Internet:* http://www.massageprogram.com
Program Administrator: Lisa Helbig, Dir. *Admissions Contact:* Carry Wichtendahl, Admin.
Year Established: 1993.
Staff: Part-time: 10.

Avg Enrollment: 75. *Avg Class Size:* 14. *Number of Graduates per Year:* 70.

Wheelchair Access: No.

Accreditation/Approval/Licensing: State board: NJ Dept of Ed; National Certification Board for Therapeutic Massage and Bodywork (CEUs).

Field of Study: Aromatherapy; Chair Massage; Energy Work; Geriatric Massage; Massage Therapy*; Pregnancy Massage; Reflexology; Reiki; Sports Massage. *Program Name/Length:* Massage and Bodywork Studies, 8 mos.

Degrees Offered: CEUs; Certificate.

License/Certification Preparation: National Certification Board for Therapeutic Massage and Bodywork.

Admission Requirements: Min age: 18; High school diploma/GED.

Application Deadline(s): Fall; Winter; Summer.

Tuition and Fees: $4000 + $275 books and supplies.

Financial Aid: Vocational rehabilitation; Payment plan.

Career Services: Career counseling; Career information.

Red Bank

517. SAMI (Swedish American Massage Institute)

120 Maple Ave, Red Bank, NJ 07701

Phone: (908) 530-1188; *Fax:* (908) 530-1919

E-mail: sami@monmouth.com *Internet:* http://www.monmouth.com/~SAMI

Program Administrator: Sharyn Ross, RN, Dir. *Admissions Contact:* Dean Ross, Asst Dir.

Year Established: 1991.

Staff: Full-time: 2; Part-time: 3.

Avg Enrollment: 60. *Avg Class Size:* 12. *Number of Graduates per Year:* 52.

Wheelchair Access: No.

Accreditation/Approval/Licensing: State board: NJ Dept of Vocational Ed.

Field of Study: Aromatherapy; Massage Therapy*; Neuromuscular Therapy; On-Site Massage; Reflexology; Sports Massage; Swedish Massage*. *Program Name/Length:* Massage Therapy, 200 hrs, 4 mos; 500 hrs, 10 mos; Brookdale Community College course for nurses.

Degrees Offered: CEUs; Certificate.

License/Certification Preparation: National Certification Board for Therapeutic Massage and Bodywork.

Admission Requirements: Min age: 18; High school diploma/GED; RN required for Brookdale course.

Tuition and Fees: $1500 (200 hrs); $4500 (500 hrs); $650 (Brookdale).

Financial Aid: State government aid; Job Training Partnership Act.

Career Services: Career information; Interview set up; Job information.

River Vale

518. MotherLove, Doula Training

584 Echo Glen Ave, River Vale, NJ 07675

Phone: (201) 358-2703; *Fax:* (201) 664-4405

E-mail: motherlove@cwix.com

Program Administrator: Debra Pascali-Bonaro, Pres. *Admissions Contact:* Debra Pascali-Bonaro.

Year Established: 1987.

Staff: Full-time: 1; Part-time: 2.

Avg Enrollment: 90. *Avg Class Size:* 15. *Number of Graduates per Year:* 90.

Wheelchair Access: Yes.

Accreditation/Approval/Licensing: Doulas of North America.

Field of Study: Doula*. *Program Name/Length:* Labor Support Doula Training, 16 hrs; Postpartum Doula Training, 18 hrs or 30 hrs/Internet; Seminars given in various locations; Home study/Correspondence.

Degrees Offered: Certificate.

License/Certification Preparation: Certification, Doulas of North America.

Admission Requirements: Min age: 18; Pretraining day course or background in maternal/child health.

Tuition and Fees: $275-$695.

Financial Aid: Payment plan; Barter.

Somers Point

519. Seashore Healing Arts Center

Integrated Massage

505 New Rd, Stes 5 and 7, Somers Point, NJ 08244

Phone: (609) 601-9272

Program Administrator: Edward Smith, Pres. *Admissions Contact:* Edward Smith; Kathy Smith.

Year Established: 1989.

Staff: Full-time: 1; Part-time: 2.

Avg Enrollment: 18. *Avg Class Size:* 18.

Wheelchair Access: No.

Accreditation/Approval/Licensing: State board: NJ Dept of Ed.

Field of Study: Acupressure; Deep Tissue Massage*; Energy Work; Massage Therapy*; Meditation; Polarity Therapy; Qigong; Reflexology; Reiki; Yoga. *Program Name/Length:* Integrated Massage, 510 hrs, 18 mos.

Degrees Offered: Certificate.

License/Certification Preparation: National Certification Board for Therapeutic Massage and Bodywork.

Admission Requirements: Min age: 18; High school diploma/GED.

Tuition and Fees: $4750.

Financial Aid: Payment plan.

Career Services: Career information; Referral service.

Somerset

520. Somerset School of Massage Therapy

7 Cedar Grove Ln, Somerset, NJ 08873
Phone: (732) 356-0787; *Fax:* (732) 469-3494
E-mail: ssmt@massagecareer.com *Internet:* http://
www.massagecareer.com
Program Administrator: Christopher Froelich,
Pres. *Admissions Contact:* Deborah Scarpitto,
Dean of Students.
Year Established: 1987.
Staff: Full-time: 6; Part-time: 12.
Avg Enrollment: 200. *Avg Class Size:* 25. *Number
of Graduates per Year:* 170.
Wheelchair Access: Yes.
Accreditation/Approval/Licensing: State board: NJ
Dept of Vocational Ed; Commission on Massage
Therapy Accreditation; National Certification
Board for Therapeutic Massage and Bodywork
(CEUs).
Field of Study: Massage Therapy*; Neuromuscular
Therapy; Reflexology; Shiatsu*. *Program
Name/Length:* Massage Therapy, 6
mos/full-time or 1 yr/part-time; Shiatsu, 6
mos/part-time.
Degrees Offered: Diploma.
License/Certification Preparation: State: FL, IA
Licensed Massage Therapist; National Certifica-
tion Board for Therapeutic Massage and Body-
work.
Admission Requirements: Min age: 18; High
school diploma/GED.
Application Deadline(s): Fall: Sep 15; Winter: Jan
15; Spring: Mar 31; Summer: May 15.
Tuition and Fees: $5590, includes books (Massage
Therapy).
Financial Aid: State government aid; VA ap-
proved; Vocational rehabilitation.
Career Services: Career counseling; Career infor-
mation; Interview set up.

Summit

521. Polarity Energy Healing Center

Associate Polarity Practitioner Training
Interweave-31 Woodland and DeForest Ave, Sum-
mit, NJ 07901
Mailing Address: 134 Graybar Dr, North Plainfield,
NJ 07062
Phone: (908) 668-1991; *Fax:* (908) 668-1738
E-mail: clio@wholenet1.com *Internet:* http://
www.wholenet1.com/pehc
Program Administrator: Clio Elizabeth Perez, RPP,
Dir. *Admissions Contact:* Clio Elizabeth Perez.
Year Established: 1996.
Staff: Part-time: 2-3.
Avg Enrollment: 10. *Avg Class Size:* 10. *Number
of Graduates per Year:* 7.
Wheelchair Access: No.
Accreditation/Approval/Licensing: American Po-
larity Therapy Association.

Field of Study: Polarity Therapy*. *Program
Name/Length:* Associate Polarity Practitioner, 6
mos (weekend seminars and practicum).
License/Certification Preparation: APP; American
Polarity Therapy Association.
Admission Requirements: Min age: 18.
Application Deadline(s): Winter: Nov.
Tuition and Fees: $235-$525 per module; $1850
total.
Financial Aid: Payment plan.
Career Services: Career information.

Toms River

522. Body, Mind and Spirit Learning Alliance

917-2 N Main St (Rte 166), Toms River, NJ 08753
Phone: (908) 349-7153
Program Administrator: Cathy Connelly, Co-Dir;
Dianne O'Brien, Co-Dir. *Admissions Contact:*
Cathy Connelly; Dianne O'Brien.
Year Established: 1996.
Staff: Full-time: 2; Part-time: 4.
Avg Enrollment: 28. *Avg Class Size:* 14. *Number
of Graduates per Year:* 14.
Wheelchair Access: Yes.
Field of Study: Aromatherapy; CranioSacral Ther-
apy; Massage Therapy*; Reflexology; Reiki;
Shiatsu; Swedish Massage*. *Program
Name/Length:* Massage Therapy Certification,
1 yr.
Degrees Offered: Certificate.
License/Certification Preparation: National Certif-
ication Board for Therapeutic Massage and
Bodywork.
Admission Requirements: Min age: 18; High
school diploma/GED.
Application Deadline(s): Fall: Sep; Spring: Feb.
Tuition and Fees: $4725 + $170 books.

523. Ocean County Vo-Tech

500 Hour Massage Therapy Program
1299 Old Freehold Rd, Toms River, NJ 08753
Phone: (732) 349-8444
Program Administrator: Frank Folinus, Dir. *Ad-
missions Contact:* Sharon Spaziani, Instr.
Year Established: 1996.
Staff: Part-time: 2.
Avg Enrollment: 18. *Avg Class Size:* 18. *Number
of Graduates per Year:* 18.
Wheelchair Access: Yes.
Accreditation/Approval/Licensing: Accrediting
Council for Continuing Education and Training;
Accrediting Commission of Career Schools and
Colleges of Technology.
Field of Study: Deep Tissue Massage; Massage
Therapy*. *Program Name/Length:* 500 hrs,
four 12-wk semesters (3 evenings per wk), 2 yrs.
Degrees Offered: Certificate.

License/Certification Preparation: National Certification Board for Therapeutic Massage and Bodywork.
Admission Requirements: Min age: 18; High school diploma/GED.
Application Deadline(s): Fall.
Tuition and Fees: $330 per semester.
Career Services: Career information.

Union

524. Academy of Professional Hypnosis
1358 Burnet Ave, Union, NJ 07083
Phone: (908) 964-4417; *Fax:* (908) 810-0255
Program Administrator: Dr. John Gatto, Pres. *Admissions Contact:* Dr. John Gatto.
Year Established: 1991.
Staff: Part-time: 4.
Avg Enrollment: 60. *Avg Class Size:* 10. *Number of Graduates per Year:* 60.
Wheelchair Access: Yes.
Accreditation/Approval/Licensing: State board: NJ Dept of Ed.
Field of Study: Hypnotherapy*. *Program Name/Length:* Certification, 100 hrs.
Degrees Offered: Certificate.
Admission Requirements: Min age: 18.
Tuition and Fees: $495.

West Orange

525. Unlimited Potential
Hypnotherapy Training; Reiki Training
623 Eagle Rock Ave, West Orange, NJ 07052
Mailing Address: PO Box 64, Roseland, NJ 07068
Phone: (973) 325-0900; *Fax:* (973) 403-9789
Program Administrator: Roxanne Louise, CHt, Dir. *Admissions Contact:* Roxanne Louise, Dir.
Year Established: 1989.
Staff: Full-time: 1; Part-time: 3.
Avg Enrollment: 50. *Avg Class Size:* 8. *Number of Graduates per Year:* 50.
Wheelchair Access: No.
Accreditation/Approval/Licensing: American Board of Hypnotherapy; International Medical and Dental Hypnotherapy Association.
Field of Study: Hypnotherapy*; Reiki*. *Program Name/Length:* Basic Hypnosis, 4 weekends; Advanced Hypnosis, weekends; Reiki I, II, III, and Master Apprenticeship.
Degrees Offered: Diploma; Certificate.
License/Certification Preparation: International Medical and Dental Hypnotherapy Association.
Admission Requirements: Min age: 18; Interview.
Tuition and Fees: $1000 (Basic Hypnosis); $150 (Reiki I); $225 (Reiki II, III); $1000 (Reiki Master).
Financial Aid: Payment plan; Work study.
Career Services: Career counseling; Career information; Referral service.

Westwood

526. Healing Hands Institute for Massage Therapy
Massage Therapy Certification
41 Bergenline Ave, Westwood, NJ 07675
Phone: (201) 722-0099; *Fax:* (201) 722-0690
E-mail: hhi@aol.com *Internet:* http://www. healinghandsinstitute.com
Program Administrator: Eva Carey, Admin. *Admissions Contact:* Eva Carey.
Year Established: 1990.
Staff: Full-time: 3; Part-time: 18.
Avg Enrollment: 100. *Avg Class Size:* 20. *Number of Graduates per Year:* 60.
Wheelchair Access: No.
Accreditation/Approval/Licensing: State board: NJ Dept of Ed; Commission on Massage Therapy Accreditation; National Certification Board for Therapeutic Massage and Bodywork (CEUs).
Field of Study: Acupressure; Aromatherapy; CranioSacral Therapy; Massage Therapy*; Medical Massage; Reflexology; Reiki; Shiatsu; Sports Massage; Swedish Massage*; Traditional Chinese Medicine. *Program Name/Length:* Therapeutic Massage, 6 mos or 1 yr; Therapeutic Massage for NY Students, 15 mos.
Degrees Offered: Diploma; Certificate.
License/Certification Preparation: State: NJ Certified Massage Therapist, NY Licensed Massage Therapist; National Certification Board for Therapeutic Massage and Bodywork.
Admission Requirements: Min age: 18; High school diploma/GED.
Tuition and Fees: $4750.
Career Services: Career counseling; Career information; Resume service.

Woodbridge

527. Academy of Natural Health Sciences
Massage and Bodywork Therapy; Nutrition and Holistic Health
102 Green St, Woodbridge, NJ 07095
Phone: (732) 634-2155; *Fax:* (732) 634-2155
Program Administrator: Dr. Frank Auriemma, Dir. *Admissions Contact:* Dr. Frank Auriemma.
Year Established: 1991.
Staff: Full-time: 1; Part-time: 2.
Avg Class Size: 12. *Number of Graduates per Year:* 28.
Wheelchair Access: No.
Accreditation/Approval/Licensing: State board: NJ Dept of Ed.
Field of Study: Acupressure; Aromatherapy; Energy Work; Herbal Medicine*; Holistic Health*; Homeopathy; Hypnotherapy; Massage Therapy*; Neuromuscular Therapy; Nutrition; Polarity Therapy; Reflexology; Reiki; Shiatsu; Sports

Massage. *Program Name/Length:* Massage, 12 mos; Nutrition and Holistic Health, 8 mos.
Degrees Offered: MH; Certificate.
License/Certification Preparation: National Certification Board for Therapeutic Massage and Bodywork.
Admission Requirements: High school diploma/GED.

Tuition and Fees: $4995 (Massage); $1995 (Nutrition).
Financial Aid: Vocational rehabilitation.
Career Services: Career counseling; Career information; Job information; Referral service.

NEW MEXICO

Albuquerque

528. The Ayurvedic Institute
11311 Menaul NE, Ste A, Albuquerque, NM 87112
Mailing Address: PO Box 23445, Albuquerque, NM 87192-1445
Phone: (505) 291-9698; *Fax:* (505) 294-7572
Internet: http://www.ayurveda.com
Program Administrator: Wynn Werner, Admin.
   Admissions Contact: Barbara Cook, Programs Admin.
Year Established: 1984.
Staff: Full-time: 3; Part-time: 6.
Avg Enrollment: 80. *Avg Class Size:* 30. *Number of Graduates per Year:* 30.
Wheelchair Access: Yes.
Field of Study: Anatomy and Physiology; Ayurvedic Medicine*; Yoga. *Program Name/Length:* Ayurvedic Studies, 8 mos.
Degrees Offered: Certificate.
Admission Requirements: High school diploma/GED.
Tuition and Fees: 4500.
Financial Aid: Work study.
Career Services: Career information.

529. Crystal Mountain Apprenticeship in the Healing Arts
Massage Therapy Licensure Program
118 Dartmouth SE, Albuquerque, NM 87106
Phone: (505) 268-4411, (800) 967-5678; *Fax:* (505) 268-4007
Program Administrator: Lori Ponge, Dir. *Admissions Contact:* Rebecca Solomon, Mgr.
Year Established: 1988.
Staff: Part-time: 18.
Avg Enrollment: 100. *Avg Class Size:* 24. *Number of Graduates per Year:* 95.
Wheelchair Access: Yes.
Accreditation/Approval/Licensing: State board: NM Board of Massage Therapy.
Field of Study: Anatomy and Physiology; Aromatherapy; CranioSacral Therapy; Energy Work; Esalen Massage; Herbal Medicine; Hydrotherapy; Kinesiology; LomiLomi Massage; Massage Therapy*; Movement Education; Neuromuscular Therapy; Polarity Therapy; Reflexology; Shiatsu; Sports Massage; Traditional Chinese Medicine. *Program Name/Length:* Massage Therapy Licensure, 6 mos, days or evenings.
Degrees Offered: Diploma.
License/Certification Preparation: NM Licensed Massage Therapist; National Certification Board for Therapeutic Massage and Bodywork.
Admission Requirements: Min age: 18; High school diploma/GED.
Tuition and Fees: $5000.
Financial Aid: Loans; Work study; Discount for prepayment.
Career Services: Career information; 150 hr in-house clinical internship.

530. Maharishi College of Vedic Medicine
2721 Arizona St NE, Albuquerque, NM 87110
Phone: (505) 830-0435; *Fax:* (505) 830-0538
E-mail: desmithmd@aol.com
Program Administrator: D. Edwards Smith, MD, Dean. *Admissions Contact:* D. Edwards Smith.
Year Established: 1996.
Staff: Full-time: 3; Part-time: 6.
Wheelchair Access: No.
Accreditation/Approval/Licensing: State board: NM Commission on Higher Ed.
Field of Study: Ayurvedic Medicine*; Maharishi Vedic Medicine. *Program Name/Length:* Assistant in Maharishi Vedic Approach to Health, 12 mos; AA in Maharishi Vedic Approach to Health, 24 mos.
Degrees Offered: AA; Diploma; Certificate.
Admission Requirements: Min age: 18; High school diploma/GED.
Tuition and Fees: $22,000 per yr.
Financial Aid: Loans; Scholarships.
Career Services: Career counseling; Career information.

531. The National College of Phytotherapy
Bachelor of Science in Herbal Medicine
3030 Isleta Blvd SW, Albuquerque, NM 87105

Phone: (505) 452-3468; *Fax:* (505) 452-3468
E-mail: phyto@swcp.com *Internet:* http://www.
nmia.com/~arken
Program Administrator: Teresa Merriken, Exec
Dir. *Admissions Contact:* Teresa Merriken.
Year Established: 1996.
Staff: Part-time: 20.
Avg Enrollment: 22. *Avg Class Size:* 14.
Wheelchair Access: Yes.
Accreditation/Approval/Licensing: State board:
NM Commission of Higher Ed.
Field of Study: Herbal Medicine*. *Program
Name/Length:* Foundations in Herbalism, 9
mos; Bachelor of Science, 3 yrs.
Degrees Offered: BS; Certificate.
Admission Requirements: Min age: 18; High
school diploma/GED; Some college (1 yr); Spe-
cific course prerequisites: biology, chemistry,
English.
Application Deadline(s): Summer.
Tuition and Fees: $1095 (Foundations); $4500 per
yr (BS).
Financial Aid: Payment plan.
Career Services: Career counseling; Career infor-
mation; Internships; Resume service.

532. New Mexico School of Natural Therapeutics

202 Morningside SE, Albuquerque, NM 87108
Phone: (505) 268-6870, (800) 654-1675; *Fax:* (505)
268-0818
E-mail: jpendry@swcp.com *Internet:* http://www.
nmsnt.org/nathealth
Program Administrator: Robert Stevens, Dir. *Ad-
missions Contact:* Alison Owens, Admin.
Year Established: 1974.
Staff: Full-time: 2; Part-time: 18.
Avg Enrollment: 95. *Avg Class Size:* 30. *Number
of Graduates per Year:* 95.
Wheelchair Access: Yes.
Accreditation/Approval/Licensing: State board:
NM Massage Therapy Board; TX and WA
Depts of Health.
Field of Study: Deep Tissue Massage; Flower Es-
sences; Herbal Medicine; Massage Therapy*;
Polarity Therapy; Pregnancy Massage;
Reflexology; Shiatsu; Sports Massage; Swedish
Massage*. *Program Name/Length:* 750 hrs, 6
mos/days or 1 yr/nights.
Degrees Offered: Certificate.
License/Certification Preparation: State: NM Li-
censed Massage Therapist; National Certifica-
tion Board for Therapeutic Massage and Body-
work; American Polarity Therapy Association.
Admission Requirements: Min age: 18; High
school diploma/GED.
Tuition and Fees: $6300.
Financial Aid: Work study; VA approved; Voca-
tional rehabilitation; Payment plan.
Career Services: Career information; Job information; Business counseling.

533. Southwest Acupuncture College, Albuquerque

Master of Science in Oriental Medicine
4308 Carlisle NE, Ste 205, Albuquerque, NM
87107
Phone: (505) 888-8898
E-mail: swaca@compuserve.com *Internet:* http://
www.swacupuncture.com
Program Administrator: Skya Gardner Abbate,
Exec Dir. *Admissions Contact:* Dr. Jim
Ventresca, Academic Dean.
Year Established: 1993.
Staff: Full-time: 24; Part-time: 1.
Avg Enrollment: 60. *Avg Class Size:* 30. *Number
of Graduates per Year:* 28.
Wheelchair Access: Yes.
Accreditation/Approval/Licensing: State board:
NM Board of Acupuncture and Oriental Medi-
cine; CA Acupuncture Board; Accreditation
Commission for Acupuncture and Oriental Med-
icine.
Field of Study: Acupuncture*; Herbal Medicine*;
Oriental Medicine*; Qigong; Shiatsu; Tradi-
tional Chinese Medicine. *Program
Name/Length:* Master of Science in Oriental
Medicine, 4 yrs.
Degrees Offered: MSOM.
License/Certification Preparation: State: NM Doc-
tor of Oriental Medicine; National Certification
Commission for Acupuncture and Oriental Med-
icine.
Admission Requirements: Min age: 20; Some col-
lege (2 yrs).
Application Deadline(s): Fall: Aug 20; Winter: Jan
10.
Tuition and Fees: $8000 per yr.
Financial Aid: Federal government aid; Loans;
Scholarships.

534. Universal Therapeutic Massage Institute, Inc

3410 Aztec Rd NE, Albuquerque, NM 87107
Phone: (800) 557-0020; *Fax:* (505) 881-0749
Program Administrator: Stacey Townsend, Admin.
Admissions Contact: Stacey Townsend.
Year Established: 1993.
Staff: Part-time: 12.
Avg Enrollment: 100. *Avg Class Size:* 25. *Number
of Graduates per Year:* 100.
Wheelchair Access: Yes.
Accreditation/Approval/Licensing: State board:
NM Board of Massage Therapy.
Field of Study: CranioSacral Therapy; Massage
Therapy*; Myofascial Release; Neuromuscular
Therapy; Polarity Therapy; Reflexology;
Shiatsu; Sports Massage; Traditional Chinese
Medicine. *Program Name/Length:* 670 hrs, 6
mos/days or 9 mos/evenings.
Degrees Offered: Diploma.
License/Certification Preparation: State: NM Li-
censed Massage Therapist; National Certifica-

tion Board for Therapeutic Massage and Body-work.

Admission Requirements: Min age: 18; High school diploma/GED.

Tuition and Fees: $3850.

Financial Aid: Payment plan.

Career Services: Career information; Internships; Job information; Referral service.

535. University of New Mexico, College of Nursing

Nurse-Midwifery Program
Nursing/Pharmacy Bldg, Albuquerque, NM 87131-1061

Phone: (505) 272-1184

E-mail: sheilar@unm.edu

Program Administrator: Barbara A. Overman, PhD, Dir.

Accreditation/Approval/Licensing: American College of Nurse-Midwives, Division of Accreditation.

Field of Study: Midwifery*.

Degrees Offered: MSN.

License/Certification Preparation: Certified Nurse-Midwife, American College of Nurse-Midwives.

Admission Requirements: Bachelor's degree; RN.

Aztec

536. Westbrook University

College of Natural Health Sciences
400 University Plaza, Aztec, NM 87410

Phone: (505) 334-1115, (800) 447-6496; *Fax:* (505) 334-7583

E-mail: admissions@cyberport.com *Internet:* http://www.westbrooku.edu

Program Administrator: Nita Resler, Pres. *Admissions Contact:* DeeAnn Greene, Dean of Students.

Year Established: 1989.

Staff: Part-time: 71.

Avg Enrollment: 650. *Number of Graduates per Year:* 230.

Wheelchair Access: Yes.

Accreditation/Approval/Licensing: State board: CA Board of Registered Nursing; NM Commission on Higher Ed; International Medical and Dental Hypnotherapy Association.

Field of Study: Acupressure; Aromatherapy; Ayurvedic Medicine; Energy Work; Flower Essences; Herbal Medicine; Homeopathy*; Iridology*; Midwifery; Naturopathic Medicine*; Polarity Therapy; Reflexology. *Program Name/Length:* Homeopathic Medicine, 20-34 credits; Iridology, 38-107 credits; Bachelor of Science in Natural Health Sciences, 70-93 credits; Doctor of Naturopathy, 275 credits; Home study/Correspondence.

Degrees Offered: BS; MS; ND; Diploma.

Admission Requirements: Min age: 18; High school diploma/GED; Min GPA: 2.0; Bachelor's degree for Naturopathy.

Tuition and Fees: $72 per credit + $750 fees.

Financial Aid: Payment plan.

Clovis

537. Eastern New Mexico School of Massage Therapy

PO Box 2142, Clovis, NM 88101

Phone: (505) 763-0551; *Fax:* (505) 763-1405

Program Administrator: Sue Pierce, Dir.

Year Established: 1996.

Staff: Full-time: 3; Part-time: 7.

Avg Class Size: 15. *Number of Graduates per Year:* 15.

Wheelchair Access: Yes.

Accreditation/Approval/Licensing: State board: NM Board of Massage Therapy.

Field of Study: CranioSacral Therapy; Energy Work; Herbal Medicine; Infant Massage; Manual Lymph Drainage; Massage Therapy*; Polarity Therapy; Reflexology; Shiatsu. *Program Name/Length:* 650 hrs, 2 semesters.

Degrees Offered: Diploma; Certificate.

License/Certification Preparation: State: NM Licensed Massage Therapist; National Certification Board for Therapeutic Massage and Bodywork.

Admission Requirements: Min age: 18; High school diploma/GED.

Application Deadline(s): Winter: Dec 30.

Tuition and Fees: $4500.

Financial Aid: VA approved; Vocational rehabilitation.

Career Services: Career information.

Espanola

538. KRI

Teacher Training in Kundalini Yoga as Taught by Yogi Bhajan
Rte 2, Box 4 Shady Lane, Espanola, NM 87532

Phone: (505) 753-0423; *Fax:* (505) 753-5982

E-mail: ikyta@3ho.org *Internet:* http://www.kundaliniyoga.com

Program Administrator: Nam K. Khalsa, Admin. *Admissions Contact:* Nam K. Khalsa.

Year Established: 1989.

Staff: Part-time: 80.

Avg Enrollment: 500. *Avg Class Size:* 35. *Number of Graduates per Year:* 400.

Accreditation/Approval/Licensing: Kundalini Research Institute.

Field of Study: Yoga Teacher Training*. *Program Name/Length:* 130 hrs, 3 mos-2 yrs; Seminars given in various locations; New Mexico summer program, 110 hrs, 2 wk intensive with home study.

Degrees Offered: Certificate.
Admission Requirements: Min age: 18; Kundalini yoga classes or assigned reading.
Tuition and Fees: $1200-$1600.
Financial Aid: Payment plan; Early registration discount.

Farmington

539. The Medicine Wheel—A School of Holistic Therapies

Licensed Massage Therapist; Holistic Health Practitioner
1243 W Apache, Farmington, NM 87401
Phone: (888) 327-1914; *Fax:* (505) 327-2234
E-mail: medicinewheel@acrnet.com
Program Administrator: Randy Barnes, Admin Dir. *Admissions Contact:* Susan Barnes, Prog Dir.
Year Established: 1992.
Staff: Full-time: 3; Part-time: 6.
Avg Enrollment: 30. *Avg Class Size:* 12. *Number of Graduates per Year:* 10.
Wheelchair Access: No.
Accreditation/Approval/Licensing: State board: NM Board of Massage Therapy; International Massage and Somatic Therapies Accreditation Council; National Certification Board for Therapeutic Massage and Bodywork (CEUs).
Field of Study: Acupressure; Aromatherapy; CranioSacral Therapy; Herbal Medicine; Holistic Health*; Massage Therapy*; Neuromuscular Therapy; Polarity Therapy; Qigong; Traditional Chinese Medicine; Tui Na. *Program Name/Length:* Massage Arts, 735 hrs, 8 mos; Associate of Occupational Studies/Holistic Health Practitioner, 1200 hrs, 18 mos.
Degrees Offered: Diploma; Certificate; AOS.
License/Certification Preparation: State: NM Licensed Massage Therapist; American Oriental Bodywork Therapy Association; National Certification Board for Therapeutic Massage and Bodywork.
Admission Requirements: Min age: 18; High school diploma/GED.
Application Deadline(s): Fall: Aug 15.
Tuition and Fees: $4875 (Massage); $9000 (AOS).
Financial Aid: Loans; VA approved; Vocational rehabilitation.

Las Cruces

540. Mesilla Valley School of Therapeutic Arts

741 N Alameda, Ste 15, Las Cruces, NM 88005
Mailing Address: PO Box 1227, Mesilla, NM 88046
Phone: (505) 527-1239

Program Administrator: Wanita Thompson, Owner/Dir. *Admissions Contact:* Wanita Thompson.
Year Established: 1986.
Staff: Full-time: 1; Part-time: 4.
Avg Enrollment: 24. *Avg Class Size:* 24. *Number of Graduates per Year:* 20.
Wheelchair Access: Yes.
Accreditation/Approval/Licensing: State board: NM Board of Massage Therapy.
Field of Study: Massage Therapy*. *Program Name/Length:* Massage Therapy Certification, 10 mos.
Degrees Offered: Diploma.
License/Certification Preparation: State: NM Licensed Massage Therapist; National Certification Board for Therapeutic Massage and Bodywork.
Admission Requirements: Min age: 18; High school diploma/GED.
Application Deadline(s): Spring: Apr.
Tuition and Fees: $3500.
Financial Aid: State government aid; Payment plan.
Career Services: Career counseling; Career information.

Ruidoso

541. White Mountain School of Applied Healing

1204 Mechem, Ste 10, Ruidoso, NM 88345
Phone: (505) 258-3046
Internet: http://www.drbartnett.com
Program Administrator: Beatrice Bartnett, DC, Dir. *Admissions Contact:* Rev. Pablo Falcon.
Year Established: 1997.
Staff: Full-time: 2.
Avg Enrollment: 20. *Avg Class Size:* 8. *Number of Graduates per Year:* 20.
Wheelchair Access: Yes.
Accreditation/Approval/Licensing: State board: NM Board of Massage Therapy; Accrediting Council for Continuing Education and Training; National Certification Board for Therapeutic Massage and Bodywork (CEUs).
Field of Study: Acupressure; Aromatherapy; Deep Tissue Massage; Energy Work; Manual Lymph Drainage; Massage Therapy*; Reflexology; Reiki; Shiatsu. *Program Name/Length:* 654 hrs, 1 yr (every other weekend).
Degrees Offered: Certificate.
License/Certification Preparation: State: NM Licensed Massage Therapist; National Certification Board for Therapeutic Massage and Bodywork.
Admission Requirements: Min age: 18; High school diploma/GED.
Tuition and Fees: $4070.
Financial Aid: VA approved; Vocational rehabilitation.

Santa Fe

542. American Institute of Vedic Studies

1701 Santa Fe River Rd, Santa Fe, NM 87501

Mailing Address: PO Box 8357, Santa Fe, NM 87504-8357

Phone: (505) 983-9385; *Fax:* (505) 982-5807

E-mail: vedicinst@aol.com *Internet:* http://www. vedanet.com

Program Administrator: Dr. David Frawley, Dir. *Admissions Contact:* Dr. Mira Foung.

Year Established: 1988.

Staff: Part-time: 2.

Avg Enrollment: 150. *Number of Graduates per Year:* 50.

Field of Study: Ayurvedic Medicine*. *Program Name/Length:* Ayurvedic Healing Correspondence Course, 250 hrs.

Degrees Offered: Certificate.

Tuition and Fees: $300-$370.

543. International Institute of Chinese Medicine

Master of Oriental Medicine

4884 La Junta del Alamo, Santa Fe, NM 87505

Mailing Address: PO Box 29988, Santa Fe, NM 87592-9988

Phone: (505) 473-5233, (800) 377-4561; *Fax:* (505) 473-9279

E-mail: 102152.3463@compuserve.com *Internet:* http://www.thuntek.net/iicm

Program Administrator: Dr. Michael Zeng, Pres. *Admissions Contact:* Admissions Dir.

Year Established: 1984.

Staff: Full-time: 20; Part-time: 20.

Avg Enrollment: 140. *Avg Class Size:* 20. *Number of Graduates per Year:* 25.

Wheelchair Access: Yes.

Accreditation/Approval/Licensing: State board: NM Board of Acupuncture and Oriental Medicine; CA Acupuncture Board; Accreditation Commission for Acupuncture and Oriental Medicine.

Field of Study: Acupuncture*; Oriental Medicine*; Qigong; Traditional Chinese Medicine*; Tui Na. *Program Name/Length:* Master of Oriental Medicine, 4 yrs.

Degrees Offered: MOM.

License/Certification Preparation: State: NM Doctor of Oriental Medicine; National Certification Commission for Acupuncture and Oriental Medicine; American Oriental Bodywork Therapy Association.

Admission Requirements: Some college (2 yrs); Min GPA: 2.5.

Application Deadline(s): Fall: Aug; Winter: Jan; Summer: May.

Tuition and Fees: $6532 per yr.

Financial Aid: Federal government aid; Scholarships; Work study; VA approved; Payment plan.

Career Services: Job information.

544. New Mexico Academy of Healing Arts

Massage and Polarity Therapy Certification

501 Franklin Ave, Santa Fe, NM 87501

Mailing Address: PO Box 932, Santa Fe, NM 87504

Phone: (505) 982-6271, (888) 808-5188; *Fax:* (505) 988-2621

E-mail: nmaha@trail.com *Internet:* http://www. nmaha.com

Program Administrator: Lorin Parrish, Dir. *Admissions Contact:* Janet Rose, Admissions Counselor.

Year Established: 1981.

Staff: Full-time: 12; Part-time: 14.

Avg Enrollment: 100. *Avg Class Size:* 24. *Number of Graduates per Year:* 78.

Wheelchair Access: Yes.

Accreditation/Approval/Licensing: State board: NM Board of Massage Therapy; American Polarity Therapy Association; National Certification Board for Therapeutic Massage and Bodywork (CEUs).

Field of Study: Aromatherapy; CranioSacral Therapy; Feldenkrais; Massage Therapy*; Polarity Therapy*; Reflexology; Shiatsu; Sports Massage; Swedish Massage. *Program Name/Length:* Massage Certification, 650 hrs (6 mos/days or 1 yr/evenings) or 1000 hrs (10 mos); Associate Polarity Practitioner, 2 mos; Registered Polarity Practitioner, 7 mos; Dual Program: Certification in Massage and Polarity, 1000 hrs.

Degrees Offered: Diploma; Certificate.

License/Certification Preparation: State: NM Licensed Massage Therapist; National Certification Board for Therapeutic Massage and Bodywork; APP and RPP; American Polarity Therapy Association.

Admission Requirements: Min age: 18; High school diploma/GED.

Application Deadline(s): Fall: Aug; Winter: Jan; Summer: Jun.

Tuition and Fees: $6000 (650 hr Massage); $8000 (1000 hr Massage); $1550 (APP); $5000 (RPP); $8500 (Dual Program).

Financial Aid: Scholarships; Payment plan.

545. Rosen Method Center Southwest

PO Box 344, Santa Fe, NM 87504

Phone: (505) 982-7149; *Fax:* (510) 254-7048

E-mail: sw.touch@ix.netcom.com *Internet:* http:// www.mcn.org/ b/rosen

Program Administrator: Sandra Wooten, MA, Dir. *Admissions Contact:* Sandra Wooten.

Year Established: 1990.

Staff: Full-time: 3; Part-time: 3.

Avg Enrollment: 40. *Avg Class Size:* 15. *Number of Graduates per Year:* 3.

Wheelchair Access: No.

Accreditation/Approval/Licensing: National Certification Board for Therapeutic Massage and Bodywork (CEUs).
Field of Study: Rosen Method Bodywork. *Program Name/Length:* Certification, 4 yrs; Personal Growth Intensives, 1+ semesters.
Degrees Offered: Certificate.
Admission Requirements: Min age: 25; Specific course prerequisites: Rosen Method weekend workshop or 10 private Rosen Method 1 hr sessions.
Application Deadline(s): Fall: Sep 1; Winter: Feb 1; Spring: May 1.
Tuition and Fees: $9500 (Certification); $850 per semester (Intensives).
Financial Aid: Work study; Scholarships for advanced students.
Career Services: Career information.

546. Scherer Institute of Natural Healing

935 Alto St, Santa Fe, NM 87501
Phone: (505) 982-8398; *Fax:* (505) 982-1825
E-mail: tsi@rt66.com *Internet:* http://www.newmexiconet.com/scher.htm
Program Administrator: Lonnie Howard, MA, Dir. *Admissions Contact:* Beth Nichols, Admin.
Year Established: 1979.
Staff: Part-time: 20.
Avg Class Size: 24. *Number of Graduates per Year:* 75.
Wheelchair Access: Yes.
Accreditation/Approval/Licensing: State board: NM Board of Massage Therapy.
Field of Study: Aromatherapy; CranioSacral Therapy; Energy Work; Herbal Medicine; Massage Therapy*; Polarity Therapy; Reflexology; Shiatsu; Sports Massage. *Program Name/Length:* Massage Therapy and Bodywork, 6 mos or 1 yr.
Degrees Offered: Diploma; Certificate.
License/Certification Preparation: State: NM Licensed Massage Therapist; National Certification Board for Therapeutic Massage and Bodywork.
Admission Requirements: Min age: 18; High school diploma/GED.
Tuition and Fees: $6000.
Financial Aid: Scholarships; Work study; Payment plan.
Career Services: Career counseling; Career information; Job information.

547. Southwest Acupuncture College, Santa Fe

Oriental Medicine
2960 Rodeo Park Dr W, Santa Fe, NM 87505
Phone: (505) 438-8884; *Fax:* (505) 438-8883
E-mail: 105315.3010@compuserve.com *Internet:* http://www.swacupuncture.com
Program Administrator: Skya Gardner Abbate, Exec Dir. *Admissions Contact:* Dr. Jim Ventresca, Academic Dean.
Year Established: 1980.
Staff: Full-time: 5; Part-time: 50.
Avg Enrollment: 80. *Avg Class Size:* 30. *Number of Graduates per Year:* 35.
Wheelchair Access: Yes.
Accreditation/Approval/Licensing: State board: NM Board of Acupuncture and Oriental Medicine; CA Acupuncture Board; Accreditation Commission for Acupuncture and Oriental Medicine.
Field of Study: Acupuncture*; Herbal Medicine; Oriental Medicine*; Qigong; Traditional Chinese Medicine*. *Program Name/Length:* Master of Science in Oriental Medicine, 3 yrs (accelerated program) or 4 yrs.
Degrees Offered: MSOM.
License/Certification Preparation: State: NM Doctor of Oriental Medicine; National Certification Commission for Acupuncture and Oriental Medicine.
Admission Requirements: Min age: 20; Some college (2 yrs).
Application Deadline(s): Fall: Aug 20.
Tuition and Fees: $9500 per yr (full-time).
Financial Aid: Federal government aid; Loans; Scholarships.

Silver City

548. New Mexico College of Natural Healing

Massage Therapy; Herbal Medicine
310 W 6th St, Silver City, NM 88062
Mailing Address: PO Box 211, Silver City, NM 88062
Phone: (505) 538-0050
Program Administrator: Gwynne Unruh, Co-Dir; John Deckebach, Co-Dir. *Admissions Contact:* Gwynne Unruh.
Year Established: 1996.
Avg Enrollment: 24. *Avg Class Size:* 12. *Number of Graduates per Year:* 12.
Wheelchair Access: No.
Accreditation/Approval/Licensing: State board: NM Board of Massage Therapy.
Field of Study: Herbal Medicine*; Massage Therapy*. *Program Name/Length:* Massage Therapy, 800 hrs, 9 mos; Herbal Medicine, 500 hrs, 9 mos.
Degrees Offered: Certificate.
License/Certification Preparation: State: NM Licensed Massage Therapist; National Certification Board for Therapeutic Massage and Bodywork.
Admission Requirements: Min age: 18; High school diploma/GED.
Application Deadline(s): Fall: Sep 10.
Tuition and Fees: $5500 (Massage Therapy); $3500 (Herbal Medicine).
Financial Aid: Work study.

Career Services: Career counseling; Career information; Internships.

Taos

549. Body-Mind Centering
Box 4552, Taos, NM 87571
Phone: (505) 758-1711; *Fax:* (505) 751-0331
E-mail: zijibg@hotmail.com *Internet:* http://www.
freeyellow.com/members4/zijibg
Program Administrator: Ziji Beth Goren, Dir. *Admissions Contact:* Ziji Beth Goren.
Year Established: 1987.
Staff: Full-time: 1; Part-time: 1.
Avg Enrollment: 20. *Avg Class Size:* 8.
Wheelchair Access: Yes.
Accreditation/Approval/Licensing: Accrediting Council for Continuing Education and Training; National Certification Board for Therapeutic Massage and Bodywork (CEUs); Body-Mind Centering Association.
Field of Study: Body-Mind Centering*. *Program Name/Length:* Voice-Movement Improvisation/Composition, 2 mos (spring and fall); BodySystems and Developmental Movement, 4 yrs; Summer Intensive, 2 wks; Winter Intensive, 2 wks (Hawaii) or 2 mos (Taos).
Degrees Offered: CEUs.
License/Certification Preparation: State: NM; National Certification Board for Therapeutic Massage and Bodywork; Body-Mind Centering.
Admission Requirements: Min age: 18; Some college (2 yrs); Specific course prerequisites: basic anatomy and physiology; Dance or movement background.
Application Deadline(s): Fall: Sep 10; Winter: Jan 10; Spring: Apr 1; Summer: Jun 10.
Tuition and Fees: $200-$500 per course.
Financial Aid: Work study.
Career Services: Career information.

550. Taos School of Massage
1021 Salazar, Taos, NM 87571
Mailing Address: 5112 NDCBU, Taos, NM 87571
Phone: (505) 758-2725
E-mail: tsm@taosnet.com
Program Administrator: Eric Ritchie, Dir. *Admissions Contact:* Eric Ritchie.

Year Established: 1994.
Staff: Full-time: 1; Part-time: 10.
Avg Enrollment: 9. *Avg Class Size:* 9. *Number of Graduates per Year:* 9.
Wheelchair Access: No.
Accreditation/Approval/Licensing: State board: NM Board of Massage Therapy.
Field of Study: Acupressure; Applied Kinesiology; Ayurvedic Medicine; Body-Mind Clearing; Energy Work; Massage Therapy*; Neuromuscular Therapy; Qigong; Reflexology; Shiatsu; Sports Massage; Traditional Chinese Medicine. *Program Name/Length:* 650 hrs, 6 mos or 1 yr.
Degrees Offered: Diploma.
License/Certification Preparation: State: NM Licensed Massage Therapist; National Certification Board for Therapeutic Massage and Bodywork.
Admission Requirements: Min age: 18; High school diploma/GED.
Application Deadline(s): Fall: Sep; Winter: Jan; Spring: May; Summer: Aug.
Tuition and Fees: $4400.
Financial Aid: Work study.
Career Services: Career information; Internships; Job information; Referral service.

551. Wellness Institute
PO Box 2843, Taos, NM 87571
Phone: (505) 776-1590, (888) 253-6331 ext 3137
E-mail: wellness@laplaza.taos.nm.us
Program Administrator: Roger Gilchrist, MA, Pres.
Year Established: 1990.
Staff: Full-time: 2; Part-time: 5.
Avg Enrollment: 50. *Avg Class Size:* 10. *Number of Graduates per Year:* 25.
Wheelchair Access: Yes.
Accreditation/Approval/Licensing: American Polarity Therapy Association.
Field of Study: Polarity Therapy*. *Program Name/Length:* Associate Polarity Practitioner, 3 wks; Registered Polarity Practitioner, 3 mos.
Degrees Offered: Diploma; Certificate.
License/Certification Preparation: APP and RPP; American Polarity Therapy Association.
Admission Requirements: Min age: 18; High school diploma/GED; Bachelor's degree preferred.

NEW YORK

Bayville
552. Ayurveda Holistic Center
2-Year Certification

82 A0 Bayville Ave, Bayville, NY 11709
Phone: (516) 628-8200
E-mail: mail@ayurvedahc.com *Internet:* http://
www.ayurvedahc.com

Program Administrator: Swami Sada Shiva Tirtha, Pres. *Admissions Contact:* Swami Sada Shiva Tirtha.
Year Established: 1988.
Staff: Full-time: 1.
Avg Enrollment: 15. *Avg Class Size:* 5. *Number of Graduates per Year:* 6.
Wheelchair Access: Yes.
Field of Study: Ayurvedic Medicine*. *Program Name/Length:* Ayurveda Certification, 2 yrs, classroom or correspondence.
Degrees Offered: Certificate.
Admission Requirements: Must be in or entering the health profession; Interview; Ayurvedic consultation, with recommendations followed for 1 mo.
Tuition and Fees: $4000.
Career Services: Career counseling; Career information; Referral service.
Comments: Credits accepted by Empire College of New York and Westbrook University.

Brooklyn

553. The Atlantic Academy of Classical Homeopathy

c/o John McCourt, 399 6th Ave, Ste 3D, Brooklyn, NY 11215
Phone: (718) 768-3811
Program Administrator: Gerald Gewiss, RS Hom (NA), Dean. *Admissions Contact:* John McCourt, Sec.
Year Established: 1989.
Staff: Part-time: 7.
Avg Enrollment: 40. *Avg Class Size:* 25. *Number of Graduates per Year:* 18.
Field of Study: Homeopathy*. *Program Name/Length:* Acute Homeopathy, 1 yr; Certificate in Classical Homeopathy, 3 yrs; Advanced Seminars, 3 days.
Degrees Offered: Certificate; CHom.
License/Certification Preparation: Council for Homeopathic Certification; North American Society of Homeopaths.
Admission Requirements: Bachelor's degree preferred; Specific course prerequisites: anatomy and physiology, pathology required for certification.
Application Deadline(s): Fall: Sep.
Tuition and Fees: $1875 per yr.
Financial Aid: Work study.

554. State University of New York, Health Science Center at Brooklyn

Midwifery Education Program, College of Health Related Professions
450 Clarkson Ave, Box 1227, Brooklyn, NY 11203-2908
Phone: (718) 270-7740/7741; *Fax:* (718) 270-7634
E-mail: chrish02@hscbklyn.edu *Internet:* http://www.hscbklyn.edu

Program Administrator: Lily Hsia, CNM, Dir. *Admissions Contact:* Liliana Montano, Dir of Admissions.
Year Established: 1932.
Staff: Full-time: 5; Part-time: 2.
Avg Enrollment: 45. *Avg Class Size:* 22. *Number of Graduates per Year:* 18.
Wheelchair Access: Yes.
Accreditation/Approval/Licensing: American College of Nurse-Midwives, Division of Accreditation.
Field of Study: Midwifery*. *Program Name/Length:* Full-time, 4 semesters, 2 yrs; Part-time, 6 semesters, 3 yrs.
Degrees Offered: MS; Certificate; Post-master's certificate.
License/Certification Preparation: State: NY; Certified Nurse-Midwife, American College of Nurse-Midwives.
Admission Requirements: Bachelor's degree; Min GPA: 3.0; Specific course prerequisites: RN, or biology, chemistry, microbiology, anatomy, physiology, human development, psychology, sociology, statistics, pathophysiology, nutrition; GRE combined score of 1000; Maternal and child health or other professional and life experiences relevant to Midwifery practice required for non-nurses.
Application Deadline(s): Fall: Apr 1.
Tuition and Fees: $2550 per semester/state resident or $4230 per semester/out of state (Full-time); $213 per credit/state resident or $351 per credit/out of state (Part-time); + $685 health insurance, $50/semester health service fee, $22-$45/semester student activities fee.
Financial Aid: Federal government aid; Loans; Scholarships; State government aid; Work study.
Career Services: Job information; Referral service.

Dobbs Ferry

555. Mercy College

Graduate Program in Acupuncture and Oriental Medicine
555 Broadway, Dobbs Ferry, NY 10522
Phone: (914) 674-7401; *Fax:* (914) 674-7374
E-mail: acupuncture@mercynet.edu *Internet:* http://mercy2.mercynet.edu/programs/graduate/acupuncture
Program Administrator: William Prensky, OMD, Dir. *Admissions Contact:* Douglas McDaniel, LAc, Associate Prog Dir.
Year Established: 1996.
Staff: Full-time: 5; Part-time: 12.
Avg Enrollment: 20.
Wheelchair Access: No.
Accreditation/Approval/Licensing: State board: NY Board of Regents; Middle States Association of Colleges and Schools; Candidate, Accreditation Commission for Acupuncture and Oriental Medicine.

Field of Study: Acupuncture*; Oriental Medicine*.
  Program Name/Length: 9 semesters, 3 yrs.
Degrees Offered: BS; MPS.
License/Certification Preparation: National Certif-
  ication Commission for Acupuncture and Orien-
  tal Medicine.
Admission Requirements: Min age: 20; High
  school diploma/GED; Some college (2 yrs), 3.0
  GPA; Specific course prerequisites: general biol-
  ogy 1 and 2 with lab, general chemistry 1 and 2
  with lab, developmental psychology, additional
  bioscience.
Application Deadline(s): Spring: Mar 1.
Tuition and Fees: $13,050 per yr.
Financial Aid: Federal government aid; Grants;
  Loans; Scholarships; State government aid;
  Work study; VA approved.
Career Services: Career counseling; Job informa-
  tion.

East Hampton

556. Barbara Brennan School of Healing
Professional Certification Program in Brennan
  Healing Science
PO Box 2005, East Hampton, NY 11937
Phone: (516) 329-0951; *Fax:* (516) 324-9745
E-mail: bbshoffice@barbarabrennan.com *Internet:*
  http://www.barbarabrennan.com
Program Administrator: Laurie Keene, Dean. *Ad-
  missions Contact:* Kay Conboy.
Year Established: 1982.
Staff: Part-time: 114.
Avg Enrollment: 750. *Number of Graduates per
  Year:* 160.
Wheelchair Access: Yes.
Field of Study: Brennan Healing Science*; Energy
  Work. *Program Name/Length:* Professional
  Certification, 5 yrs (5-day sessions/5 times per
  yr with home study).
Degrees Offered: Diploma; Certificate.
Admission Requirements: Min age: 18 with paren-
  tal consent.
Application Deadline(s): Fall.
Tuition and Fees: $5200 per yr + $100 application
  fee, $100 student workbook fee.
Financial Aid: Payment plan.
Career Services: Listing in International Directory
  of Graduate Healers.

Flushing

557. Reflexhollogy—The Science, Art and Heart
143-24 Poplar Ave, Flushing, NY 11355
Phone: (718) 961-2786
Program Administrator: Holly Papa, Prog Dir. *Ad-
  missions Contact:* Jessica Papa, Office Admin.
Year Established: 1983.
Staff: Part-time: 2.

Avg Enrollment: 20. *Avg Class Size:* 8. *Number of
  Graduates per Year:* 15.
Wheelchair Access: No.
Field of Study: Reflexology*. *Program
  Name/Length:* Reflexhollogy (includes intro-
  duction to Aromatherapy, Energy Balancing,
  Yoga), 150 hrs, 10 mos.
Degrees Offered: Certificate.
License/Certification Preparation: American
  Reflexology Certification Board.
Admission Requirements: Private session with in-
  structor.
Tuition and Fees: $1800.
Career Services: Career information.

Gardiner

558. Hudson Valley School of Classical Homeopathy
321 McKinstry Rd, Gardiner, NY 12525
Phone: (914) 255-6241; *Fax:* (914) 255-6241
E-mail: hvsch95@aol.com
Program Administrator: David Kramer, Dir. *Ad-
  missions Contact:* David Kramer.
Year Established: 1995.
Wheelchair Access: Yes.
Field of Study: Homeopathy*. *Program
  Name/Length:* 600 hrs, 4 yrs.

Hunter

559. R. J. Buckle Associates, LLC
Aromatherapy for Health Professionals
PO Box 868, Hunter, NY 12442
Phone: (518) 263-4402; *Fax:* (518) 263-4031
E-mail: rjbuckle@delphi.com
Program Administrator: Jane Buckle, RN, Dir. *Ad-
  missions Contact:* Jane Buckle.
Year Established: 1994.
Staff: Part-time: 18.
Avg Enrollment: 100. *Avg Class Size:* 14. *Number
  of Graduates per Year:* 40.
Wheelchair Access: No.
Accreditation/Approval/Licensing: National Certif-
  ication Board for Therapeutic Massage and
  Bodywork (CEUs); National Association of Ho-
  listic Aromatherapy.
Field of Study: Aromatherapy*. *Program
  Name/Length:* The 'M' Technique, 18 mos (5
  modular weekends + home study); Seminars
  given in various locations.
Degrees Offered: Certificate.
Admission Requirements: Licensed health profes-
  sional.
Tuition and Fees: $250 per module + $400 exam.

Ithaca

560. Finger Lakes School of Massage

Therapeutic Massage Certification Program
1251 Trumansburg Rd, Ithaca, NY 14850
Phone: (607) 272-9024; *Fax:* (607) 272-4271
E-mail: admissions@flsm.com *Internet:* http://
www.flsm.com
Program Administrator: Cindy Black, Co-Owner;
Andrea Butje, Co-Owner; Shirley Adams,
Co-Dir; Donna Holt, Co-Dir; Amy Whitney,
Co-Dir. *Admissions Contact:* Shirley Adams.
Year Established: 1994.
Staff: Full-time: 6; Part-time: 12.
Avg Enrollment: 140. *Avg Class Size:* 72. *Number
of Graduates per Year:* 140.
Wheelchair Access: Yes.
Accreditation/Approval/Licensing: State board:
NY Board of Ed; National Certification Board
for Therapeutic Massage and Bodywork (CEUs).
Field of Study: Aromatherapy; Energy Work; Mas-
sage Therapy*; Neuromuscular Therapy; Polar-
ity Therapy; Reflexology; Shiatsu; Sports Mas-
sage; Thai Massage; Trager. *Program
Name/Length:* 5 1/2 mos/full-time or 2
yrs/part-time.
Degrees Offered: CEUs; Certificate.
License/Certification Preparation: State: NY Li-
censed Massage Therapist; National Certification Board for Therapeutic Massage and Bodywork.
Admission Requirements: Min age: 18; High
school diploma/GED; Interview.
Tuition and Fees: $7100 (850 hrs); $9500 (1000
hrs).
Financial Aid: VA approved; NY Vocational Ed
Services for Individuals with Disabilities; Job
Training Partnership Act and other local and
federal job retraining programs.
Career Services: Career information; Job information.

561. Northeast School of Botanical Medicine

PO Box 6626, Ithaca, NY 14851
Phone: (607) 564-1023
Program Administrator: 7Song, Dir. *Admissions
Contact:* 7Song, Dir.
Year Established: 1992.
Staff: Full-time: 1; Part-time: 7.
Avg Enrollment: 16. *Avg Class Size:* 16. *Number
of Graduates per Year:* 16.
Wheelchair Access: No.
Field of Study: Herbal Medicine*. *Program
Name/Length:* 100 hrs (includes Clinical Evalu-
ation, Plant Identification, Herbal Pharmacy,
Wildcrafting, Student Clinic), 7 mos (1 week-
end/mo); 360 hrs, 6 mos (3 days/wk); Advanced
Western Clinical Herbalism, 70 hrs.
Tuition and Fees: $875 (100 hrs); $1650 (360 hrs);
$600 (Advanced).

Career Services: Business practicum.

Malverne

562. Yoga and Polarity Center

32 Church St, Malverne, NY 11565
Phone: (516) 596-0397; *Fax:* (516) 887-4747
E-mail: medcinflwr@aol.com
Program Administrator: Heather Principe, Dir. *Ad-
missions Contact:* Amy Bubser.
Year Established: 1994.
Staff: Full-time: 5; Part-time: 11.
Avg Enrollment: 35. *Avg Class Size:* 15. *Number
of Graduates per Year:* 18.
Wheelchair Access: Yes.
Accreditation/Approval/Licensing: American Po-
larity Therapy Association.
Field of Study: Energy Work; Polarity Therapy*;
Reflexology; Yoga Teacher Training*. *Program
Name/Length:* Associate Polarity Practitioner,
165 hrs; Registered Polarity Practitioner, 3 yrs.
Degrees Offered: Certificate.
License/Certification Preparation: APP; RPP;
American Polarity Therapy Association.
Admission Requirements: Min age: 18.
Application Deadline(s): Fall: Sep; Winter: Nov;
Spring: Jan.
Financial Aid: Work study.
Career Services: Internships.

New York

563. Academy of Natural Healing

40 W 72nd St, Ste 117, New York, NY 10023
Phone: (212) 724-8782; *Fax:* (212) 724-2535
E-mail: chihealer@mindspring.com
Program Administrator: Lewis Harrison, Dir. *Ad-
missions Contact:* Lewis Harrison.
Year Established: 1974.
Staff: Full-time: 1; Part-time: 15.
Avg Enrollment: 40. *Avg Class Size:* 10. *Number
of Graduates per Year:* 14.
Wheelchair Access: Yes.
Accreditation/Approval/Licensing: American Po-
larity Therapy Association.
Field of Study: Acupressure; Aromatherapy;
CranioSacral Therapy; Energy Work; Herbal
Medicine; Homeopathy; Polarity Therapy*;
Qigong; Reflexology; Shiatsu. *Program
Name/Length:* Polarity Therapy, 154 hrs; Body-
work, 154 hrs; Natural Healing, 154 hrs.
License/Certification Preparation: American Po-
larity Therapy Association.
Admission Requirements: Min age: 18; High
school diploma/GED.
Tuition and Fees: $2995.
Financial Aid: Scholarships; Work study; Payment
plan.
Career Services: Career counseling; Career infor-
mation; Internships.

564. American Center for the Alexander Technique

129 W 67th St, New York, NY 10023
Phone: (212) 799-0468; *Fax:* (212) 799-0468
Program Administrator: Barbara Kent, Dir. *Admissions Contact:* Joan Frost, Asst Dir.
Year Established: 1964.
Staff: Part-time: 10.
Avg Enrollment: 15. *Avg Class Size:* 10. *Number of Graduates per Year:* 6.
Wheelchair Access: Yes.
Accreditation/Approval/Licensing: State board: NY Bureau of Proprietary School Supervision; American Society for the Alexander Technique.
Field of Study: Alexander Technique*. *Program Name/Length:* Teacher Certification, 3 yrs.
Degrees Offered: Certificate.
License/Certification Preparation: American Society for the Alexander Technique.
Admission Requirements: Some college (3 yrs); Specific course prerequisites: 26 lessons in the Alexander Technique.
Application Deadline(s): Fall: Jun 1; Winter: Nov 1.
Tuition and Fees: $7200 per yr.
Career Services: Career counseling; Career information.

565. American Taoist Healing Center

396 Broadway, Ste 502, New York, NY 10013-3500
Phone: (212) 274-0999; *Fax:* (212) 274-9879
Program Administrator: Nan Lu, Dir. *Admissions Contact:* Louise Di Bello, Admin.
Year Established: 1991.
Staff: Full-time: 6.
Avg Enrollment: 100. *Avg Class Size:* 20.
Wheelchair Access: Yes.
Field of Study: Acupressure*; Acupuncture*; Qigong*; Traditional Chinese Medicine*. *Program Name/Length:* Qigong Meridian Therapy, 246 hrs, 9 mos; Qigong, ongoing.
Degrees Offered: Certificate.
Admission Requirements: Min age: 18 for Qigong Meridian Therapy.

566. Biofeedback Training Associates

255 W 98th St, New York, NY 10025
Phone: (212) 222-5665; *Fax:* (212) 222-5667
E-mail: ac@inx.net *Internet:* http://www.biof.com/biofeedback.html
Program Administrator: Dr. Philip Brotman, Dir. *Admissions Contact:* Dr. Philip Brotman.
Year Established: 1972.
Staff: Full-time: 2; Part-time: 5.
Avg Enrollment: 100. *Avg Class Size:* 7. *Number of Graduates per Year:* 80.
Wheelchair Access: Yes.
Accreditation/Approval/Licensing: Biofeedback Certification Institute of America; American Psychological Association.

Field of Study: Biofeedback*; Hypnotherapy; Neurofeedback. *Program Name/Length:* 80 hrs, 8-9 days; Weekend training; 1 day programs.
Degrees Offered: Certificate.
Admission Requirements: High school diploma/GED.
Tuition and Fees: $200-$350 per day.
Career Services: Referral service.

567. Body Logic Institute

Body Logic and Body Rolling Certification
295 W 11th St, Ste 1F, New York, NY 10014
Phone: (212) 633-2143, (800) 877-8429; *Fax:* (212) 633-6190
E-mail: yzake@aol.com *Internet:* http://www.bodylogic.com
Program Administrator: Yamuna Zake, Dir. *Admissions Contact:* Yamuna Zake.
Year Established: 1991.
Staff: Full-time: 1; Part-time: 4.
Avg Enrollment: 10. *Avg Class Size:* 10. *Number of Graduates per Year:* 7.
Wheelchair Access: Yes.
Accreditation/Approval/Licensing: Accrediting Council for Continuing Education and Training.
Field of Study: Body Logic*; Body Rolling*. *Program Name/Length:* Certification, 2 yrs (3 wk intensive/1st yr and four 5-day intensives/2nd yr); Continuing Education, annual 4-day intensive.
Degrees Offered: Diploma; Certificate.
Admission Requirements: Min age: 25; Some college; Specific course prerequisites: anatomy and physiology; Massage or physical therapy license, yoga teacher's certification, movement kinesiology training, or fitness degree.
Tuition and Fees: $2900 per yr (Body Logic); $1500 per yr (Body Rolling).
Career Services: Internships; Interview set up; Job information.

568. Flynn's School of Herbology

60 E 4th St, New York, NY 10003
Phone: (212) 677-8140
Program Administrator: Arcus Flynn, Owner. *Admissions Contact:* Arcus Flynn.
Year Established: 1980.
Staff: Full-time: 1.
Avg Enrollment: 105. *Avg Class Size:* 9. *Number of Graduates per Year:* 100.
Field of Study: Herbal Medicine*. *Program Name/Length:* Beginner/Intermediate Herbology, 2 mos; Advanced Herbology, 2 mos.
Degrees Offered: Certificate.
Admission Requirements: Min age: 16.
Tuition and Fees: $250 (includes books).

569. The Hypnosis Institute

139 Fulton St, Ste 304, New York, NY 10038
Phone: (212) 227-8643; *Fax:* (212) 791-9517
E-mail: hypno1@interport.net *Internet:* http://www.infaith.com

Program Administrator: Barry Seedman, PhD, Dir.
Admissions Contact: Barry Seedman.
Year Established: 1991.
Staff: Full-time: 2; Part-time: 4.
Avg Enrollment: 800. *Avg Class Size:* 30. *Number of Graduates per Year:* 750.
Wheelchair Access: Yes.
Field of Study: Hypnotherapy*; Reiki*. *Program Name/Length:* Basic Hypnotherapy Certification, weekend workshop; Career Hypnotherapy Certification, 100 hrs; Reiki Training, weekend intensive.
Degrees Offered: Certificate.
License/Certification Preparation: International Association of Counselors and Therapists; International Board of Hypnotists.
Admission Requirements: Min age: 18.
Tuition and Fees: $395 (Basic); $1495 (Career); $470 (Reiki).

570. Institute for the Alexander Technique

853 Broadway, Ste 1007, New York, NY 10003
Phone: (212) 529-3211
Program Administrator: Thomas Lemens, Head Trainer. *Admissions Contact:* Michael Ostrow, Dir.
Year Established: 1983.
Staff: Full-time: 2; Part-time: 2.
Avg Class Size: 8. *Number of Graduates per Year:* 2.
Wheelchair Access: Yes.
Accreditation/Approval/Licensing: American Society for the Alexander Technique.
Field of Study: Alexander Technique*. *Program Name/Length:* Teacher Training, 4 1/3 yrs.
Degrees Offered: Certificate.
License/Certification Preparation: American Society for the Alexander Technique.
Admission Requirements: Min age: 18; High school diploma/GED; Specific course prerequisites: series of private lessons with instructor.
Tuition and Fees: $2900 per semester.

571. Jivamukti Yoga Center

Teacher Training
404 Lafayette St, 3rd Fl, New York, NY 10003
Phone: (212) 353-0214; *Fax:* (212) 995-1313
Program Administrator: Adrienne Burke, Dir of Teaching Programs. *Admissions Contact:* Adrienne Burke.
Year Established: 1993.
Staff: Full-time: 8; Part-time: 4.
Avg Enrollment: 40. *Avg Class Size:* 40. *Number of Graduates per Year:* 35.
Field of Study: Yoga Teacher Training*. *Program Name/Length:* Levels I-III, 2000 hrs, 3 yrs.
Degrees Offered: Certificate.
Application Deadline(s): Winter: Feb.
Tuition and Fees: $2500 (Level I); $2500 (Level II); $3000 (Level III).
Career Services: Career counseling; Career information; Job information; Referral service.

572. Diana Kalfayan

Polarity Therapy
150 W 80th St, Apt 6C, New York, NY 10024
Phone: (212) 877-9626
E-mail: dkpolarity@aol.com
Program Administrator: Diana Kalfayan, Dir. *Admissions Contact:* Diana Kalfayan.
Year Established: 1997.
Staff: Full-time: 1.
Avg Enrollment: 3.
Wheelchair Access: Yes.
Accreditation/Approval/Licensing: American Polarity Therapy Association.
Field of Study: Esoteric Healing; Polarity Therapy*. *Program Name/Length:* Associate Polarity Practitioner, 165 hrs, 6 mos (7 weekends); Weekend Seminars in Esoteric Healing, 20 hrs; Seminars given in various locations.
Degrees Offered: Certificate.
License/Certification Preparation: APP; American Polarity Therapy Association.
Tuition and Fees: $1700 (APP); $250 (Weekend Seminars).

573. The Kundalini Yoga Center

419 Lafayette St, New York, NY 10003
Mailing Address: 225 E 5th St, Ste 4D, New York, NY 10003
Phone: (212) 475-0212
E-mail: ravi@ziplink.net *Internet:* http://www.ziplink.net/~ravi
Program Administrator: Ravi Singh, Dir. *Admissions Contact:* Mr. Hackman, Mktg Mgr.
Year Established: 1987.
Staff: Full-time: 4.
Avg Enrollment: 750.
Wheelchair Access: Yes.
Accreditation/Approval/Licensing: 3HO Foundation/International Kundalini Yoga Teachers Association; Accrediting Council for Continuing Education and Training.
Field of Study: Yoga Teacher Training*. *Program Name/Length:* Kundalini Yoga Teacher Training, 8 mos and home study.
Degrees Offered: Certificate.
Admission Requirements: Min age: 18; Specific course prerequisites: Kundalini Yoga classes.
Financial Aid: Payment plan.
Career Services: Career counseling.

574. Kundalini Yoga East, Inc

873 Broadway, Ste 614, New York, NY 10003
Phone: (212) 995-0521, 982-5959 voice
Program Administrator: Sat Jivan Kaur Khalsa, Dir. *Admissions Contact:* Sat Jivan Kaur Khalsa.
Year Established: 1972.
Staff: Full-time: 3; Part-time: 4.
Avg Enrollment: 30. *Avg Class Size:* 20. *Number of Graduates per Year:* 20.
Wheelchair Access: Yes.

Field of Study: Energy Work; Yoga Teacher Training*. *Program Name/Length:* Kundalini Yoga Teacher Training Certification, 130 hrs, 6 mos and home study; Sat Nam Rasayan Training (healing branch of Kundalini Yoga), ongoing.
Degrees Offered: Certificate.
License/Certification Preparation: Certification, International Kundalini Yoga Teachers' Association; Kundalini Research Institute.
Admission Requirements: Min age: 18 or parental consent; High school diploma/GED; Specific course prerequisites: Kundalini Yoga classes.
Tuition and Fees: $1600.
Career Services: Career counseling; Internships.

575. The Mathews School of the Alexander Technique

74 MacDougal St, New York, NY 10012
Phone: (212) 473-3247; *Fax:* (212) 473-0341
E-mail: irdeat@mindspring.com
Program Administrator: Troup Mathews, Co-Dir; Christine Batten, Co-Dir; Ann Mathews, Co-Dir. *Admissions Contact:* Christine Batten, Co-Dir.
Year Established: 1983.
Staff: Full-time: 3; Part-time: 1.
Avg Enrollment: 5-12. *Avg Class Size:* 11. *Number of Graduates per Year:* 5.
Wheelchair Access: No.
Accreditation/Approval/Licensing: American Society for the Alexander Technique.
Field of Study: Alexander Technique*. *Program Name/Length:* Teacher Training, 1600 hrs, 9 terms, 3 yrs.
Degrees Offered: Certificate.
License/Certification Preparation: American Society for the Alexander Technique.
Admission Requirements: Bachelor's degree or equivalent life experience; Specific course prerequisites: course of lessons in the Alexander Technique; Interview and lesson with director.
Application Deadline(s): Fall: Aug 1; Winter: Dec 1; Spring: Mar 1.
Tuition and Fees: $5460 per yr or $1820 per term.

576. MotherMassage: Massage During Pregnancy

108 E 16th St, Ste 401, New York, NY 10003
Phone: (212) 533-3188; *Fax:* (212) 533-3148
Program Administrator: Elaine Stillerman, LMT, Instr. *Admissions Contact:* Elaine Stillerman.
Year Established: 1980.
Staff: Full-time: 1.
Avg Enrollment: 250. *Avg Class Size:* 20. *Number of Graduates per Year:* 250.
Wheelchair Access: No.
Accreditation/Approval/Licensing: State board: CA Board of Registered Nursing; FL Board of Massage; American College of Nurse-Midwives, Division of Accreditation; National Certification Board for Therapeutic Massage and Bodywork (CEUs); International Childbirth Education Association; Lamaze International.

Field of Study: Postpartum Massage*; Prenatal Massage*. *Program Name/Length:* MotherMassage: Massage During Pregnancy, 16 1/2 hrs, 2 1/2 days; Seminars given in various locations.
Degrees Offered: Certificate.
License/Certification Preparation: American College of Nurse-Midwives; International Childbirth Education Association; Lamaze International.
Admission Requirements: Min age: 18; High school diploma/GED; Specific course prerequisites: basic Swedish massage training required for non-massage professionals; Licensed massage therapist, childbirth educator, nurse-midwife, doula, or advanced massage student.
Tuition and Fees: $295.

577. New York Open Center

83 Spring St, New York, NY 10012
Phone: (212) 274-1829; *Fax:* (212) 226-4056
Admissions Contact: Lisa Schimski, RPP, Polarity Therapy; Elaine Koelmel, Reflexology; Jeffrey Migdow, MD, Yoga Teacher Training.
Avg Class Size: 20.
Wheelchair Access: Yes.
Accreditation/Approval/Licensing: American Polarity Therapy Association.
Field of Study: Polarity Therapy*; Reflexology*; Yoga Teacher Training*. *Program Name/Length:* Associate Polarity Practitioner, 165 hrs, 6 mos; Prana Yoga Teacher Training, 9 mos (1 weekend per mo).
Degrees Offered: Certificate.
License/Certification Preparation: APP; American Polarity Therapy Association.

578. New York University, Division of Nursing/School of Education

Nurse-Midwifery Education Program
50 W 4th St, 429 Shimkin Hall, New York, NY 10012
Phone: (212) 998-5895
Program Administrator: Patricia Burkhardt, Coord/Assoc Clinical Professor.
Year Established: 1994.
Staff: Full-time: 2; Part-time: 4.
Avg Enrollment: 20. *Avg Class Size:* 20. *Number of Graduates per Year:* 20.
Wheelchair Access: Yes.
Accreditation/Approval/Licensing: American College of Nurse-Midwives, Division of Accreditation.
Field of Study: Midwifery*. *Program Name/Length:* Master's in Midwifery, 48 credits, 2 yrs and 1 semester; Post-Master's Certificate, 1 yr and 1 semester.
Degrees Offered: MA.
License/Certification Preparation: State: NY State Professional Midwifery License; Certified Nurse-Midwife, American College of Nurse-Midwives.

Admission Requirements: Bachelor's degree in Nursing.
Financial Aid: Fellowships; Grants; Scholarships; State government aid; Work study.
Career Services: Career information.

579. NLP Center of New York
24 E 12th St, Ste 402, New York, NY 10003
Phone: (212) 647-0860; *Fax:* (973) 509-2326
E-mail: nlp@earthlink.net *Internet:* http://www.nlptraining.com
Program Administrator: Steven Leeds, Co-Dir. *Admissions Contact:* Rachel Hott, Co-Dir.
Year Established: 1986.
Staff: Full-time: 2; Part-time: 2.
Avg Enrollment: 60. *Avg Class Size:* 20. *Number of Graduates per Year:* 20.
Wheelchair Access: Yes.
Accreditation/Approval/Licensing: International Association of Neuro-Linguistic Programming.
Field of Study: Hypnotherapy*; Neuro-Linguistic Programming*. *Program Name/Length:* Ericksonian Hypnosis, 42 hrs, 7 days; Neuro-Linguistic Programming Practitioner, 1 yr; Master Practitioner, 1 yr; Trainer, 2-4 yrs.
License/Certification Preparation: American Board of Hypnotherapy; National Board for Certified Clinical Hypnotherapists.
Tuition and Fees: $795 (Ericksonian Hypnosis); $2295 (Practitioner).
Financial Aid: Work study.
Career Services: Internships.

580. Laura Norman Reflexology Training Center
41 Park Ave, Ste 8A, New York, NY 10016
Phone: (212) 532-4404; *Fax:* (212) 532-4504
E-mail: reflexologist.com@cwixmail.com *Internet:* http://www.lauranormanreflexology.com
Program Administrator: Laura Norman, Dir. *Admissions Contact:* Judine Simpson, Admissions Dir.
Year Established: 1980.
Staff: Part-time: 6.
Avg Enrollment: 1500. *Avg Class Size:* 25. *Number of Graduates per Year:* 450.
Wheelchair Access: Yes.
Field of Study: Reflexology*. *Program Name/Length:* Laura Norman Method of Reflexology, 8 hrs-365 hrs, 1-day workshops to 9 mos.
Degrees Offered: Certificate.
Tuition and Fees: $100-$2700.
Financial Aid: Work study.

581. The Ohashi Institute
12 W 27th St, 9th Fl, New York, NY 10001
Phone: (800) 810-4190; *Fax:* (212) 447-5819
E-mail: ohashiinst@aol.com *Internet:* http://www.ohashi.com
Program Administrator: Ohashi, Founder.
Year Established: 1974.

Staff: Part-time: 40.
Avg Enrollment: 2000. *Avg Class Size:* 15. *Number of Graduates per Year:* 100.
Wheelchair Access: No.
Field of Study: Shiatsu*. *Program Name/Length:* Ohashiatsu Curriculum, 6 levels, 2 yrs; Ohashiatsu Instructor Training, 12-18 mos.
Degrees Offered: Certificate.
Admission Requirements: Min age: 18; High school diploma/GED; Specific course prerequisites: Curriculum required for Instructor Training.
Application Deadline(s): Fall: Sep 15; Winter: Jan 15; Spring: Apr 10; Summer: Jul 15.
Tuition and Fees: $395-$910 per level.
Financial Aid: Work study.

582. Pacific College of Oriental Medicine, New York
915 Broadway, 3rd Fl, New York, NY 10010
Phone: (212) 982-3456, (800) 729-3468; *Fax:* (212) 982-6514
Internet: http://www.ormed.edu
Program Administrator: Reine S. Deming. *Admissions Contact:* Jennifer Park, Alma Zengotita, Admissions Counselors.
Year Established: 1993.
Staff: Full-time: 4; Part-time: 41.
Avg Enrollment: 210. *Number of Graduates per Year:* 50.
Wheelchair Access: Yes.
Accreditation/Approval/Licensing: State board: CA Acupuncture Board; Accreditation Commission for Acupuncture and Oriental Medicine.
Field of Study: Acupuncture*; Oriental Medicine*; Traditional Chinese Medicine*. *Program Name/Length:* Bachelor of Professional Studies/Master of Science in Acupuncture, 3 yrs + 3 mos; Bachelor of Professional Studies/Master of Science in Oriental Medicine, 3 yrs + 7 mos.
Degrees Offered: MS; BPS/MS Dual degree.
License/Certification Preparation: National Certification Commission for Acupuncture and Oriental Medicine.
Admission Requirements: High school diploma/GED; Some college (Associate's degree or 60 credits).
Application Deadline(s): Fall; Winter; Spring.
Tuition and Fees: $10,000 per yr.
Financial Aid: Grants; Loans; Scholarships; State government aid; Work study.

583. The Rubenfeld Synergy Center
115 Waverly Pl, New York, NY 10011
Phone: (800) 747-6897; *Fax:* (212) 254-1174
E-mail: rubenfeld@aol.com
Program Administrator: Ilana Rubenfeld, PhD, Dir; Alreta Turner, Admin. *Admissions Contact:* Peggy Shaw-Rosato, Dir of Ed.
Year Established: 1977.
Staff: Full-time: 5; Part-time: 8.

Avg Enrollment: 80.
Wheelchair Access: Yes.
Field of Study: Rubenfeld Synergy Method*. *Program Name/Length:* Professional Certification, 4 yrs (3 wks/yr).

584. The School of Homeopathy, New York

964 Third Ave, 8th Fl, New York, NY 10155-0003
Phone: (212) 570-2576; *Fax:* (212) 758-4079
E-mail: kathy@homeopathyschool.com *Internet:* http://www.homeopathyschool.com
Program Administrator: Kathleen A. Lukas, Dir.
   Admissions Contact: Kathleen A. Lukas.
Year Established: 1981.
Avg Enrollment: 200.
Field of Study: Homeopathy*. *Program Name/Length:* Comprehensive Professional Training, 4 yrs (1 weekend per mo).
Degrees Offered: Diploma.
License/Certification Preparation: Council for Homeopathic Certification; Homeopathic Academy of Naturopathic Physicians; North American Society of Homeopaths; National Board of Homeopathic Examiners.
Admission Requirements: Some college (2 yrs).
Application Deadline(s): Fall: Sep.
Tuition and Fees: $3050.
Financial Aid: Payment plan.
Career Services: Case supervision internships.

585. Swedish Institute, Inc

Massage Therapy; Acupuncture and Oriental Studies
226 W 26th St, 5th Fl, New York, NY 10001
Phone: (212) 924-5900; *Fax:* (212) 924-7600
Accreditation/Approval/Licensing: Accrediting Commission of Career Schools and Colleges of Technology; National Certification Board for Therapeutic Massage and Bodywork (CEUs); Candidate, Accreditation Commission for Acupuncture and Oriental Medicine; American Oriental Bodywork Therapy Association.
Field of Study: Acupressure; Acupuncture*; Massage Therapy*; Oriental Medicine*; Shiatsu*. *Program Name/Length:* Massage Therapy, 1224 hrs; Diploma in Acupuncture, 2713 hrs, 3 yrs.
Degrees Offered: Diploma.
License/Certification Preparation: State: NY Licensed Massage Therapist, NY Licensed Acupuncturist; National Certification Commission for Acupuncture and Oriental Medicine; National Certification Board for Therapeutic Massage and Bodywork.

586. Teleosis School of Homeopathy

61 W 62nd St, New York, NY 10023
Phone: (212) 707-8481; *Fax:* (212) 707-8481
E-mail: teleosis@igc.org
Program Administrator: Joel Kreisberg, DC, Dir.
   Admissions Contact: Kim Kalina, Office Mgr.
Year Established: 1995.

Staff: Full-time: 1; Part-time: 5.
Avg Enrollment: 15. *Avg Class Size:* 15. *Number of Graduates per Year:* 5.
Wheelchair Access: Yes.
Field of Study: Homeopathy*. *Program Name/Length:* Certificate program, 2 yrs (10 weekends/yr); Clinical program, 2 yrs (10 weekends/yr).
Degrees Offered: Certificate.
License/Certification Preparation: American Board of Homeotherapeutics; Council for Homeopathic Certification; Homeopathic Academy of Naturopathic Physicians.
Admission Requirements: Licensed medical provider.
Application Deadline(s): Fall: Jun 30.
Tuition and Fees: $2500 per yr (certificate); $3000 per yr (clinical).
Financial Aid: Work study; Payment plan.

587. Tri-State Institute of Traditional Chinese Acupuncture

80 8th Ave, Ste 400, New York, NY 10024
Phone: (212) 242-2255; *Fax:* (212) 242-2920
Program Administrator: Mark D. Seem, PhD, Pres.
   Admissions Contact: Audrey Hartmann, Registrar.
Year Established: 1979.
Staff: Full-time: 3; Part-time: 13.
Avg Enrollment: 125. *Avg Class Size:* 38. *Number of Graduates per Year:* 32.
Wheelchair Access: Yes.
Accreditation/Approval/Licensing: Accreditation Commission for Acupuncture and Oriental Medicine.
Field of Study: Acupuncture*; Herbal Medicine*; Traditional Chinese Medicine*. *Program Name/Length:* Traditional Chinese Herbal Program, 450 hrs, 2 yrs; Master's-Level Diploma in Acupuncture, 3 yrs; Program for Physicians and Dentists, 300 hrs, 1 yr.
Degrees Offered: Diploma; Certificate.
License/Certification Preparation: State: NY Licensed Acupuncturist; National Certification Commission for Acupuncture and Oriental Medicine.
Admission Requirements: Min age: 21; High school diploma/GED; Min GPA: 2.0; Some college (60 credits or 2 yrs); Min GPA: 2.0.
Application Deadline(s): Fall: Jul 1.
Tuition and Fees: $7700 per yr.
Financial Aid: Federal government aid; Loans.
Career Services: Career information.

588. Reese Williams

Polarity Therapy
270 Lafayette St, Ste 805, New York, NY 10012
Phone: (212) 343-9382
Program Administrator: Reese Williams, Dir. *Admissions Contact:* Reese Williams.
Year Established: 1991.
Staff: Part-time: 3.

Avg Enrollment: 20. *Avg Class Size:* 10. *Number of Graduates per Year:* 8.
Wheelchair Access: Yes.
Accreditation/Approval/Licensing: American Polarity Therapy Association.
Field of Study: CranioSacral Therapy*; Polarity Therapy*. *Program Name/Length:* Associate Polarity Practitioner, 161 hrs; Registered Polarity Practitioner, 523 hrs.
Degrees Offered: Diploma.
License/Certification Preparation: APP and RPP; American Polarity Therapy Association.
Admission Requirements: Specific course prerequisites: APP or equivalent required for RPP.
Financial Aid: Payment plan.
Career Services: Career information; Instruction in basic business skills.

Port Jefferson

589. Long Island Reflexology Center
14 E Broadway, Port Jefferson, NY 11777
Phone: (516) 474-3137; *Fax:* (516) 287-3127
Program Administrator: Geraldine Brill, RN, Dir. *Admissions Contact:* Geraldine Brill.
Year Established: 1985.
Staff: Full-time: 1.
Avg Enrollment: 18. *Avg Class Size:* 6.
Wheelchair Access: No.
Field of Study: Reflexology*; Therapeutic Touch. *Program Name/Length:* 110 hrs, 3 semesters, 8 mos.
Degrees Offered: Certificate.
License/Certification Preparation: American Reflexology Certification Board.
Admission Requirements: Min age: 18; High school diploma/GED.
Tuition and Fees: $500 per semester.
Financial Aid: Payment plan.
Career Services: Career counseling; Career information; Job information; Referral service.

Poughkeepsie

590. The Linden Tree Center for Holistic Health
8 Noxon Rd, Poughkeepsie, NY 12603-2926
Phone: (914) 471-8000
E-mail: rgsiegel@igc.apc.org
Program Administrator: Gary Seigel, Dir.
Wheelchair Access: Yes.
Accreditation/Approval/Licensing: American Polarity Therapy Association.
Field of Study: CranioSacral Therapy; Polarity Therapy*. *Program Name/Length:* Associate Polarity Practitioner, 165 hrs (1 weekend per mo, Sep-Jun).
License/Certification Preparation: APP; American Polarity Therapy Association.

Rhinebeck

591. Omega Institute for Holistic Studies
260 Lake Dr, Rhinebeck, NY 12572
Phone: (914) 266-4444; *Fax:* (914) 266-4828
Internet: http://omega-inst.org
Program Administrator: Greg Zelonka, Dir of Programming. *Admissions Contact:* Laurie Zollo, Registrar.
Year Established: 1978.
Staff: Part-time: 300.
Avg Enrollment: 15,000. *Avg Class Size:* 30.
Wheelchair Access: Yes.
Accreditation/Approval/Licensing: Accrediting Council for Continuing Education and Training; National Certification Board for Therapeutic Massage and Bodywork (CEUs); National Board for Certified Counselors.
Field of Study: Energy Work; Healing Touch; Massage Therapy*; Mind-Body Medicine*; Qigong; Reflexology; Yoga Teacher Training*. *Program Name/Length:* Professional Training in Massage Therapy, Healing Touch, Yoga, DansKinetics, 1 mo; Workshops in Acupressure, Aromatherapy, Ayurvedic Medicine, CranioSacral Therapy, Feldenkrais, Herbal Medicine, Homeopathy, Hypnosis, Massage Therapy, Myotherapy, Qigong, Reflexology, Shiatsu, Traditional Chinese Medicine, 2-12 days.
Degrees Offered: Certificate.
Admission Requirements: Min age: 18.
Tuition and Fees: $2300 (Professional Training); $195-$1050 (Workshops).
Financial Aid: Scholarships; Work study.

Ruby

592. Rainbow Reiki Center
Reiki I, II, and III
1330 Main St, Ruby, NY 12475
Mailing Address: PO Box 110, Ruby, NY 12475
Phone: (914) 336-4609
E-mail: rainbow@ulster.net *Internet:* http://www.rainbowcrystal.com
Program Administrator: Joyce Kaessinger, Co-Dir; Constance Sohodski, Co-Dir. *Admissions Contact:* Joyce Kaessinger; Constance Sohodski.
Year Established: 1990.
Staff: Full-time: 2.
Avg Enrollment: 90. *Avg Class Size:* 6. *Number of Graduates per Year:* 90.
Wheelchair Access: No.
Accreditation/Approval/Licensing: National Certification Board for Therapeutic Massage and Bodywork (CEUs).
Field of Study: Reiki*. *Program Name/Length:* Reiki I, 7 hrs; Reiki II, 7 hrs; Reiki III, 14 hrs; Seminars given in various locations.
Degrees Offered: Certificate.

Tuition and Fees: $100 (Reiki I); $350 (Reiki II); $600 Reiki (III).

Saugerties

593. Wise Woman Center

416 Fishcreek, Saugerties, NY 12477
Mailing Address: PO Box 64, Woodstock, NY 12498
Phone: (914) 246-8081; *Fax:* (941) 246-8081
Program Administrator: Susun S. Weed, Dir. *Admissions Contact:* Susun S. Weed.
Year Established: 1982.
Staff: Full-time: 1; Part-time: 20.
Avg Enrollment: 75. *Avg Class Size:* 13. *Number of Graduates per Year:* 30.
Wheelchair Access: No.
Field of Study: Animal Therapy*; Energy Work; Herbal Medicine*. *Program Name/Length:* Live-in Apprentice, 3-7 mos; Live-out Apprentice, 1-2 yrs; Correspondence course, 2-4 yrs.
Degrees Offered: Certificate.
Admission Requirements: Min age: 16; Written application.
Application Deadline(s): Fall: May 1; Spring: Dec 1; Summer: Feb 1.
Tuition and Fees: $5400 per semester.
Financial Aid: Scholarships; Work study.
Career Services: Career counseling; Internships.

Seneca Falls

594. New York Chiropractic College

2360 SR 89, Seneca Falls, NY 13148-0800
Phone: (315) 568-3000; *Fax:* (315) 568-3015
E-mail: enrolnow@nycc.edu *Internet:* http://www.nycc.edu
Program Administrator: Kenneth W. Padgett, Pres. *Admissions Contact:* Michael P. Pynch, Dir of Admissions.
Year Established: 1919.
Staff: Full-time: 52; Part-time: 48.
Avg Enrollment: 1000. *Number of Graduates per Year:* 100.
Wheelchair Access: Yes.
Accreditation/Approval/Licensing: State board: NY State Board of Regents; Council on Chiropractic Education; Middle States Association of Colleges and Schools.
Field of Study: Chiropractic*. *Program Name/Length:* Doctor of Chiropractic, 10 trimesters.
Degrees Offered: DC.
License/Certification Preparation: State: NY State Boards of Chiropractic; National Board of Chiropractic Examiners.
Admission Requirements: High school diploma/GED; Some college (75 semester hrs); Min GPA: 2.25, science GPA: 2.0; Specific course prerequisites: 24 hrs science, 24 hrs social sciences/humanities.
Tuition and Fees: $5150 per trimester.
Financial Aid: Federal government aid; Loans; Scholarships; State government aid; Work study.
Career Services: Career counseling; Career information; Employment opportunities database; Internships; Interview set up; Resume service.

Stone Ridge

595. Woodstock Polarity Retreat Center

872 Buck Rd, Stone Ridge, NY 12484
Phone: (914) 687-4767, (800) 925-0159; *Fax:* (212) 327-4049
E-mail: johnb310@aol.com
Program Administrator: John Beaulieu, PhD, Dir.
Year Established: 1981.
Staff: Full-time: 10; Part-time: 14.
Avg Enrollment: 100. *Avg Class Size:* 20. *Number of Graduates per Year:* 25.
Accreditation/Approval/Licensing: American Polarity Therapy Association.
Field of Study: Polarity Therapy*. *Program Name/Length:* Associate Polarity Practitioner, weekend modules; Registered Polarity Practitioner, weekend modules.
Degrees Offered: Certificate.
License/Certification Preparation: APP, RPP; American Polarity Therapy Association.
Admission Requirements: Min age: 19; High school diploma/GED.
Financial Aid: Work study.

Stony Brook

596. State University of New York at Stony Brook, School of Nursing

Pathways to Midwifery
Health Sciences Center, Stony Brook, NY 11794-8240
Phone: (516) 444-2879; *Fax:* (516) 444-6049
E-mail: ronnie.lichtman@sunysb.edu
Program Administrator: Ronnie Lichtman, PhD, Dir. *Admissions Contact:* Linda Sacino, Admin Asst.
Year Established: 1995.
Staff: Full-time: 8.
Avg Enrollment: 120. *Avg Class Size:* 20 (Jan), 50 (Aug). *Number of Graduates per Year:* 70.
Wheelchair Access: Yes.
Accreditation/Approval/Licensing: American College of Nurse-Midwives, Division of Accreditation.
Field of Study: Midwifery*. *Program Name/Length:* 4 semesters.
Degrees Offered: MS.
License/Certification Preparation: Certified Nurse-Midwife, American College of Nurse-Midwives.

Admission Requirements: Bachelor's degree; RN.
Tuition and Fees: $9885/resident, $15,795/nonresident + books, fees, insurance.
Financial Aid: Federal government aid; State government aid.

Syosset

597. The New York College for Wholistic Health Education and Research

6801 Jericho Tpk, Ste 300, Syosset, NY 11791
Phone: (516) 364-0808; *Fax:* (516) 364-0989
Program Administrator: Steven Schenkman, Pres.
  Admissions Contact: Susan Scoboria, Assoc Dir
  of Admissions.
Year Established: 1981.
Staff: Full-time: 35; Part-time: 75.
Avg Enrollment: 600. *Avg Class Size:* 70. *Number of Graduates per Year:* 300.
Wheelchair Access: Yes.
Accreditation/Approval/Licensing: State board: NY Board of Regents; Accrediting Council for Continuing Education and Training; Accreditation Commission for Acupuncture and Oriental Medicine.
Field of Study: Acupuncture*; Herbal Medicine*; Holistic Nursing*; Massage Therapy*; Oriental Medicine*; Traditional Chinese Medicine*. *Program Name/Length:* Massage Therapy, 68 credits, 16 mos; Acupuncture, 144 credits, 3 yrs; Oriental Medicine, 170 credits, 3 1/3 yrs; Diploma in Oriental Herbal Medicine, 2750 hrs, 3 yrs; Wholistic Nursing, 805 hrs, 2 1/2 yrs.
Degrees Offered: Diploma; BPS/MS in Acupuncture or Oriental Medicine; AOS in Massage.
License/Certification Preparation: State: NY Massage Therapy and Acupuncture Licenses; American Oriental Bodywork Therapy Association; National Certification Board for Therapeutic Massage and Bodywork.
Admission Requirements: Min age: 18; High school diploma/GED; Min GPA: 2.0 for Massage; Some college (2 yrs); Min GPA: 2.0 for Acupuncture and Oriental Medicine programs; RN for Wholistic Nursing.
Tuition and Fees: $18,700 (Massage); $39,600 (Acupuncture); $46,750 (Oriental Medicine); $9660 (Wholistic Nursing).
Financial Aid: Federal government aid; Loans; State government aid.
Career Services: Career counseling; Career information.

Syracuse

598. The Onondaga School of Therapeutic Massage

220 Walton St, Syracuse, NY 13202
Phone: (315) 424-1159; *Fax:* (315) 424-0796
E-mail: ostm@dreamscape.com *Internet:*
http://www.massage-school.com
Program Administrator: Douglas Delia, Owner/Dir. *Admissions Contact:* Jean Vatter, Admissions Dir.
Year Established: 1997.
Avg Enrollment: 150. *Avg Class Size:* 25. *Number of Graduates per Year:* 140.
Wheelchair Access: No.
Accreditation/Approval/Licensing: State board: NY Board of Regents.
Field of Study: Massage Therapy*. *Program Name/Length:* 6 mos/full-time or 13 mos/part-time.
Degrees Offered: Certificate.
License/Certification Preparation: State: NY Licensed Massage Therapist; National Certification Board for Therapeutic Massage and Bodywork.
Admission Requirements: Min age: 18; High school diploma/GED; Interview.
Application Deadline(s): Fall: Oct; Winter: Apr.
Tuition and Fees: $9800.
Career Services: Career counseling; Career information.

Treadwell

599. The Traditional Reiki Network

Fire No 602, Case Hill Rd, Treadwell, NY 13846-0262
Phone: (607) 829-3702; *Fax:* (914) 254-4835
E-mail: ellensokolow@usa.nct
Program Administrator: Ellen Sokolow, Traditional Reiki Master, Dir. *Admissions Contact:* Brian Streett, Traditional Reiki Master.
Year Established: 1984.
Staff: Full-time: 22.
Avg Enrollment: 1000. *Avg Class Size:* 25.
Wheelchair Access: Yes.
Field of Study: Reiki*. *Program Name/Length:* First Degree, 12-15 hrs; Second Degree, 15-22 hrs; Reiki Master/Teacher, 1-3 yrs; Practitioner Apprenticeship, 6 mos-2 yrs.
Admission Requirements: For First Degree: None; for Second Degree: Completion of First Degree at least 100 days previously, audit additional class, complete 50 full-body treatments and regular self-treatments; for Reiki Master/Teacher: Min age: 38, high school diploma (Min GPA: 3.0), some college, 3 years of Reiki practice, giving and receiving treatments, attend min of 8 First and Second Degree classes, Interview.
Tuition and Fees: $150-$200 (First Degree); $350-$500 (Second Degree); $10,000 (Reiki Master/Teacher).
Financial Aid: Fellowships; Grants; Loans; Scholarships; Work study.
Career Services: Career counseling; Internships; Resume service; Apprenticeship; Residential Reiki clinic in Israel.

Williamsville

600. New York Institute of Massage
4701 Transit Rd, Williamsville, NY 14221
Mailing Address: PO Box 645, Buffalo, NY 14231
Phone: (716) 633-0355, (800) 884-6946; *Fax:* (716) 633-0213
E-mail: nyim@compuserve.com *Internet:* http://www.massage-ny.com
Program Administrator: David Kasprzyk, Dir. *Admissions Contact:* Sharon Boyd, Admissions Dir.
Year Established: 1994.
Staff: Part-time: 25.
Avg Enrollment: 130. *Avg Class Size:* 40. *Number of Graduates per Year:* 130.
Wheelchair Access: Yes.
Accreditation/Approval/Licensing: State board: NY Board of Massage.
Field of Study: Massage Therapy*. *Program Name/Length:* 1000 hrs + 60 hrs Clinic and 20 hrs Community Service, 1 yr.
Degrees Offered: Diploma.
License/Certification Preparation: State: NY Licensed Massage Therapist; National Certification Board for Therapeutic Massage and Bodywork.
Admission Requirements: Min age: 17; High school diploma/GED.
Tuition and Fees: $8000 + $400 books.
Financial Aid: VA approved; NY Vocational Ed Services for Individuals with Disabilities.
Career Services: Career counseling; Career information; Interview set up.

Woodbourne

601. Sivananda Yoga Ranch
Sivananda Yoga Teachers Training Course
PO Box 195, Woodbourne, NY 12788
Phone: (914) 436-6492; *Fax:* (914) 434-1032
E-mail: yogaranch@sivananda.org *Internet:* http://www.sivananda.org/ranch.htm
Program Administrator: Srinivasan, Dir. *Admissions Contact:* Srinivasan, Dir; Laksmi, Asst Dir.
Year Established: 1974.
Staff: Full-time: 4; Part-time: 3.
Avg Enrollment: 40. *Avg Class Size:* 40. *Number of Graduates per Year:* 38.
Wheelchair Access: No.
Accreditation/Approval/Licensing: International Sivananda Yoga Vedanta Centers.
Field of Study: Yoga Teacher Training*. *Program Name/Length:* Hatha Yoga Teacher Training (includes Basic Anatomy and Physiology, Yoga Asana, Bhagavad Gita, Mantra Chanting, Vedanta Philosophy), 1 mo intensive/10 hrs per day instruction and practice.
Degrees Offered: Certificate.
License/Certification Preparation: International Sivananda Yoga Vedanta Centers.
Admission Requirements: Min age: 18 or special approval.
Tuition and Fees: $1450 + $300 dormitory accommodations.
Financial Aid: 1 yr as full-time staff for work study.
Career Services: Internships; Sivananda Yoga Teacher Listing in Yoga Life magazine; Volunteer positions in yoga centers and ashrams.

NORTH CAROLINA

Apex

602. Doula Training
1007 W Lady Diana Ct, Apex, NC 27502
Phone: (919) 362-5517; *Fax:* (919) 387-6273
E-mail: atumblin@aol.com
Program Administrator: Ann Tumblin, FACCE, Dir. *Admissions Contact:* Ann Tumblin.
Year Established: 1996.
Staff: Full-time: 1.
Avg Enrollment: 120. *Avg Class Size:* 5-40. *Number of Graduates per Year:* 120.
Accreditation/Approval/Licensing: Doulas of North America.
Field of Study: Doula*. *Program Name/Length:* Doula Training, 2-3 days; Seminars given in various locations.
Degrees Offered: Certificate.
License/Certification Preparation: Fulfills one step toward certification with Doulas of North America or International Childbirth Education Association.
Admission Requirements: Audit childbirth education course unless experienced as labor and delivery nurse, midwife, or certified childbirth educator; required reading list available from instructor or Doulas of North America.
Tuition and Fees: $175-$300.
Career Services: Referral service through DONA.

Asheville

603. The Asheville School of Massage, Inc
Massage Therapy Certification
729 Haywood Rd, Asheville, NC 28806
Phone: (828) 236-9977; *Fax:* (828) 254-5613
E-mail: massage@earthaven.org *Internet:* http://
www.earthaven.org/massage
Program Administrator: Stephanie Keach, Dir. *Admissions Contact:* Tracy McMahon, Asst Dir.
Year Established: 1998.
Staff: Full-time: 4; Part-time: 10.
Avg Class Size: 16.
Wheelchair Access: No.
Field of Study: Acupressure*; Aromatherapy*;
CranioSacral Therapy*; Deep Tissue Massage*;
Energy Work*; Manual Lymph Drainage*; Massage Therapy*; Polarity Therapy*;
Reflexology*; Shiatsu*; Yoga Teacher
Training*. *Program Name/Length:* Massage
Therapy Certification, 6 mos, 10 mos or 12 mos;
Weekend workshops, 12 hrs.
Degrees Offered: CEUs; Certificate.
License/Certification Preparation: State: NC Licensed Massage Therapist; National Certification Board for Therapeutic Massage and Bodywork.
Admission Requirements: Min age: 18; High
school diploma/GED.
Application Deadline(s): Fall: Aug 30; Winter: Jan
1; Spring: Mar 10; Summer: Jul 1.
Tuition and Fees: $4750 + $250 books.
Financial Aid: Loans; Scholarships; Work study.
Career Services: Career information.

604. Lighten Up Yoga Center
60 Biltmore Ave, Asheville, NC 28801
Phone: (828) 254-7756; *Fax:* (828) 254-3797
E-mail: lightupyog@aol.com
Program Administrator: Lillah Schwartz, Pres. *Admissions Contact:* Alice Dawson, Office Mgr.
Year Established: 1996.
Staff: Full-time: 1; Part-time: 3.
Avg Enrollment: 24. *Avg Class Size:* 24. *Number
of Graduates per Year:* 16.
Wheelchair Access: No.
Field of Study: Yoga Teacher Training*. *Program
Name/Length:* 1 yr intensive (meets 6 times per
yr with home study).
Degrees Offered: Certificate.
Admission Requirements: Min age: 20; High
school diploma/GED.
Application Deadline(s): Fall: Aug-Nov.

605. North Carolina School of Natural Healing
20 Battery Park Ave, Rm 570, Asheville, NC 28801
Phone: (704) 252-7096
Program Administrator: Craig Ellis, Dir. *Admissions Contact:* Craig Ellis.
Year Established: 1991.

Staff: Full-time: 2; Part-time: 6.
Avg Enrollment: 60. *Avg Class Size:* 16. *Number
of Graduates per Year:* 16.
Wheelchair Access: Yes.
Field of Study: Acupressure; Aromatherapy;
CranioSacral Therapy; Energy Work*; Herbal
Medicine*; Massage Therapy*; Meditation*;
Polarity Therapy; Reiki; Shiatsu. *Program
Name/Length:* Massage Therapy, 9 1/2 mos;
Herbal Studies, 9 mos; Meditation Instructor and
Energy Healing, 9 1/2 mos.
Degrees Offered: Certificate.
License/Certification Preparation: State: NC Licensed Massage Therapist; National Certification Board for Therapeutic Massage and Bodywork.
Admission Requirements: Min age: 18; High
school diploma/GED.
Application Deadline(s): Fall: Aug 1.
Tuition and Fees: $4450-$4950 (Massage Therapy).
Financial Aid: Payment plan.
Career Services: Career counseling; Career information.

606. The Wellness Training Center
Hypnosis Training and Certification for the Health
Care Professional
231 Erwin Hills Rd, Asheville, NC 28806
Mailing Address: PO Box 599, Leicester, NC
28748
Phone: (828) 683-3369
Program Administrator: Robert Luka, RN, Dir.
Admissions Contact: Robert Luka.
Year Established: 1996.
Staff: Full-time: 1.
Avg Enrollment: 40. *Avg Class Size:* 18. *Number
of Graduates per Year:* 40.
Wheelchair Access: No.
Accreditation/Approval/Licensing: Accrediting
Council for Continuing Education and Training;
International Medical and Dental Hypnotherapy
Association.
Field of Study: Hypnotherapy*. *Program
Name/Length:* Classroom, 60-80 hrs, weekends;
Home study, 40-60 hrs.
Degrees Offered: CEUs.
License/Certification Preparation: International
Medical and Dental Hypnotherapy Association.
Admission Requirements: Health care professional.
Application Deadline(s): Fall; Spring.
Tuition and Fees: $250-$295 per weekend.

Carrboro

607. Listening Hands Polarity
605 Jones Ferry Rd, EE2, Carrboro, NC 27510
Phone: (919) 942-1819
E-mail: jyotigt@mindspring.com
Program Administrator: Gabriella Tal, Dir.

Accreditation/Approval/Licensing: American Polarity Therapy Association.
Field of Study: Polarity Therapy*. *Program Name/Length:* Associate Polarity Practitioner, 7 weekends.
License/Certification Preparation: APP; American Polarity Therapy Association.
Application Deadline(s): Fall: Oct; Spring: Mar.

Charlotte

608. Southeastern School of Neuromuscular and Massage Therapy, Inc, Charlotte

Clinical Massage Therapy
4 Woodlawn Green, Ste 200, Charlotte, NC 28217
Phone: (704) 527-4979; *Fax:* (704) 527-3104
E-mail: massage@clt.mindspring.com *Internet:* http://www.se-massage.com
Program Administrator: Kimberly Williams, Dir.
 Admissions Contact: Kimberly Williams.
Year Established: 1994.
Staff: Part-time: 10.
Avg Enrollment: 110. *Avg Class Size:* 24. *Number of Graduates per Year:* 100.
Wheelchair Access: Yes.
Field of Study: Massage Therapy*; Neuromuscular Therapy*. *Program Name/Length:* Clinical Massage Therapy, 6 mos; Neuromuscular Therapy, 6 mos.
Degrees Offered: Certificate.
License/Certification Preparation: State: FL Licensed Massage Therapist; National Certification Board for Therapeutic Massage and Bodywork.
Admission Requirements: Min age: 18; High school diploma/GED.
Application Deadline(s): Fall: Aug 15; Winter: Nov 15; Spring: Feb 15; Summer: May 15.
Tuition and Fees: $5300.
Financial Aid: Loans; VA approved; Vocational rehabilitation; Division of Services for the Blind.
Career Services: Career counseling; Career information.

609. Therapeutic Massage Training Institute

Professional Certification
726 East Blvd, Charlotte, NC 28203
Phone: (704) 338-9660; *Fax:* (704) 523-4389
E-mail: asktmti@aol.com *Internet:* http://www.massagetraining.com
Program Administrator: Lynda L. Clay, Dir. *Admissions Contact:* Cynthia Calvin, Admin Asst.
Year Established: 1987.
Staff: Full-time: 1; Part-time: 13.
Avg Enrollment: 50. *Avg Class Size:* 14. *Number of Graduates per Year:* 40.
Wheelchair Access: No.
Accreditation/Approval/Licensing: State board: NC State Board of Proprietary Schools.

Field of Study: Massage Therapy*. *Program Name/Length:* Therapeutic Massage Professional Certification, 16 mos.
Degrees Offered: Diploma; Certificate.
License/Certification Preparation: State: NC Licensed Massage Therapist; National Certification Board for Therapeutic Massage and Bodywork.
Admission Requirements: Min age: 18; High school diploma/GED.
Tuition and Fees: $5135.
Financial Aid: Work study; VA approved.
Career Services: Career information; Job information.

Columbus

610. The G-Jo Institute

Master of G-Jo Acupressure/Instructor of G-Jo Acupressure Home-Study Certification Program
PO Box 1460, Columbus, NC 28722
Phone: (828) 863-4660
E-mail: office@g-jo.com *Internet:* http://www.g-jo.com
Program Administrator: Michael Blate, Exec Dir.
 Admissions Contact: Barbara Gail Watson, Admin Dir.
Year Established: 1976.
Avg Enrollment: 750.
Field of Study: Acupressure; Reflexology. *Program Name/Length:* Master of G-Jo Acupressure Certification, home study; Instructor of G-Jo Acupressure, home study.
Degrees Offered: Certificate.
Admission Requirements: Specific course prerequisites: Master Certification required for Instructor of G-Jo Acupressure.

Greensboro

611. Natural Touch School of Massage Therapy, Greensboro

4007 W Wendover, Greensboro, NC 24007
Phone: (877) 799-0060
Program Administrator: Wanda Adkins, LMT, Dir.
 Admissions Contact: Wanda Adkins.
Year Established: 1998.
Wheelchair Access: Yes.
Accreditation/Approval/Licensing: State board: VA Dept of Ed, Div of Proprietary Schools.
Field of Study: Acupressure; CranioSacral Therapy; Energy Work*; Massage Therapy*; Myofascial Release; Polarity Therapy; Shiatsu.
 Program Name/Length: Massage Therapy, 600 hrs, 7 mos/days or 15 mos/nights (includes 100 hr internship).
Degrees Offered: Diploma; Certificate.
License/Certification Preparation: State: VA Certified Massage Therapist; National Certification Board for Therapeutic Massage and Bodywork.

Admission Requirements: Min age: 18; High
school diploma/GED.
Application Deadline(s): Fall: Sep 21; Spring: Mar
21.
Tuition and Fees: $4500.
Financial Aid: Work study; Payment plan.
Career Services: Career counseling; Career infor-
mation; Internships.

Greenville

612. East Carolina University, School of Nursing
Nurse-Midwifery Program
Greenville, NC 27858
Phone: (919) 328-4298
E-mail: numoss@ecuvm.cis.ecu.edu
Program Administrator: Nancy Moss, CNM, PhD,
Dir.
Accreditation/Approval/Licensing: American Col-
lege of Nurse-Midwives, Division of Accredita-
tion.
Field of Study: Midwifery*.
Degrees Offered: MSN.
License/Certification Preparation: Certified
Nurse-Midwife, American College of
Nurse-Midwives.
Admission Requirements: Bachelor's degree; RN.

Marshall

613. Academy of Natural Therapies
5 Piney View Estates, Marshall, NC 28753
Mailing Address: PO Box 9223, Asheville, NC
28815
Phone: (828) 683-1737; *Fax:* (828) 683-0265
E-mail: angelap@earthlink.net
Program Administrator: Rev. Angela Plum, PhD,
RPP, Dir. *Admissions Contact:* Rev. Angela
Plum.
Year Established: 1994.
Staff: Full-time: 2.
Avg Enrollment: 10. *Avg Class Size:* 10. *Number
of Graduates per Year:* 10.
Wheelchair Access: No.
Accreditation/Approval/Licensing: American Po-
larity Therapy Association.
Field of Study: Acupressure; Aromatherapy;
CranioSacral Therapy; Polarity Therapy*. *Pro-
gram Name/Length:* Associate Polarity Practi-
tioner, 155 hrs.
License/Certification Preparation: APP; American
Polarity Therapy Association.
Admission Requirements: Min age: 20.
Application Deadline(s): Spring: Mar 15.
Tuition and Fees: $1550.

Raleigh

614. Medical Arts Massage School
Professional Massage Therapy Program
2321 Blue Ridge Rd, Raleigh, NC 27607
Phone: (919) 783-9290; *Fax:* (919) 785-9081
Program Administrator: Tien Sydnor-Campbell,
Prog Dir. *Admissions Contact:* Margaret
Bowden, Dean of Admissions.
Year Established: 1996.
Staff: Part-time: 14.
Avg Enrollment: 50. *Avg Class Size:* 12. *Number
of Graduates per Year:* 48.
Wheelchair Access: No.
Accreditation/Approval/Licensing: State board: NC
Community Colleges; Pending, Accrediting
Council for Continuing Education and Training.
Field of Study: Deep Tissue Massage; Massage
Therapy*; Sports Massage. *Program
Name/Length:* 600 hrs.
Degrees Offered: Certificate.
License/Certification Preparation: State: NC Li-
censed Massage Therapist; National Certifica-
tion Board for Therapeutic Massage and Body-
work.
Admission Requirements: Min age: 18; High
school diploma/GED.
Application Deadline(s): Fall: Aug; Winter: Dec;
Spring: Feb.
Tuition and Fees: $5500 + $395 books, $400-$600
massage table.
Financial Aid: Work study; VA approved; Voca-
tional rehabilitation.
Career Services: Resume service; Job information.

Rutherfordton

615. The Whole You School of Massage and Bodywork
525-Hour Certification
143 Woodview Dr, Rutherfordton, NC 28139
Phone: (828) 287-0955; *Fax:* (828) 287-0067
E-mail: institute@blueridge.net *Internet:* http://
www.blueridge.net/~wholeyou/
Program Administrator: Cheryl Shew, Dir of Ed.
Admissions Contact: Kenneth Shew.
Year Established: 1990.
Staff: Full-time: 3; Part-time: 4.
Avg Enrollment: 50. *Avg Class Size:* 25. *Number
of Graduates per Year:* 25.
Wheelchair Access: Yes.
Accreditation/Approval/Licensing: State board: NC
Community College Proprietary School; Ac-
crediting Commission of Career Schools and
Colleges of Technology.
Field of Study: Acupressure*; Aromatherapy*;
CranioSacral Therapy*; Deep Tissue Massage*;
Massage Therapy*; Neuromuscular Therapy*;
Reflexology*; Reiki*. *Program Name/Length:*
Massage and Bodywork, 525 hrs.

Degrees Offered: Certificate.
License/Certification Preparation: State: NC Licensed Massage Therapist; National Certification Board for Therapeutic Massage and Bodywork.
Admission Requirements: Min age: 18; High school diploma/GED.
Application Deadline(s): Fall; Spring.
Tuition and Fees: $3900.
Financial Aid: Payment plan.
Career Services: Career counseling; Career information.

Salisbury

616. New Life Empowerment Center

129 S Long St, Salisbury, NC 28144
Phone: (704) 633-2700; *Fax:* (704) 633-2046
E-mail: hypnosis@salisbury.net
Program Administrator: Thomas Hartman, Dir.
   Admissions Contact: Thomas Hartman.
Year Established: 1998.
Staff: Full-time: 1; Part-time: 1.
Avg Class Size: 8.
Wheelchair Access: Yes.
Accreditation/Approval/Licensing: American Board of Hypnotherapy; International Medical and Dental Hypnotherapy Association.
Field of Study: Acupressure*; Aromatherapy*; Energy Work*; Hypnotherapy*; Qigong*; Reflexology*; Reiki*. *Program Name/Length:* Seminars given in various locations.
Degrees Offered: Certificate.
License/Certification Preparation: International Medical and Dental Hypnotherapy Association.
Admission Requirements: Min age: 18; High school diploma/GED.

Saxapahaw

617. Tree of Life Polarity Center

PO Box 281, Saxapahaw, NC 27340
Phone: (336) 376-8186
E-mail: jmdchi@mindspring.com
Program Administrator: Janice Durand, Dir. *Admissions Contact:* Janice Durand.
Year Established: 1997.
Staff: Full-time: 1; Part-time: 2.
Avg Enrollment: 20. *Avg Class Size:* 8. *Number of Graduates per Year:* 18.

Accreditation/Approval/Licensing: American Polarity Therapy Association.
Field of Study: Energy Work; Polarity Therapy*.
   Program Name/Length: Associate Polarity Practitioner, 215 hrs; Registered Polarity Practitioner, 215 hrs; Seminars given in various locations.
Degrees Offered: Certificate.
License/Certification Preparation: American Polarity Therapy Association.
Tuition and Fees: $2150 per course.
Financial Aid: Work study; Payment plan.
Career Services: Career counseling; Career information; Internships; Job information.

Siler City

618. The Body Therapy Institute

300 S Wind Rd, Siler City, NC 27344
Phone: (919) 663-3111, (888) 500-4500; *Fax:* (919) 663-0369
Program Administrator: Rick Rosen, Co-Dir; Carey Smith, Co-Dir. *Admissions Contact:* Ivonne Eiseman, Admin.
Year Established: 1983.
Staff: Full-time: 8; Part-time: 6.
Avg Enrollment: 64. *Avg Class Size:* 32. *Number of Graduates per Year:* 64.
Wheelchair Access: Yes.
Accreditation/Approval/Licensing: State board: NC Community College System, Proprietary School License; Accrediting Council for Continuing Education and Training.
Field of Study: Massage Therapy*. *Program Name/Length:* Certification, 8 mos/days or 11 mos/evenings and weekends.
Degrees Offered: Diploma.
License/Certification Preparation: State: NC Licensed Massage Therapist; National Certification Board for Therapeutic Massage and Bodywork.
Admission Requirements: Min age: 21; High school diploma/GED; Specific course prerequisites: introductory course in massage therapy.
Tuition and Fees: $7500.
Financial Aid: Work study.
Career Services: Career information; Job information.

NORTH DAKOTA

Fargo

619. Sister Rosalind Gefre School of Professional Massage, Fargo
McMerty Ctr, 619 7th St N, Ste L, Fargo, ND 58102
Phone: (701) 297-5993
Staff: Part-time: 80 over 4 campuses.
Accreditation/Approval/Licensing: International Massage and Somatic Therapies Accreditation Council; National Certification Board for Therapeutic Massage and Bodywork (CEUs).
Field of Study: Deep Tissue Massage; Massage Therapy*; Reflexology. *Program Name/Length:* Intro class; Professional Massage Therapy, 650 hrs.
Degrees Offered: CEUs; Certificate.
License/Certification Preparation: National Certification Board for Therapeutic Massage and Bodywork.
Admission Requirements: Min age: 18; High school diploma/GED.
Application Deadline(s): Fall: Aug; Winter: Feb.
Tuition and Fees: $495 (Intro); $5554 (Professional).
Financial Aid: VA approved; Vocational rehabilitation; Payment plan.
Career Services: Career information.

620. Professional Institute of Massage Therapy, Fargo
4553 9th Ave SW, Ste 2, Fargo, ND 58103
Phone: (701) 281-5078
E-mail: pimt@fargocity.com
Program Administrator: Michael Stafford, Admin. *Admissions Contact:* Michael Stafford.
Year Established: 1998.
Staff: Full-time: 1; Part-time: 1.
Avg Enrollment: 16. *Avg Class Size:* 16.
Wheelchair Access: Yes.
Accreditation/Approval/Licensing: State board: ND Board of Massage.
Field of Study: Massage Therapy*. *Program Name/Length:* Massage Therapy, 1100 hrs, 1 yr; Advanced Massage Therapy, 2200 hrs, 2 yrs.
Degrees Offered: Diploma.
License/Certification Preparation: State: ND Licensed Massage Therapist; National Certification Board for Therapeutic Massage and Bodywork.
Admission Requirements: Min age: 18; High school diploma/GED; Specific course prerequisites: biology.
Application Deadline(s): Fall: May.
Tuition and Fees: $5750 per yr + $50 registration.
Financial Aid: Loans.
Career Services: Career counseling; Career information.

OHIO

Akron

621. National Institute of Massotherapy, Akron
2110 Copley Rd, Akron, OH 44320
Phone: (330) 867-1996; *Fax:* (330) 869-6422
Program Administrator: Stephen Perkinson, Dir/Curriculum Coord. *Admissions Contact:* Ewa Perkinson, Admissions Dir.
Year Established: 1991.
Staff: Full-time: 5; Part-time: 15.
Avg Enrollment: 100. *Avg Class Size:* 12. *Number of Graduates per Year:* 100.
Wheelchair Access: Yes.
Accreditation/Approval/Licensing: State board: OH Medical Board.
Field of Study: Acupressure; CranioSacral Therapy; Massage Therapy*; Neuromuscular Therapy; Polarity Therapy; Reflexology; Reiki; Shiatsu. *Program Name/Length:* Massotherapy, 1 yr/full-time or 2 yrs/part-time.
Degrees Offered: Diploma; Certificate.
License/Certification Preparation: State: OH Licensed Massage Therapist.
Admission Requirements: Min age: 18; High school diploma/GED.
Application Deadline(s): Fall: Sep; Spring: Mar.
Tuition and Fees: $7450.
Financial Aid: Loans; Work study; VA approved; Vocational rehabilitation.
Career Services: Career information.

622. Ohio College of Massotherapy
Associate of Applied Science in Massotherapy
225 Heritage Woods Dr, Akron, OH 44321
Phone: (330) 665-1084; *Fax:* (330) 665-5021
E-mail: jeff@ocm.edu *Internet:* http://www.ocm.
edu
Program Administrator: Ann K. Morrow, Pres. *Admissions Contact:* Sue Whitlam, Admissions
Mgr.
Year Established: 1973.
Staff: Full-time: 5; Part-time: 5.
Avg Enrollment: 300. *Avg Class Size:* 20. *Number of Graduates per Year:* 140.
Wheelchair Access: Yes.
Accreditation/Approval/Licensing: State board: OH Medical Board; Accrediting Commission of Career Schools and Colleges of Technology.
Field of Study: Acupressure; Aromatherapy; CranioSacral Therapy; Massage Therapy*; Myofascial Release*; Neuromuscular Therapy*; Reflexology; Sports Massage*. *Program Name/Length:* Massotherapy, 18 mos or 2 yrs.
Degrees Offered: CEUs; Diploma; Associate of Applied Science.
License/Certification Preparation: State: OH Licensed Massage Therapist; National Certification Board for Therapeutic Massage and Bodywork; Myofascial Release, Neuromuscular Therapy, and Sports Massage Certification.
Admission Requirements: Min age: 18; High school diploma/GED.
Application Deadline(s): Fall: Sep 1; Spring: Mar 1.
Tuition and Fees: $6875 (18 mos); $9108 (2 yrs).
Financial Aid: Federal government aid; Grants; Loans; Scholarships; State government aid; VA approved; Vocational rehabilitation.
Career Services: Career information; Interview set up; Job placement.

Beavercreek

623. Ohio Academy of Holistic Health, Inc
3033 Dayton-Xenia Rd, Beavercreek, OH 45434
Phone: (937) 427-0506, (800) 833-8122; *Fax:* (937) 426-8883
Program Administrator: Jedidiah Smith, Dir. *Admissions Contact:* Kim Gorka, Admissions Clerk.
Year Established: 1987.
Staff: Full-time: 3; Part-time: 8.
Avg Enrollment: 200. *Avg Class Size:* 24. *Number of Graduates per Year:* 176.
Wheelchair Access: Yes.
Accreditation/Approval/Licensing: State board: OH Board of Proprietary School Registration.
Field of Study: Aromatherapy; Energy Work; Herbal Medicine; Hypnotherapy*; Iridology; NeuroLinguistic Programming; Reflexology*; Reiki; Touch For Health. *Program Name/Length:* Clinical Hypnotherapy, 2 yrs; Reflexology, 2 yrs.
Degrees Offered: Certificate.
License/Certification Preparation: American Board of Hypnotherapy.
Admission Requirements: Min age: 18; High school diploma/GED; Professional and personal recommendations; Interview.
Financial Aid: Loans; Scholarships; Vocational rehabilitation.
Career Services: Career counseling; Career information.

Berlin Heights

624. Retha J. Martin School of Hypnotherapy
5018 Mason Rd, Berlin Heights, OH 44814
Phone: (419) 433-5440/2912
Program Administrator: Retha J. Martin, Owner/Founder. *Admissions Contact:* Retha J. Martin.
Year Established: 1989.
Staff: Full-time: 1.
Avg Class Size: 10.
Wheelchair Access: No.
Accreditation/Approval/Licensing: International Medical and Dental Hypnotherapy Association.
Field of Study: Energy Work; Hypnotherapy*; Reiki. *Program Name/Length:* Basic, 15 wks (1 night/wk); Advanced, 15 wks (1 night/wk); Clinical, 15 wks (1 night/wk).
Degrees Offered: Certificate.
License/Certification Preparation: American Board of Hypnotherapy; International Medical and Dental Hypnotherapy Association.
Admission Requirements: High school diploma/GED; Specific course prerequisites: Basic required for Advanced, Advanced required for Clinical.
Tuition and Fees: $495.

Cincinnati

625. Alexander Technique of Cincinnati
Certification as Teachers of the Alexander Technique
954 W Northbend Rd, Cincinnati, OH 45224
Phone: (513) 542-1010
Program Administrator: Vivien Schapera, Co-Dir; Neil Schapera, Co-Dir. *Admissions Contact:* Vivien Schapera; Neil Schapera.
Year Established: 1991.
Staff: Full-time: 2; Part-time: 1.
Avg Enrollment: 10. *Avg Class Size:* 10. *Number of Graduates per Year:* 3.
Wheelchair Access: No.
Accreditation/Approval/Licensing: American Society for the Alexander Technique.

Field of Study: Alexander Technique*. *Program Name/Length:* Teacher Training, 3 yrs.
Degrees Offered: Certificate.
License/Certification Preparation: American Society for the Alexander Technique.
Admission Requirements: Min age: 26; Some college (2 yrs).
Application Deadline(s): Fall: Aug 10; Winter: Dec 10.
Tuition and Fees: $6600 per yr.
Career Services: Career counseling; Career information.

626. International Academy for Reflexology Studies

4759 Cornell Rd, Ste D, Cincinnati, OH 45241
Phone: (513) 489-9328; *Fax:* (513) 489-9354
Program Administrator: Marcia L. Aschendorf, Naturopathic Medical Doctor, Dir of Studies. *Admissions Contact:* Jay E. Aschendorf, Naturopathic Medical Doctor, Registrar.
Year Established: 1992.
Staff: Full-time: 3; Part-time: 7.
Avg Enrollment: 10. *Avg Class Size:* 8. *Number of Graduates per Year:* 8.
Wheelchair Access: Yes.
Accreditation/Approval/Licensing: State board: OH Board of Proprietary School Registration; International Massage and Somatic Therapies Accreditation Council.
Field of Study: Reflexology*. *Program Name/Length:* Reflexology Practitioner, 780 hrs, 13 mos.
Degrees Offered: Diploma.
License/Certification Preparation: American Reflexology Certification Board.
Admission Requirements: Min age: 18; High school diploma/GED; Min GPA: 2.5.
Application Deadline(s): Fall.
Tuition and Fees: $5000-$5600 per yr.
Financial Aid: Loans; State government aid.
Career Services: Career counseling; Interview set up.

627. University of Cincinnati, College of Nursing and Health

Nurse-Midwifery Education Program
PO Box 210038, Cincinnati, OH 45221-0038
Phone: (513) 558-5282/5380 (applicant info)
E-mail: mary.akers@uc.edu *Internet:* http://www.cu.edu/www/nursing
Program Administrator: Mary Carol Akers, CNM, Dir.
Field of Study: Midwifery*.
Degrees Offered: MSN.

Circleville

628. Integrated Touch Therapy, Inc, for Animals

7041 Zane Trail Rd, Circleville, OH 43113

Phone: (740) 474-6436; *Fax:* (740) 474-2625
E-mail: wshaw1@bright.net
Program Administrator: Patricia Whalen-Shaw, MA, LMT, NCTMB, Dir. *Admissions Contact:* Patricia Whalen-Shaw.
Year Established: 1998.
Staff: Full-time: 1; Part-time: 2.
Avg Enrollment: 110. *Avg Class Size:* 5. *Number of Graduates per Year:* 110.
Wheelchair Access: Yes.
Accreditation/Approval/Licensing: National Certification Board for Therapeutic Massage and Bodywork (CEUs).
Field of Study: Acupressure; Animal Therapy*; CranioSacral Therapy; Energy Work; Equine Massage*; Herbal Medicine; Massage Therapy*; Polarity Therapy. *Program Name/Length:* Equine Massage, 2 levels, 48 hrs and 40 hrs; Canine Massage, 2 levels, 24 hrs each; Feline Massage, 24 hrs.
Degrees Offered: Certificate.
Admission Requirements: High school diploma/GED; Animal care or massage therapy experience helpful.
Tuition and Fees: $299-$899.
Comments: Formerly Optissage, Inc.

Cleveland

629. Bhumi's Yoga and Wellness Center

King James Plaza, 25068 Center Ridge Rd, Cleveland, OH 44145
Phone: (440) 899-9569; *Fax:* (440) 899-9569
E-mail: healingbreath@mediaone.net *Internet:* http://www.junior.apk.net/~BHUMI
Program Administrator: Harriet L. Russell, Dir, CEO. *Admissions Contact:* Harriet L. Russell.
Year Established: 1995.
Staff: Full-time: 1; Part-time: 6.
Avg Enrollment: 10. *Avg Class Size:* 10. *Number of Graduates per Year:* 10.
Wheelchair Access: No.
Field of Study: Acupressure; Energy Work; Meditation; Polarity Therapy; Reiki; Shiatsu; Yoga Teacher Training*. *Program Name/Length:* Level 1, 7 mos; Home study course available.
Degrees Offered: Certificate.
Admission Requirements: Min age: 18; Specific course prerequisites: 1 yr yoga at approved school.
Tuition and Fees: $1600.
Career Services: Career information; Interview set up; Job information; Referral service.

630. Case Western Reserve University, Frances Payne Bolton School of Nursing

Nurse-Midwifery Program
10900 Euclid Ave, Cleveland, OH 44106-4904
Phone: (216) 368-2532
Program Administrator: Marcia Riegger, CNM, Dir.

Accreditation/Approval/Licensing: American College of Nurse-Midwives, Division of Accreditation.
Field of Study: Midwifery*.
Degrees Offered: MSN.
License/Certification Preparation: Certified Nurse-Midwife, American College of Nurse-Midwives.
Admission Requirements: Bachelor's degree; RN.

Columbus

631. Central Ohio School of Massage
1120 Morse Rd, Ste 250, Columbus, OH 43229
Phone: (614) 841-1122; *Fax:* (614) 841-0387
E-mail: admissions@cosm.org *Internet:* http://www.cosm.org
Program Administrator: Peg Thompson, Dir.
Field of Study: Massage Therapy*. *Program Name/Length:* 18 mos (1 day or 2 evenings per wk).
Tuition and Fees: $6300.

632. Columbus Polarity Therapy Institute
An Educational Center for Natural Healing Therapies and Energy Medicine
170 W 5th Ave, Columbus, OH 43201
Phone: (614) 299-9438; *Fax:* (614) 291-7252
E-mail: maryjo@columbuspolarity.com *Internet:* http://www.columbuspolarity.com
Program Administrator: Mary Jo Ruggieri, PhD, Dir. *Admissions Contact:* Mary Jo Ruggieri.
Year Established: 1992.
Staff: Full-time: 6; Part-time: 5.
Avg Enrollment: 600. *Avg Class Size:* 28. *Number of Graduates per Year:* 450.
Wheelchair Access: Yes.
Accreditation/Approval/Licensing: State board: OH Dept of Ed; American Polarity Therapy Association.
Field of Study: Acupressure; Aromatherapy; Ayurvedic Medicine; CranioSacral Therapy; Energy Work*; Naturopathic Medicine; Polarity Therapy*; Reflexology. *Program Name/Length:* Associate Polarity Practitioner, 8 mos; Registered Polarity Practitioner, 18 mos; Seminars given in various locations; Home study/Correspondence.
Degrees Offered: CEUs; Certificate.
License/Certification Preparation: American Polarity Therapy Association; APP, RPP.
Admission Requirements: Min age: 18; High school diploma/GED.
Application Deadline(s): Fall: Oct 30; Winter: Jan 30; Spring: Jun 30; Summer: Sep 30.
Tuition and Fees: $1500 (APP); $5000 (RPP).
Financial Aid: Scholarships; Work study; Payment plan.
Career Services: Internships.

633. Massage Away, Inc, School of Therapy
Massage Technician; Licensed Massage Therapist
6685 Doubletree Ave, Columbus, OH 43229
Phone: (614) 825-6278; *Fax:* (614) 825-6279
E-mail: massageawayinc@netscape.com *Internet:* http://www.massageaway.com
Program Administrator: Linda Fleming-Willis, Dir. *Admissions Contact:* Gail Quinn, Education Coord.
Year Established: 1994.
Staff: Part-time: 15.
Avg Enrollment: 78. *Avg Class Size:* 25. *Number of Graduates per Year:* 40.
Wheelchair Access: Yes.
Accreditation/Approval/Licensing: State board: OH Board of Proprietary School Registration; OH Medical Board.
Field of Study: Massage Therapy*. *Program Name/Length:* Relaxation Massage Technician, 160 hrs, 6 mos; Licensed Massage Therapist, 710 hrs, 12 mos or 19 mos.
Degrees Offered: Diploma; Certificate.
License/Certification Preparation: State: OH Licensed Massage Therapist.
Admission Requirements: Min age: 18; High school diploma/GED; Min GPA: 2.5; Health certificate.
Application Deadline(s): Fall: Jul; Winter: Dec; Spring: Jan; Summer: May.
Tuition and Fees: $2000 (Massage Technician); $6000 (Massage Therapist).
Financial Aid: Payment plan.
Career Services: Job information.

634. Ohio State University, College of Nursing
Nurse-Midwifery Graduate Program
1585 Neil Ave, Columbus, OH 43210-1289
Phone: (614) 292-4041
E-mail: nursing@osu.edu *Internet:* http://www.con.ohio.state.edu/
Program Administrator: Nancy K. Lowe, PhD, Dir.
Accreditation/Approval/Licensing: Pre-accreditation status, American College of Nurse-Midwives.
Field of Study: Midwifery*.
Degrees Offered: MS.

635. Reflexology Science Institute
Reflexology Certification; Polarity Therapy
1170 Old Henderson Rd, Ste 206, Columbus, OH 43220
Phone: (614) 457-5783; *Fax:* (614) 442-0133
E-mail: beritnils@aol.com *Internet:* http://www.reflexologyscience.com
Program Administrator: Berit Nilsson, Dir of Ed. *Admissions Contact:* Eileen Motok, Student Service Dir.
Year Established: 1983.
Staff: Full-time: 1; Part-time: 3.

Avg Enrollment: 50. *Avg Class Size:* 10. *Number of Graduates per Year:* 50.
Wheelchair Access: Yes.
Accreditation/Approval/Licensing: American Polarity Therapy Association.
Field of Study: Acupressure; CranioSacral Therapy; Energy Work*; Polarity Therapy*; Reflexology*; Reiki*. *Program Name/Length:* Reflexology Certification, 200 hrs; Polarity Therapy, 155 hrs; Energy Release Somatic Therapy, 32 hrs; Seminars given in various locations.
Degrees Offered: Certificate.
License/Certification Preparation: American Reflexology Certification Board; American Polarity Therapy Association.
Admission Requirements: Min age: 18; High school diploma/GED.
Application Deadline(s): Fall; Winter; Spring.
Financial Aid: State government aid.

Garfield Heights

636. National Institute of Massotherapy, Garfield Heights

12684 Rockside Rd, Garfield Heights, OH 44125
Phone: (216) 662-6955; *Fax:* (216) 662-6980
Program Administrator: Stephen Perkinson, Dir. *Admissions Contact:* Ewa Perkinson, Dean.
Year Established: 1991.
Staff: Full-time: 10; Part-time: 7.
Avg Enrollment: 250. *Avg Class Size:* 10. *Number of Graduates per Year:* 250.
Wheelchair Access: Yes.
Accreditation/Approval/Licensing: State board: OH Medical Board.
Field of Study: Massage Therapy*; Neuromuscular Therapy*; Ortho-Bionomy; Polarity Therapy; Shiatsu. *Program Name/Length:* Massotherapy, 740 hrs, 1 yr/full-time or 2 yrs/part-time; Seminars given in various locations.
Degrees Offered: Certificate.
License/Certification Preparation: State: OH Licensed Massage Therapist.
Admission Requirements: Min age: 18; High school diploma/GED.
Application Deadline(s): Fall; Spring.
Financial Aid: VA approved; Vocational rehabilitation.

Highland Hills

637. Cuyahoga Community College

Massotherapy Program
4250 Richmond Rd, Highland Hills, OH 44122-6195
Phone: (216) 987-2426; *Fax:* (216) 987-2450
E-mail: sheila.batheja@tri-c.cc.oh.us
Program Administrator: Sheila Batheja, MS, Prog Mgr.
Year Established: 1998.

Staff: Full-time: 3; Part-time: 1.
Avg Enrollment: 50. *Avg Class Size:* 25.
Accreditation/Approval/Licensing: State board: OH Board of Regents; OH Medical Board; North East Bureau of Higher Ed.
Field of Study: Massage Therapy*. *Program Name/Length:* Associate Degree in Massotherapy, 5 semesters (including summer), 2 yrs.
Degrees Offered: Associate of Applied Science.
License/Certification Preparation: National Certification Board for Therapeutic Massage and Bodywork.
Admission Requirements: Min age: 18; High school diploma/GED; Min GPA: 2.5; Specific course prerequisites: English, biology, psychology.
Application Deadline(s): Fall; Spring.
Tuition and Fees: $4305 + lab fees.
Financial Aid: Federal government aid; Grants; Loans; Scholarships; State government aid; Work study; VA approved.
Career Services: Career counseling; Career information; Internships; Interview set up; Resume service.

Hilliard

638. Columbus Academy of Medical Massage

3600 Main St, Hilliard, OH 43026
Phone: (614) 777-1161; *Fax:* (614) 336-8478
Program Administrator: Jennifer Hastings-Schunn, Admin. *Admissions Contact:* Tonya Gioffre-Buoni, Dean of Students.
Year Established: 1993.
Staff: Part-time: 8.
Avg Enrollment: 12. *Avg Class Size:* 12. *Number of Graduates per Year:* 12.
Wheelchair Access: No.
Accreditation/Approval/Licensing: State board: OH Medical Board.
Field of Study: Aromatherapy; Massage Therapy*; Medical Massage*; Myofascial Release*; Trigger Point Therapy. *Program Name/Length:* Basic Massage Therapy, 650 hrs; Advanced Myofascial, 6 mos.
Degrees Offered: Diploma; Certificate.
License/Certification Preparation: State: OH Licensed Massage Therapist.
Admission Requirements: Min age: 18; High school diploma/GED; Specific course prerequisites: Basic Massage required for Advanced Myofascial.
Application Deadline(s): Fall: Aug 1; Spring: Mar 1.
Tuition and Fees: $6000 (Basic); $1500 (Advanced).
Career Services: Career counseling; Career information.

Lebanon

639. SHI, Integrative Medical Massage School

130 Cook Rd, Lebanon, OH 45036
Mailing Address: PO Box 474, Lebanon, OH 45036
Phone: (513) 932-8712; *Fax:* (513) 932-8180
Program Administrator: Sharon L. Barnes, PhD, Dir. *Admissions Contact:* Brenda Rae Long, Asst Dir of Student Svcs.
Year Established: 1980.
Staff: Full-time: 4; Part-time: 12.
Avg Enrollment: 200. *Avg Class Size:* 40. *Number of Graduates per Year:* 175.
Wheelchair Access: Yes.
Accreditation/Approval/Licensing: State board: OH Medical Board; National Certification Board for Therapeutic Massage and Bodywork (CEUs).
Field of Study: Alexander Technique; Biofeedback; CranioSacral Therapy; Energy Work; Feldenkrais; Massage Therapy*; Medical Massage*; Myofascial Release; Neuromuscular Therapy; Polarity Therapy; Somatic Education; Therapeutic Touch. *Program Name/Length:* Massage Therapy, 18 mos; Accelerated Massage Therapy, 12 mos.
Degrees Offered: CEUs; Diploma; Certificate; Bachelor's degree available through Cincinnati State.
License/Certification Preparation: State: OH Licensed Massage Therapist; National Certification Board for Therapeutic Massage and Bodywork.
Admission Requirements: Min age: 18; High school diploma/GED; Min GPA: 2.5; Science background required for Accelerated program; Understanding of medical massage; Letters of recommendation; College experience desirable.
Application Deadline(s): Fall: Sep 1; Winter: Feb 15.
Tuition and Fees: $6750 + $450 books.
Financial Aid: VA approved; Vocational rehabilitation; Payment plan.
Career Services: Career information; Instruction in business practices.
Comments: Will increase from 600 hrs to 1000 hrs (18-mo and 2-yr programs) in year 2000.

Maumee

640. Northwest Academy of Massotherapy

Massage Therapy
1910 Indian Wood Circle, Ste 301, Maumee, OH 43537
Phone: (419) 893-6464
Program Administrator: Patricia A. West, Pres. *Admissions Contact:* Patricia A. West.
Year Established: 1995.
Staff: Full-time: 3.
Avg Enrollment: 45. *Avg Class Size:* 20. *Number of Graduates per Year:* 45.

Wheelchair Access: Yes.
Accreditation/Approval/Licensing: State board: OH Medical Board.
Field of Study: Massage Therapy*; Reflexology; Sports Massage. *Program Name/Length:* Massage Therapy, 18 mos.
Degrees Offered: Diploma.
License/Certification Preparation: State: OH Licensed Massage Therapist.
Admission Requirements: Min age: 18; High school diploma/GED; Specific course prerequisites: medical terminology.
Tuition and Fees: $6000.
Financial Aid: VA approved.
Career Services: Job information.

Rutland

641. Healing Heart Herbals

36254 McCumber Rd, Rutland, OH 45775
Phone: (740) 742-8901
E-mail: cindyp@eurekanet.com
Program Administrator: Cindy Parker, Dir. *Admissions Contact:* Cindy Parker.
Year Established: 1986.
Staff: Part-time: 10.
Avg Enrollment: 12. *Number of Graduates per Year:* 8.
Wheelchair Access: No.
Field of Study: Aromatherapy*; Ayurvedic Medicine; Energy Work; Herbal Medicine*; Homeopathy; Oriental Medicine; Polarity Therapy; Reflexology; Traditional Chinese Medicine. *Program Name/Length:* Apprenticeship (includes Rosemary Gladstar's correspondence course), 6 mos; Beyond Herbology Advanced Workshops, weekends.
Degrees Offered: Certificate.
Tuition and Fees: $900 (Apprenticeship).
Financial Aid: Scholarships; Work study.
Comments: Classes run Mar-Oct.

Struthers

642. The Youngstown College of Massotherapy

14 Highland Ave, Struthers, OH 44471
Phone: (330) 755-1406; *Fax:* (330) 755-1605
E-mail: yocm@aol.com *Internet:* http://www.yocm.com
Program Administrator: Douglas M. Shodd Sr, Owner/Pres. *Admissions Contact:* Mary Shodd, VP/Dir of Student Relations.
Year Established: 1995.
Staff: Full-time: 2; Part-time: 2.
Avg Enrollment: 100. *Avg Class Size:* 12. *Number of Graduates per Year:* 95.
Wheelchair Access: Yes.
Accreditation/Approval/Licensing: State board: OH Medical Board.

Field of Study: Massage Therapy*. *Program Name/Length:* Massotherapy, 18 mos.
Degrees Offered: Diploma; Certificate.
License/Certification Preparation: State: OH Licensed Massage Therapist; National Certification Board for Therapeutic Massage and Bodywork.
Admission Requirements: Min age: 18; High school diploma/GED.
Application Deadline(s): Fall: Aug; Spring: Feb.
Tuition and Fees: $2100 per semester + books.
Financial Aid: VA approved; Vocational rehabilitation; Payment plan; GM; WCI Steel.
Career Services: Job postings at school and on Web page.

Twinsburg

643. Cleveland School of Massage/Advanced Bodywork Institute
Ethical Massage Practitioner Certification
10683 Ravenna Rd, Twinsburg, OH 44087
Phone: (330) 405-1933

Program Administrator: Jeff Kates, LMT, Dir. *Admissions Contact:* Jeff Kates.
Year Established: 1996.
Staff: Full-time: 2; Part-time: 1.
Avg Enrollment: 50. *Avg Class Size:* 8. *Number of Graduates per Year:* 50.
Accreditation/Approval/Licensing: State board: OH Board of Proprietary School Registration.
Field of Study: Aromatherapy; Deep Tissue Massage; Energy Work; Myofascial Release; Polarity Therapy*; Reflexology*; Swedish Massage*. *Program Name/Length:* 4-100 hrs, 4 mos (1 day per wk); Seminars.
Degrees Offered: Certificate; Ethical Massage Practitioner.
Admission Requirements: Min age: 18; High school diploma/GED.
Application Deadline(s): Fall: Sep 7; Winter: Jan 7; Spring: May 7.
Tuition and Fees: $2450 includes books, materials.
Financial Aid: Payment plan.
Career Services: Career counseling; Career information; Interview set up; Job placement.

OKLAHOMA

Oklahoma City

644. Praxis College of Health Arts and Sciences
808 NW 88, Oklahoma City, OK 73114
Phone: (405) 949-2244; *Fax:* (405) 946-7040
Program Administrator: Andre F. Fountain, BSN, Dir. *Admissions Contact:* Linda Young.
Year Established: 1987.
Staff: Full-time: 7; Part-time: 5.
Avg Enrollment: 100. *Avg Class Size:* 16. *Number of Graduates per Year:* 8.
Wheelchair Access: Yes.
Accreditation/Approval/Licensing: State board: OK Board of Private Vocational Schools.
Field of Study: Acupressure; Acupuncture*; Aromatherapy; CranioSacral Therapy; Energy Work; Herbal Medicine; Hydrotherapy; Massage Therapy*; Oriental Medicine; Polarity Therapy; Qigong; Reflexology; Shiatsu; Sports Massage; Traditional Chinese Medicine. *Program Name/Length:* Associate Massage Technician, 6 mos; Certified Massage Therapist, 2 yrs; Certified Acupuncturist, 3 yrs; Medical Hydrologist, 3 yrs.
Degrees Offered: CEUs; Certificate.
License/Certification Preparation: National Certification Commission for Acupuncture and Orien-

tal Medicine; National Certification Board for Therapeutic Massage and Bodywork.
Admission Requirements: Min age: 25; Some college.
Application Deadline(s): Fall: Aug 15; Spring: Feb 15.
Tuition and Fees: $500 (Associate Massage); $2800 (Certified Massage); $3000 (Hydrologist).
Financial Aid: Grants; Loans; Scholarships; Work study; Payment plan.
Career Services: Career counseling; Career information; Internships; Interview set up; Resume service; Job information; Referral service; Business financing.

Tulsa

645. Massage Therapy Institute of Oklahoma
9433 E 51st St, Ste H, Tulsa, OK 74145
Phone: (918) 622-6644; *Fax:* (918) 622-3401
E-mail: mtio@swbell.net
Program Administrator: Xerlan Geiser, NCTMB, Dir. *Admissions Contact:* Xerlan Geiser.
Year Established: 1992.
Staff: Part-time: 3.

Avg Enrollment: 32. *Avg Class Size:* 8. *Number of Graduates per Year:* 30.

Wheelchair Access: Yes.

Accreditation/Approval/Licensing: State board: OK Board of Private Vocational Schools; National Certification Board for Therapeutic Massage and Bodywork (CEUs).

Field of Study: Acupressure; Aromatherapy; CranioSacral Therapy; Massage Therapy*; Oriental Medicine; Reflexology; Shiatsu; Sports Massage. *Program Name/Length:* Clinical Massage Therapy, 2 semesters.

Degrees Offered: Certificate.

License/Certification Preparation: National Certification Board for Therapeutic Massage and Bodywork.

Admission Requirements: Min age: 18; High school diploma/GED.

Application Deadline(s): Fall: Aug 15; Winter: Jan 5; Summer: May 15.

Tuition and Fees: $2200 per semester.

Financial Aid: Scholarships; Work study.

Career Services: Career counseling; Career information; Interview set up.

646. The Oklahoma School of Natural Healing

1660 E 71st, Ste 2-O, Tulsa, OK 74136-5191
Phone: (918) 496-9401; *Fax:* (918) 496-4461
E-mail: healing01@sprynet.com
Program Administrator: Dr. Robert L. Groves, Dir.
  Admissions Contact: Dr. Robert L. Groves.

Year Established: 1980.

Staff: Full-time: 1; Part-time: 8.

Avg Enrollment: 30. *Avg Class Size:* 15. *Number of Graduates per Year:* 25.

Wheelchair Access: Yes.

Accreditation/Approval/Licensing: State board: OK Board of Private Vocational Schools.

Field of Study: Acupressure*; CranioSacral Therapy; Energy Work*; Herbal Medicine*; Homeopathy; Massage Therapy*; Naturopathic Medicine; Neuromuscular Therapy*; Ortho-Bionomy*; Polarity Therapy*; Qigong; Reflexology*; Reiki; Shiatsu; Sports Massage; Traditional Chinese Medicine. *Program Name/Length:* Technician, 250 hrs; Therapist, 650 hrs; Master Therapist, 1000 hrs; Instructor, 1500 hrs.

Degrees Offered: Diploma.

License/Certification Preparation: National Certification Board for Therapeutic Massage and Bodywork; American Polarity Therapy Association; Ortho-Bionomy Society.

Admission Requirements: Min age: 18; High school diploma/GED.

Application Deadline(s): Fall: Aug 15; Winter: Dec 15.

Tuition and Fees: $2223 (Technician); $4705 (Therapist) includes table, books, materials.

Financial Aid: Loans; State government aid; Vocational rehabilitation.

Career Services: Career counseling; Internships.

OREGON

Ashland

647. Ashland Massage Institute

PO Box 1233, Ashland, OR 97520
Phone: (541) 482-5134
E-mail: massage@jeffnet.org
Program Administrator: Beth Hoffman, LMT, Dir.
  Admissions Contact: Beth Hoffman.
Year Established: 1988.
Staff: Part-time: 12.
Avg Enrollment: 30. *Avg Class Size:* 22. *Number of Graduates per Year:* 18.
Wheelchair Access: Yes.
Accreditation/Approval/Licensing: State board: OR Dept of Ed; OR Board of Massage.
Field of Study: Massage Therapy*. *Program Name/Length:* 10 mos.
Degrees Offered: Certificate.
License/Certification Preparation: State: OR Licensed Massage Technician.

Admission Requirements: Min age: 18; Transcripts; Interview.

Tuition and Fees: $4850.

Financial Aid: Loans; VA approved; Payment plan.

Career Services: Informal networking.

Eugene

648. Cascade Institute of Massage and Body Therapies

1250 Charnelton St, Eugene, OR 97401
Phone: (541) 687-8101; *Fax:* (541) 687-0285
Program Administrator: Wendy Doran, Admin.
  Admissions Contact: Wendy Doran.
Year Established: 1988.
Staff: Part-time: 15.
Avg Enrollment: 45. *Avg Class Size:* 15. *Number of Graduates per Year:* 45.
Wheelchair Access: No.

Accreditation/Approval/Licensing: State board: OR Dept of Ed; OR and WA Boards of Massage.
Field of Study: Acupressure; Energy Work; Massage Therapy*; Shiatsu; Swedish Massage*.
Program Name/Length: Pre-licensing Massage, 1 yr.
Degrees Offered: Certificate.
License/Certification Preparation: State: OR Licensed Massage Technician, WA Licensed Massage Practitioner; National Certification Board for Therapeutic Massage and Bodywork.
Admission Requirements: Min age: 18; High school diploma/GED.
Tuition and Fees: $5125.
Financial Aid: VA approved; Vocational rehabilitation.

649. Friends Landing International Centers for Conscious Living, Eugene

Hypnotherapy Certification; Spherical Reality Certification
492 E 13th St, Ste 101, Eugene, OR 97401
Phone: (541) 484-6004; *Fax:* (541) 741-1705
E-mail: office@friendslanding.net *Internet:* http://www.friendslanding.net
Program Administrator: Whitewind Swan Fisher, Exec Dir. *Admissions Contact:* Whitewind Swan Fisher.
Year Established: 1996.
Staff: Full-time: 2; Part-time: 7.
Avg Enrollment: 90. *Avg Class Size:* 20. *Number of Graduates per Year:* 60.
Wheelchair Access: Yes.
Accreditation/Approval/Licensing: American Association of Professional Hypnotherapists.
Field of Study: Hypnotherapy*. *Program Name/Length:* Hypnotherapy Certification, 100 hrs, 5 mos or intensive format; Spherical Reality Certification, 10 mos (1 weekend per month and retreats); Seminars given in various locations; Friends Practitioner Certification, 4 levels, up to 8 yrs.
Degrees Offered: Certificate.
Application Deadline(s): Fall: Aug 15 for Hypnotherapy and Spherical Reality; Spring: Feb 15 for Hypnotherapy; Summer: May 15 for Hypnotherapy.
Tuition and Fees: $1635 (Hypnotherapy); $7500 (Spherical Reality).
Financial Aid: Scholarships.
Career Services: Business support.

650. Northwest Acupressure Institute

966 Lorane Hwy, Eugene, OR 97405
Phone: (503) 345-2220
Program Administrator: Kamala Quale, MSOM, Dir. *Admissions Contact:* Kamala Quale.
Year Established: 1985.
Staff: Part-time: 2.
Avg Enrollment: 12. *Avg Class Size:* 8. *Number of Graduates per Year:* 10.
Wheelchair Access: Yes.

Accreditation/Approval/Licensing: Jin Shin Do Foundation.
Field of Study: Acupressure*; Jin Shin Do*; Oriental Medicine; Qigong. *Program Name/Length:* Jin Shin Do and Body-Mind Studies, 2 yrs.
Degrees Offered: Certificate; Registered Jin Shin Do Practitioner.
License/Certification Preparation: American Oriental Bodywork Therapy Association.
Admission Requirements: Min age: 18; High school diploma/GED.
Tuition and Fees: $1000 per yr.
Financial Aid: Payment plan.
Career Services: Career counseling; Career information.

651. Northwest Center for Herbal Studies

2-Year Certification Program
86437 Lorane Hwy, Eugene, OR 97405
Phone: (541) 484-6708
E-mail: herbs@ordata.com *Internet:* http://www.ordata.com/~herbs.com
Program Administrator: Cherie Capps, Dir. *Admissions Contact:* Cherie Capps.
Year Established: 1992.
Staff: Full-time: 1.
Avg Enrollment: 40. *Avg Class Size:* 10. *Number of Graduates per Year:* 10.
Wheelchair Access: Yes.
Field of Study: Herbal Medicine*. *Program Name/Length:* Herbal Studies Units I and II and Clinical Studies Units I and II, 2 yrs, classroom or correspondence.
Degrees Offered: Certificate; Certified Herbalist Diploma.
Application Deadline(s): Fall: Aug 30 for Herbal Studies I; Winter: Nov 1 for Clinical Studies I; Spring: Mar 1 for Herbal Studies II.
Tuition and Fees: $960 includes tapes, manuals, exams.
Career Services: Interview set up.
Comments: Units may be taken in any combination..

652. Oregon School of Midwifery

342 E 12th Ave, Eugene, OR 97401
Phone: (541) 338-9778; *Fax:* (541) 338-9783
E-mail: daphnetree@aol.com *Internet:* http://www.efn.org/~osm
Program Administrator: Daphne Singingtree, LM, Exec Dir. *Admissions Contact:* Daphne Singingtree.
Year Established: 1995.
Staff: Part-time: 6.
Avg Enrollment: 13. *Avg Class Size:* 13.
Wheelchair Access: No.
Accreditation/Approval/Licensing: Midwifery Education Accreditation Council.
Field of Study: Midwifery*. *Program Name/Length:* Direct Entry Midwife, 3 yrs.
Degrees Offered: Certificate.

License/Certification Preparation: State: OR Licensed Direct Entry Midwife; Certified Professional Midwife, North American Registry of Midwives.
Admission Requirements: Min age: 18; High school diploma/GED.
Application Deadline(s): Fall: May 1.
Tuition and Fees: $9495 per yr.
Financial Aid: Loans; Scholarships; Work study.

653. Professional Course in Veterinary Homeopathy

1283 Lincoln St, Eugene, OR 97401
Phone: (541) 342-7665; *Fax:* (541) 344-5356
E-mail: anhc@pacinfo.com
Program Administrator: Richard Pitcairn, DVM, Dir. *Admissions Contact:* Susan Pitcairn, MS, Admin.
Year Established: 1992.
Staff: Full-time: 2.
Avg Enrollment: 45. *Avg Class Size:* 45. *Number of Graduates per Year:* 45.
Wheelchair Access: Yes.
Accreditation/Approval/Licensing: State board: OR; Academy of Veterinary Homeopathy.
Field of Study: Animal Therapy*; Homeopathy*. *Program Name/Length:* 130 hrs, five 4-day sessions,1 yr.
Degrees Offered: Certificate.
License/Certification Preparation: Academy of Veterinary Homeopathy.
Admission Requirements: Licensed veterinarian, DVM.
Application Deadline(s): Fall: Sep-Nov.
Tuition and Fees: $2500.
Career Services: Career information.

Lake Oswego

654. Australasian College of Herbal Studies

530 1st St, Ste A, Lake Oswego, OR 97034
Mailing Address: PO Box 57, Lake Oswego, OR 97034
Phone: (503) 635-6652; *Fax:* (503) 636-0706
E-mail: achs@herbed.com *Internet:* http://www.herbed.com
Program Administrator: Dorene Petersen, ND, DiplAc, Principal. *Admissions Contact:* Dorene Petersen.
Year Established: 1979.
Staff: Full-time: 3; Part-time: 7.
Avg Enrollment: 1000.
Accreditation/Approval/Licensing: State board: OR Office of Educational Policy and Planning.
Field of Study: Aromatherapy*; Flower Essences; Herbal Medicine*; Homeobotanical Therapy*; Homeopathy*; Iridology. *Program Name/Length:* Diploma of Herbal Studies, 2 yrs; Diploma in Homeobotanicals, 2 yrs; Certificate in Aromatherapy, 1 yr; Certificate in

Iridology, Homeopathy, and Flower Essences, 1 yr; Home study/Correspondence.
Degrees Offered: Diploma; Certificate.
Tuition and Fees: $288-$2768.
Financial Aid: Scholarships; Work study.
Career Services: Career counseling; Career information.

Lincoln City

655. Oregon Coast School of Massage

Pre-License Certification; Continuing Education
1845 SW Hwy 101, Ste 2, Lincoln City, OR 97367
Phone: (541) 994-2728
E-mail: ocsm@wcn.net
Program Administrator: Margaret Welch, LMT, Owner. *Admissions Contact:* Margaret Welch.
Year Established: 1997.
Staff: Full-time: 2; Part-time: 6.
Avg Enrollment: 12. *Avg Class Size:* 12. *Number of Graduates per Year:* 10.
Wheelchair Access: No.
Accreditation/Approval/Licensing: State board: OR Board of Massage; OR Licensed Private Vocational School.
Field of Study: Deep Tissue Massage; Energy Work; Massage Therapy*; Shiatsu; Tai Chi. *Program Name/Length:* 500 hrs, 18 mos/part-time.
License/Certification Preparation: State: OR Licensed Massage Technician.
Admission Requirements: Min age: 18; High school diploma/GED; Some college preferred.
Application Deadline(s): Fall: Aug.
Tuition and Fees: $5500.
Financial Aid: Vocational rehabilitation.
Career Services: Career information.

O'Brien

656. Sage Femme Midwifery School

Midwifery; Childbirth Arts; Doula Training
PO Box 91, O'Brien, OR 97534
Phone: (541) 596-2543; (800) 247-8422; *Fax:* (541) 596-2543
E-mail: wisearth@cdsnet.net *Internet:* http://www.sagefemme.net
Program Administrator: Patricia Downing, Operations Dir. *Admissions Contact:* Patricia Downing; Kim Garret, Minneapolis Dir; Cynthia Feinberg, Portland Dir; Paula Tipton-Healy, San Diego Dir.
Year Established: 1984.
Staff: Full-time: 1 per location; Part-time: 4 per location.
Avg Enrollment: 6 per location. *Avg Class Size:* 6.
Wheelchair Access: Yes.
Accreditation/Approval/Licensing: State board: OR Direct Entry Midwifery Board; Midwifery Education Accreditation Council.

Field of Study: Childbirth Education*; Doula*; Herbal Medicine; Homeopathy; Midwifery*. *Program Name/Length:* Childbirth Arts, 1 yr; Complete Midwifery Training, 3-5 yrs; Doula Training, 3 days; Seminars given in various locations.

Degrees Offered: CEUs; Diploma; Certificate.

License/Certification Preparation: State: CA, MN, OR, WA Licensed Midwife; Certified Professional Midwife, North American Registry of Midwives.

Admission Requirements: Min age: 18; High school diploma/GED; Specific course prerequisites: Childbirth Arts required for Midwifery Training.

Application Deadline(s): Fall: Sep 1; Winter: Feb 1.

Tuition and Fees: $4862 (Childbirth Arts); $16,830 (Midwifery).

Financial Aid: Work study; Vocational rehabilitation; County vocational training.

Career Services: Career counseling; Career information; Internships; Interview set up; Resume service.

Comments: Campuses in Minneapolis, San Diego, and Portland, OR.

Portland

657. Birthingway Midwifery Center

4620 N Maryland Ave, Portland, OR 97217
Phone: (503) 282-5729; *Fax:* (503) 282-5729
E-mail: holmar@spiretech.com *Internet:* http://www.gurlpages.com/nolabel/birthingway
Program Administrator: Holly Scholles, CPM, Dir.
Year Established: 1992.
Staff: Full-time: 1; Part-time: 6.
Avg Enrollment: 9. *Avg Class Size:* 9. *Number of Graduates per Year:* 4.
Wheelchair Access: No.
Accreditation/Approval/Licensing: Midwifery Education Accreditation Council.
Field of Study: Midwifery*. *Program Name/Length:* 3 yrs.
Degrees Offered: BS; Diploma.
License/Certification Preparation: State: OR Licensed Midwife; Certified Professional Midwife, North American Registry of Midwives.
Admission Requirements: High school diploma/GED; Specific course prerequisites: human anatomy and physiology; Min GPA: 3.0 ; Proficiency in English.
Application Deadline(s): Winter: Nov 10.
Tuition and Fees: $5000 (1st yr); $4000 (2nd yr); $3000 (3rd yr); + $200 annual enrollment fee.
Financial Aid: Work study.
Career Services: Career counseling; Career information.

658. East-West College of the Healing Arts

4531 SE Belmont St, Portland, OR 97215-1635

Phone: (503) 231-1500, (800) 635-9141; *Fax:* (503) 232-4087
E-mail: ewcha@aol.com *Internet:* http://www.ewcha.com
Program Administrator: Richard Martin, Dir of Admissions and Mktg. *Admissions Contact:* Richard Martin; Elizabeth Halsey, Admissions Office.
Year Established: 1972.
Staff: Part-time: 15.
Avg Enrollment: 300. *Avg Class Size:* 14. *Number of Graduates per Year:* 275.
Wheelchair Access: Yes.
Accreditation/Approval/Licensing: State board: OR Dept of Ed; OR and WA Boards of Massage; Commission on Massage Therapy Accreditation.
Field of Study: Energy Work; Massage Therapy*; Polarity Therapy; Shiatsu; Sports Massage. *Program Name/Length:* Professional Massage Training, 529 hrs, 1 yr; 661 hrs, 15 mos.
Degrees Offered: Diploma.
License/Certification Preparation: National Certification Board for Therapeutic Massage and Bodywork.
Admission Requirements: Min age: 18; High school diploma/GED; Min GPA: 2.0.
Application Deadline(s): Fall: Oct 1; Winter: Jan 1; Spring: Apr 1; Summer: Jul 1.
Tuition and Fees: $5500 (529 hrs); $6900 (661 hrs).
Financial Aid: Loans; Scholarships; State government aid; VA approved; Vocational rehabilitation.
Career Services: Career information; Interview set up; Referral service.

659. International Loving Touch Foundation, Inc

Certified Infant Massage Instructor Training
PO Box 16374, Portland, OR 97292
Phone: (503) 253-8482; *Fax:* (503) 256-6753
E-mail: children@lovingtouch.com *Internet:* http://www.lovingtouch.com
Program Administrator: Diana Moore, MS, Founder. *Admissions Contact:* Diana Moore.
Year Established: 1992.
Avg Class Size: 20. *Number of Graduates per Year:* 200.
Field of Study: Infant Massage*. *Program Name/Length:* 24 hrs, 3 days; Seminars given in various locations.
Degrees Offered: Certificate; Certified Infant Massage Instructor.
Admission Requirements: Min age: 18; High school diploma/GED; Specific course prerequisites: anatomy, early childhood, or massage preferred.
Tuition and Fees: $400.

660. National College of Naturopathic Medicine

049 SW Porter, Portland, OR 97201

Phone: (503) 499-4343
Internet: http://www.ncnm.edu
Program Administrator: Clyde Jensen, PhD, Pres.
  Admissions Contact: Glen D. Young, Dir of Admissions.
Year Established: 1956.
Staff: Full-time: 14; Part-time: 60.
Avg Enrollment: 375. *Avg Class Size:* 120. *Number of Graduates per Year:* 100.
Wheelchair Access: Yes.
Accreditation/Approval/Licensing: State board: OR Office of Educational Policy and Planning; Council on Naturopathic Medicine Education.
Field of Study: Herbal Medicine*; Homeopathy*; Naturopathic Medicine*; Oriental Medicine*; Traditional Chinese Medicine*. *Program Name/Length:* Doctorate in Naturopathic Medicine, 4-5 yrs; Master of Science in Oriental Medicine, 2 yrs (concurrent with ND program).
Degrees Offered: ND; MSOM.
License/Certification Preparation: State: OR Naturopathic Physician; Homeopathic Academy of Naturopathic Physicians; Naturopathic Physicians Licensing Exam.
Admission Requirements: Bachelor's degree; Min GPA: 3.0.
Application Deadline(s): Winter: Feb.
Tuition and Fees: $14,300 per yr + $2300-$2500 supplies per yr.
Financial Aid: Federal government aid.
Career Services: Career counseling; Career information; Internships.

661. Oregon College of Oriental Medicine
10525 SE Cherry Blossom Dr, Portland, OR 97216
Phone: (503) 253-3443; *Fax:* (503) 253-2701
E-mail: lpowell@teleport.com *Internet:* http://www.infinite.org/oregon.acupuncture
Program Administrator: Elizabeth Goldblatt, PhD, Pres. *Admissions Contact:* Linda Powell, Admissions/Financial Aid Officer.
Year Established: 1983.
Staff: Full-time: 6; Part-time: 25.
Avg Enrollment: 185. *Avg Class Size:* 60. *Number of Graduates per Year:* 45.
Wheelchair Access: Yes.
Accreditation/Approval/Licensing: State board: CA Acupuncture Board; Accreditation Commission for Acupuncture and Oriental Medicine.
Field of Study: Acupressure; Acupuncture*; Herbal Medicine; Oriental Medicine*; Qigong; Shiatsu; Traditional Chinese Medicine*. *Program Name/Length:* Master of Acupuncture and Oriental Medicine, 3 yrs.
Degrees Offered: MAcOM.
License/Certification Preparation: All licensed states; National Certification Commission for Acupuncture and Oriental Medicine.
Admission Requirements: High school diploma/GED; Some college (3 yrs); Specific course prerequisites: chemistry, biology, psychology.

Tuition and Fees: $8500 per yr.
Financial Aid: Federal government aid; Loans; Work study; VA approved.
Career Services: Career information.

662. Oregon Health Sciences University, School of Nursing
Nurse-Midwifery Program
3181 SW Sam Jackson Park Rd, Portland, OR 97210
Phone: (503) 494-3114; *Fax:* (503) 494-3878
E-mail: howec@ohsu.edu
Program Administrator: Carol Howe, CNM, Dir.
Year Established: 1981.
Staff: Full-time: 5; Part-time: 2.
Avg Enrollment: 10. *Avg Class Size:* 10. *Number of Graduates per Year:* 10.
Wheelchair Access: Yes.
Accreditation/Approval/Licensing: American College of Nurse-Midwives, Division of Accreditation.
Field of Study: Midwifery*. *Program Name/Length:* Nurse-Midwifery, 6 qtrs.
Degrees Offered: MS; Post-Master's Certificate.
License/Certification Preparation: State: OR Licensed Midwife; Certified Nurse-Midwife, American College of Nurse-Midwives.
Admission Requirements: Bachelor's degree in Nursing; Min GPA: 3.0; RN.
Financial Aid: Federal government aid.

663. Oregon School of Massage, Portland
555 Hour Massage Certificate Program
9500 SW Barbur Blvd, Ste 100, Portland, OR 97219
Phone: (800) 844-3420, (503) 244-3420; *Fax:* (503) 244-1815
E-mail: osmlbg@teleport.com *Internet:* http://www.oregonschoolofmassage.com
Program Administrator: Ray Siderius, Pres. *Admissions Contact:* Lisa Garofalo, Dir of Ed.
Year Established: 1984.
Staff: Full-time: 1; Part-time: 20.
Avg Enrollment: 210. *Avg Class Size:* 16. *Number of Graduates per Year:* 75.
Wheelchair Access: Yes.
Accreditation/Approval/Licensing: State board: OR Dept of Ed; OR and WA Boards of Massage.
Field of Study: Acupressure; Alexander Technique; CranioSacral Therapy; Energy Work; Massage Therapy*; Neuromuscular Therapy; Oriental Medicine; Polarity Therapy; Reflexology; Reiki; Shiatsu*; Traditional Chinese Medicine. *Program Name/Length:* Professional Massage Training, 555 hrs, 15 mos.
Degrees Offered: Certificate.
License/Certification Preparation: State: OR Licensed Massage Technician; WA Licensed Massage Practitioner; National Certification Board for Therapeutic Massage and Bodywork.

Admission Requirements: Min age: 18 or parental consent; High school diploma/GED.
Application Deadline(s): Fall: Sep 20; Winter: Dec 30; Spring: Mar 15; Summer: Jun 15.
Tuition and Fees: $6290.
Financial Aid: Loans; VA approved; Vocational rehabilitation.
Career Services: Career counseling; Career information; Marketing events.

664. Western States Chiropractic College
2900 NE 132nd St, Portland, OR 97009
Phone: (503) 251-5734; *Fax:* (503) 251-5723
E-mail: admissions@wschiro.edu *Internet:* http://www.wschiro.edu
Program Administrator: William Dallas, DC, Pres.
   Admissions Contact: Randall Hand, Admissions Dir.
Year Established: 1904.
Staff: Full-time: 45; Part-time: 53.
Avg Enrollment: 500. *Number of Graduates per Year:* 120.
Accreditation/Approval/Licensing: Council on Chiropractic Education; Northwest Association of Schools and Colleges.
Field of Study: Chiropractic*. *Program Name/Length:* Doctor of Chiropractic, 12 qtrs.
Degrees Offered: BS; DC.
License/Certification Preparation: State: OR Doctor of Chiropractic.
Admission Requirements: High school diploma/GED; Some college (2 yrs); Min GPA: 2.5.
Tuition and Fees: $4710 per qtr.
Financial Aid: Federal government aid; Scholarships; Work study; ChiroLoan.

Salem

665. The American Herbal Institute
Modern Herbal Studies Course
3056 Lancaster Dr NE, Salem, OR 97305
Phone: (503) 364-7242
Program Administrator: Constance Walker, MH, Pres.
Year Established: 1991.
Staff: Part-time: 6.
Avg Enrollment: 15. *Avg Class Size:* 15. *Number of Graduates per Year:* 8.
Field of Study: Aromatherapy; Herbal Medicine*; Hypnotherapy; Nutrition; Reflexology; Traditional Chinese Medicine. *Program Name/Length:* Beginning Program (General Studies), 6 mos or home study; Advanced Program, 5 mos.
Degrees Offered: Certificate.
Admission Requirements: Min age: 18.
Application Deadline(s): Fall: Sep 20; Winter: Jan 20.
Career Services: Internships.

666. Oregon School of Massage, Salem
440 Ferry St NE, Salem, OR 97302-3605
Mailing Address: PO Box 2779, Salem, OR 97308-2779
Phone: (800) 844-3420, (503) 585-8912; *Fax:* (503) 585-0988
E-mail: osm@teleport.com *Internet:* http://www.oregonschoolofmassage.com
Program Administrator: Ray Siderius, Owner/Pres.
   Admissions Contact: Lisa Barck Garofalo, Dir of Ed.
Year Established: 1989.
Staff: Part-time: 6.
Avg Class Size: 15.
Wheelchair Access: Yes.
Accreditation/Approval/Licensing: State board: OR and WA Boards of Massage; OR Dept of Ed.
Field of Study: Alexander Technique; Anatomy and Physiology; Energy Work; Kinesiology; Massage Therapy*; Polarity Therapy; Reflexology; Reiki; Shiatsu; Sports Massage; Traditional Chinese Medicine. *Program Name/Length:* 555 hrs, 1-2 yrs.
Degrees Offered: Certificate.
License/Certification Preparation: State: OR Licensed Massage Technician; WA Licensed Massage Practitioner.
Admission Requirements: Min age: 18; High school diploma/GED.
Application Deadline(s): Fall: Sep; Winter: Dec; Spring: Mar; Summer: Jun.
Tuition and Fees: $6290.
Financial Aid: Loans; VA approved; Payment plan.
Career Services: Career information; Job information.

667. Polarity Center of Salem
1940 Breyman NE, Salem, OR 97301
Phone: (503) 581-6512
Program Administrator: Ann Watters, LMT, Dir.
   Admissions Contact: Ann Watters.
Year Established: 1995.
Staff: Full-time: 1; Part-time: 1.
Avg Enrollment: 4. *Avg Class Size:* 4. *Number of Graduates per Year:* 2.
Wheelchair Access: No.
Accreditation/Approval/Licensing: State board: OR Board of Massage; Accrediting Council for Continuing Education and Training; American Polarity Therapy Association.
Field of Study: Polarity Therapy*. *Program Name/Length:* Associate Polarity Practitioner, 4-12 mos.
Degrees Offered: CEUs; Certificate.
License/Certification Preparation: APP; American Polarity Therapy Association.
Admission Requirements: Min age: 21; High school diploma/GED; Min GPA: 2.0.
Application Deadline(s): Winter: Feb; Summer: Aug.
Tuition and Fees: $1500 + $500 books, sessions.

Financial Aid: Scholarships; Payment options.
Career Services: Career counseling; Career information; Internships.

PENNSYLVANIA

Conshohocken

668. A Rose Therapeutics
Basic Massage: Integrated Technique Approach;
Reiki: All Levels
352 E 6th Ave, Conshohocken, PA 19428
Phone: (610) 834-8140
Program Administrator: Aura Rose, Dir. *Admissions Contact:* Aura Rose.
Year Established: 1989.
Staff: Full-time: 1; Part-time: 2.
Avg Class Size: 7.
Wheelchair Access: Yes.
Field of Study: Acupressure; CranioSacral Therapy;
Energy Work*; Feldenkrais; Herbal Medicine;
Hypnotherapy; Massage Therapy*;
Neuromuscular Therapy; Reflexology; Reiki*;
Shiatsu; Sports Massage; Swedish Massage;
Yoga*. *Program Name/Length:* Basic Massage
Therapy (includes Reiki I), 42 hrs; Reiki I,
weekend; Reiki II, weekend; Reiki Master.
Degrees Offered: Certificate.
Financial Aid: Scholarships; Work study; Trades.
Career Services: Career counseling; Career information; Internships; Interview set up; Referral
service.

Doylestown

669. Feldenkrais Professional Training Programs
59 Pebble Woods Dr, Doylestown, PA 18901
Phone: (215) 230-9208; *Fax:* (215) 230-9086
Program Administrator: David Zemach-Bersin,
Educational Dir. *Admissions Contact:* David
Zemach-Bersin.
Year Established: 1994.
Avg Enrollment: 100. *Avg Class Size:* 45. *Number
of Graduates per Year:* 45 every 2 yrs.
Wheelchair Access: Yes.
Accreditation/Approval/Licensing: Feldenkrais
Guild.
Field of Study: Feldenkrais*. *Program
Name/Length:* 4 yrs (200 hrs/40 days per yr);
Seminars given in various locations.
Degrees Offered: Diploma; Certificate.
License/Certification Preparation: Certified
Feldenkrais Practitioner, Feldenkrais Guild.
Tuition and Fees: $3600 per yr.

Financial Aid: Scholarships.
Career Services: Career information.

670. International School of Shiatsu
10 S Clinton St, Ste 300, Doylestown, PA 18901
Phone: (215) 340-9918; *Fax:* (215) 340-9181
Internet: http://www.shiatsubo.com
Program Administrator: Saul Goodman, Dir. *Admissions Contact:* Megan Wilson, Admissions
Dir.
Year Established: 1978.
Staff: Full-time: 4; Part-time: 4.
Avg Enrollment: 45. *Avg Class Size:* 15. *Number
of Graduates per Year:* 20.
Accreditation/Approval/Licensing: State board: PA
Board of Private Licensed Schools; American
Oriental Bodywork Therapy Association.
Field of Study: Acupressure*; Shiatsu*. *Program
Name/Length:* Shiatsu Foundation Program,
243 hrs, 9 mos; Practitioner Program, 386 hrs,
15 mos.
Degrees Offered: Diploma; Certificate.
Admission Requirements: Min age: 18; High
school diploma/GED; Specific course prerequisites: Shiatsu Foundation required for Practitioner Program.
Tuition and Fees: $2850 (Foundation); $7365
(Practitioner).

Emmaus

671. Lehigh Valley Healing Arts Academy
5412 Shimerville Rd, Emmaus, PA 18049
Phone: (610) 965-6165; *Fax:* (610) 965-6165
E-mail: lvhaa@fast.net *Internet:* http://www.illion/
lvhaa.com
Program Administrator: Bonita A.
Cassel-Beckwith, Dir. *Admissions Contact:*
Bonita A. Cassel-Beckwith.
Year Established: 1984.
Staff: Full-time: 1; Part-time: 10.
Avg Enrollment: 30. *Avg Class Size:* 12. *Number
of Graduates per Year:* 20.
Wheelchair Access: No.
Accreditation/Approval/Licensing: State board: PA
Board of Private Licensed Schools; National
Certification Board for Therapeutic Massage
and Bodywork (CEUs).

Field of Study: Acupressure; Alexander Technique; Aromatherapy; Ayurvedic Medicine; CranioSacral Therapy; Energy Work; Feldenkrais; Herbal Medicine; Homeopathy; Massage Therapy*; Meditation; Oriental Medicine; Polarity Therapy; Reflexology; Reiki; Shiatsu; Sports Massage; Therapeutic Touch; Traditional Chinese Medicine; Trager; Yoga. *Program Name/Length:* Professional Integrated Bodywork Training: Level I, 150 hrs, 3 mos; Level II, 150 hrs, 3 mos; Level III, 200 hrs, 6 mos; Whole Program, 500 hrs, 1-2 yrs.

Degrees Offered: Diploma.

License/Certification Preparation: National Certification Board for Therapeutic Massage and Bodywork.

Admission Requirements: Min age: 18; High school diploma/GED; Proficiency in English.

Application Deadline(s): Fall: Sep; Winter: Jan; Spring: Mar; Summer: Jun.

Tuition and Fees: $1500 (Levels I and II); $2000 (Level III); $4500 (500 hrs).

Financial Aid: State government aid.

Career Services: Career counseling.

Factoryville

672. Endless Mountain School of Shiatsu

RR1, Box 1741, Factoryville, PA 18419

Phone: (570) 942-4481; *Fax:* (570) 942-6139

Program Administrator: Samuel R. Kupetsky, Dir. *Admissions Contact:* Samuel R. Kupetsky.

Year Established: 1991.

Staff: Full-time: 1; Part-time: 1.

Avg Enrollment: 25. *Avg Class Size:* 6. *Number of Graduates per Year:* 10.

Wheelchair Access: Yes.

Accreditation/Approval/Licensing: National Certification Board for Therapeutic Massage and Bodywork (CEUs).

Field of Study: Acupressure; Energy Work; Herbal Medicine; Oriental Medicine; Shiatsu*; Traditional Chinese Medicine*; Visualization*. *Program Name/Length:* Shiatsu, Courses One-Six, 1 1/2 yrs; Seminars given in various locations; Traditional Chinese Medicine, weekend workshops, 2 yrs; Seminars given in various locations; Home study/Correspondence.

Degrees Offered: CEUs; Certificate.

License/Certification Preparation: National Certification Commission for Acupuncture and Oriental Medicine; National Certification Board for Therapeutic Massage and Bodywork.

Admission Requirements: Min age: 18.

Application Deadline(s): Fall: Aug; Spring: Feb; Summer: May.

Tuition and Fees: $250-$320 per course (Shiatsu); $195 first workshop, successive workshops discounted (TCM).

Financial Aid: Work study; Payment plan.

Career Services: Career information; Referral service.

Harrisburg

673. Academy of Medical Arts and Business

Professional Massage Therapist

2301 Academy Dr, Harrisburg, PA 17112-1012

Phone: (717) 545-4747; *Fax:* (717) 901-9090

Internet: http://www.acadcampus.com

Program Administrator: Gary Kay, Pres. *Admissions Contact:* Gary Kay.

Year Established: 1980.

Staff: Full-time: 3; Part-time: 2.

Avg Enrollment: 100. *Avg Class Size:* 15. *Number of Graduates per Year:* 100.

Wheelchair Access: Yes.

Accreditation/Approval/Licensing: State board: PA Board of Private Licensed Schools; Accrediting Commission of Career Schools and Colleges of Technology; National Certification Board for Therapeutic Massage and Bodywork (CEUs).

Field of Study: Acupressure; Aromatherapy; CranioSacral Therapy; Deep Tissue Massage*; Hypnotherapy; Massage Therapy*; Prenatal Massage; Reflexology; Reiki; Shiatsu; Yoga Teacher Training. *Program Name/Length:* Massage Therapy, 740 hrs, 7 mos; Seminars given in various locations.

Degrees Offered: CEUs; Diploma.

License/Certification Preparation: American Board of Clinical Hypnosis; American Council of Hypnotist Examiners; National Certification Board for Therapeutic Massage and Bodywork.

Admission Requirements: Min age: 18; High school diploma/GED.

Application Deadline(s): Fall; Winter; Spring; Summer.

Financial Aid: Federal government aid; Grants; Loans; Scholarships; Work study; VA approved; Vocational rehabilitation.

Career Services: Career counseling; Career information; Internships; Interview set up; Resume service.

Honesdale

674. Himalayan Institute

Hatha Yoga Teachers Training

RR 1, Box 400, Honesdale, PA 18431

Phone: (570) 253-5551 ext 1305, (800) 822-4547; *Fax:* (570) 253-9078

E-mail: hita@himalayaninstitute.org *Internet:* http://www.himalayaninstitute.org

Field of Study: Meditation; Yoga Teacher Training*. *Program Name/Length:* Residential intensive, 2 wks and six home-study courses.

Admission Requirements: Ongoing hatha yoga practice.

Tuition and Fees: $950 + $650 room and board.
Career Services: Referral service.

Lancaster

675. Esthetic Training Institute
Advanced Educational Division
702 Fountain Ave, Lancaster, PA 17601
Phone: (800) 446-2260; *Fax:* (610) 292-0299
E-mail: esthetic@aol.com *Internet:* http://www.
purelight.com/esthe-tec/home.htm
Program Administrator: Rose Ann
Acuazzo-Linkens. *Admissions Contact:*
Kathleen Martorelli.
Year Established: 1984.
Staff: Full-time: 2; Part-time: 3.
Avg Enrollment: 10. *Avg Class Size:* 8. *Number of
Graduates per Year:* 10.
Wheelchair Access: Yes.
Field of Study: Aromatherapy*; Massage Therapy;
Reflexology; Reiki. *Program Name/Length:*
Certification, 1 mo; Correspondence course.
Degrees Offered: Certificate.
Admission Requirements: High school di-
ploma/GED.
Tuition and Fees: $450 (Certification); $350 (Cor-
respondence).

676. Lancaster School of Massage
317 N Queen St, Lancaster, PA 17603
Phone: (717) 293-9698
E-mail: lsmassage@redrose.net
Program Administrator: Winona F. Bontrager,
LMT, Owner/Dir. *Admissions Contact:* Winona
F. Bontrager.
Year Established: 1991.
Staff: Part-time: 7.
Avg Enrollment: 40. *Avg Class Size:* 20. *Number
of Graduates per Year:* 40.
Wheelchair Access: No.
Accreditation/Approval/Licensing: State board: PA
Board of Private Licensed Schools.
Field of Study: Connective Tissue Massage;
CranioSacral Therapy; Massage Therapy*;
Neuromuscular Therapy; Polarity Therapy;
Reflexology; Sports Massage; Swedish Mas-
sage*. *Program Name/Length:* 500 hrs, 6
mos/days or 9 mos/evenings.
Degrees Offered: Certificate.
License/Certification Preparation: National Certif-
ication Board for Therapeutic Massage and
Bodywork.
Admission Requirements: Min age: 18; High
school diploma/GED; Min GPA: 2.0.
Application Deadline(s): Fall: Aug; Spring: Feb.
Tuition and Fees: $4500 + books.

Langhorne

677. Professional School of Massage
131 E Maple Ave, Langhorne, PA 19047
Phone: (215) 750-0700
Admissions Contact: David Scott, LMT,
Founder/Dir.
Year Established: 1996.
Staff: Part-time: 7.
Avg Enrollment: 40. *Avg Class Size:* 16. *Number
of Graduates per Year:* 40.
Wheelchair Access: No.
Accreditation/Approval/Licensing: State board: PA
Board of Private Licensed Schools.
Field of Study: Acupressure; Herbal Medicine;
Massage Therapy*; Polarity Therapy; Qigong;
Reflexology*; Reiki; Shiatsu*. *Program
Name/Length:* Massage Therapy, 300 hrs, 6
mos; Advanced Massage Therapy, 200 hrs; Ad-
vanced Hand and Foot Reflexology, 6 mos;
Shiatsu Practitioner, 1 yr.
Degrees Offered: Diploma.
Admission Requirements: Min age: 19; High
school diploma/GED.
Application Deadline(s): Winter: Dec; Summer:
Jun.
Tuition and Fees: $3000 (Massage Therapy);
$1750 (Advanced Massage Therapy); $1600
Reflexology); $5000 (Shiatsu).
Career Services: Career counseling; Career infor-
mation.

678. School of Body Therapies
931 Langhorne-Yardley Rd, Langhorne, PA
19047-1368
Phone: (215) 752-7666; *Fax:* (215) 752-1909
Program Administrator: Joan L. Stocker, Dir. *Ad-
missions Contact:* Joan L. Stocker.
Year Established: 1989.
Staff: Part-time: 15.
Avg Enrollment: 15. *Avg Class Size:* 8. *Number of
Graduates per Year:* 10.
Wheelchair Access: No.
Field of Study: Deep Muscle Massage*; Massage
Therapy*; Thai Massage. *Program
Name/Length:* Deep Muscle Therapeutic Mas-
sage and Bodywork, 500 hrs.
Degrees Offered: Diploma; Certificate.
License/Certification Preparation: National Certif-
ication Board for Therapeutic Massage and
Bodywork.
Admission Requirements: Min age: 18; High
school diploma/GED.
Application Deadline(s): Fall: Aug 1; Spring: Dec
1.
Tuition and Fees: $5000.

Lemoyne

679. The Alternative Conjunction Clinic and School of Massage Therapy

716 State St, Lemoyne, PA 17043
Phone: (717) 737-6001; *Fax:* (717) 737-6607
E-mail: melmassag1@aol.com
Program Administrator: Melodie A. Adinolfi, Owner/Dir. *Admissions Contact:* Melodie A. Adinolfi.
Year Established: 1994.
Staff: Full-time: 6; Part-time: 4.
Avg Enrollment: 75. *Avg Class Size:* 14. *Number of Graduates per Year:* 55.
Wheelchair Access: Yes.
Accreditation/Approval/Licensing: State board: PA Board of Private Licensed Schools; National Accrediting Commission of Cosmetology Arts and Sciences.
Field of Study: Aromatherapy; Chair Massage; Esalen Massage; Massage Therapy*; Neuromuscular Therapy; Russian Massage; Swedish Massage*. *Program Name/Length:* 604 hrs, 7 mos.
Degrees Offered: Diploma; Certificate.
License/Certification Preparation: State: FL, IA Licensed Massage Therapist; National Certification Board for Therapeutic Massage and Bodywork.
Admission Requirements: Min age: 18; High school diploma/GED; Interview with director; Physical exam; 3 letters of reference.
Application Deadline(s): Fall; Winter; Spring; Summer.
Tuition and Fees: $3921.
Financial Aid: Federal government aid; Grants; Loans; State government aid; VA approved; Vocational rehabilitation; Private finance companies.
Career Services: Career counseling; Career information; Interview set up.

Monroeville

680. Career Training Academy, Monroeville

Expo Mart, 105 Mall Blvd, Ste 300W, Monroeville, PA 15146
Phone: (412) 372-3900, (800) 491-3470; *Fax:* (412) 373-4262
E-mail: jreddy@careerta.com *Internet:* http://www.careerta.com
Program Administrator: Maryagnes Luczak, Dir. *Admissions Contact:* Diana Kocinski, Admissions Rep.
Year Established: 1992.
Staff: Full-time: 5; Part-time: 3 (2 campuses).
Avg Enrollment: 125. *Avg Class Size:* 15. *Number of Graduates per Year:* 120.
Wheelchair Access: Yes.
Accreditation/Approval/Licensing: State board: PA Board of Private Licensed Schools; Commission on Massage Therapy Accreditation; Accrediting Commission of Career Schools and Colleges of Technology; International Massage and Somatic Therapies Accreditation Council.
Field of Study: Acupressure; Aromatherapy; Massage Therapy*; Reflexology; Shiatsu*; Sports Massage; Swedish Massage*. *Program Name/Length:* Swedish Massage Practitioner, 4 mos; Therapeutic Massage Technician, 7 1/2 mos; Basic Shiatsu Technician, 4 mos; Advanced Shiatsu Technician, 7 1/2 mos; Comprehensive Massage Therapist, 11 mos; Advanced Bodyworker, 18 mos.
Degrees Offered: Diploma.
License/Certification Preparation: National Certification Board for Therapeutic Massage and Bodywork.
Admission Requirements: Min age: 18; High school diploma/GED.
Tuition and Fees: $1900-$9500.
Financial Aid: Federal government aid; Grants; Loans; State government aid; Vocational rehabilitation.
Career Services: Career information; Listing service.

New Kensington

681. Career Training Academy, New Kensington

703 5th Ave, New Kensington, PA 15068-6301
Phone: (724) 337-1000, (800) 600-3470; *Fax:* (724) 335-7140
E-mail: jreddy@careerta.com *Internet:* http://www.careerta.com
Program Administrator: John Reddy, Pres. *Admissions Contact:* Deborah Athey-Ducar.
Year Established: 1989.
Staff: Full-time: 8; Part-time: 3.
Avg Enrollment: 125. *Avg Class Size:* 15. *Number of Graduates per Year:* 120.
Wheelchair Access: Yes.
Accreditation/Approval/Licensing: State board: PA Board of Private Licensed Schools; Commission on Massage Therapy Accreditation; Accrediting Commission of Career Schools and Colleges of Technology; International Massage and Somatic Therapies Accreditation Council.
Field of Study: Acupressure*; Aromatherapy; Massage Therapy*; Reflexology; Shiatsu*; Swedish Massage*. *Program Name/Length:* Swedish Massage Practitioner, 5 mos; Therapeutic Massage Technician, 9 1/2 mos; Basic Shiatsu Technician, 5 mos; Advanced Shiatsu Technician, 9 1/2 mos.
Degrees Offered: Diploma.
License/Certification Preparation: National Certification Board for Therapeutic Massage and Bodywork.

Admission Requirements: Min age: 18; High school diploma/GED; Health release; Essay.
Tuition and Fees: $3145-$5274.
Financial Aid: Federal government aid; Grants; Loans; Scholarships; State government aid; Vocational rehabilitation.
Career Services: Career counseling; Career information; Listing service.

Norristown

682. Northeastern School of Medical Massage, Inc

2525 W Main, 2nd Fl, Norristown, PA 19403
Phone: (610) 631-5188
Program Administrator: Constance J. Perry, RN, Massage Practitioner, Dir of Ed. *Admissions Contact:* Constance J. Perry.
Year Established: 1991.
Staff: Full-time: 4; Part-time: 2.
Avg Enrollment: 100. *Avg Class Size:* 18. *Number of Graduates per Year:* 75.
Wheelchair Access: No.
Field of Study: Acupressure*; Aromatherapy; Infant Massage; Massage Therapy*; Medical Massage*; Neuromuscular Therapy*; Pregnancy Massage; Reflexology; Sports Massage; Swedish Massage*. *Program Name/Length:* Therapeutic Massage, 150 hrs, 3 mos; Medical Massage, 550 hrs, 5 mos/full-time or 10 mos/part-time; Neuromuscular Therapy, 200 hrs, 6 mos/part-time (1 weekend/mo).
Degrees Offered: Diploma; Certificate.
License/Certification Preparation: National Certification Board for Therapeutic Massage and Bodywork.
Admission Requirements: Min age: 18; High school diploma/GED; Min GPA: 3.0; Health care professional or 500 hr massage course for Neuromuscular Therapy.
Application Deadline(s): Fall: Aug 15; Winter: Jan 7.
Tuition and Fees: $995 (Therapeutic); $4500 (Medical); $1800 (Neuromuscular).
Financial Aid: Loans; Scholarships; Payment plan.
Career Services: Career counseling; Career information; Internships.

Northampton

683. Health Options Institute

Massage Therapy
1410 Main St, Northampton, PA 18067
Phone: (610) 261-0880; *Fax:* (610) 261-2964
E-mail: massage8@aol.com *Internet:* http://www.members.aol.com/massage8
Program Administrator: Elizabeth Bieber, Dir. *Admissions Contact:* Elizabeth Bieber.
Year Established: 1984.
Staff: Part-time: 25.

Avg Enrollment: 135. *Avg Class Size:* 15. *Number of Graduates per Year:* 130.
Wheelchair Access: No.
Accreditation/Approval/Licensing: State board: PA Board of Private Licensed Schools.
Field of Study: Acupressure; Aromatherapy; Deep Muscle Massage*; Herbal Medicine*; Massage Therapy*; Neuromuscular Therapy; Reflexology*; Reiki; Shiatsu. *Program Name/Length:* Massage Therapy, 500 hrs, 12-18 mos; Advanced Massage Therapy, 1 yr; Reflexology, 1 yr; Deep Muscle Massage, 3 mos; Nutrition/Herbology, 2 mos.
Degrees Offered: Diploma; Certificate.
License/Certification Preparation: American Reflexology Certification Board; National Certification Board for Therapeutic Massage and Bodywork.
Admission Requirements: Min age: 18 or parental consent.
Tuition and Fees: $5200 (500 hr Massage).
Financial Aid: Payment plan.

Paoli

684. Myofascial Release Seminars

222 W Lancaster Ave, Paoli, PA 19301
Phone: (800) 327-2425; *Fax:* (610) 644-1662
E-mail: fascia@erols.com *Internet:* http://www.vll.com/mfr/
Program Administrator: Sandra Levengood, Seminar Dir.
Accreditation/Approval/Licensing: National Certification Board for Therapeutic Massage and Bodywork (CEUs); American Speech-Language-Hearing Association; National Athletic Trainers Association Board of Certification.
Field of Study: Myofascial Release*. *Program Name/Length:* Myofascial Release I, 20 hrs; Myofascial Release II, 20 hrs; Myofascial Unwinding, 20 hrs; Fascial-Pelvis Myofascial/Osseous Release, 20 hrs; Cervical-Thoracic Myofascial/Osseous Release, 20 hrs; Myofascial Mobilization, 12 hrs; Pediatric Myofascial Release, 12 hrs; Myofascial Freedom, 20 hrs.
Degrees Offered: CEUs.
Tuition and Fees: $350-$400 (12 hrs); $595-$650 (20 hrs).
Comments: Licensed by 40 state boards of physical therapy, massage therapy, occupational therapy. Seminars taught around the country.

Philadelphia

685. Center for Human Integration

8400 Pine Rd, Philadelphia, PA 19111
Phone: (215) 742-3505; *Fax:* (215) 742-3507
Program Administrator: Sr. Mary Em McGlone, BSN, Dir. *Admissions Contact:* Kathy Schival, Office Mgr.

Year Established: 1981.
Avg Class Size: 20.
Accreditation/Approval/Licensing: State board:
Pending, PA Board of Private Licensed Schools.
Field of Study: Acupressure; Aromatherapy;
CranioSacral Therapy; Energy Work; Herbal
Medicine; Hypnotherapy; Massage Therapy; Po-
larity Therapy; Reflexology; Reiki; Therapeutic
Touch; Touch for Health; Zero Balancing. *Pro-
gram Name/Length:* Basic Massage, 11 days;
Foot Reflexology: Level 1 & 2, 5 days each;
Aromatherapy, 10 hrs, 5 days; Polarity Therapy,
4 daysg Introduction to Herbal Medicine, 8 hrs,
4 daysh Process Acupressure, 4 daysi Core Zero
Balancing 1 & 2, 50 hrs (two 25-hr segments, 4
days each)j Clinical Hypnotherapy Certification,
30 hrs, 4 daysk Reiki: Levels 1 & 2, 2 days eachl
Reiki: Level 3, Master/Teacherm Touch for
Health 1, 3 daysn Touch for Health 2 & 3, 2
days eacho Touch for Health 4, 1 day.
Tuition and Fees: $900 (Basic Massage);
$150-$175 (Reflexology Level 1); $175-$200
(Reflexology Level 2); $125-$150 per course
(Therapeutic Touch); $250 (Aromatherapy);
$475 (Polarity Therapy); $150 (Herbal Medi-
cine); $495 per course (Process Acupressure;
Zero Balancing 1 & 2); $595 (Clinical
Hypnotherapy); $125-$150 (Reiki Level 1);
$250-$275 (Reiki Level 2); $175-$200 per
course (Touch for Health 1-3); $110 (Touch for
Health 4).

686. Institute of Midwifery, Women, and Health

222 Hayward Hall, School House Ln and Henry
Ave, Philadelphia, PA 19144
Phone: (215) 843-5775; *Fax:* (215) 951-2526
E-mail: imwah@bbs.acnm.org *Internet:* http://
www.instituteofmidwifery.org
Program Administrator: Kate McHugh, Dir. *Ad-
missions Contact:* Kate Siegrist, Admissions
Coord.
Year Established: 1996.
Staff: Full-time: 2; Part-time: 6.
Avg Enrollment: 40. *Avg Class Size:* 10. *Number
of Graduates per Year:* 30.
Wheelchair Access: Yes.
Accreditation/Approval/Licensing: American Col-
lege of Nurse-Midwives, Division of Accredita-
tion.
Field of Study: Midwifery*. *Program
Name/Length:* Distance Learning Program in
Nurse-Midwifery, 21 mos.
Degrees Offered: Diploma.
License/Certification Preparation: Certified
Nurse-Midwife, American College of
Nurse-Midwives.
Admission Requirements: Bachelor's degree; Min
GPA: 3.0; RN; Specific course prerequisites:
physical assessment.
Tuition and Fees: $16,000.
Financial Aid: Loans.

687. Massage Arts and Sciences Center of Philadelphia

1515 Locust St, 2nd Fl, Philadelphia, PA 19102
Phone: (215) 985-0674; *Fax:* (215) 985-0175
E-mail: rglaser@ix.netcom.com *Internet:* http://
www.mascp.com
Program Administrator: Rosemarie Glaser,
Owner/Dir. *Admissions Contact:* Rosemarie
Glaser.
Year Established: 1984.
Staff: Part-time: 12.
Avg Enrollment: 50. *Avg Class Size:* 14. *Number
of Graduates per Year:* 50.
Wheelchair Access: Yes.
Accreditation/Approval/Licensing: State board: PA
Dept of Ed; National Certification Board for
Therapeutic Massage and Bodywork (CEUs).
Field of Study: Massage Therapy*; Reiki*; Shiatsu;
Sports Massage. *Program Name/Length:* Mas-
sage Certification, 5 mos; Massage Practitioner,
1 yr.
Degrees Offered: CEUs; Diploma; Certificate.
License/Certification Preparation: National Certif-
ication Board for Therapeutic Massage and
Bodywork.
Admission Requirements: Min age: 18; High
school diploma/GED.
Application Deadline(s): Fall: Sep; Spring: Feb.
Tuition and Fees: $3500 (Certification); $6500
(Practitioner).
Financial Aid: Loans; State government aid; Pay-
ment plan.
Career Services: Career counseling; Career infor-
mation; Job information.

688. University of Pennsylvania, School of Nursing

Nurse-Midwifery Program
Nursing Education Bldg, 420 Guardian Dr, Phila-
delphia, PA 19104-6096
Phone: (215) 898-4335
Internet: http://www.nursing.upenn.edu/
midwifery/
Program Administrator: Joyce E. Thompson,
DrPH, Dir. *Admissions Contact:* Dr. William
McCool.
Year Established: 1980.
Staff: Full-time: 2; Part-time: 6.
Avg Enrollment: 20. *Avg Class Size:* 20. *Number
of Graduates per Year:* 20.
Wheelchair Access: Yes.
Accreditation/Approval/Licensing: American Col-
lege of Nurse-Midwives, Division of Accredita-
tion.
Field of Study: Midwifery*. *Program
Name/Length:* 16 mos, full-time.
Degrees Offered: MS; Certificate; MSN; Post-Mas-
ter's Certificate in Nurse-Midwifery.
License/Certification Preparation: Certified
Nurse-Midwife, American College of
Nurse-Midwives.

Admission Requirements: Bachelor's degree; RN.
Application Deadline(s): Spring: Feb 15.
Tuition and Fees: $44,260 + $630 technology fee.
Financial Aid: Fellowships; Federal government
   aid; Loans.
Career Services: Career counseling; Career infor-
   mation; Resume service; Job information.

Phoenixville

689. Valley Forge Institute of Muscle Therapy

808 Valley Forge Rd, Phoenixville, PA 19460
Phone: (610) 935-3554
Program Administrator: Thomas V. O'Ancona,
   Dir. *Admissions Contact:* Thomas V.
   O'Ancona.
Year Established: 1995.
Staff: Full-time: 3; Part-time: 2.
Avg Enrollment: 12. *Avg Class Size:* 12. *Number
   of Graduates per Year:* 12.
Wheelchair Access: Yes.
Accreditation/Approval/Licensing: State board: PA
   Dept of Ed.
Field of Study: Chair Massage; Neuromuscular
   Therapy*; Polarity Therapy; Reflexology; Reiki;
   Sports Massage*; Swedish Massage*. *Program
   Name/Length:* Swedish Massage, 505 hrs, 6-7
   mos; Neuromuscular Therapy, 95 hrs, 5 ses-
   sions; Sports Massage, 28 hrs, 4 days;
   Reflexology, 16 hrs, 2 days; Seated Massage, 16
   hrs, 2 days.
Degrees Offered: Diploma; Certificate.
License/Certification Preparation: National Certif-
   ication Board for Therapeutic Massage and
   Bodywork.
Admission Requirements: Min age: 18; High
   school diploma/GED.
Application Deadline(s): Fall: Aug; Spring: Feb.

Pittsburgh

690. Academy for Myofascial Trigger Point Therapy

1312 E Carson St, Pittsburgh, PA 15203
Phone: (412) 481-2553; *Fax:* (412) 481-3279
E-mail: amtpt@bellatlantic.net
Program Administrator: Richard Finn, Dir. *Admis-
   sions Contact:* Joe Erdos, Admin Asst.
Year Established: 1994.
Staff: Full-time: 1; Part-time: 4.
Avg Enrollment: 10. *Avg Class Size:* 10. *Number
   of Graduates per Year:* 10.
Wheelchair Access: No.
Accreditation/Approval/Licensing: State board: PA
   Board of Private Licensed Schools; National As-
   sociation of Myofascial Trigger Point Thera-
   pists.

Field of Study: Trigger Point Therapy. *Program
   Name/Length:* Myofascial Trigger Point Ther-
   apy, 500 hrs.
Degrees Offered: Diploma.
License/Certification Preparation: Certification
   Board for Trigger Point Myotherapists.
Admission Requirements: High school di-
   ploma/GED; Specific course prerequisites: col-
   lege or trade school anatomy and physiology.
Tuition and Fees: $7400.

691. Pittsburgh School of Massage Therapy

10989 Frankstown Rd, Pittsburgh, PA 15235
Phone: (800) 860-1114; *Fax:* (412) 241-4933
E-mail: pghschmass@aol.com *Internet:* http://
   www.pghschmass.com
Program Administrator: Robert Jantsch, Dir. *Ad-
   missions Contact:* Robert Jantsch.
Year Established: 1986.
Staff: Part-time: 21.
Avg Enrollment: 100. *Avg Class Size:* 14. *Number
   of Graduates per Year:* 90.
Wheelchair Access: Yes.
Accreditation/Approval/Licensing: State board: PA
   Board of Private Licensed Schools.
Field of Study: Acupressure; Alexander Technique;
   Aromatherapy; Energy Work; Massage Ther-
   apy*; Neuromuscular Therapy*; Reflexology;
   Shiatsu; Sports Massage; Swedish Massage*.
   Program Name/Length: Massage Therapy
   Training, 308 hrs, 6 mos; Advanced Massage
   Therapy Training, 308 hrs, 6 mos.
Degrees Offered: Diploma.
License/Certification Preparation: National Certif-
   ication Board for Therapeutic Massage and
   Bodywork.
Admission Requirements: Min age: 18; High
   school diploma/GED; 2 letters of reference; In-
   terview; Autobiography.
Tuition and Fees: $2200.
Financial Aid: Loans; Scholarships; Vocational re-
   habilitation.

692. Somatic Institute, Pittsburgh

8600 W Barkhurst Dr, Pittsburgh, PA 15237
Phone: (412) 366-5580; *Fax:* (412) 367-1029
Program Administrator: Kay Miller, Exec Dir. *Ad-
   missions Contact:* Rosanne Minich, Admin Dir.
Year Established: 1984.
Staff: Full-time: 6.
Avg Enrollment: 18. *Avg Class Size:* 18. *Number
   of Graduates per Year:* 18.
Wheelchair Access: Yes.
Accreditation/Approval/Licensing: State board: PA
   Chemical Abuse Certification Board.
Field of Study: Alexander Technique; Core
   Somatics*; Feldenkrais; Somatic Education*.
   Program Name/Length: coreSomatics Profes-
   sional Intensive Training, 2 yrs; coreSomatics
   Mastery and Associates Program, 1 yr;
   coreSomatics Internships, 1-2 1/2 yrs.
Degrees Offered: Certificate.

Admission Requirements: Min age: 25; Some college (2 yrs); Understanding of Alexander Technique, Feldenkrais, Gestalt psychology, body therapies.
Application Deadline(s): Fall: Jul 1.
Tuition and Fees: $3000 per yr.
Financial Aid: Scholarships.
Career Services: Practice development support.

Point Pleasant

693. Unergi School of Holistic Therapy
PO Box 335, Point Pleasant, PA 18950
Phone: (215) 297-8006; *Fax:* (215) 297-8199
E-mail: unergi@aol.com *Internet:* http://www. unergi.com
Program Administrator: Ute Arnold, Dir. *Admissions Contact:* Siobhan Royak, Office Mgr.
Year Established: 1992.
Staff: Full-time: 3; Part-time: 6.
Avg Class Size: 15-20.
Wheelchair Access: No.
Accreditation/Approval/Licensing: Feldenkrais Guild; Alexander Technique International; Candidate, Accrediting Council for Continuing Education and Training.
Field of Study: Alexander Technique; Energy Work; Feldenkrais; Hypnotherapy; Unergi Integrated Therapy*. *Program Name/Length:* Unergi Training, 1 yr; Unergi Certification, nine 6-day modules, 3 yrs.
Degrees Offered: Certificate.
Admission Requirements: Min age: 22; High school diploma/GED; Interview with director; Workshop participation recommended.
Application Deadline(s): Fall; Winter; Summer.
Tuition and Fees: $3300 per yr.
Financial Aid: Work study for PA students; Payment plan.
Career Services: Career counseling; Career information; Internships; Resume service.

Quakertown

694. Pennsylvania Institute of Massage Therapy
93 SW End Blvd, Ste 102, Quakertown, PA 18951-1150
Phone: (215) 538-5339; *Fax:* (215) 538-8896
E-mail: drbob@fast.net
Program Administrator: Robert Tosh, DC, Co-Owner; Terry Tosh, Co-Owner. *Admissions Contact:* Robert Tosh; Terry Tosh.
Accreditation/Approval/Licensing: International Massage and Somatic Therapies Accreditation Council.
Field of Study: Animal Therapy; CPR/First Aid; Massage Therapy*; Reflexology; Shiatsu*; Tai Chi. *Program Name/Length:* Massage Therapy, 520 hrs; Shiatsu, 110 hrs; Continuing Education.

State College

695. Central Pennsylvania School of Massage, Inc
336 S Fraser St, State College, PA 16801
Phone: (814) 234-4900; *Fax:* (814) 234-0440
Internet: http://www.schoolofmassage.com
Program Administrator: Julie Wolin, Pres. *Admissions Contact:* Tom Broeren.
Year Established: 1994.
Staff: Full-time: 8; Part-time: 10.
Avg Enrollment: 75. *Avg Class Size:* 8. *Number of Graduates per Year:* 75.
Wheelchair Access: Yes.
Accreditation/Approval/Licensing: State board: PA Board of Private Licensed Schools.
Field of Study: Acupressure; Aromatherapy; Ayurvedic Medicine; Deep Tissue Massage; Energy Work; Geriatric Massage; Infant Massage; Massage Therapy*; Oriental Medicine; Prenatal Massage; Qigong; Reflexology; Reiki; Shiatsu; Sports Massage; Traditional Chinese Medicine; Yoga Teacher Training. *Program Name/Length:* Massage Therapy, 1080 hrs.
Degrees Offered: CEUs; Diploma.
License/Certification Preparation: National Certification Board for Therapeutic Massage and Bodywork.
Admission Requirements: Min age: 18; High school diploma/GED; Min GPA: 2.0; Interview.
Tuition and Fees: $12,246 + $1600 supplies, equipment.
Financial Aid: Loans; VA approved; Vocational rehabilitation.
Career Services: Career counseling; Career information; Interview set up; Resume service.

696. Mount Nittany Institute of Natural Health
301 Shiloh Rd, State College, PA 16801
Phone: (814) 238-1121; *Fax:* (814) 238-8145
E-mail: mail2@mtnittanyinstitute.com *Internet:* http://www.mtnittanyinstitute.com
Program Administrator: Anne Mascelli, Dir. *Admissions Contact:* Jennifer Welch.
Year Established: 1995.
Staff: Part-time: 12.
Avg Enrollment: 60. *Avg Class Size:* 20. *Number of Graduates per Year:* 40.
Wheelchair Access: Yes.
Accreditation/Approval/Licensing: State board: PA Board of Private Licensed Schools.
Field of Study: Acupressure; Anatomy and Physiology; Aromatherapy; Connective Tissue Massage; Energy Work*; Herbal Medicine*; Holistic Health*; Massage Therapy*; Neuromuscular Therapy; Polarity Therapy; Reflexology*; Shiatsu; Sports Massage; Swedish Massage*; Tai Chi; Yoga*. *Program Name/Length:* Massage Therapist, 17 mos; Relaxation Massage, 4 mos; Energy Work, 5 mos; Herbal Studies, 1 yr;

Reflexology, 1 yr; Holistic Health Educator, 1 yr.

Degrees Offered: Diploma; Certificate.

License/Certification Preparation: American Reflexology Certification Board; National Certification Board for Therapeutic Massage and Bodywork.

Admission Requirements: Min age: 19; High school diploma/GED; Specific course prerequisites: Background in health or helping profession for Holistic Health Educator; Interview, in person or by phone.

Tuition and Fees: $5535 + $115 books (Massage Therapist); $930 (Herbal Studies); $1885 (Reflexology); $2535 (Holistic Health).

Financial Aid: Payment plan.

Career Services: Career counseling; Career information; Job information.

Wayne

697. Meridian Shiatsu Institute
Five Element Shiatsu Certification
998 Old Eagle School Rd, Ste 1212, Wayne, PA 19087
Phone: (610) 293-4030; *Fax:* (610) 971-9860
E-mail: caroleepf@aol.com
Program Administrator: Carolee Parker, Dir. *Admissions Contact:* George Fleck, VP.
Year Established: 1984.
Staff: Full-time: 3; Part-time: 3.
Avg Enrollment: 45. *Avg Class Size:* 12. *Number of Graduates per Year:* 40.
Wheelchair Access: Yes.
Accreditation/Approval/Licensing: State board: PA Dept of Ed; National Certification Board for Therapeutic Massage and Bodywork (CEUs); American Oriental Bodywork Therapy Association.
Field of Study: Acupressure*; Qigong; Reflexology; Reiki; Shiatsu*; Traditional Chinese Medicine. *Program Name/Length:* Five Element Shiatsu Certification, 540 hrs, 2 yrs.
Degrees Offered: Certificate.
License/Certification Preparation: American Oriental Bodywork Therapy Association.
Admission Requirements: Min age: 18; High school diploma/GED.
Tuition and Fees: $5600.
Financial Aid: Loans.

698. Pennsylvania School of Muscle Therapy, Ltd
994C Old Eagle School Rd, Ste 1005, Wayne, PA 19087
Phone: (610) 687-0888; *Fax:* (610) 687-4726
E-mail: psmt@psmt.com *Internet:* http://www.psmt.com
Program Administrator: MaryJo Myers, CEO. *Admissions Contact:* Jennifer A. Oetzel, Admissions Dir.

Year Established: 1982.
Staff: Full-time: 6 office staff; Part-time: 21.
Avg Enrollment: 175. *Avg Class Size:* 18. *Number of Graduates per Year:* 175.
Wheelchair Access: Yes.
Accreditation/Approval/Licensing: State board: PA Dept of Ed; Commission on Massage Therapy Accreditation; International Massage and Somatic Therapies Accreditation Council; National Certification Board for Therapeutic Massage and Bodywork (CEUs).
Field of Study: Aromatherapy; Deep Muscle Massage; Massage Therapy*; Qigong; Reflexology; Shiatsu; Sports Massage; Swedish Massage*; Traditional Chinese Medicine. *Program Name/Length:* Swedish Massage, 9 mos; Advanced Corrective Muscle Therapy, 1 yr.
Degrees Offered: Diploma; Certificate.
License/Certification Preparation: State: FL, NY Licensed Massage Therapist; DE Massage Practitioner; American Oriental Bodywork Therapy Association; American Reflexology Certification Board; National Certification Board for Therapeutic Massage and Bodywork.
Admission Requirements: Min age: 18; High school diploma/GED.
Application Deadline(s): Fall: Sep; Spring: Jan.
Tuition and Fees: $5150-$9600.
Financial Aid: Loans; VA approved.
Career Services: Career counseling; Career information; Internships; Instruction in business skills; Job placement assistance.

Wyomissing

699. Berks Technical Institute
Professional Massage Therapy
2205 Ridgewood Dr, Wyomissing, PA 19610
Phone: (610) 372-1722; *Fax:* (610) 376-4684
Internet: http://www.berkstech.com
Program Administrator: Tony Dooley, Dir of Ed. *Admissions Contact:* Tony Dooley.
Staff: Part-time: 7.
Avg Enrollment: 55. *Avg Class Size:* 10. *Number of Graduates per Year:* 55.
Wheelchair Access: Yes.
Accreditation/Approval/Licensing: State board: PA Dept of Ed; Accrediting Commission of Career Schools and Colleges of Technology.
Field of Study: Massage Therapy*; Swedish Massage*. *Program Name/Length:* Day, 9 mos; Evening, 18 mos.
Degrees Offered: Certificate.
License/Certification Preparation: National Certification Board for Therapeutic Massage and Bodywork.
Admission Requirements: High school diploma/GED.
Financial Aid: Grants; Loans; Scholarships; VA approved; Vocational rehabilitation; Payment plan.

Career Services: Career counseling; Career information; Internships; Interview set up; Resume service; Job information; Referral service.

700. East-West School of Massage Therapy
Massage Therapy and Bodywork Training; Shiatsu
504 Park Rd N, Wyomissing, PA 19610
Phone: (610) 375-7520; *Fax:* (610) 375-7554
E-mail: ewsmt@talon.net *Internet:* http://www.
ewsmt.com
Program Administrator: Elizabeth Brubaker, Dir.
   Admissions Contact: Elizabeth Brubaker.
Year Established: 1995.
Staff: Part-time: 9.
Avg Enrollment: 25. *Avg Class Size:* 6. *Number of
   Graduates per Year:* 25.
Wheelchair Access: No.
Accreditation/Approval/Licensing: State board: PA
   Dept of Ed; International Massage and Somatic
   Therapies Accreditation Council; National Cer-
   tification Board for Therapeutic Massage and
   Bodywork (CEUs).

Field of Study: Acupressure; Aromatherapy; Energy Work; Massage Therapy*; Polarity Ther-
   apy; Reflexology; Reiki; Shiatsu*; Sports Massage. *Program Name/Length:* Massage Therapy
   and Bodywork Training, 520 hrs, 11 mos;
   Shiatsu, 545 hrs.
Degrees Offered: Diploma.
License/Certification Preparation: National Certif-
   ication Board for Therapeutic Massage and
   Bodywork.
Admission Requirements: Min age: 18; High
   school diploma/GED; Physician's form; Letters
   of reference.
Application Deadline(s): Fall: Sep; Winter: Dec;
   Summer: Jun.
Tuition and Fees: $4490 + $238 books (Massage);
   $4700 + $75 books (Shiatsu).
Financial Aid: Vocational rehabilitation; Berks
   Employment and Training.
Career Services: Career counseling; Career infor-
   mation; Resume service.

PUERTO RICO

San Juan

701. University of Puerto Rico, Medical Sciences Campus
Graduate School of Public Health, Nurse-Midwifery
   Education Program
PO Box 365067, San Juan, PR 00936
Phone: (787) 759-6546; *Fax:* (787) 759-6719
Program Administrator: Irene G. dela Torre, CNM,
   Prog Dir. *Admissions Contact:* Irene G. dela
   Torre.
Year Established: 1998.
Staff: Full-time: 4; Part-time: 2.
Avg Enrollment: 10. *Avg Class Size:* 10. *Number
   of Graduates per Year:* 10.
Wheelchair Access: Yes.
Accreditation/Approval/Licensing: American Col-
   lege of Nurse-Midwives, Division of Accredita-
   tion.

Field of Study: Midwifery*. *Program
   Name/Length:* Master of Public Health—
   Nurse-Midwifery, 2 yrs; Certificate in
   Nurse-Midwifery, 1 yr.
Degrees Offered: Certificate; MPH.
License/Certification Preparation: State: Puerto
   Rico; Certified Nurse-Midwife, American Col-
   lege of Nurse-Midwives.
Admission Requirements: Bachelor's degree; Min
   GPA: 2.75; 2 yrs experience in maternal-child
   health.
Application Deadline(s): Fall: Mar 15.
Tuition and Fees: $1800-$2500 per yr.
Financial Aid: Loans; Scholarships.
Career Services: Career information.

RHODE ISLAND

Kingston

702. University of Rhode Island, College of Nursing

Graduate Program in Nurse-Midwifery
2 Heathman Rd, Kingston, RI 02881
Phone: (401) 874-5328; *Fax:* (401) 874-2061
Program Administrator: Holly Kennedy, PhD, Dir.
Wheelchair Access: Yes.
Accreditation/Approval/Licensing: American College of Nurse-Midwives, Division of Accreditation.
Field of Study: Midwifery*. *Program Name/Length:* 2 yrs/full-time.
Degrees Offered: MS.
License/Certification Preparation: Certified Nurse-Midwife, American College of Nurse-Midwives.
Admission Requirements: Bachelor's degree; RN.
Application Deadline(s): Fall; Spring.
Financial Aid: Federal government aid; Loans.
Career Services: Career counseling; Career information.

SOUTH CAROLINA

Boiling Springs

703. Sherman College of Straight Chiropractic

2020 Springfield Rd, Boiling Springs, SC 29316
Mailing Address: PO Box 1452, Spartanburg, SC 29304
Phone: (864) 578-8770; *Fax:* (864) 599-7145
E-mail: admissions@sherman.edu *Internet:* http://www.sherman.edu
Program Administrator: Dr. David B. Koch, Pres. *Admissions Contact:* Susan S. Newlin, VP for Enrollment Svcs.
Year Established: 1973.
Staff: Full-time: 26; Part-time: 15.
Avg Enrollment: 160. *Avg Class Size:* 40. *Number of Graduates per Year:* 100.
Wheelchair Access: Yes.
Accreditation/Approval/Licensing: Council on Chiropractic Education.
Field of Study: Chiropractic*. *Program Name/Length:* Doctor of Chiropractic, 3 1/4 yrs.
Degrees Offered: DC.
License/Certification Preparation: State: SC; National Board of Chiropractic Examiners.
Admission Requirements: Some college (2 yrs); Min GPA: 2.25; Specific course prerequisites: contact admission office for specific requirements.
Tuition and Fees: $20,133 per yr.
Financial Aid: Federal government aid; Loans; Scholarships; Work study.
Career Services: Career information; Career placement.

Charleston

704. Charleston School of Massage, Inc

Clinical Massage Therapy
778 Folly Rd, Ste 3, Charleston, SC 29412
Phone: (843) 762-7727; *Fax:* (843) 762-1392
Program Administrator: Mark Hendler, PhD, Clinical Dir. *Admissions Contact:* Mark Hendler.
Year Established: 1997.
Staff: Full-time: 2.
Avg Class Size: 14.
Wheelchair Access: Yes.
Accreditation/Approval/Licensing: State board: SC Commission on Higher Ed; SC Division of Professional Licensing.
Field of Study: Acupressure; Aromatherapy; Ayurvedic Medicine; Deep Tissue Massage; Energy Work; Herbal Medicine; Massage Therapy*; Reflexology; Reiki; Shiatsu; Spa Therapies. *Program Name/Length:* Clinical Massage Therapy, 6 mos/full-time or 1 yr/part-time; Specialization programs.
Degrees Offered: Certificate.
License/Certification Preparation: State: FL and SC Licensed Massage Therapist; National Certification Board for Therapeutic Massage and Bodywork.
Admission Requirements: Min age: 18; High school diploma/GED; Physical exam.
Tuition and Fees: $4775.
Financial Aid: Loans; Vocational rehabilitation; Payment plan.
Career Services: Career information.

705. Medical University of South Carolina, College of Nursing

Nurse-Midwifery Program
99 Jonathan Lucas St, Charleston, SC 29403
Phone: (843) 792-2051
E-mail: bearem@musc.edu *Internet:* http://www.
musc.edu
Program Administrator: Deborah Williamson,
CNM, Interim Prog Dir.
Accreditation/Approval/Licensing: American College of Nurse-Midwives, Division of Accreditation.
Field of Study: Midwifery*.
Degrees Offered: MSN.
License/Certification Preparation: Certified
Nurse-Midwife, American College of
Nurse-Midwives.
Admission Requirements: Bachelor's degree; RN.

Greenville

706. Massage School of MTA, Inc

Therapeutic Massage
1901 Laurens Rd, Ste H, Greenville, SC 29607
Phone: (864) 232-9001
Program Administrator: Kenn Elrod, LMT,
Owner.
Year Established: 1997.
Staff: Full-time: 3; Part-time: 1.
Avg Enrollment: 20. *Avg Class Size:* 10. *Number
of Graduates per Year:* 20.
Wheelchair Access: Yes.
Accreditation/Approval/Licensing: State board: SC
Commission on Higher Ed.
Field of Study: Acupressure; Aromatherapy;
CranioSacral Therapy; Deep Tissue Massage;
Energy Work; Massage Therapy*; Polarity
Therapy; Reflexology; Reiki; Shiatsu. *Program
Name/Length:* 500 hrs, 6 mos.
Degrees Offered: Certificate.
License/Certification Preparation: State: SC Licensed Massage Therapist; National Certification Board for Therapeutic Massage and Bodywork.
Admission Requirements: Min age: 18; High
school diploma/GED.
Application Deadline(s): Fall; Summer.
Tuition and Fees: $3700.
Career Services: Career information.

Hilton Head Island

707. Dovestar Institute, Hilton Head Island

4C Northridge Dr, Hilton Head Island, SC 29928
Phone: (803) 342-3361, (888) 222-5603; *Fax:* (803)
342-3639
Internet: http://www.dovestar.edu
Program Administrator: Kamala Renner, Dir.
Year Established: 1973.

Staff: Full-time: 3; Part-time: 12.
Avg Class Size: 12.
Wheelchair Access: Yes.
Accreditation/Approval/Licensing: State board: SC
Commission on Higher Ed.
Field of Study: Acupressure; Breathwork; Colon
Hydrotherapy; Energy Work*; Hypnotherapy*;
Kriya Massage*; Massage Therapy*; Qigong;
Reflexology; Reiki*; Shiatsu; Yoga Teacher
Training*. *Program Name/Length:* Colon
Hydrotherapy, 2 mos; Reiki-Alchemia, 3 mos;
Alchemical Synergy/Hypnotherapy, 6 mos;
Kriya Massage, 9 mos; Alchemia Yoga Teacher
Training, 1 yr.
Degrees Offered: Certificate.
License/Certification Preparation: American
Council of Hypnotist Examiners; American Oriental Bodywork Therapy Association; National
Certification Board for Therapeutic Massage and
Bodywork.
Tuition and Fees: $2000-$6000.
Financial Aid: State government aid; Work study;
Vocational rehabilitation.
Career Services: Career counseling; Career information; Internships.

Myrtle Beach

708. Horry Georgetown Technical College

Massage Therapy
743 Hemlock Ave, Myrtle Beach, SC 29577
Phone: (843) 477-0808; *Fax:* (843) 477-0775
Program Administrator: Angelique Fahy, Instr.
Admissions Contact: Lisa Aglietti, Counselor.
Year Established: 1997.
Staff: Full-time: 7.
Avg Enrollment: 40. *Avg Class Size:* 16. *Number
of Graduates per Year:* 40.
Wheelchair Access: Yes.
Accreditation/Approval/Licensing: State board: SC
Board of Massage; Southern Association of Colleges and Schools.
Field of Study: Massage Therapy*. *Program
Name/Length:* 600 hrs, 3 semesters.
Degrees Offered: Certificate.
License/Certification Preparation: State: SC Licensed Massage Therapist; National Certification Board for Therapeutic Massage and Bodywork.
Admission Requirements: Min age: 18; High
school diploma/GED; Physical exam.
Application Deadline(s): Fall: Aug 1.
Financial Aid: Federal government aid; Loans;
State government aid; Work study; VA approved.
Career Services: Career counseling; Career information; Internships.

Spartanburg

709. Southeastern School of Neuromuscular and Massage Therapy Inc, Spartanburg

Clinical Neuromuscular Massage
7000 N Pine St, Ste 2B Pinewood Mall,
   Spartanburg, SC 29303
Phone: (864) 591-1134; *Fax:* (864) 582-7805
E-mail: sesptg@aol.com *Internet:* http://www.
   se-massage.com
Program Administrator: Harold Privette, DC, Dir.
   Admissions Contact: Janice Schuelke, Asst Dir.
Year Established: 1991.
Staff: Full-time: 5; Part-time: 2.
Avg Enrollment: 64. *Avg Class Size:* 16. *Number
   of Graduates per Year:* 64.
Wheelchair Access: Yes.
Accreditation/Approval/Licensing: State board: SC
   Commission on Higher Ed; International Mas-
sage and Somatic Therapies Accreditation
Council.
Field of Study: Aromatherapy; Massage Therapy*;
   Myofascial Release; Neuromuscular Therapy*;
   Swedish Massage*. *Program Name/Length:*
   500 hrs, 6 mos/full-time or 1 yr/part-time.
Degrees Offered: Certificate.
License/Certification Preparation: State: SC Li-
   censed Massage Therapist; National Certifica-
   tion Board for Therapeutic Massage and Body-
   work.
Admission Requirements: Min age: 18; High
   school diploma/GED.
Tuition and Fees: $5300.
Financial Aid: Loans; VA approved; Vocational
   rehabilitation.
Career Services: Career counseling; Career information; Internships.

SOUTH DAKOTA

Mitchell

710. Carrie's Kadesh and School of Massage

Massage Theory and Practice
112 E 3rd Ave, Mitchell, SD 57301
Phone: (605) 996-3916
Program Administrator: Carrie Badker, Owner/Dir.
   Admissions Contact: Carrie Badker.
Year Established: 1980.
Staff: Full-time: 2.
Avg Enrollment: 10. *Avg Class Size:* 10. *Number
   of Graduates per Year:* 10.
Wheelchair Access: Yes.
Field of Study: Acupressure; Aromatherapy; Mas-
   sage Therapy*; Polarity Therapy; Reflexology;
   Sports Massage. *Program Name/Length:* Anat-
   omy and Basic Massage Techniques, 5 mos.
Degrees Offered: Diploma.
License/Certification Preparation: National Certif-
   ication Board for Therapeutic Massage and
   Bodywork.
Admission Requirements: Min age: 18; High
   school diploma/GED; Interview; Health release.
Application Deadline(s): Fall: Feb 1; Summer:
   Aug 1.
Tuition and Fees: $4500.
Financial Aid: VA approved.
Career Services: Career information.

Rapid City

711. Scientific Massage Institute

1523 1/2 Deadwood Ave, Rapid City, SD 57702
Mailing Address: 3213 W Main, Box 258, Rapid
   City, SD 57702
Phone: (605) 341-5402; *Fax:* (605) 342-0554
E-mail: scimas@aol.com
Program Administrator: Sandy Feist, RN, Dir. *Ad-
   missions Contact:* Sandy Feist.
Year Established: 1980.
Staff: Full-time: 1; Part-time: 1-3.
Avg Enrollment: 22. *Avg Class Size:* 8. *Number of
   Graduates per Year:* 18.
Wheelchair Access: Yes.
Field of Study: Acupressure; Chair Massage; Infant
   Massage; Massage Therapy*; Reflexology. *Pro-
   gram Name/Length:* Basic Massage (including
   Anatomy, Physiology, Pathology), 500 hrs.
Degrees Offered: Certificate.
License/Certification Preparation: National Certif-
   ication Board for Therapeutic Massage and
   Bodywork.
Admission Requirements: Min age: 18; High
   school diploma/GED.
Application Deadline(s): Fall: Aug 15; Winter: Dec
   15; Spring: Apr 15.
Tuition and Fees: $3250 + books, lab fees.
Financial Aid: Payment plan.
Career Services: Job information.

Sioux Falls

712. South Dakota School of Massage Therapy

902 W 22nd St, Sioux Falls, SD 57105
Phone: (605) 334-4422; *Fax:* (605) 334-4422
Program Administrator: Robin Jensen, Dir. *Admissions Contact:* Robin Jensen.
Year Established: 1987.
Staff: Full-time: 2; Part-time: 2.
Avg Enrollment: 40. *Avg Class Size:* 20. *Number of Graduates per Year:* 38.
Wheelchair Access: No.
Field of Study: Acupressure; Anatomy and Physiology; Aromatherapy; Deep Tissue Massage; Hydrotherapy; Kinesiology; Massage Therapy*; Qigong; Rebirthing; Reflexology; Shiatsu; Sports Massage; Swedish Massage*; Yoga. *Program Name/Length:* 6 mos.
Degrees Offered: Certificate.
License/Certification Preparation: National Certification Board for Therapeutic Massage and Bodywork.
Admission Requirements: Min age: 18; High school diploma/GED.
Tuition and Fees: $4800.
Career Services: Career information; Business class.

713. Stress Management Services, Inc, Sioux Falls School of Massage Therapy

317 S Cleveland Ave, Sioux Falls, SD 57103
Phone: (605) 330-0175
Program Administrator: Kristie R. Knudtson, Pres. *Admissions Contact:* Kristie R. Knudtson.
Year Established: 1995.
Staff: Full-time: 3; Part-time: 2.
Avg Enrollment: 30. *Avg Class Size:* 6. *Number of Graduates per Year:* 30.
Wheelchair Access: Yes.
Field of Study: Massage Therapy*. *Program Name/Length:* 200 hrs, 10 wks; Seminars given in various locations; 500 hrs, 20 wks.
Degrees Offered: Diploma.
License/Certification Preparation: National Certification Board for Therapeutic Massage and Bodywork.
Admission Requirements: Min age: 18; High school diploma/GED.
Tuition and Fees: $2350 (200 hrs); $5800 (500 hrs).
Financial Aid: VA approved.
Career Services: Career counseling; Career information.

TENNESSEE

Brentwood

714. Cumberland Institute for Wellness Education

500 Wilson Pike Cir, Ste 121, Brentwood, TN 37027
Mailing Address: PO Box 1527, Brentwood, TN 37024-1527
Phone: (615) 370-9794; *Fax:* (615) 370-5869
E-mail: cumberinst@aol.com
Program Administrator: Chad Porter, Dir. *Admissions Contact:* Sharrye Taylor, Admin.
Year Established: 1987.
Staff: Full-time: 3; Part-time: 21.
Avg Enrollment: 120. *Avg Class Size:* 25. *Number of Graduates per Year:* 60.
Wheelchair Access: Yes.
Accreditation/Approval/Licensing: State board: TN Higher Ed Commission.
Field of Study: Acupressure; Aromatherapy; CranioSacral Therapy; Lymphatic Massage; Massage Therapy*; Sports Massage. *Program Name/Length:* Massage Therapist, 500 hrs, 9 mos.
Degrees Offered: Certificate.
License/Certification Preparation: State: TN Licensed Massage Therapist; National Certification Board for Therapeutic Massage and Bodywork.
Admission Requirements: Min age: 18; High school diploma/GED.
Application Deadline(s): Fall: Aug; Winter: Dec; Spring: Mar; Summer: May.
Tuition and Fees: $7000.
Financial Aid: Loans; State government aid; Vocational rehabilitation.
Career Services: Career counseling; Career information; Job lists.

Chattanooga

715. Tennesee Institute of Healing Arts

5779 Brainerd Rd, Chattanooga, TN 37411
Phone: (423) 892-9882, (800) 735-1910; *Fax:* (423) 892-5006
E-mail: tiha@aol.com *Internet:* http://www.tiha.com

Program Administrator: Alan Jordan, Exec Dir.
Admissions Contact: Mary Ringenberg, Dir.
Year Established: 1989.
Staff: Full-time: 3; Part-time: 16.
Avg Enrollment: 60. *Avg Class Size:* 18. *Number of Graduates per Year:* 45.
Wheelchair Access: Yes.
Accreditation/Approval/Licensing: State board: TN Higher Ed Commission; Commission on Massage Therapy Accreditation; Accrediting Commission of Career Schools and Colleges of Technology; National Certification Board for Therapeutic Massage and Bodywork (CEUs).
Field of Study: Massage Therapy*; Neuromuscular Therapy. *Program Name/Length:* 1 yr.
Degrees Offered: Diploma.
License/Certification Preparation: National Certification Board for Therapeutic Massage and Bodywork.
Admission Requirements: Min age: 18; High school diploma/GED.
Tuition and Fees: $7500.
Financial Aid: Federal government aid; Loans; VA approved; Vocational rehabilitation.
Career Services: Career information.

Hendersonville

716. Middle Tennessee Institute of Therapeutic Massage
394 W Main St, Ste A-15, Hendersonville, TN 37075
Phone: (615) 826-9500; *Fax:* (615) 826-9527
E-mail: mtitm@bellsouth.net *Internet:* http://www.mtitm.com
Program Administrator: Tami Mercer, Dir. *Admissions Contact:* Shannon Dickson, Exec Admin.
Year Established: 1994.
Staff: Full-time: 10; Part-time: 2.
Avg Enrollment: 125. *Avg Class Size:* 15. *Number of Graduates per Year:* 30.
Wheelchair Access: Yes.
Accreditation/Approval/Licensing: Accrediting Council for Continuing Education and Training; TN Board of Massage.
Field of Study: Aromatherapy*; CranioSacral Therapy*; Massage Therapy*; Neuromuscular Therapy*; Polarity Therapy*; Reflexology*; Shiatsu*; Sports Massage*. *Program Name/Length:* 500 hrs, 12-15 mos.
Degrees Offered: CEUs; Certificate.
License/Certification Preparation: State: TN Licensed Massage Therapist; National Certification Board for Therapeutic Massage and Bodywork.
Admission Requirements: Min age: 18; High school diploma/GED.
Application Deadline(s): Fall: Sep; Winter: Jan; Spring: Apr; Summer: Jul.
Tuition and Fees: $6100 + $500 table.

Financial Aid: Loans; Scholarships; Vocational rehabilitation.
Career Services: Job information; Referral service.

Memphis

717. American Academy of Medical Hypnoanalysts
Clinical Training Program
5628 Murray Rd, Ste 4, Memphis, TN 38119-3876
Phone: (800) 344-9766; *Fax:* (901) 683-1224
Program Administrator: David Leistikow, MD, Dir. *Admissions Contact:* David Leistikow.
Year Established: 1974.
Staff: Part-time: 12.
Avg Enrollment: 100. *Number of Graduates per Year:* 100.
Wheelchair Access: No.
Field of Study: Hypnotherapy*. *Program Name/Length:* Basic Practical Hypnosis; Postgraduate Clinical Training, 3 mos-2 yrs; Seminars given in various locations.
Degrees Offered: Certificate.
Admission Requirements: Master's degree in health or behavioral sciences; Specific course prerequisites: Basic course required for Clinical Training.
Tuition and Fees: $4800 (Clinical Training).

718. The Massage Institute of Memphis
3445 Poplar, Ste 4, Memphis, TN 38111
Phone: (901) 324-4411; *Fax:* (901) 324-4470
E-mail: massinst@bellsouth.net *Internet:* http://www.themassageinstitute.com
Program Administrator: Karen E. Craig, Owner/Dir. *Admissions Contact:* Karen E. Craig.
Year Established: 1987.
Staff: Full-time: 1; Part-time: 14.
Avg Enrollment: 30. *Avg Class Size:* 15. *Number of Graduates per Year:* 26.
Wheelchair Access: Yes.
Accreditation/Approval/Licensing: State board: TN Higher Ed Commission; National Certification Board for Therapeutic Massage and Bodywork (CEUs).
Field of Study: Energy Work; Healing Touch; Massage Therapy*; Reflexology; Sports Massage; Trigger Point Therapy. *Program Name/Length:* Massage Therapy, 550 hrs, 6 mos/days or 1 yr/evenings.
Degrees Offered: Diploma.
License/Certification Preparation: State: TN, AR Licensed Massage Therapist; National Certification Board for Therapeutic Massage and Bodywork.
Admission Requirements: Min age: 18; High school diploma/GED.
Application Deadline(s): Fall: Sep 27; Winter: Dec 31; Summer: Jun 1.
Tuition and Fees: $4830.

Financial Aid: VA approved; Vocational rehabilitation.
Career Services: Career information.

719. Tennessee School of Massage
Professional Massage Therapy
4726 Poplar, Ste 4, Memphis, TN 38117
Phone: (901) 767-8484
E-mail: relax@touchofhealth.com *Internet:* http://www.touchofhealth.com
Program Administrator: Cissie Pryor, RN, Dir. *Admissions Contact:* Cissie Pryor.
Year Established: 1988.
Staff: Full-time: 3; Part-time: 2.
Avg Enrollment: 50. *Avg Class Size:* 10. *Number of Graduates per Year:* 48.
Wheelchair Access: Yes.
Accreditation/Approval/Licensing: State board: TN Higher Ed Commission.
Field of Study: Acupressure; Aromatherapy; Hypnotherapy; Massage Therapy*; Polarity Therapy; Reflexology; Shiatsu; Spa Therapies; Swedish Massage*. *Program Name/Length:* Professional Massage Therapy, 9 mos.
Degrees Offered: Diploma.
License/Certification Preparation: State: TN Licensed Massage Therapist; National Certification Board for Therapeutic Massage and Bodywork.
Admission Requirements: Min age: 18; High school diploma/GED.
Application Deadline(s): Fall: Aug; Winter: Sep; Spring: Mar; Summer: May.
Tuition and Fees: $4200 + $150 books.
Financial Aid: Work study; Payment plan.
Career Services: Job information.

Nashville

720. Institute of Therapeutic Massage and Movement, Inc
1161 Murfreesboro Rd, Ste 405, Nashville, TN 37217
Phone: (615) 360-8554
E-mail: itmm@aol.com *Internet:* http://www.citysearch.com/nas/itmm
Program Administrator: Fran Cegelka, Pres. *Admissions Contact:* Angela Wood, VP.
Year Established: 1995.
Staff: Full-time: 2.
Avg Enrollment: 90. *Avg Class Size:* 15. *Number of Graduates per Year:* 90.
Wheelchair Access: Yes.
Accreditation/Approval/Licensing: State board: TN Higher Ed Commission; National Certification Board for Therapeutic Massage and Bodywork (CEUs).
Field of Study: Deep Tissue Massage*; Massage Therapy*. *Program Name/Length:* 500 hrs, 7 1/2 mos.
Degrees Offered: Diploma.

License/Certification Preparation: State: TN Licensed Massage Therapist; National Certification Board for Therapeutic Massage and Bodywork.
Admission Requirements: Min age: 18; High school diploma/GED.
Tuition and Fees: $5000 + $200 books, supplies.
Financial Aid: State government aid; Vocational rehabilitation; Payment plan.
Career Services: Career counseling; Career information.

721. Natural Health Institute
209 10th Ave S, Ste 212, Nashville, TN 37203
Phone: (615) 242-6811; *Fax:* (615) 242-6288
Program Administrator: Jaya Judy Seeley, Exec Steward. *Admissions Contact:* Angela Schlitt, Exec Asst.
Year Established: 1996.
Staff: Full-time: 12; Part-time: 4.
Avg Enrollment: 50. *Avg Class Size:* 14. *Number of Graduates per Year:* 30.
Wheelchair Access: Yes.
Accreditation/Approval/Licensing: State board: TN Board of Massage; TN Commission of Higher Ed.
Field of Study: Acupressure; Ayurvedic Massage; Feldenkrais; Herbal Medicine*; Hypnotherapy*; Massage Therapy*; Polarity Therapy; Reflexology; Reiki*; Somatic Education*. *Program Name/Length:* Massage Therapy, 500 hrs, 7 mos; Seminars given in various locations; Herbal Studies, 180 hrs, 1 yr; Clinical Hypnotherapy, 250 hrs, 1 yr; Somatic Education, 250 hrs, 2 yrs.
Degrees Offered: CEUs; Diploma; Certificate.
License/Certification Preparation: State: TN Licensed Massage Therapist; American Board of Clinical Hypnosis; National Certification Board for Therapeutic Massage and Bodywork.
Admission Requirements: Min age: 18; High school diploma/GED; Some college for Somatic Education.
Application Deadline(s): Fall: Sep 5; Winter: Jan 5; Summer: May 15.
Tuition and Fees: $5000 (Massage Therapy); $1800 (Herbal Studies); $2500 (Hypnotherapy; Somatic Education).
Financial Aid: Loans; State government aid; Work study; Vocational rehabilitation.
Career Services: Career counseling; Career information; Internships.

722. Vanderbilt University, School of Nursing
Nurse-Midwifery Program
102 Godchaux Hall, Nashville, TN 37240-0008
Phone: (615) 322-3800
E-mail: vusn_admissions@mcmail.vanderbilt.edu
Internet: http://www.mc.vanderbilt.edu/nursing/
Program Administrator: Barbara Petersen, CNM, Dir.

Accreditation/Approval/Licensing: American College of Nurse-Midwives, Division of Accreditation.
Field of Study: Midwifery*.
Degrees Offered: MSN.

License/Certification Preparation: Certified Nurse-Midwife, American College of Nurse-Midwives.
Admission Requirements: Bachelor's degree; RN.

TEXAS

Austin

723. Academy of Oriental Medicine, Austin
2700 W Anderson Ln, Ste 117, Austin, TX 78757
Phone: (512) 454-1188; *Fax:* (512) 454-7001
E-mail: info@aoma.edu *Internet:* http://www.aoma.edu
Program Administrator: Stuart Watts, LAc, President. *Admissions Contact:* Jim Coombes, Exec Dir.
Year Established: 1993.
Staff: Full-time: 5; Part-time: 19.
Avg Enrollment: 28. *Avg Class Size:* 26. *Number of Graduates per Year:* 18.
Wheelchair Access: Yes.
Accreditation/Approval/Licensing: State board: CA Acupuncture Board; NM Board of Acupuncture and Oriental Medicine; TX Board of Acupuncture and Oriental Medicine; Accreditation Commission for Acupuncture and Oriental Medicine; American Oriental Bodywork Therapy Association.
Field of Study: Acupressure; Acupuncture*; Herbal Medicine; Jin Shin Do; Oriental Medicine*; Qigong*; Shiatsu*; Tai Chi; Traditional Chinese Medicine; Tui Na*. *Program Name/Length:* Shiatsu, 600 hrs, 1 yr; Tui Na, 600 hrs, 1 yr; Chi Nei Tsang, 600 hrs, 1 yr; Master of Science in Oriental Medicine, 2880 hrs, 3 yrs; Post Graduate Training in Oriental Medicine, 400 hrs, 2 yrs; Teacher Training in Oriental Medicine.
Degrees Offered: CEUs; MSOM; Certificate in Oriental Bodywork; Teacher Training Certificate.
License/Certification Preparation: State: CA, NM, TX Boards of Acupuncture and Oriental Medicine; National Certification Commission for Acupuncture and Oriental Medicine; American Oriental Bodywork Therapy Association.
Admission Requirements: High school diploma/GED; Some college (2 yrs); Min GPA: 2.0.
Application Deadline(s): Fall: Sep; Winter: Jan; Summer: Jul.
Tuition and Fees: $7750 (1-yr programs); $26,500 (MSOM).
Financial Aid: Federal government aid; Loans; Scholarships; VA approved; Vocational rehabilitation.

Career Services: Career counseling; Career information; Internships; Job information.

724. The Lauterstein-Conway Massage School
4701-B Burnet Rd, Austin, TX 78756
Phone: (512) 374-9222, (800) 474-0852; *Fax:* (512) 374-9812
E-mail: info@tlcschool.com *Internet:* http://www.tlcschool.com
Program Administrator: John Conway, Co-Dir; David Lauterstein, Pres. *Admissions Contact:* Donna Jarrett, Admissions Counselor.
Year Established: 1989.
Staff: Part-time: 25.
Avg Enrollment: 180. *Avg Class Size:* 26 (practical), 50 (lecture). *Number of Graduates per Year:* 150.
Wheelchair Access: Yes.
Accreditation/Approval/Licensing: State board: TX Dept of Health; Commission on Massage Therapy Accreditation; National Certification Board for Therapeutic Massage and Bodywork (CEUs).
Field of Study: Acupressure; CranioSacral Therapy; Energy Work; Massage Therapy*; Reflexology; Shiatsu; Sports Massage; Swedish Massage*; Zero Balancing* Deep Tissue Massage. *Program Name/Length:* Professional Massage Therapy Training: Semester One, 300 hrs, 5-8 mos; Semester Two, 250 hrs, 5 mos; Semester Three, 200 hrs, 5 mos.
Degrees Offered: Diploma.
License/Certification Preparation: State: TX Registered Massage Therapist; National Certification Board for Therapeutic Massage and Bodywork; Zero Balancing Association.
Admission Requirements: Min age: 18; High school diploma/GED; Interview.
Application Deadline(s): Fall: Sep 1; Winter: Oct 20; Spring: Mar 1; Summer: May 15.
Tuition and Fees: $2550 per semester (Semesters One and Two); $2200 (Semester Three).
Financial Aid: Scholarships; Payment plan.
Career Services: Career counseling; Career information; Internships.

725. National Institute for Health Sciences and The Austin School of Massage Therapy

2600 W Stassney, Austin, TX 78745
Phone: (512) 462-3005, (800) 276-2768; *Fax:* (512) 462-3265
Internet: http://www.asmt.com
Program Administrator: Idar Dart, Dir. *Admissions Contact:* Bob Brock, Admissions Dir.
Year Established: 1985.
Staff: Part-time: 26.
Avg Enrollment: 750. *Avg Class Size:* 27. *Number of Graduates per Year:* 650.
Wheelchair Access: Yes.
Accreditation/Approval/Licensing: State board: TX Dept of Health; International Massage and Somatic Therapies Accreditation Council.
Field of Study: Holistic Health*; Massage Therapy*; Neuromuscular Therapy*; Polarity Therapy; Reflexology; Shiatsu. *Program Name/Length:* 6 mos.
License/Certification Preparation: State: TX Registered Massage Therapist.
Admission Requirements: Min age: 18; High school diploma/GED.
Tuition and Fees: $2850.
Financial Aid: Loans; Scholarships; Work study; VA approved.
Career Services: Career counseling; Career information; Internships; Job placement.

726. Texas College of Traditional Chinese Medicine

Master of Science in Oriental Medicine
4005 Manchaca Rd, Ste 102, Austin, TX 78704
Phone: (512) 444-8082, (800) 252-5088; *Fax:* (512) 444-6345
E-mail: texastcm@texastcm.edu *Internet:* http://www.texastcm.edu
Program Administrator: Lisa P.H. Lin, Dir. *Admissions Contact:* Kermit Heimann, Dir of Admin.
Year Established: 1990.
Staff: Full-time: 5; Part-time: 7.
Avg Enrollment: 50. *Avg Class Size:* 25. *Number of Graduates per Year:* 15.
Wheelchair Access: Yes.
Accreditation/Approval/Licensing: State board: TX Board of Acupuncture Examiners; Accreditation Commission for Acupuncture and Oriental Medicine.
Field of Study: Acupuncture*; Herbal Medicine; Oriental Medicine*; Qigong; Traditional Chinese Medicine*. *Program Name/Length:* 6 semesters, 3 yrs (day or evening classes).
Degrees Offered: MS.
License/Certification Preparation: State: TX Licensed Acupuncturist; National Certification Commission for Acupuncture and Oriental Medicine.
Admission Requirements: Min age: 18; Some college (2 yrs); Min GPA: 2.25.

Application Deadline(s): Fall: Aug 1; Spring: Feb 1.
Tuition and Fees: $3500 per semester.
Financial Aid: Federal government aid; Scholarships; VA approved; TX Rehabilitation Commission.
Career Services: Career counseling; Career information; Job information.

727. Texas Healing Arts Institute, LLC and School of Massage

2704 Rio Grande, Ste 11, Austin, TX 78705
Phone: (512) 236-8424; *Fax:* (512) 236-1040
E-mail: school@thaisom.com *Internet:* http://www.thaisom.com
Program Administrator: Dr. Kirsten Kern, Co-Dir; Dr. Eri Weinstein, Co-Dir. *Admissions Contact:* Jo Bunny, Admin.
Year Established: 1997.
Staff: Full-time: 2; Part-time: 2.
Avg Enrollment: 80. *Avg Class Size:* 16. *Number of Graduates per Year:* 70.
Wheelchair Access: Yes.
Accreditation/Approval/Licensing: State board: TX Dept of Health.
Field of Study: CranioSacral Therapy; Deep Tissue Massage*; Hydrotherapy; Massage Therapy*; Myofascial Release; Reflexology; Shiatsu. *Program Name/Length:* Massage Therapy, 300 hrs, 4-6 mos; Advanced Seminars in Anatomy and Physiology, CranioSacral Therapy, Hydrotherapy, Myofascial Release, Reflexology, and Shiatsu.
Degrees Offered: Certificate.
License/Certification Preparation: State: TX Registered Massage Therapist.
Admission Requirements: Min age: 18; High school diploma/GED.
Tuition and Fees: $1950 + $200 books, $39 insurance.
Financial Aid: Payment plan.
Career Services: Career information; Internships.

Beaumont

728. Greater Beaumont School of Massage

229 Dowlen Rd, Ste 15A, Beaumont, TX 77706
Phone: (409) 866-8661; *Fax:* (409) 866-4371
Program Administrator: Jennifer Smith, Dir. *Admissions Contact:* Jennifer Smith.
Year Established: 1996.
Staff: Part-time: 4.
Avg Enrollment: 25. *Avg Class Size:* 10. *Number of Graduates per Year:* 25.
Wheelchair Access: Yes.
Accreditation/Approval/Licensing: State board: TX Dept of Health.
Field of Study: Massage Therapy*. *Program Name/Length:* Basic Massage Therapy, 300 hrs.
Degrees Offered: Diploma.

License/Certification Preparation: State: TX Registered Massage Therapist.
Admission Requirements: Min age: 18; High school diploma/GED.
Tuition and Fees: $2600 includes books, supplies.
Financial Aid: Payment plan.

Boerne

729. Anne King's Hypnosis Training
109 Smokey River N, Boerne, TX 78006
Phone: (830) 537-5411; Fax: (830) 537-5404
E-mail: akhypno@gvtc.com
Program Administrator: Anne King, Owner. Admissions Contact: Anne King.
Year Established: 1992.
Staff: Full-time: 1.
Avg Enrollment: 90. Avg Class Size: 15. Number of Graduates per Year: 90.
Wheelchair Access: No.
Accreditation/Approval/Licensing: International Medical and Dental Hypnotherapy Association.
Field of Study: Hypnotherapy*. Program Name/Length: Basic, 40 hrs; Intermediate, 40 hrs; Advanced, 40 hrs; Marketing, 22 hrs.
Degrees Offered: CEUs; Certificate.
License/Certification Preparation: International Medical and Dental Hypnotherapy Association.
Tuition and Fees: $400 per course (40 hrs).

Colleyville

730. The Institute of Natural Healing Sciences, Inc
4100 Felps Dr, Ste E, Colleyville, TX 76034
Phone: (817) 498-0716; Fax: (817) 281-1414
E-mail: hmmj@nkn.net Internet: http://www.body-mind-spirit.com
Program Administrator: Hollis M. Morrow, Jr., Admin. Admissions Contact: Hollis M. Morrow, Jr.
Year Established: 1986.
Staff: Full-time: 4; Part-time: 4.
Avg Enrollment: 120. Avg Class Size: 30. Number of Graduates per Year: 118.
Wheelchair Access: Yes.
Accreditation/Approval/Licensing: State board: TX Dept of Health.
Field of Study: Acupressure; Chair Massage; CranioSacral Therapy; Massage Therapy*; Polarity Therapy; Reflexology; Shiatsu; Sports Massage. Program Name/Length: Basic Class, 300 hrs, 4-8 mos; Advanced Class, 290 hrs, 8 mos.
Degrees Offered: Certificate.
License/Certification Preparation: State: TX Registered Massage Therapist.
Admission Requirements: Min age: 18; High school diploma/GED; References; Health release.

Tuition and Fees: $2150 per semester.
Financial Aid: Loans; Payment plan.
Career Services: Career information; Internships.

Dallas

731. Heartsong Hypnotherapy Training Center
4314 W Lovers Ln, Dallas, TX 75209
Mailing Address: PO Box 7972, Dallas, TX 75209
Phone: (214) 358-3633; Fax: (241) 352-1338
E-mail: hypnosis@heartsong.com Internet: http://www.heartsong.com
Program Administrator: Bette Epstein, Owner/Co-Dir. Admissions Contact: Bette Epstein; Francisco Philibert, Co-Dir.
Year Established: 1989.
Staff: Full-time: 2; Part-time: 5.
Avg Enrollment: 50. Avg Class Size: 15. Number of Graduates per Year: 50.
Wheelchair Access: Yes.
Accreditation/Approval/Licensing: Accrediting Council for Continuing Education and Training; American Society of Hypnotists.
Field of Study: Aromatherapy; Biofeedback; Energy Work; Hypnotherapy*; Reiki. Program Name/Length: Clinical Hypnotherapist Certification, 250 hrs.
License/Certification Preparation: American Board of Clinical Hypnosis; American Council of Hypnotist Examiners.
Admission Requirements: High school diploma/GED; Interview and test.
Application Deadline(s): Fall: Sep; Winter: Jan; Spring: May; Summer: Jul.
Tuition and Fees: $3000.
Financial Aid: State government aid; Vocational rehabilitation; Payment plan.
Career Services: Career counseling; Career information; Job information; Referral service.

732. Parker College of Chiropractic
2500 Walnut Hill Lane, Dallas, TX 75229
Phone: (214) 438-6932, (800) 438-6932; Fax: (214) 357-3620
E-mail: nstern@parkercc.edu Internet: http://www.parkercc.edu
Program Administrator: Neil Stern, DC, Acting Pres. Admissions Contact: Reba Sexton, Admissions Dir.
Year Established: 1982.
Staff: Full-time: 130; Part-time: 8.
Avg Enrollment: 350. Avg Class Size: 110. Number of Graduates per Year: 280.
Wheelchair Access: Yes.
Accreditation/Approval/Licensing: State board: TX Board of Chiropractic; Council on Chiropractic Education; Southern Association of Colleges and Schools.

Field of Study: Chiropractic*. *Program Name/Length:* Doctor of Chiropractic, 9 trimesters, 3 yrs.
Degrees Offered: BS; DC.
License/Certification Preparation: State: TX Doctor of Chiropractic.
Admission Requirements: Min age: 18; Some college (2 yrs); Min GPA: 2.5; Specific course prerequisites: 6 hrs English, 18 hrs humanities/social sciences, biology, inorganic chemistry, organic chemistry, physics.
Tuition and Fees: $4400 per trimester.
Financial Aid: Federal government aid; Grants; Loans; Scholarships; State government aid; Work study.
Career Services: Career counseling; Career information; Internships.

733. Parkland School of Nurse-Midwifery
Parkland Memorial Hospital, UTSW Medical Center at Dallas
5201 Harry Hines Blvd, MS 6107A, Dallas, TX 75235
Phone: (214) 590-2580
Internet: http://www.swmed/edu/home_pages/parkland/midwifery/midwifehome.html
Program Administrator: Mary C. Brucker, CNM, Dir.
Accreditation/Approval/Licensing: American College of Nurse-Midwives, Division of Accreditation.
Field of Study: Midwifery*. *Program Name/Length:* Nurse-Midwifery Certificate.
Degrees Offered: Certificate.
License/Certification Preparation: Certified Nurse-Midwife, American College of Nurse-Midwives.
Admission Requirements: RN.

734. Sterling Health Center
Massage Therapy
15070 Beltwood Pkwy, Dallas, TX 75244
Phone: (972) 991-9293; *Fax:* (972) 991-3292
E-mail: sterlinghc@juno.com *Internet:* http://www.flash.net/~STERCHC
Program Administrator: Sterling Mansoori, Dir. *Admissions Contact:* Dianna Lee.
Year Established: 1991.
Staff: Full-time: 2; Part-time: 7.
Avg Enrollment: 250. *Avg Class Size:* 20. *Number of Graduates per Year:* 220.
Wheelchair Access: Yes.
Accreditation/Approval/Licensing: State board: TX Dept of Health.
Field of Study: Anatomy and Physiology; Aromatherapy; Chair Massage; Deep Tissue Massage; Manual Lymph Drainage; Massage Therapy*; Myofascial Release; Pregnancy Massage; Reflexology; Shiatsu; Sports Massage; Trigger Point Therapy. *Program Name/Length:* Massage Therapy Level I, 300 hrs, 3 mos;

Reflexology and other Advanced Classes, 5-75 hrs, Sundays.
Degrees Offered: Certificate.
License/Certification Preparation: State: TX Registered Massage Therapist.
Tuition and Fees: $1985 (Massage Therapy).
Financial Aid: Payment plan.
Career Services: Career information; Internships; Interview set up.

735. Wellness Skills, Inc, Dallas
6102 E Mockingbird Ln, Ste 401, Dallas, TX 75214-2620
Phone: (214) 828-4000; *Fax:* (214) 828-0065
E-mail: infowsi@aol.com *Internet:* http://www.wellnessskills.com
Program Administrator: Catherine Morris, Dir. *Admissions Contact:* Richard Nottingham, Dir of Admissions.
Year Established: 1985.
Staff: Full-time: 10 (2 campuses); Part-time: 10 (2 campuses).
Avg Enrollment: 350 (2 campuses). *Avg Class Size:* 20. *Number of Graduates per Year:* 300 (2 campuses).
Wheelchair Access: Yes.
Accreditation/Approval/Licensing: State board: TX Dept of Health.
Field of Study: Aromatherapy; Massage Therapy*; Polarity Therapy; Reflexology; Shiatsu; Trigger Point Therapy*. *Program Name/Length:* Basic Semester 1300 hrs, 4-7 mos; Advanced courses, 300 hrs.
Degrees Offered: Certificate.
License/Certification Preparation: State: TX Registered Massage Therapist; National Certification Board for Therapeutic Massage and Bodywork.
Admission Requirements: Min age: 18.
Application Deadline(s): Fall: Aug; Winter: Dec; Spring: Mar; Summer: May.
Tuition and Fees: $2385 (Basic); $2655 (Advanced).
Financial Aid: Work study; VA approved.

Denton

736. University of North Texas
Counselor Education
PO Box 311337, Denton, TX 76203-1337
Phone: (940) 565-2910; *Fax:* (940) 565-2905
E-mail: chandler@coefs.coe.unt.edu *Internet:* http://www.coe.unt.edu/cdhe/biofeedback1.htm
Program Administrator: Dr. Cynthia K. Chandler, Associate Prof. *Admissions Contact:* Dr. Michael Attekruse, Chair of Dept.
Staff: Full-time: 14.
Avg Enrollment: 75. *Avg Class Size:* 15. *Number of Graduates per Year:* 20.
Wheelchair Access: Yes.

Accreditation/Approval/Licensing: Biofeedback Certification Institute of America.

Field of Study: Biofeedback*; Mental Health Counseling*. *Program Name/Length:* Master's, 2 yrs; Doctorate, 2 yrs.

Degrees Offered: MS; PhD.

License/Certification Preparation: State: Licensed Professional Counselor; Biofeedback Certification Institute of America.

Admission Requirements: Bachelor's degree; Min GPA: 3.0.

Application Deadline(s): Fall: Sep 15; Winter: Feb 15; Spring: Mar 1.

Financial Aid: Fellowships; Grants; Loans; Scholarships.

Career Services: Career counseling; Career information; Internships.

El Paso

737. El Paso Community College

Massage Therapy/Continuing Education for Health
100 W Rio Grande, El Paso, TX 79902

Mailing Address: PO Box 20500, El Paso, TX 79998

Phone: (915) 831-4116; *Fax:* (915) 831-4131

E-mail: martadlf@epcc.edu

Program Administrator: Marta de la Fuente, Dir. *Admissions Contact:* Marta de la Fuente.

Year Established: 1996.

Staff: Part-time: 4.

Avg Enrollment: 24. *Avg Class Size:* 12. *Number of Graduates per Year:* 20.

Wheelchair Access: Yes.

Accreditation/Approval/Licensing: State board: TX Dept of Health.

Field of Study: Massage Therapy*; Reflexology. *Program Name/Length:* Massage Therapy, 5 mos.

Degrees Offered: CEUs.

License/Certification Preparation: State: TX Registered Massage Therapist.

Admission Requirements: High school diploma/GED; 10th grade reading level.

Application Deadline(s): Spring: Dec; Summer: May.

Tuition and Fees: $978.

738. El Paso School of Massage

Professional Massage Therapy Program
661 S Mesa Hills Dr, Ste 100, El Paso, TX 79912

Phone: (915) 833-2935; *Fax:* (915) 833-3094

Program Administrator: Hilda L. Chavez, ND, Dir/Instr. *Admissions Contact:* Hilda L. Chavez.

Year Established: 1986.

Staff: Full-time: 3.

Avg Enrollment: 30. *Avg Class Size:* 12. *Number of Graduates per Year:* 28.

Wheelchair Access: Yes.

Accreditation/Approval/Licensing: State board: TX Dept of Health.

Field of Study: Hydrotherapy; Massage Therapy*; Neuromuscular Therapy; Swedish Massage*. *Program Name/Length:* Professional Massage Therapy (includes Clinical Internship), 17-wk intensive.

Degrees Offered: Diploma.

License/Certification Preparation: State: TX Registered Massage Therapist.

Admission Requirements: Min age: 18; High school diploma/GED; Min GPA: 3.0.

Application Deadline(s): Winter: Nov 30; Spring: Mar 30; Summer: May 30.

Tuition and Fees: $2700.

Financial Aid: Payment plan.

Career Services: Internships; Instruction in business practices.

739. Maternidad La Luz—The Birth Place

1308 Magoffin, El Paso, TX 79901

Phone: (915) 532-5895; *Fax:* (915) 532-7127

Program Administrator: Deborah Kaley, Educational Dir. *Admissions Contact:* Deborah Kaley.

Year Established: 1987.

Staff: Full-time: 5; Part-time: 6.

Avg Enrollment: 15. *Avg Class Size:* 15. *Number of Graduates per Year:* 15.

Wheelchair Access: No.

Accreditation/Approval/Licensing: Midwifery Education Accreditation Council.

Field of Study: Midwifery*. *Program Name/Length:* 1 wk-3 yrs.

Degrees Offered: Certificate.

License/Certification Preparation: State: TX Registered Midwife; Certified Professional Midwife, North American Registry of Midwives.

Admission Requirements: Min age: 18; High school diploma/GED; Specific course prerequisites: CPR; Negative TB and syphilis.

Tuition and Fees: $250 per wk, $1125 per qtr.

Financial Aid: 1 woman-of-color scholarship.

740. University of Texas at El Paso/Texas Tech University

Collaborative Nurse-Midwifery Program
Texas Tech Univ HSC, Dept of OB/GYN, 4800 Alberta Ave, El Paso, TX 79905

Phone: (915) 545-6490

E-mail: obegcr@ttuhsc.edu

Program Administrator: Carolyn Simmons, CNM, Dir.

Accreditation/Approval/Licensing: American College of Nurse-Midwives, Division of Accreditation.

Field of Study: Midwifery*.

Degrees Offered: MSN.

License/Certification Preparation: Certified Nurse-Midwife, American College of Nurse-Midwives.

Admission Requirements: Bachelor's degree; RN.

Fort Worth

741. Beijing School of Acupuncture and Oriental Medicine
4109 Cagle Dr, Ste F, Fort Worth, TX 76107
Phone: (817) 284-3037; *Fax:* (817) 284-1047
E-mail: 1us@ibm.net
Program Administrator: Dr. Hadi Kareem, Pres.
  Admissions Contact: Dr. Hadi Kareem.
Year Established: 1988.
Staff: Full-time: 2; Part-time: 8.
Avg Enrollment: 15. *Avg Class Size:* 15.
Wheelchair Access: Yes.
Field of Study: Acupuncture*; Oriental Medicine*.
  Program Name/Length: Oriental Medicine, 4
  yrs.
Degrees Offered: Certificate.
License/Certification Preparation: State: TX Li-
  censed Acupuncturist; National Certification
  Commission for Acupuncture and Oriental Med-
  icine.
Admission Requirements: Min age: 21; Some col-
  lege (60 hrs/2 yrs).
Tuition and Fees: $14,000.

742. Fort Worth School of Massage
2929 Cleburne Rd, Fort Worth, TX 76110
Phone: (817) 923-9944; *Fax:* (817) 923-9944
Program Administrator: Joetta Payne, School Dir.
  Admissions Contact: Joetta Payne.
Year Established: 1997.
Staff: Full-time: 1; Part-time: 4.
Avg Enrollment: 36.
Field of Study: CranioSacral Therapy; Massage
  Therapy*; Reflexology; Reiki.
Degrees Offered: Certificate.
License/Certification Preparation: State: TX Reg-
  istered Massage Therapist.
Admission Requirements: Min age: 18; High
  school diploma/GED.
Application Deadline(s): Fall: Sep; Winter: Feb;
  Spring: May; Summer: Aug.
Tuition and Fees: $2300 + $140 supplies.
Financial Aid: Loans; Vocational rehabilitation.
Career Services: Career information.

743. Wellness Skills, Inc, Fort Worth
6301 Airport Fwy, Ste 200, Fort Worth, TX
  76117-5360
Phone: (817) 838-3800; *Fax:* (817) 838-2933
E-mail: infowsi@aol.com *Internet:* http://www.
  wellnessskills.com
Program Administrator: Kelli Eager, Dir. *Admis-
  sions Contact:* Terri/Diane.
Year Established: 1985.
Staff: Full-time: 10 (2 campuses); Part-time: 10 (2
  campuses).
Avg Enrollment: 350 (2 campuses). *Avg Class
  Size:* 20. *Number of Graduates per Year:* 300
  (2 campuses).
Wheelchair Access: Yes.

Accreditation/Approval/Licensing: State board: TX
  Dept of Health.
Field of Study: Aromatherapy; Massage Therapy*;
  Polarity Therapy; Reflexology; Reiki; Shiatsu;
  Sports Massage; Trigger Point Therapy*. *Pro-
  gram Name/Length:* Basic: Semester 1, 300 hrs,
  4-7 mos; Core Training, 100 hrs; Trigger Point
  Therapy, 100 hrs; East-West Healing Arts, 100
  hrs.
Degrees Offered: Certificate.
License/Certification Preparation: State: TX Reg-
  istered Massage Therapist; National Certifica-
  tion Board for Therapeutic Massage and Body-
  work.
Admission Requirements: Min age: 18; High
  school diploma/GED.
Application Deadline(s): Fall: Aug; Winter: Dec;
  Spring: Mar; Summer: May.
Tuition and Fees: $2485 (Basic); $885 (100 hr pro-
  grams).
Financial Aid: State government aid; Work study;
  VA approved; Vocational rehabilitation.
Career Services: Career counseling; Career infor-
  mation; Internships.

Galveston

744. University of Texas at Galveston, School of Nursing
Nurse-Midwifery Program
1100 Mechanic, Galveston, TX 77555-1029
Phone: (409) 772-8347; *Fax:* (409) 772-3770
E-mail: jkvale@utmb.edu *Internet:* http://www.
  utmb.edu
Program Administrator: Janice Keller Kvale, Aca-
  demic Program Dir. *Admissions Contact:* JoAnn
  Mahoney, Admissions Coord.
Year Established: 1993.
Avg Enrollment: 10. *Avg Class Size:* 10. *Number
  of Graduates per Year:* 10.
Wheelchair Access: Yes.
Accreditation/Approval/Licensing: State board: TX
  Board of Nurse Examiners; Southern Associa-
  tion of Colleges and Schools; American College
  of Nurse-Midwives, Division of Accreditation.
Field of Study: Midwifery*. *Program
  Name/Length:* Nurse-Midwifery, 5 semesters,
  21 mos.
Degrees Offered: MSN.
License/Certification Preparation: Certified
  Nurse-Midwife, American College of
  Nurse-Midwives.
Admission Requirements: Bachelor's degree; Min
  GPA: 3.0; RN; Specific course prerequisites:
  statistics; Experience as nurse or midwife pre-
  ferred.
Application Deadline(s): Fall: Feb 1.
Tuition and Fees: $36/resident per credit,
  $278/nonresident per credit.
Financial Aid: Federal government aid; Scholar-
  ships; Work study.

Career Services: Career counseling.

Houston

745. American College of Acupuncture and Oriental Medicine
Master of Science in Oriental Medicine
9100 Park West Dr, Houston, TX 77063
Phone: (713) 780-9777; *Fax:* (713) 781-5781
E-mail: 102657.1730@compuserve.com *Internet:* http://www.acaom.edu
Program Administrator: Minmay Liang, Exec Dir. *Admissions Contact:* Scott Cotlar, Assistant Executive Director.
Year Established: 1991.
Staff: Full-time: 3; Part-time: 12.
Avg Enrollment: 60. *Avg Class Size:* 15. *Number of Graduates per Year:* 10.
Wheelchair Access: Yes.
Accreditation/Approval/Licensing: State board: TX Board of Medical Examiners, Acupuncture Division; Accreditation Commission for Acupuncture and Oriental Medicine.
Field of Study: Acupuncture*; Herbal Medicine; Homeopathy; Oriental Medicine*; Traditional Chinese Medicine. *Program Name/Length:* Master of Science in Acupuncture and Oriental Medicine, 145 credits, 8 semesters.
Degrees Offered: MS.
License/Certification Preparation: State: TX Licensed Acupuncturist; National Certification Commission for Acupuncture and Oriental Medicine.
Admission Requirements: Some college (60 semester hrs).
Application Deadline(s): Fall: Sep; Spring: Jan; Summer: May.
Tuition and Fees: $21,025 (full-time), $21,750 (part-time).
Financial Aid: Federal government aid; Loans.
Career Services: Job information.

746. Baylor College of Medicine
6550 Fannin, Ste 901, Houston, TX 77030
Phone: (713) 798-7594; *Fax:* (713) 798-3579
E-mail: swente@bcm.tmc.edu
Program Administrator: Betty Carter, CNM, Interim Dir.
Year Established: 1985.
Wheelchair Access: Yes.
Accreditation/Approval/Licensing: American College of Nurse-Midwives, Division of Accreditation.
Field of Study: Midwifery*. *Program Name/Length:* Master of Science in Nurse-Midwifery, 2 yrs.
Degrees Offered: MS.
License/Certification Preparation: State: TX Registered Nurse; Certified Nurse-Midwife, American College of Nurse-Midwives.

Admission Requirements: Bachelor's degree; Min GPA: 3.0; RN; Specific course prerequisites: biochemistry recommended; GRE required.
Application Deadline(s): Winter: Jan.
Tuition and Fees: $8400 per yr.
Financial Aid: Grants; Loans; Scholarships.

747. Hypnosis Institute of Houston
13700 Veterans Memorial, Ste 230, Houston, TX 77014
Phone: (281) 587-1055; *Fax:* (281) 379-3153
E-mail: gschoon1@pdq.net *Internet:* http://www.hypnosisconsultant.com
Program Administrator: Gerald L. Schoonover, Dir. *Admissions Contact:* Gerald L. Schoonover.
Year Established: 1989.
Staff: Full-time: 1; Part-time: 2.
Avg Enrollment: 40. *Avg Class Size:* 8. *Number of Graduates per Year:* 25.
Wheelchair Access: No.
Accreditation/Approval/Licensing: International Medical and Dental Hypnotherapy Association.
Field of Study: Hypnotherapy*. *Program Name/Length:* 27 hrs, 3 days; 120 hrs (three 40-hr courses); Seminars given in various locations; Home study/Correspondence.
Degrees Offered: Diploma; Certificate.
License/Certification Preparation: American Council of Hypnotist Examiners; International Medical and Dental Hypnotherapy Association.
Admission Requirements: Min age: 18.
Tuition and Fees: $400 (40 hrs).

748. Massage Therapy Clinic and School
Swedish Massage, Levels I and II
2045 Space Park Dr, Ste 200, Houston, TX 77058
Phone: (281) 333-0400; *Fax:* (281) 333-9010
Internet: http://www.wxs.com/massageschool
Program Administrator: Charline L. Utley, PhD, Owner/Dir. *Admissions Contact:* Charline L. Utley.
Year Established: 1990.
Staff: Full-time: 4; Part-time: 8.
Avg Enrollment: 100. *Avg Class Size:* 12. *Number of Graduates per Year:* 88.
Wheelchair Access: Yes.
Accreditation/Approval/Licensing: State board: TX Dept of Health; National Certification Board for Therapeutic Massage and Bodywork (CEUs).
Field of Study: Deep Tissue Massage; Energy Work; Massage Therapy*; Polarity Therapy; Reflexology; Shiatsu; Swedish Massage*. *Program Name/Length:* Basic Swedish Massage: Level I, 300 hrs, 3-6 mos; Level II, 500-600 hrs, 6-10 mos.
Degrees Offered: Certificate.
License/Certification Preparation: State: TX Registered Massage Therapist; National Certification Board for Therapeutic Massage and Bodywork.

Admission Requirements: Min age: 18; High school diploma/GED recommended.
Tuition and Fees: $2750 + $225 books (Level I).
Financial Aid: VA approved; Vocational rehabilitation; TX Commission for the Blind.
Career Services: Career counseling; Career information; Internships.

749. MRC School of Massage
2990 Richmond, Ste 142, Houston, TX 77098
Phone: (713) 522-1423; *Fax:* (713) 522-1446
Program Administrator: Robert I. Garza, Owner/Dir. *Admissions Contact:* Imelda Garcia.
Year Established: 1985.
Staff: Full-time: 3.
Avg Enrollment: 150. *Avg Class Size:* 18.
Wheelchair Access: Yes.
Accreditation/Approval/Licensing: State board: TX Dept of Health; Accrediting Council for Continuing Education and Training.
Field of Study: Massage Therapy*; Swedish Massage*. *Program Name/Length:* 5 1/2 mos/days or 6 1/2 mos/evenings.
Degrees Offered: Diploma.
License/Certification Preparation: State: TX Registered Massage Therapist.
Admission Requirements: Min age: 16; Reading comprehension.
Tuition and Fees: $2400 + books.
Financial Aid: Texas Commission for the Blind.
Career Services: Internships.

750. The Winters School, Inc
Massage Therapy Programs
4625 Southwest Fwy, Ste 142, Houston, TX 77027
Phone: (713) 626-2200; *Fax:* (713) 626-2230
E-mail: twschool@aol.com
Program Administrator: Cari Denson West, RMT, Dir.
Year Established: 1984.
Staff: Part-time: 15.
Avg Enrollment: 120. *Avg Class Size:* 20. *Number of Graduates per Year:* 100.
Wheelchair Access: Yes.
Accreditation/Approval/Licensing: State board: TX Dept of Health; National Certification Board for Therapeutic Massage and Bodywork (CEUs).
Field of Study: Deep Tissue Massage; Massage Therapy*; Polarity Therapy; Reflexology; Shiatsu. *Program Name/Length:* 250 hrs, 5 mos; 300 hrs, 4-8 mos.
Degrees Offered: CEUs; Certificate.
License/Certification Preparation: State: TX Registered Massage Therapist; National Certification Board for Therapeutic Massage and Bodywork.
Application Deadline(s): Fall: Aug; Winter: Dec; Spring: Mar; Summer: Apr.
Tuition and Fees: $2500-$2700.

751. The Yoga Institute and Bookshop
3830 Villanova St, Houston, TX 77005-3640

Phone: (800) 524-6674
Program Administrator: Lex Gillan, Owner. *Admissions Contact:* Lex Gillan.
Year Established: 1974.
Staff: Full-time: 3; Part-time: 8.
Avg Enrollment: 100. *Avg Class Size:* 20.
Wheelchair Access: Yes.
Field of Study: Yoga Teacher Training*. *Program Name/Length:* 9 days; Seminars given in various locations.
Career Services: Career counseling; Career information; Internships.

Kingwood

752. The PATH Foundation, Kingwood
1006 Burning Tree, Kingwood, TX 77339
Phone: (281) 358-3700, 359-7284; *Fax:* (281) 359-5700
E-mail: email@pathfoundation.com *Internet:* http://www.pathfoundation.com
Program Administrator: Ed R. Martin, PhD, Exec Dir. *Admissions Contact:* Cheryl Martin, LMSW, Records Admin.
Year Established: 1984.
Staff: Full-time: 2.
Avg Enrollment: 35. *Avg Class Size:* 18. *Number of Graduates per Year:* 35.
Wheelchair Access: No.
Field of Study: Hypnotherapy*. *Program Name/Length:* Certified Hypnotherapist, 1 yr.
Degrees Offered: Certificate.
License/Certification Preparation: American Board of Clinical Hypnosis; American Council of Hypnotist Examiners; International Medical and Dental Hypnotherapy Association; National Guild of Hypnotists.
Admission Requirements: High school diploma/GED.
Application Deadline(s): Fall: Sep 15; Spring: Feb 15.
Tuition and Fees: $2340.

753. The Relax Station School of Massage Therapy
1409 Kingwood Dr, Kingwood, TX 77339
Phone: (281) 358-0600; *Fax:* (281) 358-4089
Internet: http://www.therelaxstation.com
Program Administrator: Allen Boxman, Owner/Dir. *Admissions Contact:* Allen Boxman.
Year Established: 1994.
Staff: Full-time: 1; Part-time: 3.
Avg Enrollment: 62. *Avg Class Size:* 12. *Number of Graduates per Year:* 60.
Wheelchair Access: Yes.
Accreditation/Approval/Licensing: State board: TX Dept of Health.
Field of Study: Acupressure; Aromatherapy; CranioSacral Therapy; Massage Therapy*; Neuromuscular Therapy; Sports Massage. *Pro-*

gram Name/Length: 4 mos/days or 6 mos/nights.
Degrees Offered: Certificate.
License/Certification Preparation: State: TX Registered Massage Therapist.
Admission Requirements: Min age: 17.
Application Deadline(s): Fall: Sep; Winter: Jan, nights; Spring: Feb, days.
Financial Aid: TX Rehabilitation Commission.
Career Services: Internships; Job information; Referral service.

Lubbock

754. Healing Arts Institute, Lubbock
Massage Therapy; Myofascial Program
5601 Aberdeen, Ste G, Lubbock, TX 79414
Phone: (806) 797-0034
Program Administrator: David Goyette, Owner.
   Admissions Contact: Kay Nash.
Year Established: 1996.
Staff: Full-time: 6.
Avg Enrollment: 60. Avg Class Size: 20. Number of Graduates per Year: 60.
Wheelchair Access: No.
Accreditation/Approval/Licensing: State board: TX Dept of Health.
Field of Study: Aromatherapy; Deep Tissue Massage; Energy Work*; Hydrotherapy; Massage Therapy*; Polarity Therapy; Reflexology; Shiatsu. Program Name/Length: Massage Therapy Basic, 7 mos; Myofascial Program, 5 mos; Seminars given in various locations.
Degrees Offered: Diploma; Certificate.
License/Certification Preparation: State: TX Registered Massage Therapist.
Admission Requirements: Min age: 18; High school diploma/GED.
Tuition and Fees: $2400-$2700.
Financial Aid: Work study; VA approved; Vocational rehabilitation; Commission for the Blind.
Career Services: Career counseling; Career information; Internships.

McAllen

755. School of Natural Therapy
Massage Therapy
4309 N 10th, Stes A, B, C, McAllen, TX 78504
Phone: (956) 630-0928; Fax: (956) 630-6103
E-mail: school @acnet.net
Program Administrator: Naomi Morton, Co-Dir; Carol Jackson, Co-Dir. Admissions Contact: Lorena Granados.
Year Established: 1988.
Staff: Full-time: 2; Part-time: 5.
Wheelchair Access: Yes.
Accreditation/Approval/Licensing: State board: TX Dept of Health.

Field of Study: Deep Tissue Massage; Massage Therapy*; Reflexology. Program Name/Length: Basic Massage Therapy, 300 hrs, 6-8 mos; Advanced Program, 305 hrs, 6-8 mos.
License/Certification Preparation: State: TX Registered Massage Therapist; National Certification Board for Therapeutic Massage and Bodywork.
Admission Requirements: Min age: 16; High school diploma/GED.
Application Deadline(s): Fall: Sep; Winter: Nov; Spring: Mar; Summer: Jun.
Financial Aid: VA approved; Vocational rehabilitation; Payment plan.

Midland

756. Midland College Health Sciences Continuing Education
Massage Therapy School
3600 N Garfield, Midland, TX 79705
Phone: (915) 685-6440
E-mail: bprichard@midland.cc.tx.us
Program Administrator: Beverly B. Prichard, Dir.
   Admissions Contact: Norma Chavez, Sec.
Year Established: 1996.
Staff: Part-time: 3.
Avg Enrollment: 40. Avg Class Size: 20. Number of Graduates per Year: 40.
Wheelchair Access: Yes.
Accreditation/Approval/Licensing: State board: TX Higher Ed Commission; Southern Association of Colleges and Schools.
Field of Study: Massage Therapy*. Program Name/Length: 300 hrs, 4 mos.
Degrees Offered: CEUs; Certificate.
License/Certification Preparation: State: TX Registered Massage Therapist.
Admission Requirements: Min age: 18; High school diploma/GED.
Application Deadline(s): Fall; Spring.
Tuition and Fees: $1000 + $150 books.
Financial Aid: State government aid.
Career Services: Career counseling; Career information.

Nacogdoches

757. Giving Tree Cottage
Massage Therapy
1808 South St, Nacogdoches, TX 75964
Phone: (409) 560-6299; Fax: (409) 569-9400
Program Administrator: Nancy Lemberger, Dir.
   Admissions Contact: Jo Harbison, Coord.
Year Established: 1995.
Staff: Full-time: 4; Part-time: 3.
Avg Enrollment: 16. Avg Class Size: 16. Number of Graduates per Year: 14.
Wheelchair Access: No.

Accreditation/Approval/Licensing: State board: TX Dept of Health.
Field of Study: Massage Therapy*. *Program Name/Length:* 6 mos.
Degrees Offered: Diploma.
License/Certification Preparation: State: TX Registered Massage Therapist.
Admission Requirements: Min age: 18; High school diploma/GED.
Application Deadline(s): Summer: Aug.
Tuition and Fees: $2500.
Financial Aid: Vocational rehabilitation; Payment plan.
Career Services: Career counseling; Career information.

Pasadena

758. Texas Chiropractic College

5912 Spencer Hwy, Pasadena, TX 77505-1699
Phone: (281) 487-1170, (800) 468-6839; *Fax:* (281) 991-4871
E-mail: gabbygreen@aol.com *Internet:* http://www.txchiro.edu
Program Administrator: S. M. Elliott, DC, Pres. *Admissions Contact:* Robert Cooper, Admissions Dir.
Year Established: 1908.
Staff: Full-time: 30; Part-time: 20.
Avg Enrollment: 500. *Avg Class Size:* 50. *Number of Graduates per Year:* 150.
Wheelchair Access: Yes.
Accreditation/Approval/Licensing: Council on Chiropractic Education; Southern Association of Colleges and Schools.
Field of Study: Chiropractic*. *Program Name/Length:* Bachelor of Science in Human Biology, 6 trimesters, 2 yrs; Doctor of Chiropractic, 10 trimesters, 3 1/3 yrs.
Degrees Offered: BS; DC.
License/Certification Preparation: State: TX Doctor of Chiropractic.
Admission Requirements: High school diploma/GED; Some college (60 semester hrs); Min GPA: 2.5, 2.0 in sciences; Specific course prerequisites: 2 semesters each (with labs): biology, general chemistry, organic chemistry, general physics; 1 semester general psychology; 2 semesters English; 5 semesters social sciences/humanities; also required for BS: 2 semesters math, 2 semesters of electives.
Tuition and Fees: $4600 per trimester.
Financial Aid: ChrioLoan; Federal government aid; Grants; Scholarships; State government aid; VA approved; Work study.
Career Services: Career counseling; Career information; Internships; Interview set up; Practice information; Resume service.

Richardson

759. Asten Center of Natural Therapeutics

797 N Grove Rd, Ste 101, Richardson, TX 75081
Phone: (972) 669-3245; *Fax:* (972) 669-1191
Program Administrator: Lisa Mumford, Admin. *Admissions Contact:* Jill Townsend.
Year Established: 1983.
Staff: Part-time: 12.
Avg Enrollment: 150. *Avg Class Size:* 15. *Number of Graduates per Year:* 140.
Wheelchair Access: Yes.
Accreditation/Approval/Licensing: State board: TX Dept of Health; National Certification Board for Therapeutic Massage and Bodywork (CEUs).
Field of Study: Massage Therapy*; Polarity Therapy; Reflexology; Sports Massage; Swedish Massage*; Trigger Point Therapy. *Program Name/Length:* Basic: Semester I, 300 hrs; Advanced: Semester II, 250 hrs.
Degrees Offered: Certificate.
License/Certification Preparation: State: TX Registered Massage Therapist; National Certification Board for Therapeutic Massage and Bodywork.
Tuition and Fees: $2630 (Basic); $2420 (Advanced).
Career Services: Job information.

Richland Hills

760. Texas College of Oriental Medicine, Inc

3917 Booth Calloway Rd, Richland Hills, TX 76118
Phone: (817) 595-2339; *Fax:* (817) 284-1047
E-mail: 1us@ibm.net *Internet:* http://www.acupuncture-schools.com
Program Administrator: Dr. Hadi Kareem, Pres. *Admissions Contact:* Dr. Hadi Kareem.
Year Established: 1998.
Staff: Full-time: 2; Part-time: 3.
Avg Class Size: 10.
Wheelchair Access: Yes.
Field of Study: Acupuncture*; Herbal Medicine; Oriental Medicine*; Traditional Chinese Medicine. *Program Name/Length:* Acupuncture, 3 yrs; Seminars given in various locations; Home study/Correspondence.
Degrees Offered: Certificate.
Admission Requirements: Min age: 21; Some college (60 hrs).
Application Deadline(s): Fall; Winter; Spring; Summer.
Tuition and Fees: $3600 per yr.

San Antonio

761. European Massage Therapy Institute

7220 Louis Pasteur, Ste 140, San Antonio, TX 78229

Phone: (210) 615-8207; *Fax:* (210) 614-3732
Program Administrator: Rosario Perez Garza, Co-Dir/Instr. *Admissions Contact:* Leigh J. Kuder, Dir of Student Affairs.
Year Established: 1988.
Staff: Full-time: 2; Part-time: 3.
Avg Enrollment: 75. *Avg Class Size:* 26. *Number of Graduates per Year:* 72.
Wheelchair Access: Yes.
Accreditation/Approval/Licensing: State board: TX Dept of Health.
Field of Study: Aromatherapy; Manual Lymph Drainage; Massage Therapy*; Postural Analysis; Reflexology. *Program Name/Length:* Basic Massage Therapy, 9 mos; Advanced Massage Therapy: Treatment of Upper Extremities, 6 mos.
Degrees Offered: Certificate.
License/Certification Preparation: State: TX Registered Massage Therapist.
Admission Requirements: Min age: 18; High school diploma/GED; Interview with director; TB release.
Tuition and Fees: $2459 (Basic); $1000 (Advanced); includes supplies, uniform.
Financial Aid: VA approved; Payment plan; TX Rehabilitation Commission.
Career Services: Career information; Internships; Job information.

762. Mind Body Naturopathic and Holistic Health Institute

10911 West Ave, San Antonio, TX 78213
Phone: (210) 308-8888; *Fax:* (210) 349-5679
E-mail: libbe9@mail.idt.net *Internet:* http://www. colon-hydrotherapy.com
Program Administrator: Jeri C. Tiller, ND. *Admissions Contact:* Dick Hoenninger, ND; Tom Tiller III.
Year Established: 1989.
Staff: Full-time: 5; Part-time: 2.
Avg Enrollment: 65. *Avg Class Size:* 15. *Number of Graduates per Year:* 65.
Wheelchair Access: Yes.
Accreditation/Approval/Licensing: State board: TX Dept of Health; International Association for Colon Hydrotherapy.
Field of Study: Aromatherapy; Colon Hydrotherapy*; Massage Therapy*; Reflexology; Reiki; Yoga. *Program Name/Length:* Massage Therapy, 300 hrs; Colon Hydrotherapy, 100 hrs.
Degrees Offered: Certificate.
License/Certification Preparation: State: TX Registered Massage Therapist; National Certification Board for Therapeutic Massage and Body-work; International Association for Colon Hydrotherapy.
Admission Requirements: Min age: 18; High school diploma/GED; Specific course prerequisites: anatomy and physiology recommended.
Tuition and Fees: $2200, includes books (Massage); $800 (Colon Hydrotherapy).
Financial Aid: State government aid; Payment plan; TX Rehabilitation Commission.
Career Services: Career counseling; Career information; Internships; Referral service.

763. NeuroMuscular Concepts School of Massage

8607 Wurzbach Rd, Bldg Q, Ste 101, San Antonio, TX 78240
Phone: (210) 558-3148; *Fax:* (210) 558-3114
E-mail: nmpnc@sanantonio.net
Program Administrator: Jana Miller, Co-Dir; Paul Frizzell, Co-Dir. *Admissions Contact:* Paul Frizzell.
Year Established: 1984.
Staff: Full-time: 2; Part-time: 3.
Avg Enrollment: 30. *Avg Class Size:* 15. *Number of Graduates per Year:* 20.
Wheelchair Access: Yes.
Accreditation/Approval/Licensing: State board: TX Dept of Health.
Field of Study: Acupressure; Aromatherapy; Ayurvedic Medicine; CranioSacral Therapy; Energy Work; Feldenkrais; Herbal Medicine; Homeopathy; Massage Therapy*; Naturopathic Medicine; Neuromuscular Therapy*; Oriental Medicine; Polarity Therapy; Qigong; Reflexology; Reiki; Shiatsu; Sports Massage; Traditional Chinese Medicine; Yoga Teacher Training. *Program Name/Length:* Massage Therapy, 300 hrs; Integrated Therapies, workshops; Seminars given in various locations.
Degrees Offered: Certificate.
License/Certification Preparation: State: TX Registered Massage Therapist.
Admission Requirements: Min age: 18; High school diploma/GED; Min GPA: 2.0.
Application Deadline(s): Fall: Sep 1; Spring: Mar 1.
Tuition and Fees: $2500 includes books (Massage Therapy); $25-$1000 (Workshops).
Financial Aid: Payment plan; TX Rehabilitation Commission; Pending, VA approval.
Career Services: Internships; Job information; Referral service.

764. Saint Philip's College

Massage Therapy Program
1801 Martin Luther King Blvd, San Antonio, TX 78203
Phone: (210) 531-4770; *Fax:* (210) 531-4774
Program Administrator: Barbara Witte-Howell, Continuing Ed Specialist. *Admissions Contact:* Barbara Witte-Howell.
Year Established: 1985.

Staff: Part-time: 8.
Avg Enrollment: 100. *Avg Class Size:* 22. *Number of Graduates per Year:* 95.
Wheelchair Access: Yes.
Accreditation/Approval/Licensing: State board: TX Dept of Health; Southern Association of Colleges and Schools.
Field of Study: Massage Therapy*. *Program Name/Length:* 300 hrs, 5 mos.
Degrees Offered: Certificate.
License/Certification Preparation: State: TX Registered Massage Therapist.
Admission Requirements: Min age: 18; High school diploma/GED.
Tuition and Fees: $2000.
Financial Aid: Federal government aid.

765. The South Texas Educational Center for Classical Homeopathy
13526 George Rd, Ste 101, San Antonio, TX 78230-3002
Phone: (310) 493-0561; *Fax:* (310) 492-8013
E-mail: benchmarkpub@stic.net
Program Administrator: Sandra J. Perko, PhD, Dir.
Year Established: 1986.
Staff: Full-time: 3; Part-time: guest instructors.
Avg Enrollment: 60. *Avg Class Size:* 30. *Number of Graduates per Year:* 40.
Wheelchair Access: Yes.
Field of Study: Clinical Nutrition; Herbal Medicine; Homeopathy*. *Program Name/Length:* 6 mos; Seminars given in various locations.
Degrees Offered: Certificate.

766. Therapeutic Body Concepts
6162 Wurzbach Rd, San Antonio, TX 78238
Phone: (210) 684-6563; *Fax:* (210) 680-2782
Program Administrator: Jeanie Esciksen; Leon Gosset. *Admissions Contact:* Jeanie Esciksen; Leon Gosset.
Year Established: 1994.
Staff: Full-time: 2.
Avg Enrollment: 25. *Avg Class Size:* 7. *Number of Graduates per Year:* 22.
Wheelchair Access: Yes.
Accreditation/Approval/Licensing: State board: TX Dept of Health.

Field of Study: Massage Therapy*. *Program Name/Length:* Massage Therapy Level I, 300 hrs, 7 1/2 mos.
Degrees Offered: Certificate.
License/Certification Preparation: State: TX Registered Massage Therapist.
Admission Requirements: Min age: 18; High school diploma/GED.
Application Deadline(s): Fall: Sep; Winter: Jan; Spring: May.
Tuition and Fees: $2400.
Career Services: Referral service.

Tyler

767. Hands-On Therapy School of Massage
1101 E 5th St, Tyler, TX 75701
Phone: (903) 535-7733; *Fax:* (903) 535-7799
Program Administrator: Jeannine Martin, School Admin. *Admissions Contact:* Jeannine Martin.
Year Established: 1995.
Staff: Full-time: 4.
Avg Enrollment: 95. *Avg Class Size:* 14. *Number of Graduates per Year:* 90.
Wheelchair Access: Yes.
Accreditation/Approval/Licensing: State board: TX Dept of Health; National Certification Board for Therapeutic Massage and Bodywork (CEUs).
Field of Study: Aromatherapy; Massage Therapy*; Reflexology; Shiatsu; Swedish Massage* Deep Tissue Massage. *Program Name/Length:* Basic Swedish Massage, 300 hrs, 4-7 mos; Advanced Program, 200 hrs; Seminars given in various locations.
Degrees Offered: CEUs; Certificate.
License/Certification Preparation: State: TX Registered Massage Therapist; National Certification Board for Therapeutic Massage and Bodywork.
Admission Requirements: Min age: 16.
Tuition and Fees: $2300 (Basic Swedish).
Financial Aid: Loans; Work study; VA approved; Vocational rehabilitation.
Career Services: Career information; Internships.

UTAH

Lindon

768. Utah College of Massage Therapy, Utah Valley Campus
135 S State St, Ste 12, Lindon, UT 84042
Phone: (801) 796-0300; *Fax:* (801) 796-0309

Program Administrator: Aimee Huhtala, Campus Mgr. *Admissions Contact:* Karyn Grant, Admissions Representative.
Year Established: 1997.
Staff: Part-time: 33.

Avg Enrollment: 320. *Avg Class Size:* 38. *Number of Graduates per Year:* 300.
Wheelchair Access: Yes.
Accreditation/Approval/Licensing: Accrediting Council for Continuing Education and Training.
Field of Study: Acupressure; CranioSacral Therapy; Energy Work; Feldenkrais; Massage Therapy*; Neuromuscular Therapy; Reflexology; Shiatsu; Sports Massage*. *Program Name/Length:* Professional Massage Therapy, 6 mos/days or 1 yr/evenings.
Degrees Offered: Diploma; Certificate.
License/Certification Preparation: State: UT Licensed Massage Technician; National Certification Board for Therapeutic Massage and Bodywork.
Admission Requirements: Min age: 16; High school diploma/GED.
Tuition and Fees: $5700-$6250 + $1042 books, fees, table.
Financial Aid: Federal government aid; Grants; Loans; Vocational rehabilitation; Payment plan.
Career Services: Career information; Internships; Interview set up; Resume service; Job information.

Ogden

769. Ogden Institute of Massage Therapy
3500 Harrison Blvd, Ogden, UT 84403
Phone: (801) 627-8227; *Fax:* (801) 627-2228
Program Administrator: Craig S. Anderson, LMT, Dir. *Admissions Contact:* Craig S. Anderson.
Year Established: 1997.
Staff: Part-time: 12.
Avg Enrollment: 20. *Avg Class Size:* 8. *Number of Graduates per Year:* 14.
Wheelchair Access: Yes.
Accreditation/Approval/Licensing: State board: UT Board of Regents.
Field of Study: CranioSacral Therapy; Deep Tissue Massage; Massage Therapy*; Shiatsu. *Program Name/Length:* 1 yr.
Degrees Offered: Certificate.
License/Certification Preparation: State: UT Licensed Massage Technician; National Certification Board for Therapeutic Massage and Bodywork.
Admission Requirements: Min age: 17; High school diploma/GED.
Application Deadline(s): Fall: Aug; Winter: Mar.
Tuition and Fees: $6500.
Financial Aid: Grants; Loans.
Career Services: Career information; Interview set up.

Orem

770. Utah College of Midwifery
230 W 170 N, Orem, UT 84057

Phone: (801) 764-9068, (888) 489-1238
E-mail: midwife@uswest.net
Program Administrator: Dianne Bjarnson, Exec Dir. *Admissions Contact:* Suzanne Smith, Registrar.
Year Established: 1980.
Staff: Part-time: 10.
Avg Enrollment: 35. *Avg Class Size:* 10. *Number of Graduates per Year:* 7.
Accreditation/Approval/Licensing: Midwifery Education Accreditation Council.
Field of Study: Childbirth Educator; Doula*; Midwifery*. *Program Name/Length:* Associate of Science in Midwifery, 3 yrs; Bachelor of Science in Midwifery, 4 yrs; Doula, 1 wk + experience; Childbirth Educator, 1 wk + experience.
Degrees Offered: BS; CEUs; MS; Certificate; AS in Midwifery; Certified Traditional Midwife.
License/Certification Preparation: Certified Professional Midwife, North American Registry of Midwives.
Admission Requirements: High school diploma/GED.
Tuition and Fees: $2000 per yr.
Career Services: Career counseling; Career information; Internships.

Saint George

771. Sensory Development Institute
Massage Therapy
1871 W Canyon View Dr, Saint George, UT 84770
Phone: (435) 652-9003; *Fax:* (435) 652-8949
Program Administrator: Pam Shelline, Administrative Dir. *Admissions Contact:* Pam Shelline.
Year Established: 1997.
Staff: Full-time: 3; Part-time: 4.
Avg Enrollment: 30. *Avg Class Size:* 30. *Number of Graduates per Year:* 25.
Wheelchair Access: Yes.
Accreditation/Approval/Licensing: State board: UT Board of Massage.
Field of Study: Aromatherapy; Energy Work*; Massage Therapy*; Oriental Medicine; Reflexology; Shiatsu*; Spa Therapies. *Program Name/Length:* 3 trimesters.
Degrees Offered: Certificate.
License/Certification Preparation: State: UT Licensed Massage Technician.
Admission Requirements: Min age: 18; High school diploma/GED.
Application Deadline(s): Summer: May.
Tuition and Fees: $7000.
Financial Aid: Loans.
Career Services: Career counseling; Career information; Interview set up; Job placement.

Salt Lake City

772. Myotherapy College of Utah
Massage Therapy
1174 E 2700 S, Ste 19, Salt Lake City, UT 84106
Phone: (801) 484-7624; *Fax:* (801) 484-1928
Program Administrator: Vaughn L. Belnap, Dir.
  Admissions Contact: Sheridan Black.
Year Established: 1987.
Staff: Full-time: 2; Part-time: 15.
Avg Enrollment: 110. *Avg Class Size:* 15. *Number
  of Graduates per Year:* 56.
Wheelchair Access: Yes.
Accreditation/Approval/Licensing: State board: UT
  Board of Massage; Accrediting Commission of
  Career Schools and Colleges of Technology.
Field of Study: Aromatherapy; CranioSacral Ther-
  apy; Deep Tissue Massage; Energy Work; Ho-
  meopathy; Massage Therapy*; Polarity Therapy;
  Qigong; Reflexology; Reiki; Shiatsu. *Program
  Name/Length:* 8 mos/full-time or 15
  mos/part-time.
Degrees Offered: Certificate.
License/Certification Preparation: State: UT Li-
  censed Massage Technician; National Certifica-
  tion Board for Therapeutic Massage and Body-
  work.
Admission Requirements: Min age: 18; High
  school diploma/GED.
Application Deadline(s): Fall: Aug and Oct; Winter: Jan; Spring: Mar; Summer: Jun.
Financial Aid: Federal government aid; Grants;
  Loans; VA approved; Vocational rehabilitation.
Career Services: Career counseling; Career infor-
  mation; Interview set up; Resume service.

773. University of Utah, College of Nursing
Graduate Program in Nurse-Midwifery; Women's
  Health Nurse-Practitioner Program
10 S 2000 East Front, Salt Lake City, UT
  84112-5880
Phone: (801) 581-8274; *Fax:* (801) 581-4642
Program Administrator: Marilyn Stewart, CNM,
  Dir. *Admissions Contact:* Marilyn Stewart.
Year Established: 1965.
Staff: Full-time: 6; Part-time: 1.
Avg Class Size: 10. *Number of Graduates per
  Year:* 10.
Wheelchair Access: Yes.
Accreditation/Approval/Licensing: American Col-
  lege of Nurse-Midwives, Division of Accredita-
  tion.
Field of Study: Midwifery*. *Program
  Name/Length:* Nurse-Midwifery, 18-24 mos;
  Women's Health Nurse-Practitioner, 2 yrs.
Degrees Offered: MS.
License/Certification Preparation: State: All 50
  states; Certified Nurse-Midwife, American Col-
  lege of Nurse-Midwives.
Admission Requirements: Bachelor's degree in
  Nursing; Min GPA: 3.0.
Application Deadline(s): Winter: Feb.

Financial Aid: Federal government aid; Loans;
  Scholarships.
Career Services: Career information; Internships.

774. Utah College of Massage Therapy
25 S 300 E, Salt Lake City, UT 84111
Phone: (800) 617-3302; *Fax:* (801) 521-3339
E-mail: info@ucmt.com *Internet:* http://www.
  ucmt.com
Program Administrator: Norman Cohn,
  Owner/Dir. *Admissions Contact:* Edward
  Schwartz, Dir of Operations.
Year Established: 1986.
Staff: Full-time: 45; Part-time: 30.
Avg Class Size: 48. *Number of Graduates per
  Year:* 500.
Wheelchair Access: Yes.
Accreditation/Approval/Licensing: State board: UT
  Board of Regents; Accrediting Council for Con-
  tinuing Education and Training; Commission on
  Massage Therapy Accreditation.
Field of Study: Acupressure; CranioSacral Ther-
  apy; Deep Tissue Massage; Feldenkrais; Infant
  Massage; Injury Massage; Massage Therapy*;
  Qigong; Reflexology; Russian Massage;
  Shiatsu; Touch for Health; Trigger Point Ther-
  apy. *Program Name/Length:* Accelerated Day,
  6 mos; Clinical Accelerated Day, 9 mos; Ex-
  tended Evening, 1 yr; Clinical Extended Eve-
  ning, 18 mos.
Degrees Offered: Certificate.
License/Certification Preparation: State: UT Li-
  censed Massage Technician; National Certifica-
  tion Board for Therapeutic Massage and Body-
  work.
Admission Requirements: Min age: 18 by gradua-
  tion; High school diploma/GED.
Tuition and Fees: $5600 (Accelerated Day); $7900
  (Clinical Accelerated Day); $5400 (Extended
  Evening); $7700 (Clinical Extended Evening).
Financial Aid: Federal government aid; Grants;
  Loans; State government aid; VA approved.
Career Services: Career counseling; Career infor-
  mation; Resume service; Referral service.

Springville

775. The School of Natural Healing
25 W 200 S, Springville, UT 84663
Mailing Address: PO Box 412, Springville, UT
  84663
Phone: (800) 372-8255; *Fax:* (801) 489-8341
E-mail: snh@qi3.com *Internet:* http://www.
  homestar.net/school
Program Administrator: David W. Christopher,
  MH, Dir. *Admissions Contact:* Emma Flake,
  Registrar.
Year Established: 1953.
Staff: Full-time: 1; Part-time: 7.
Avg Enrollment: 2000. *Avg Class Size:* 25. *Num-
  ber of Graduates per Year:* 20.

Wheelchair Access: Yes.
Field of Study: Herbal Medicine*. *Program Name/Length:* Master Herbalist, 21 mos, correspondence; Master of Herbology Certification Seminar, 1 wk.
Degrees Offered: MH.
Admission Requirements: Min age: 17; Bachelor's degree for Master Herbalist; Aromatherapy and

Master Herbalist required for Master of Herbology.
Tuition and Fees: $1785-$2100 (Master Herbalist); $495 (Master of Herbology).
Financial Aid: Scholarships.

VERMONT

Barre

776. Vermont School of Professional Massage
14 Merchant St, Barre, VT 05641
Phone: (802) 479-2340
Program Administrator: Faeterri Silver, Owner/Dir. *Admissions Contact:* Faeterri Silver.
Year Established: 1989.
Staff: Full-time: 1.
Avg Enrollment: 10. *Avg Class Size:* 10. *Number of Graduates per Year:* 10.
Wheelchair Access: Yes.
Field of Study: Massage Therapy*. *Program Name/Length:* Professional Massage, 600 hrs, 2 semesters.
Degrees Offered: Certificate.
License/Certification Preparation: National Certification Board for Therapeutic Massage and Bodywork.
Application Deadline(s): Spring: May 15.
Tuition and Fees: $4100.
Financial Aid: Grants.

East Barre

777. Sage Mountain Retreat Center and Botanical Sanctuary
PO Box 420, East Barre, VT 05649
Phone: (802) 479-9825; *Fax:* (802) 476-3722
E-mail: sagemt@sover.net
Program Administrator: Rosemary Gladstar, Founder/Dir. *Admissions Contact:* Katie Pickens, Office Asst.
Year Established: 1987.
Staff: Full-time: 4; Part-time: 4.
Avg Enrollment: 175. *Avg Class Size:* 30. *Number of Graduates per Year:* 70.
Wheelchair Access: No.
Field of Study: Herbal Medicine*. *Program Name/Length:* The Science and Art of Herbalism, correspondence; Apprenticeship, 7 mos; Advanced Herbal Training Program, 7 mos.

Tuition and Fees: $350 (Correspondence); $1050 (Apprenticeship); $1300 (Advanced Herbal Training).
Financial Aid: Scholarships.

Middlesex

778. Universal Institute of Healing Arts
90 Three Mile Bridge Rd, Middlesex, VT 05602
Mailing Address: RFD 3, Box 5285, Montpelier, VT 05602
Phone: (802) 229-4844
E-mail: univinst@aol.com
Program Administrator: Bob Onne, Dir. *Admissions Contact:* Bob Onne.
Year Established: 1982.
Staff: Part-time: 2.
Avg Enrollment: 25. *Avg Class Size:* 10. *Number of Graduates per Year:* 5.
Wheelchair Access: No.
Field of Study: Acupressure*; Deep Tissue Massage*; Reflexology; Shiatsu*. *Program Name/Length:* 150 hrs, 6 semesters, 3 yrs; Apprenticeship, 20 hrs.
Degrees Offered: Certificate.
Application Deadline(s): Fall.
Tuition and Fees: $400 per semester.
Financial Aid: Grants.

Pawlet

779. Partner Earth Education Center
Apprentice Program
PO Box 298, Pawlet, VT 05761-0298
Phone: (802) 325-2121; *Fax:* (802) 325-2121, *51
E-mail: greenpam@aol.com
Program Administrator: Pam Montgomery, Dir. *Admissions Contact:* Pam Montgomery.
Year Established: 1989.
Staff: Full-time: 1; Part-time: 1.
Avg Enrollment: 18. *Avg Class Size:* 18. *Number of Graduates per Year:* 18.
Wheelchair Access: No.

Field of Study: Herbal Medicine*; Plant Spirit Medicine. *Program Name/Length:* Apprenticeship, 7 mos.
Degrees Offered: Certificate.
Admission Requirements: Min age: 16.
Tuition and Fees: $950.
Financial Aid: Work study.
Career Services: Career information.

South Burlington

780. Vermont Institute of Massage Therapy
Massage Therapist Program
10 Cottage Grove Ave, South Burlington, VT 05403
Phone: (802) 862-1111; *Fax:* (802) 660-3733
E-mail: massage@together.net *Internet:* http://www.together.net/~massage/institute.html
Program Administrator: Don Wright, Pres/Dir. *Admissions Contact:* Kathleen Wright, Asst Dir.

Year Established: 1986.
Staff: Full-time: 1; Part-time: 1.
Avg Enrollment: 30. *Avg Class Size:* 6. *Number of Graduates per Year:* 30.
Wheelchair Access: Yes.
Field of Study: Acupressure*; Energy Work*; Massage Therapy*; Reflexology*. *Program Name/Length:* 1 yr.
Degrees Offered: Diploma.
License/Certification Preparation: American Reflexology Certification Board; National Certification Board for Therapeutic Massage and Bodywork.
Admission Requirements: Min age: 16.
Tuition and Fees: $4400.
Financial Aid: State government aid; Vocational rehabilitation; Payment plan; VT Association for the Blind.
Career Services: Career counseling; Career information; Referral service.

VIRGINIA

Alexandria

781. Institute for Integrated Therapies
3708 N Rosser St, Ste 201, Alexandria, VA 22311
Phone: (703) 931-8340; *Fax:* (703) 931-8567
Program Administrator: Margaret L. D'Urso, ND, Dir. *Admissions Contact:* Margaret L. D'Urso.
Year Established: 1985.
Staff: Part-time: 2.
Avg Enrollment: 200. *Avg Class Size:* 18. *Number of Graduates per Year:* 100.
Wheelchair Access: Yes.
Accreditation/Approval/Licensing: National Certification Board for Therapeutic Massage and Bodywork (CEUs).
Field of Study: CranioSacral Therapy; Massage Therapy; Reflexology*; Vibrational Therapy. *Program Name/Length:* Basic Reflexology, 8 mos; Advanced Reflexology Series and Apprenticeship; TransFiber Therapy, 10 mos; Vibrational Therapy, 10 mos.
Degrees Offered: CEUs; Diploma; Certificate.
License/Certification Preparation: American Reflexology Certification Board; National Certification Board for Therapeutic Massage and Bodywork.
Admission Requirements: Min age: 21; High school diploma/GED; Some college; Specific course prerequisites: anatomy and physiology.
Application Deadline(s): Winter; Summer.
Tuition and Fees: $800 (Basic Reflexology); $1500 (Advanced Reflexology); $1800

(TransFiber Therapy); $1000 (Vibrational Therapy).
Financial Aid: Work study; Payment plan.
Career Services: Career counseling; Career information; Internships; Job information; Referral service.

782. National Center for Instruction of Homeopathy and Homeotherapeutics
National Center for Homeopathy Annual Summer School
801 N Fairfax St, Ste 306, Alexandria, VA 22314
Phone: (703) 548-7790; *Fax:* (703) 548-7792
E-mail: nchinfo@igc.apc.org *Internet:* http://www.homeopathic.org
Program Administrator: Stephen Messer, ND, Dean. *Admissions Contact:* National Center for Homeopathy Staff.
Year Established: 1922.
Staff: Part-time: 10.
Avg Enrollment: 275. *Avg Class Size:* 25.
Wheelchair Access: No.
Accreditation/Approval/Licensing: Council on Homeopathic Education.
Field of Study: Animal Therapy; Homeopathy*. *Program Name/Length:* Foundations in Homeopathy, 2 days; Basic Acute Homeopathy, 5 days; Intermediate Acute Homeopathy, 5 days; Understanding Chronic Prescribing, 4 days; Homeopathic Prescribing I for Professionals, 5 days; Homeopathic Prescribing II for Professionals, 5 days; Philosophy of Homeopathic

Medicine, 2 days; Introduction to Veterinary Homeopathy, 2 days; Intermediate Veterinary Homeopathy, 2 days; Advanced Veterinary Homeopathy, 2 days.

Degrees Offered: Certificate.

License/Certification Preparation: State: NV Board of Homeopathic Examiners; Council for Homeopathic Certification; Homeopathic Academy of Naturopathic Physicians; North American Society of Homeopaths; National Board of Homeopathic Examiners.

Admission Requirements: Licensed health care provider for Homeopathic Prescribing I and II; course levels must be taken in successive order.

Tuition and Fees: $180-$600 per course.

Financial Aid: Grants; Loans; Scholarships.

Blacksburg

783. Blue Ridge School of Massage and Yoga

201 S Main St, Blacksburg, VA 24060

Mailing Address: PO Box 767, Blacksburg, VA 24063

Phone: (540) 552-2177

E-mail: oha@bellatlantic.net *Internet:* http://www.ohassociates.com

Program Administrator: Jeffrey C. Tiebout, VP. Admissions Contact: Colleen A. Kelly, Coord of Ed Svcs.

Year Established: 1997.

Staff: Full-time: 1; Part-time: 1.

Avg Enrollment: 15. *Avg Class Size:* 8. *Number of Graduates per Year:* 8.

Wheelchair Access: No.

Field of Study: Acupressure*; Alexander Technique; Deep Tissue Massage*; Energy Work; Massage Therapy*; Meditation; Polarity Therapy; Qigong; Reflexology; Reiki; Shiatsu; Traditional Chinese Medicine; Yoga. *Program Name/Length:* Massage Therapy Certification, 500 hrs, 1 yr or 18 mos.

Degrees Offered: Certificate.

License/Certification Preparation: American Reflexology Certification Board; National Certification Board for Therapeutic Massage and Bodywork.

Admission Requirements: Min age: 18; High school diploma/GED.

Career Services: Career information.

784. Virginia School of Massage, Blacksburg

Southwest Decentralized Facility, 106-B Southpark Dr, Blacksburg, VA 24060

Phone: (804) 293-4031; *Fax:* (804) 293-4190

E-mail: registrar@vasom.com *Internet:* http://www.vasom.com

Program Administrator: Sue Ellis Dyar, Admin. Admissions Contact: Lori Nicolaysen, Dir of Ed.

Year Established: 1989.

Staff: Part-time: 7.

Avg Enrollment: 225. *Avg Class Size:* 16. *Number of Graduates per Year:* 90.

Wheelchair Access: Yes.

Accreditation/Approval/Licensing: State board: VA Dept of Ed, Div of Proprietary Schools; Accrediting Commission of Career Schools and Colleges of Technology; National Certification Board for Therapeutic Massage and Bodywork (CEUs).

Field of Study: Massage Therapy*. *Program Name/Length:* Massage Therapy, 510 hrs; Professional Medical Massage Therapy, 610 hrs, 8 1/2 mos/full-time.

Degrees Offered: Certificate.

License/Certification Preparation: State: VA Certified Massage Therapist; National Certification Board for Therapeutic Massage and Bodywork.

Admission Requirements: Min age: 18; High school diploma/GED.

Application Deadline(s): Fall: Sep; Spring: Apr.

Tuition and Fees: $4950 (510 hrs); $6150 (610 hrs).

Financial Aid: Federal government aid; Loans; VA approved.

Career Services: Career information; Job information.

Buckingham

785. Satchidananda Ashram—Yogaville

Rte 1, Box 1720, Buckingham, VA 23921

Phone: (804) 969-3121, (800) 858-YOGA (9642); *Fax:* (804) 969-1303

E-mail: iyi@yogaville.org *Internet:* http://www.yogaville.org

Field of Study: Yoga Teacher Training*. *Program Name/Length:* Integral Yoga Teacher Training Certification: Basic, Intermediate and Advanced.

Charlottesville

786. Virginia School for Alexander Technique

1021 Sheridan Ave, Charlottesville, VA 22901

Phone: (804) 977-7186

E-mail: dokugawa@redlt.com

Program Administrator: Daria T. Okugawa, Dir.

Year Established: 1987.

Staff: Full-time: 1; Part-time: 4.

Accreditation/Approval/Licensing: American Society for the Alexander Technique.

Field of Study: Alexander Technique. *Program Name/Length:* Teacher Training, 1600 hrs, 3 yrs.

License/Certification Preparation: American Society for the Alexander Technique.

Admission Requirements: Bachelor's degree or equivalent life experience; Specific course pre-

requisites: 10 lessons in the Alexander Technique; Interview and lesson with director.
Tuition and Fees: $4800 per yr.

787. Virginia School of Massage, Charlottesville

2008 Morton Dr, Charlottesville, VA 22903
Phone: (804) 293-4031; *Fax:* (804) 293-4190
E-mail: registrar@vasom.com *Internet:* http://www.vasom.com
Program Administrator: Sue Ellis Dyar, Admin. *Admissions Contact:* Lori Nicolaysen, Dir of Ed.
Year Established: 1989.
Staff: Part-time: 7.
Avg Enrollment: 225. *Avg Class Size:* 16. *Number of Graduates per Year:* 90.
Wheelchair Access: Yes.
Accreditation/Approval/Licensing: State board: VA Dept of Ed, Div of Proprietary Schools; Accrediting Commission of Career Schools and Colleges of Technology; National Certification Board for Therapeutic Massage and Bodywork (CEUs).
Field of Study: Massage Therapy*. *Program Name/Length:* Massage Therapy, 510 hrs, 15 mos; Professional Medical Massage Therapy, 610 hrs, 8 1/2 mos/full-time or 17 mos/part-time.
Degrees Offered: Certificate.
License/Certification Preparation: State: VA Certified Massage Therapist; National Certification Board for Therapeutic Massage and Bodywork.
Admission Requirements: Min age: 18; High school diploma/GED.
Application Deadline(s): Fall: Sep; Spring: Apr.
Tuition and Fees: $4950 (510 hrs); $6150 (610 hrs).
Financial Aid: Federal government aid; Loans; VA approved.
Career Services: Career information; Job information.

Danville

788. Natural Touch School of Massage Therapy, Danville

291 Park Ave, Danville, VA 24541
Phone: (804) 799-0060, (877) 799-0060
Program Administrator: Wanda Adkins, LMT, Dir. *Admissions Contact:* Wanda Adkins.
Year Established: 1994.
Staff: Full-time: 4; Part-time: 2.
Avg Enrollment: 25. *Avg Class Size:* 12. *Number of Graduates per Year:* 20.
Wheelchair Access: Yes.
Accreditation/Approval/Licensing: State board: VA Dept of Ed, Div of Proprietary Schools.
Field of Study: Acupressure; CranioSacral Therapy; Energy Work*; Massage Therapy*; Myofascial Release; Polarity Therapy; Shiatsu.

Program Name/Length: Massage Therapy, 500 hrs, 7 mos/days or 15 mos/nights.
Degrees Offered: Diploma; Certificate.
License/Certification Preparation: State: VA Certified Massage Therapist; National Certification Board for Therapeutic Massage and Bodywork.
Admission Requirements: Min age: 18; High school diploma/GED.
Application Deadline(s): Fall: Sep 21; Spring: Mar 21.
Tuition and Fees: $4500.
Financial Aid: Work study; Payment plan.
Career Services: Career counseling; Career information; Internships.

Goshen

789. Eastern Institute of Hypnotherapy

PO Box 249, Goshen, VA 24439-0249
Phone: (540) 997-0325, (800) 296-MIND (6463); *Fax:* (540) 997-0324
E-mail: hyptrainer@aol.com *Internet:* http://www.members.aol.com/EIH/NATH/
Program Administrator: Allen S. Chips, DCH, Exec Dir. *Admissions Contact:* Dee Chips, MHt, Admin.
Year Established: 1989.
Staff: Full-time: 2; Part-time: 8.
Avg Enrollment: 200. *Avg Class Size:* 17. *Number of Graduates per Year:* 200.
Accreditation/Approval/Licensing: State board: VA Nonproprietary School; American Board of Hypnotherapy; International Medical and Dental Hypnotherapy Association.
Field of Study: Hypnotherapy*; Neuro-Linguistic Programming*. *Program Name/Length:* Certification (CHt), 100 hrs, 1 mo; Master Certification (MHt), 135 hrs, 3 mos; Trainer, 100 hrs, 1 mo; Assistant Master Trainer, 235 hrs, 2-3 yrs; Neuro-Linguistic Programming Practitioner Certification.
Degrees Offered: CEUs; Certificate; CHt; MHt.
Admission Requirements: Min age: 18; High school diploma/GED; Min GPA: 2.0; Specific course prerequisites: CHt required for MHt.
Tuition and Fees: $950 per course ($895 pre-registered).
Financial Aid: Scholarships; Work study; Vocational rehabilitation; Payment plan.
Career Services: Internships.

790. Transpersonal Reiki Institute

A division of Eastern Institute of Hypnotherapy
956 The Knob Rd, Goshen, VA 24439-0249
Mailing Address: PO Box 249, Goshen, VA 24439-0249
Phone: (540) 997-0325, (800) 296-MIND (6463); *Fax:* (540) 997-0324
E-mail: hyptrainer@aol.com *Internet:* http://www.members.aol.com/EIH/NATH

Program Administrator: Dee Chips, CRM, Exec Dir. *Admissions Contact:* Dee Chips.
Year Established: 1995.
Staff: Full-time: 1; Part-time: 1.
Avg Enrollment: 40. *Avg Class Size:* 10. *Number of Graduates per Year:* 40.
Wheelchair Access: Yes.
Field of Study: Reiki*. *Program Name/Length:* Level I, 8 hrs, 1 day; Level II, 8 hrs, 1 day; Master Reiki, 1 yr, weekends.
Degrees Offered: CEUs; Certificate.
Admission Requirements: Min age: 18 or written parental consent; Level I required for Level II; Level II required for Master.
Tuition and Fees: $195 (Level I); $250 (Level II); $1500 (Master).
Financial Aid: Scholarships; Work study; Vocational rehabilitation; Payment plan.
Career Services: Mentorship.

Herndon

791. Applied Kinesthetic Studies School of Massage

692 Pine St, Herndon, VA 20170
Phone: (703) 464-0333; *Fax:* (703) 464-5999
E-mail: school-of-aks@erols.com *Internet:* http://www.school-of-aks.com
Program Administrator: Katharine Hunter, Dir. *Admissions Contact:* Katharine Hunter.
Year Established: 1992.
Staff: Part-time: 6.
Avg Enrollment: 54. *Avg Class Size:* 18. *Number of Graduates per Year:* 50.
Wheelchair Access: No.
Accreditation/Approval/Licensing: State board: VA Dept of Ed.
Field of Study: Swedish Massage*. *Program Name/Length:* 500 hrs, 10 mos.
Degrees Offered: Certificate.
License/Certification Preparation: National Certification Board for Therapeutic Massage and Bodywork.
Admission Requirements: Min age: 20; High school diploma/GED.
Tuition and Fees: $3300.
Financial Aid: VA approved.
Career Services: Career information; Job information; Referral service.

Lynchburg

792. Natural Touch School of Massage Therapy, Lynchburg

1202 Main St, Lynchburg, VA 24504
Phone: (804) 845-3003, (877) 799-0060
Program Administrator: Wanda Adkins, LMT, Dir. *Admissions Contact:* Wanda Adkins.
Year Established: 1998.
Wheelchair Access: Yes.

Accreditation/Approval/Licensing: State board: VA Dept of Ed, Div of Proprietary Schools.
Field of Study: Acupressure; CranioSacral Therapy; Energy Work*; Massage Therapy*; Myofascial Release; Polarity Therapy; Shiatsu.
Program Name/Length: Massage Therapy, 600 hrs, 7 mos/days or 15 mos/nights.
Degrees Offered: Diploma; Certificate.
License/Certification Preparation: State: VA Certified Massage Therapist; National Certification Board for Therapeutic Massage and Bodywork.
Admission Requirements: Min age: 18; High school diploma/GED.
Application Deadline(s): Fall: Sep 21; Spring: Mar 21.
Tuition and Fees: $4500.
Financial Aid: Work study; Payment plan.
Career Services: Career counseling; Career information; Internships.

McLean

793. Alexander Technique Center of Washington, DC

PO Box 449, McLean, VA 22101
Phone: (703) 821-2920
Program Administrator: Marian Goldberg, Dir. *Admissions Contact:* Marian Goldberg.
Year Established: 1995.
Accreditation/Approval/Licensing: American Society for the Alexander Technique.
Field of Study: Alexander Technique*. *Program Name/Length:* Teacher Training, 3 yrs.
License/Certification Preparation: American Society for the Alexander Technique.
Admission Requirements: Specific course prerequisites: 20 individual lessons in the Alexander Technique, minimum of 2 with director.

Richmond

794. Richmond Academy of Massage

2004 Bremo Rd, Ste 102, Richmond, VA 23226
Phone: (804) 282-5003; *Fax:* (804) 288-7356
Program Administrator: D. C. Ashburn, Dir. *Admissions Contact:* Kelly Meadors, Chief Admin.
Year Established: 1989.
Staff: Full-time: 3; Part-time: 5.
Avg Enrollment: 60. *Avg Class Size:* 16. *Number of Graduates per Year:* 50.
Wheelchair Access: Yes.
Accreditation/Approval/Licensing: State board: VA Board of Ed.
Field of Study: Massage Therapy*. *Program Name/Length:* 1 yr.
Degrees Offered: Certificate.
License/Certification Preparation: State: VA Certified Massage Therapist; National Certification Board for Therapeutic Massage and Bodywork.
Admission Requirements: Min age: 17.

Tuition and Fees: $3950.
Financial Aid: Federal government aid; Loans; State government aid; VA approved; Vocational rehabilitation; Payment plan.
Career Services: Career counseling; Career information; Interview set up.

Round Hill

795. Equissage, Inc
Equine Sports Massage Therapy Certificate Program
15715 Southern Cross Ln, Round Hill, VA 20141
Mailing Address: PO Box 447, Round Hill, VA 20141
Phone: (800) 843-0224; *Fax:* (540) 338-5569
E-mail: equissage@webtv.net *Internet:* http://www.equissage.com
Program Administrator: Mary Schreiber, Pres. *Admissions Contact:* Nelson R. Schreiber, VP.
Year Established: 1990.
Staff: Full-time: 2; Part-time: 2.
Avg Enrollment: 400. *Avg Class Size:* 9. *Number of Graduates per Year:* 380.
Accreditation/Approval/Licensing: International Association of Equine Sports Massage Therapists.
Field of Study: Animal Therapy*; Deep Tissue Massage*; Equine Massage*. *Program Name/Length:* 60 hrs.
Degrees Offered: Certificate.
License/Certification Preparation: International Association of Equine Sports Massage Therapists Certificate Board.
Admission Requirements: Min age: 18; High comfort level around horses.
Tuition and Fees: $875.
Career Services: National advertising support.

Virginia Beach

796. Cayce/Reilly School of Massotherapy
215 67th St, Virginia Beach, VA 23451
Phone: (757) 437-7202; *Fax:* (757) 428-0398
E-mail: are@are-cayce.com *Internet:* http://www.are-cayce.com
Program Administrator: Dwight Zieman, Admin. *Admissions Contact:* Coleen Temple, Registrar.
Year Established: 1988.
Staff: Part-time: 27.
Avg Enrollment: 100. *Avg Class Size:* 20. *Number of Graduates per Year:* 75.
Wheelchair Access: Yes.
Accreditation/Approval/Licensing: State board: VA Dept of Ed; VA Association of Proprietary Career Schools; Commission on Massage Therapy Accreditation; National Certification Board for Therapeutic Massage and Bodywork (CEUs).
Field of Study: Acupressure; Alexander Technique; Aromatherapy; CranioSacral Therapy; Hypnotherapy; Massage Therapy*; Neuromuscular Therapy; Reflexology; Reiki; Sports Massage. *Program Name/Length:* Massotherapy, 600 hrs, 6 mos; 1000 hrs, 1 yr.
Degrees Offered: Diploma.
License/Certification Preparation: State: VA Certified Massage Therapist.
Admission Requirements: High school diploma/GED; 2 letters of reference; Medical exam; Copies of transcripts.
Application Deadline(s): Fall: Aug; Winter: Dec; Summer: Apr.
Tuition and Fees: $4500 (600 hrs).
Financial Aid: Scholarships.

797. Fuller School of Massage Therapy
3500 Virginia Beach Blvd, Virginia Beach, VA 23452
Phone: (757) 340-7132; *Fax:* (757) 486-2192
Program Administrator: Nancy Bender, Dir of Ed. *Admissions Contact:* Nancy Bender.
Year Established: 1983.
Staff: Full-time: 4; Part-time: 16.
Avg Enrollment: 90. *Avg Class Size:* 20. *Number of Graduates per Year:* 70.
Wheelchair Access: Yes.
Accreditation/Approval/Licensing: State board: VA Dept of Ed; National Certification Board for Therapeutic Massage and Bodywork (CEUs).
Field of Study: Aromatherapy*; CranioSacral Therapy; Herbal Medicine; Homeopathy; Massage Therapy*; Neuromuscular Therapy; Polarity Therapy; Prenatal Massage; Qigong; Reflexology*; Reiki; Shiatsu; Sports Massage. *Program Name/Length:* Massage Practitioner, 6 mos; Certified Massage Therapist, 1 yr.
Degrees Offered: Diploma; Certificate.
License/Certification Preparation: National Certification Board for Therapeutic Massage and Bodywork.
Admission Requirements: Min age: 18; High school diploma/GED; Specific course prerequisites: massage workshop.
Application Deadline(s): Fall: Jul; Spring: Jan 31.
Tuition and Fees: $1650 per semester + $70 books, $150 financing.
Financial Aid: Work study; VA approved; Vocational rehabilitation.
Career Services: Career counseling; Career information; Internships.

Winchester

798. Shenandoah University
Nurse-Midwifery Program
1775 N Sector Ct, Winchester, VA 22611
Phone: (540) 678-4382; *Fax:* (540) 665-5519
E-mail: jfehr@su.edu
Program Administrator: Juliana Fehr, CNM, MS, Coord. *Admissions Contact:* Juliana Fehr.
Year Established: 1996.

Staff: Full-time: 1.

Avg Enrollment: 6. *Avg Class Size:* 6. *Number of Graduates per Year:* 6.

Wheelchair Access: Yes.

Accreditation/Approval/Licensing: American College of Nurse-Midwives, Division of Accreditation.

Field of Study: Midwifery*. *Program Name/Length:* Nurse-Midwifery, 5 semesters.

Degrees Offered: MSN.

License/Certification Preparation: Certified Nurse-Midwife, American College of Nurse-Midwives.

Admission Requirements: Bachelor's degree: BSN; Min GPA: 2.8; RN.

Application Deadline(s): Fall: Nov.

Tuition and Fees: $20,900.

Financial Aid: Grants; Loans; Scholarships.

Career Services: Internships.

799. Virginia School of Massage, Winchester

Winchester Decentralized Facility, 2820 Valley Ave, Winchester, VA 22601

Phone: (804) 293-4031; *Fax:* (804) 293-4190

E-mail: registrar@vasom.com *Internet:* http://www.vasom.com

Program Administrator: Sue Ellis Dyar, Admin. *Admissions Contact:* Lori Nicolaysen, Dir of Ed.

Year Established: 1989.

Staff: Part-time: 7.

Avg Enrollment: 225. *Avg Class Size:* 16. *Number of Graduates per Year:* 90.

Wheelchair Access: Yes.

Accreditation/Approval/Licensing: State board: VA Dept of Ed, Div of Proprietary Schools; Accrediting Commission of Career Schools and Colleges of Technology; National Certification Board for Therapeutic Massage and Bodywork (CEUs).

Field of Study: Massage Therapy*. *Program Name/Length:* Massage Therapy, 510 hrs; Professional Medical Massage Therapy, 610 hrs, 8 1/2 mos/full-time.

Degrees Offered: Certificate.

License/Certification Preparation: State: VA Certified Massage Therapist; National Certification Board for Therapeutic Massage and Bodywork.

Admission Requirements: Min age: 18; High school diploma/GED.

Application Deadline(s): Fall: Sep; Spring: Apr.

Tuition and Fees: $4950 (510 hrs); $6150 (610 hrs).

Financial Aid: Federal government aid; Loans; VA approved.

Career Services: Career information; Job information.

Woodbridge

800. Piedmont School of Professional Massage

12712 Directors Loop, Woodbridge, VA 22192

Phone: (703) 497-4437

Program Administrator: Alan Coyne, Jim Weiler, Co-Dirs.

Year Established: 1995.

Staff: Full-time: 2; Part-time: 3.

Avg Enrollment: 24. *Avg Class Size:* 12. *Number of Graduates per Year:* 24.

Wheelchair Access: Yes.

Accreditation/Approval/Licensing: State board: VA Dept of Ed, Div of Proprietary Schools.

Field of Study: Massage Therapy*. *Program Name/Length:* Massage Therapy, 10 mos.

Degrees Offered: Diploma; Certificate.

License/Certification Preparation: State: VA Certified Massage Therapist; National Certification Board for Therapeutic Massage and Bodywork.

Admission Requirements: Min age: 18; High school diploma/GED.

Tuition and Fees: $4500.

Financial Aid: Loans.

Career Services: Career counseling; Career information.

Yorktown

801. Virginia Academy of Massage Therapy

Certified Massage Therapist

5314 George Washington Memorial Hwy, Yorktown, VA 23692

Phone: (757) 872-0934; *Fax:* (757) 898-0620

Program Administrator: David Marker, Dir of Ed. *Admissions Contact:* Barbara Marker, Dir of Admissions.

Year Established: 1997.

Staff: Full-time: 2; Part-time: 8.

Avg Enrollment: 11. *Number of Graduates per Year:* 6.

Wheelchair Access: Yes.

Accreditation/Approval/Licensing: State board: VA Board of Ed; National Certification Board for Therapeutic Massage and Bodywork (CEUs).

Field of Study: Acupressure*; CranioSacral Therapy*; Deep Tissue Massage*; Energy Work*; Hypnotherapy*; Massage Therapy*; Reflexology*; Traditional Chinese Medicine. *Program Name/Length:* Massage Therapy, 1 yr.

Degrees Offered: CEUs; Certificate.

License/Certification Preparation: State: VA Certified Massage Therapist; National Certification Board for Therapeutic Massage and Bodywork.

Admission Requirements: Min age: 18; High school diploma/GED.

Application Deadline(s): Fall: Sep; Spring: Feb.

Tuition and Fees: $4090 + $180 books.

Financial Aid: Vocational rehabilitation; Payment plan.

Career Services: Career information.

WASHINGTON

Bellevue

802. Bellevue Massage School
16301 NE 8th St, Ste 106, Bellevue, WA 98008
Phone: (425) 641-3409; *Fax:* (425) 641-3409
Program Administrator: Kathy Schmidt, Co-Dir; James Schmidt, Co-Dir. *Admissions Contact:* Elise Hockett.
Year Established: 1977.
Staff: Full-time: 2; Part-time: 5.
Avg Enrollment: 65. *Avg Class Size:* 12. *Number of Graduates per Year:* 60.
Wheelchair Access: Yes.
Accreditation/Approval/Licensing: State board: WA Board of Massage.
Field of Study: Deep Tissue Massage; Energy Work; Massage Therapy*; Reflexology; Touch For Health. *Program Name/Length:* 513 hrs, 6 1/2 mos.
Degrees Offered: CEUs; Diploma.
License/Certification Preparation: State: WA Licensed Massage Practitioner; National Certification Board for Therapeutic Massage and Bodywork.
Admission Requirements: Min age: 18; High school diploma/GED.
Application Deadline(s): Fall: Sep 15; Winter: Jan 15; Spring: Apr 1; Summer: Jun 1.
Tuition and Fees: $5630.
Financial Aid: State government aid.
Career Services: Career counseling; Career information; Student clinic.

803. BodyMind Academy
1247 120th Ave NE, Bellevue, WA 98005
Phone: (425) 635-0145; *Fax:* (425) 635-3588
E-mail: info@bodymind-academy.com *Internet:* http://www.bodymind-academy.com
Program Administrator: Thomas J. Johnston, MEd, Dir. *Admissions Contact:* Jill Frostenson, BS, Admissions Dir.
Year Established: 1992.
Staff: Full-time: 6; Part-time: 5.
Avg Enrollment: 100. *Avg Class Size:* 16. *Number of Graduates per Year:* 80.
Wheelchair Access: Yes.
Accreditation/Approval/Licensing: State board: WA Board of Massage; Accrediting Council for Continuing Education and Training.
Field of Study: Breathwork*; Hypnotherapy*; Massage Therapy*; Shiatsu*. *Program*

Name/Length: BodyMind Shiatsu Practitioner, 6 mos; BodyMind Counseling Hypnotherapy Practitioner, 6 mos; BodyMind Massage Practitioner, 9 mos; BodyMind Breathwork Practitioner, 7 mos.
Degrees Offered: Diploma.
License/Certification Preparation: State: WA Licensed Massage Practitioner, WA Registered Counselor; American Council of Hypnotist Examiners; National Certification Board for Therapeutic Massage and Bodywork.
Admission Requirements: Min age: 18; High school diploma/GED; BodyMind Breathwork or interview for BodyMind Counseling Hypnotherapy.
Application Deadline(s): Fall: Aug 15; Winter: Dec 15; Spring: Feb 15; Summer: Jun 15.
Tuition and Fees: $2550 (Shiatsu); $2465 (Hypnotherapy); $6450 (Massage); $6000 (Breathwork).
Financial Aid: State government aid; VA approved.
Career Services: Career information.

804. Yoga Centers
2255 140th Ave NE, Stes E and F, Bellevue, WA 98003
Phone: (425) 746-7476; *Fax:* (425) 746-3961
E-mail: yoga@oz.net *Internet:* http://www.yogacenters.com
Program Administrator: Aadil B. Palkhivala, Dir. *Admissions Contact:* Mona Renner, Asst Dir.
Year Established: 1981.
Staff: Full-time: 3; Part-time: 13.
Avg Enrollment: 35. *Avg Class Size:* 35. *Number of Graduates per Year:* 20.
Wheelchair Access: Yes.
Field of Study: Aromatherapy; Energy Work; Yoga Teacher Training*. *Program Name/Length:* 3 yrs.
Degrees Offered: Certificate.
Admission Requirements: Min age: 20; Licensed massage therapist preferred.
Application Deadline(s): Fall: Aug 31.
Tuition and Fees: $1000 per semester.
Financial Aid: Work study.
Career Services: Resume service; Referral service.

Buckley

805. Soma Institute
730 Klink, Buckley, WA 98321
Phone: (360) 829-1025; *Fax:* (360) 829-2805
Internet: http://www.soma-institute.com
Program Administrator: Karen L. Bolesky, Co-Dir.
  Admissions Contact: Karen L. Bolesky.
Year Established: 1978.
Staff: Full-time: 2; Part-time: 1.
Avg Enrollment: 12. *Avg Class Size:* 12. *Number
  of Graduates per Year:* 12.
Wheelchair Access: No.
Accreditation/Approval/Licensing: State board:
  WA Board of Massage; WA Workforce Training
  and Ed Coordinating Board.
Field of Study: Soma Neuromuscular Integration.
  Program Name/Length: Foundation Program, 3
  mos; Soma Neuromuscular Integration Training,
  3 1/2 mos; Combined program, 6 mos.
Degrees Offered: Certificate.
License/Certification Preparation: State: WA Li-
  censed Massage Practitioner; National Certifica-
  tion Board for Therapeutic Massage and Body-
  work.
Admission Requirements: Min age: 25; High
  school diploma/GED; Individual assessment.
Tuition and Fees: $9500 (Combined program).
Financial Aid: Loans.

Everett

806. Ashmead College, Everett
2721 Wetmore Ave, Everett, WA 98201
Phone: (425) 339-2678; *Fax:* (425) 258-2620
Internet: http://www.ashmeadcollege.com
Program Administrator: Kathryn Young, LMP,
  Campus Mgr. *Admissions Contact:* Cheryl
  France, Admissions Rep.
Year Established: 1993.
Staff: Part-time: 17.
Avg Enrollment: 150. *Avg Class Size:* 24. *Number
  of Graduates per Year:* 120.
Wheelchair Access: Yes.
Accreditation/Approval/Licensing: State board:
  WA Workforce Training and Ed Coordinating
  Board; Accrediting Council for Continuing Edu-
  cation and Training; Commission on Massage
  Therapy Accreditation.
Field of Study: Anatomy and Physiology;
  Aromatherapy*; First Aid/CPR; Geriatric Mas-
  sage; Hydrotherapy; Kinesiology*; Massage
  Therapy*; Pregnancy Massage; Spa Therapies*;
  Sports Massage*. *Program Name/Length:*
  Comprehensive Professional Licensing, 1038
  hrs, 1 yr; Sports Massage Specialist, 243 hrs, 3
  mos; Aromatherapy and Spa Specialist, 242 hrs,
  3 mos; Hospital/Long Term Care Massage Spe-
  cialist, 247 hrs, 3 mos.
Degrees Offered: Diploma.

License/Certification Preparation: State: WA Licensed Massage Practitioner; National Certification Board for Therapeutic Massage and Bodywork.
Admission Requirements: Min age: 18; High
  school diploma/GED.
Tuition and Fees: $9874 + $1240 books, table,
  supplies (Comprehensive); $2800 + $920 books,
  table, supplies (Specialist).
Financial Aid: Federal government aid.
Career Services: Career counseling; Career information; Internships; Interview set up; Resume
  service.
Comments: Formerly Seattle Massage School.

Federal Way

807. Tacoma Community College/Continuing Professional Education
Professional Hypnosis Training Program
30640 Pacific Hwy S, Ste E, Federal Way, WA
  98003
Phone: (253) 927-8888, 566-5020 Admissions
E-mail: rhunter@halcyon.com *Internet:* http://
  www.hunter.holowww.com
Program Administrator: Roy Hunter, MS, Hypno-
  sis Training Coord. *Admissions Contact:* Con-
  tinuing Ed Dept.
Year Established: 1987.
Staff: Part-time: 2.
Avg Enrollment: 20. *Avg Class Size:* 8. *Number of
  Graduates per Year:* 16.
Wheelchair Access: Yes.
Accreditation/Approval/Licensing: International
  Medical and Dental Hypnotherapy Association.
Field of Study: Hypnotherapy*. *Program
  Name/Length:* Professional Hypnosis Training,
  9 mos; Hypnosis and Childbirth, 3 mos.
Degrees Offered: Certificate.
License/Certification Preparation: International
  Medical and Dental Hypnotherapy Association.
Admission Requirements: Min age: 18; High
  school diploma/GED.
Application Deadline(s): Fall: Sep 30; Spring: Apr.
Tuition and Fees: $450 per qtr.
Financial Aid: State government aid; Vocational
  rehabilitation.

Fife

808. Ashmead College, Tacoma Area Campus
5005 Pacific Hwy E, Ste 20, Fife, WA 98424
Phone: (253) 926-1435
Internet: http://www.ashmeadcollege.com
Program Administrator: Frank Hatstat, MBA,
  Campus Mgr. *Admissions Contact:* Julie Curri-
  er; Anna Shaw.
Staff: Part-time: 25.

Avg Enrollment: 185. *Avg Class Size:* 24. *Number of Graduates per Year:* 165.

Wheelchair Access: Yes.

Accreditation/Approval/Licensing: State board: WA Workforce Training and Ed Coordinating Board; Accrediting Council for Continuing Education and Training; Commission on Massage Therapy Accreditation.

Field of Study: Anatomy and Physiology; Aromatherapy*; First Aid/CPR; Geriatric Massage; Hydrotherapy; Kinesiology*; Massage Therapy*; Pregnancy Massage; Spa Therapies*; Sports Massage*. *Program Name/Length:* Comprehensive Professional Licensing, 1038 hrs, 1 yr; Sports Massage Specialist, 243 hrs, 3 mos; Aromatherapy and Spa Specialist, 242 hrs, 3 mos; Hospital/Long-Term Care Massage Specialist, 247 hrs, 3 mos.

Degrees Offered: Diploma.

License/Certification Preparation: State: WA Licensed Massage Practitioner; National Certification Board for Therapeutic Massage and Bodywork.

Admission Requirements: Min age: 18; High school diploma/GED.

Tuition and Fees: $9874 + $1240 books, table, supplies (Comprehensive); $2800 + $920 books, table, supplies (Specialist).

Financial Aid: Federal government aid.

Career Services: Career counseling; Career information; Internships; Interview set up; Resume service.

Comments: Formerly Seattle Massage School.

Issaquah

809. The Wellness Institute

3716 274th Ave SE, Issaquah, WA 98029

Phone: (425) 391-9716; *Fax:* (425) 391-9737

E-mail: heartcenter@wellness-institute.org

Internet: http://www.wellness-institute.org

Program Administrator: Diane Zimberoff, Dir. *Admissions Contact:* David Hartman.

Year Established: 1985.

Staff: Full-time: 2; Part-time: 7.

Avg Class Size: 25.

Wheelchair Access: Yes.

Accreditation/Approval/Licensing: State board: WA Workforce Training and Ed Coordinating Board; National Board for Certified Clinical Hypnotherapists.

Field of Study: Breathwork*; Energy Work*; Hypnotherapy*. *Program Name/Length:* Heart-Centered Hypnotherapy Certification, 60 hrs; Heart-Centered Breath Therapy Certification, 60 hrs; Seminars given in various locations.

Degrees Offered: CEUs; Certificate.

License/Certification Preparation: National Board for Certified Clinical Hypnotherapists.

Admission Requirements: Master's degree in mental health field, medical degree, or RN.

Tuition and Fees: $895 per course.

Kenmore

810. Bastyr University

14500 Juanita Dr NE, Kenmore, WA 98028-4966

Phone: (425) 823-1300; *Fax:* (425) 823-6222

E-mail: admis@bastyr.edu *Internet:* http://www.bastyr.edu

Program Administrator: Joseph Pizzorno, ND, Pres. *Admissions Contact:* Sandra Lane, Assoc Dir of Admissions.

Year Established: 1978.

Staff: Full-time: 18; Part-time: 44.

Avg Class Size: 30.

Accreditation/Approval/Licensing: Council on Naturopathic Medicine Education; Accreditation Commission for Acupuncture and Oriental Medicine; Northwest Association of Schools and Colleges.

Field of Study: Acupuncture*; Ayurvedic Medicine; Herbal Medicine*; Homeopathy; Midwifery*; Naturopathic Medicine*; Nutrition*; Qigong; Shiatsu; Traditional Chinese Medicine*. *Program Name/Length:* Bachelor of Science in Natural Health Sciences (Oriental Medicine, Nutrition or Exercise Science and Wellness), 2 yrs; Bachelor of Science in Psychology, 2 yrs; Master of Science in Acupuncture, 3 yrs; Master of Science in Acupuncture and Oriental Medicine, 3 1/2 yrs; Doctor of Naturopathic Medicine, 4 yrs; Certificate in Chinese Herbal Medicine; Midwifery Certificate; Postgraduate Certificate in Spirituality, Health, and Medicine, 1 yr.

Degrees Offered: BS; MS; ND; Certificate.

License/Certification Preparation: National Certification Commission for Acupuncture and Oriental Medicine; Naturopathic Physicians Licensing Exam.

Admission Requirements: Some college (60 semester hrs for BS, 90 semester hrs for ND); Min GPA: 2.25; Bachelor's degree for MS; Master's degree for Postgraduate Certificate in Spirituality, Health and Medicine; Naturopathic medicine or acupuncture background required for Chinese Herbal Medicine; Naturopathic medical student or physician for Midwifery Certificate.

Application Deadline(s): Fall: Feb 1 for ND; Spring: Apr 1.

Tuition and Fees: $8805 + $705 books per yr (BS Nutrition, Psychology); $11,980 + $1200 books per yr (BS Oriental Medicine); $12,340 + $1235 books per yr (MS Acupuncture); $14,300 + $1445 books per yr (ND).

Financial Aid: Federal government aid; Grants; Loans; State government aid.

Kennewick

811. Tri-City School of Massage
26 E 3rd Ave, Kennewick, WA 99336
Phone: (509) 586-6434
Program Administrator: Patty J. Kruschke, Dir.
Year Established: 1968.
Staff: Full-time: 2.
Avg Enrollment: 40. *Avg Class Size:* 20. *Number of Graduates per Year:* 40.
Wheelchair Access: No.
Accreditation/Approval/Licensing: State board: WA Workforce Training and Ed Coordinating Board.
Field of Study: Massage Therapy*. *Program Name/Length:* 6 mos.
Degrees Offered: Diploma.
License/Certification Preparation: State: WA Licensed Massage Practitioner; National Certification Board for Therapeutic Massage and Bodywork.
Admission Requirements: High school diploma/GED.
Application Deadline(s): Fall: Aug.
Tuition and Fees: $4300.

Lake Stevens

812. Spectrum Center School of Massage
Professional Massage Training
12506 18th St NE, Ste 1, Lake Stevens, WA 98258
Mailing Address: 1001 N Russell Rd, Snohomish, WA 98290
Phone: (425) 334-5409
E-mail: spctrmcntr@aol.com
Program Administrator: Barbara Collins, Owner/Dir. *Admissions Contact:* Barbara Collins.
Year Established: 1981.
Staff: Full-time: 5; Part-time: 10.
Avg Enrollment: 40. *Avg Class Size:* 18. *Number of Graduates per Year:* 34.
Wheelchair Access: Yes.
Accreditation/Approval/Licensing: State board: WA Board of Massage; WA Workforce Training and Ed Coordinating Board.
Field of Study: CranioSacral Therapy; Massage Therapy*; Polarity Therapy; Sports Massage. *Program Name/Length:* 10 mos.
Degrees Offered: Diploma.
License/Certification Preparation: State: WA Licensed Massage Practitioner; National Certification Board for Therapeutic Massage and Bodywork.
Admission Requirements: Min age: 18; High school diploma/GED.
Application Deadline(s): Fall: Aug 15.
Tuition and Fees: $6350.
Financial Aid: VA approved; Vocational rehabilitation.

Career Services: Career information; Job information.

Port Angeles

813. Peninsula College
Massage Therapy Program
1502 E Lauridsen Blvd, Port Angeles, WA 98362
Phone: (360) 417-6569
Program Administrator: Lisa Redlin, Coord. *Admissions Contact:* Dona Smasal, Asst to Dean.
Year Established: 1996.
Staff: Part-time: 4.
Avg Enrollment: 20. *Avg Class Size:* 20. *Number of Graduates per Year:* 18.
Wheelchair Access: Yes.
Accreditation/Approval/Licensing: State board: WA Dept of Health.
Field of Study: Aromatherapy; Deep Muscle Massage*; Energy Work; Massage Therapy*; Oriental Medicine; Shiatsu*. *Program Name/Length:* 850-1000 hrs, 1 yr.
Degrees Offered: Certificate.
License/Certification Preparation: State: WA Licensed Massage Practitioner; National Certification Board for Therapeutic Massage and Bodywork.
Admission Requirements: High school diploma/GED.
Application Deadline(s): Fall: Sep.
Tuition and Fees: $3600.
Financial Aid: Grants; Loans; State government aid; Work study; VA approved.
Career Services: Career information; Internships; Resume service.

Seattle

814. Ashmead College, Seattle
7120 Woodlawn Ave NE, Seattle, WA 98115
Phone: (206) 527-0807; *Fax:* (206) 527-1957
Internet: http://www.ashmeadcollege.com
Program Administrator: Jillian Orton, LMP, Campus Mgr. *Admissions Contact:* Marsha Aldinger, Admissions Rep; Sonia DeLeon, Admissions Rep.
Year Established: 1974.
Staff: Part-time: 29.
Avg Enrollment: 200. *Avg Class Size:* 22. *Number of Graduates per Year:* 150.
Wheelchair Access: Yes.
Accreditation/Approval/Licensing: State board: WA Workforce Training and Ed Coordinating Board; Accrediting Council for Continuing Education and Training; Commission on Massage Therapy Accreditation.
Field of Study: Anatomy and Physiology; Aromatherapy*; First Aid/CPR; Geriatric Massage; Hydrotherapy; Kinesiology*; Massage Therapy*; Pregnancy Massage; Spa Therapies*;

Sports Massage*. *Program Name/Length:* Comprehensive Professional Licensing, 1038 hrs, 1 yr; Sports Massage Specialist, 243 hrs, 3 mos; Aromatherapy and Spa Specialist, 242 hrs, 3 mos; Hospital/Long-Term Care Massage Specialist, 247 hrs, 3 mos.
Degrees Offered: Diploma.
License/Certification Preparation: State: WA Licensed Massage Practitioner; National Certification Board for Therapeutic Massage and Bodywork.
Admission Requirements: Min age: 18; High school diploma/GED.
Tuition and Fees: $9874 + $1240 books, table, supplies (Comprehensive); $2800 + $920 books, table, supplies (Specialist).
Financial Aid: Federal government aid.
Career Services: Career counseling; Career information; Internships; Interview set up; Resume service.
Comments: Formerly Seattle Massage School.

815. Ayur-vedic Medicine, Yoga Therapy, Ultra-Nutrition (AYU) School

819 NE 65th St, Seattle, WA 98115
Phone: (206) 729-9999; *Fax:* (206) 729-0164
Program Administrator: Vivek Shanbhag, MD, Prog Dir. *Admissions Contact:* Gaya, Prog Mgr.
Year Established: 1991.
Staff: Full-time: 3.
Avg Enrollment: 30. *Avg Class Size:* 30. *Number of Graduates per Year:* 25.
Wheelchair Access: Yes.
Field of Study: Aromatherapy; Ayurvedic Medicine*; Herbal Medicine*; Naturopathic Medicine*; Yoga Therapy*. *Program Name/Length:* Ayurveda, Yoga, and Ultra-Nutrition (AYU) Education, individualized 1-6 mos.
Degrees Offered: Certificate.
Admission Requirements: Min age: 18; High school diploma/GED; Specific course prerequisites: introductory ayur-veda, naturopathy, nutrition.
Tuition and Fees: $400-$2000.
Financial Aid: Work study.
Career Services: Internships.

816. BodyMind Energetics Institute

15832 34th Ave NE, Seattle, WA 98155
Phone: (206) 361-4700
Program Administrator: Reed Svadesh Johnson, Dir. *Admissions Contact:* Reed Svadesh Johnson.
Year Established: 1996.
Staff: Part-time: 4.
Avg Class Size: 10.
Wheelchair Access: No.
Accreditation/Approval/Licensing: National Certification Board for Therapeutic Massage and Bodywork (CEUs).
Field of Study: Orgodynamics*; Qigong; Shiatsu*; Trager*. *Program Name/Length:* Art and Technique of Deep Touching, 83 hrs, 13 wks; Orgodynamics, 14 hrs, 2 days; Orgodynamics, 56 hrs, 7 days; Orgodynamics, 10 days; Shiatsu, 25 hrs, 10 wks; Introduction to Meridians, 16 hrs; Trager, 16 hrs, 2 days.
Degrees Offered: Certificate.
Admission Requirements: Licensed health care professional for all except Orgodynamics.
Tuition and Fees: $1095 (Deep Touching); $200 (14-hr Orgodynamics; Meridians; Trager); $850 (7-day Orgodynamics) includes room and board; $1150 (10-day Orgodynamics) includes room and board; $325 (Shiatsu).

817. Brenneke School of Massage

160 Roy St, Seattle, WA 98109
Phone: (206) 282-1233; *Fax:* (206) 282-9183
E-mail: brenneke@halcyon.com *Internet:* http://www.brennekeschool.com
Program Administrator: Heida Brenneke, Dir. *Admissions Contact:* Lee Mattingly, Admissions Dir.
Year Established: 1974.
Staff: Full-time: 5; Part-time: 15.
Avg Enrollment: 125. *Avg Class Size:* 35. *Number of Graduates per Year:* 125.
Wheelchair Access: No.
Accreditation/Approval/Licensing: State board: WA Board of Massage; Accrediting Council for Continuing Education and Training; Commission on Massage Therapy Accreditation; National Certification Board for Therapeutic Massage and Bodywork (CEUs).
Field of Study: CranioSacral Therapy; Massage Therapy*; Polarity Therapy; Reflexology; Reiki; Shiatsu; Sports Massage. *Program Name/Length:* Professional Licensing, 11 mos; Expanded Professional Licensing, 11 mos or 18 mos.
Degrees Offered: Diploma.
License/Certification Preparation: State: WA Licensed Massage Practitioner; National Certification Board for Therapeutic Massage and Bodywork.
Admission Requirements: Min age: 18; High school diploma/GED; Specific course prerequisites: introductory massage class.
Application Deadline(s): Fall; Winter; Spring.
Tuition and Fees: $6950 + $700-$1000 books, table, supplies (Professional Licensing).
Financial Aid: Federal government aid.
Career Services: Career counseling; Career information; Resume service.

818. Heartspring Transformation Trainings

5404 Meridian Ave N, Seattle, WA 98103
Phone: (206) 547-4064
E-mail: byheart@wolfenet.com
Program Administrator: Pamela Grace, Dir. *Admissions Contact:* Pamela Grace.
Year Established: 1990.
Staff: Part-time: 11.

Avg Enrollment: 30. *Avg Class Size:* 15. *Number of Graduates per Year:* 20.
Wheelchair Access: Yes.
Accreditation/Approval/Licensing: National Board for Hypnotherapy and Hypnotic Anesthesiology.
Field of Study: Hypnotherapy*; Reiki*. *Program Name/Length:* TransSynthesis Transpersonal Therapy, 18 mos.
Degrees Offered: Diploma; Certificate.
License/Certification Preparation: American Council of Hypnotist Examiners.
Admission Requirements: Min age: 18; High school diploma/GED; Written biography; interview.
Financial Aid: Payment plan.
Career Services: Internships; Referral service.

819. Institute for Therapeutic Learning

9322 21st Ave NW, Seattle, WA 98117
Phone: (206) 783-1838
E-mail: jelias@sprynet.com *Internet:* http://www.home.sprynet.com/sprynet/jelias
Program Administrator: Jack Elias, Dir. *Admissions Contact:* Jack Elias.
Year Established: 1988.
Staff: Full-time: 1.
Avg Enrollment: 30. *Avg Class Size:* 10. *Number of Graduates per Year:* 30.
Wheelchair Access: No.
Accreditation/Approval/Licensing: State board: WA Workforce Training and Ed Coordinating Board.
Field of Study: Energy Work; Hypnotherapy*. *Program Name/Length:* Transpersonal Hypnotherapy Certification, 150-450+ hrs, classroom and home study.
Degrees Offered: CEUs; Certificate.
License/Certification Preparation: American Board of Clinical Hypnosis; American Council of Hypnotist Examiners.
Admission Requirements: Min age: 18; High school diploma/GED; Min GPA: 2.5.
Tuition and Fees: $1500-$3000.
Financial Aid: State government aid; Vocational rehabilitation.

820. The Institute of Dynamic Aromatherapy

2000 2nd Ave, Ste 206, Seattle, WA 98121
Phone: (206) 374-8773, (800) 260-7401; *Fax:* (206) 374-9020
E-mail: jades@accessone.com *Internet:* http://www.fragrantearth.com
Program Administrator: Jade Shutes, Pres/Head Lecturer. *Admissions Contact:* Jade Shutes.
Year Established: 1991.
Staff: Full-time: 2; Part-time: 1.
Avg Enrollment: 600. *Avg Class Size:* 15. *Number of Graduates per Year:* 500.
Wheelchair Access: Yes.
Accreditation/Approval/Licensing: National Association for Holistic Aromatherapy.

Field of Study: Aromatherapy*; Herbal Medicine*; Reflexology. *Program Name/Length:* Dynamic Aromatherapy, 9 mos; Advanced Clinical Aromatherapy, 9 mos; Aroma-Reflex Therapy, 6 mos; Modular Program, 1 yr, classroom or correspondence; Correspondence course, 6-12 mos; Day and evening workshops.
Degrees Offered: Diploma; Certificate.
Admission Requirements: Min age: 18; High school diploma/GED.
Application Deadline(s): Fall: Sep 15; Winter: Oct 15; Spring: Jan 20; Summer: Mar 15.
Tuition and Fees: $1850 (Dynamic; Advanced Clinical); $600 (Aroma-Reflex); $375 (Correspondence).
Financial Aid: Work study.
Career Services: Career counseling; Career information; Internships.

821. North American Institute of Neuro-Therapy

117 E Louisa, Ste 188, Seattle, WA 98102
Phone: (206) 322-0633
E-mail: neurother@aol.com *Internet:* http://www.members.aol.com/NeuroTher/
Program Administrator: Marilyn Michael, Admin. *Admissions Contact:* Marilyn Michael.
Year Established: 1987.
Staff: Full-time: 1.
Avg Enrollment: 40. *Number of Graduates per Year:* 35.
Accreditation/Approval/Licensing: State board: WA Workforce Training and Ed Coordinating Board.
Field of Study: Neuro-Therapy*. *Program Name/Length:* Neuro-Therapy Training Certification, home study or personal coaching.
Degrees Offered: Certificate.
Admission Requirements: Min age: 18; High school diploma/GED.
Tuition and Fees: $1250.

822. Northwest Institute of Acupuncture and Oriental Medicine

701 N 34th St, Ste 300, Seattle, WA 98103
Phone: (206) 633-2419; *Fax:* (206) 633-5578
E-mail: niaom@halcyon.com *Internet:* http://www.halcyon.com/niaom
Program Administrator: Frederick O. Lanphear, PhD, Pres. *Admissions Contact:* Mary McGhee, Admissions Advisor.
Year Established: 1981.
Staff: Full-time: 10; Part-time: 45.
Avg Enrollment: 70. *Avg Class Size:* 35. *Number of Graduates per Year:* 60.
Wheelchair Access: Yes.
Accreditation/Approval/Licensing: State board: WA Higher Ed Coordinating Board; Accreditation Commission for Acupuncture and Oriental Medicine.
Field of Study: Acupuncture*; Oriental Medicine*; Traditional Chinese Medicine*. *Program*

Name/Length: Master of Acupuncture, 3 yrs; Master of Traditional Chinese Medicine, 4 yrs.
Degrees Offered: MAc; MTCM.
License/Certification Preparation: State: WA Certified Acupuncturist; National Certification Commission for Acupuncture and Oriental Medicine.
Admission Requirements: Some college (3 yrs); Specific course prerequisites: college-level biology, psychology.
Tuition and Fees: $25, 338 (MAc); $30, 344 (MTCM).
Financial Aid: Federal government aid.
Career Services: Career information.

823. Seattle Institute of Oriental Medicine

916 NE 65th St, Ste B, Seattle, WA 98115
Phone: (206) 517-4541; *Fax:* (206) 526-1932
E-mail: info@siom.com *Internet:* http://www.siom.com
Program Administrator: Dan Bensky, Co-Dir; Paul Karsten, Co-Dir. *Admissions Contact:* Timothy Callahan, Academic Dean.
Year Established: 1994.
Staff: Full-time: 3; Part-time: 20.
Avg Enrollment: 30. *Avg Class Size:* 10. *Number of Graduates per Year:* 10.
Wheelchair Access: Yes.
Accreditation/Approval/Licensing: State board: WA Workforce Training and Ed Coordinating Board; Accreditation Commission for Acupuncture and Oriental Medicine.
Field of Study: Acupuncture*; Oriental Medicine*; Traditional Chinese Medicine*. *Program Name/Length:* Acupuncture and Oriental Medicine, 3 yrs.
Degrees Offered: Diploma.
License/Certification Preparation: State: WA Licensed Acupuncturist; National Certification Commission for Acupuncture and Oriental Medicine.
Admission Requirements: Some college (3 yrs); Specific course prerequisites: 120 hrs anatomy and physiology, and western medical terminology, and CPR/First Aid.

824. Seattle Midwifery School

2524 16th Ave S, Rm 300, Seattle, WA 98109
Phone: (206) 322-8834; *Fax:* (206) 328-280
E-mail: sms06@sprynet.com
Program Administrator: Therese Charvet, RN, Dir. *Admissions Contact:* Melissa Hicks, Asst.
Year Established: 1978.
Staff: Part-time: 17.
Avg Enrollment: 35. *Avg Class Size:* 14. *Number of Graduates per Year:* 12.
Wheelchair Access: Yes.
Accreditation/Approval/Licensing: State board: WA Workforce Training and Ed Coordinating Board; Accrediting Council for Continuing Education and Training; Midwifery Education Accreditation Council.

Field of Study: Childbirth Education; Doula*; Midwifery*. *Program Name/Length:* Midwifery Education Program, 27 mos.
Degrees Offered: Certificate.
License/Certification Preparation: State: WA Licensed Midwife.
Admission Requirements: Min age: 21; High school diploma/GED; Some college (1 yr); Specific course prerequisites: Min GPA: 3.0 and 5 qtr credits each: English, social science, anatomy and physiology, microbiology; 3 qtr credits: nutrition, math (or 2 yrs h.s.), biology (or 1 yr h.s.); Labor support course certified by Doulas of North America; Proficiency in English.
Application Deadline(s): Fall: Feb 1.
Tuition and Fees: $20,000-$30,000.
Financial Aid: Scholarships.

825. University of Washington, School of Nursing

Nurse-Midwifery Program, Dept of Family and Child Nursing
PO Box 357262, Seattle, WA 98195-7262
Phone: (206) 543-8241
E-mail: midwife@u.washington.edu *Internet:* http://www.son.washington.edu/~midwife/
Program Administrator: Aileen MacLaren, PhD, Dir.
Accreditation/Approval/Licensing: American College of Nurse-Midwives, Division of Accreditation.
Field of Study: Midwifery*.
Degrees Offered: MN.
License/Certification Preparation: Certified Nurse-Midwife, American College of Nurse-Midwives.
Admission Requirements: Bachelor's degree; RN.

826. Brian Utting School of Massage

900 Thomas St, Seattle, WA 98109
Phone: (206) 292-8055, (800) 842-8731; *Fax:* (206) 292-0113
E-mail: admissions@busm.com *Internet:* http://www.busm.com
Program Administrator: Brian Utting, Dir. *Admissions Contact:* Susan Sanford, Kelly Maloney, Admissions Counselors.
Year Established: 1982.
Staff: Full-time: 10; Part-time: 9.
Avg Class Size: 40.
Wheelchair Access: No.
Accreditation/Approval/Licensing: State board: OR and WA Boards of Massage; Accrediting Council for Continuing Education and Training; Commission on Massage Therapy Accreditation; National Certification Board for Therapeutic Massage and Bodywork (CEUs).
Field of Study: Connective Tissue Massage; Deep Tissue Massage; Hydrotherapy; Injury Treatment and Evaluation; Massage Therapy*; Neuromuscular Therapy; Sports Massage. *Pro-*

gram Name/Length: Massage Licensing, 1000 hrs, 15 mos.

Degrees Offered: Certificate.

License/Certification Preparation: State: WA Licensed Massage Practitioner; National Certification Board for Therapeutic Massage and Bodywork.

Admission Requirements: Min age: 18; High school diploma/GED; Health release; Specific course prerequisites: introductory workshop.

Tuition and Fees: $8700.

Financial Aid: Loans; State government aid; VA approved.

Career Services: Career information; Instruction in business skills; Internships; Job information.

Spokane

827. Inland Massage Institute, Inc

111 E Magnesium Rd, Ste F, Spokane, WA 99208

Phone: (509) 465-3033; Fax: (509) 326-1236

Program Administrator: Sheryl L. Storro, Admin. Admissions Contact: Sheryl L. Storro.

Year Established: 1988.

Staff: Full-time: 4.

Avg Enrollment: 60. Avg Class Size: 30. Number of Graduates per Year: 58.

Wheelchair Access: Yes.

Accreditation/Approval/Licensing: State board: WA Workforce Training and Ed Coordinating Board.

Field of Study: Massage Therapy*; Swedish Massage*. Program Name/Length: 1 yr.

Degrees Offered: Certificate.

License/Certification Preparation: State: WA Licensed Massage Practitioner.

Admission Requirements: Min age: 18; High school diploma/GED.

Application Deadline(s): Fall: Aug 1; Spring: Feb 1.

Tuition and Fees: $5000 + $500 books.

Financial Aid: VA approved; Vocational rehabilitation.

Vancouver

828. Cedar Mountain Center for Massage, Inc

5601 NE Saint John's Rd, Vancouver, WA 98661

Phone: (360) 696-2210; Fax: (360) 696-0130

E-mail: handshealr@aol.com

Program Administrator: Sandra V. Hattan, Co-Dir; Liz Addis, Co-Dir. Admissions Contact: Sandra V. Hattan; Liz Addis.

Staff: Part-time: 16.

Avg Enrollment: 60. Avg Class Size: 22. Number of Graduates per Year: 45.

Wheelchair Access: No.

Accreditation/Approval/Licensing: State board: WA Workforce Training and Ed Coordinating Board; WA and OR Boards of Massage.

Field of Study: Aromatherapy; Massage Therapy*; Polarity Therapy; Reflexology; Shiatsu; Sports Massage. Program Name/Length: Licensed Massage Therapy, 1 yr.

Degrees Offered: Certificate.

License/Certification Preparation: State: WA Licensed Massage Practitioner; OR Licensed Massage Technician; National Certification Board for Therapeutic Massage and Bodywork.

Admission Requirements: Min age: 18; High school diploma/GED.

Application Deadline(s): Fall: Oct 10; Spring: Feb 20; Summer: Jun 20.

Tuition and Fees: $6550.

Financial Aid: VA approved; Vocational rehabilitation; Private credit company for tuition financing.

Career Services: Career information.

WEST VIRGINIA

Malden

829. Mountain State School of Massage

3407 River Lane Dr, Malden, WV 25306

Mailing Address: PO Box 4487, Charleston, WV 25364

Phone: (304) 926-8822; Fax: (304) 926-8837

E-mail: info@mtnstmassage.com Internet: http://www.mtnstmassage.com

Program Administrator: Robert Rogers, LMT, Dir.

Year Established: 1995.

Staff: Full-time: 1; Part-time: 10.

Avg Enrollment: 30. Avg Class Size: 20. Number of Graduates per Year: 29.

Accreditation/Approval/Licensing: State board: WV College Systems; National Certification Board for Therapeutic Massage and Bodywork (CEUs).

Field of Study: Anatomy and Physiology; Chair Massage; Connective Tissue Massage; Hydrotherapy; Kinesiology; Massage Therapy*; Neuromuscular Therapy*; Polarity Therapy*; Reflexology*; Shiatsu*; Sports Massage*; Swedish Massage*. Program Name/Length:

Massage Therapy, 6 mos or 18 mos/home study and weekend classes.
Degrees Offered: Diploma.
License/Certification Preparation: State: WV Licensed Massage Therapist; National Certification Board for Therapeutic Massage and Bodywork.

Admission Requirements: Min age: 19; High school diploma/GED.
Tuition and Fees: $5600 (6 mos); $5200 (18 mos).
Financial Aid: State government aid; Vocational rehabilitation.
Career Services: Career information.

WISCONSIN

Appleton

830. Fox Valley School of Massage
Professional Massage Training
2003 N Meade St, Appleton, WI 54914
Mailing Address: PO Box 615, Neenah, WI 54957
Phone: (920) 722-3271; *Fax:* (920) 882-9412
Program Administrator: Stephanie Lynn Hall, Admin. *Admissions Contact:* Tom Finch, Pres.
Year Established: 1996.
Staff: Full-time: 2; Part-time: 8.
Avg Enrollment: 55. *Avg Class Size:* 16. *Number of Graduates per Year:* 55.
Wheelchair Access: Yes.
Accreditation/Approval/Licensing: State board: WI Educational Approval Board.
Field of Study: Aromatherapy; Massage Therapy*; Neuromuscular Therapy; Polarity Therapy; Qigong; Reiki. *Program Name/Length:* Massage Therapy, 600 hrs, 6 mos or 10 mos.
Degrees Offered: Certificate.
License/Certification Preparation: National Certification Board for Therapeutic Massage and Bodywork.
Admission Requirements: Min age: 18; High school diploma/GED; Essay; Medical approval; 2 letters of recommendation; 2 professional massages.
Application Deadline(s): Fall: Aug 15; Spring: Jan 15.
Tuition and Fees: $5000 + $350 books.
Financial Aid: Vocational rehabilitation; Payment plan.
Career Services: Job information.

Grafton

831. Blue Sky Educational Foundation, Professional School of Massage and Therapeutic Bodywork
220 Oak St, Grafton, WI 53024
Phone: (414) 376-1011; *Fax:* (414) 376-7707
Program Administrator: Karen Lewis, Dean. *Admissions Contact:* Vicki Chossek, Exec Dir.
Staff: Part-time: 6.

Avg Enrollment: 120. *Avg Class Size:* 36.
Wheelchair Access: Yes.
Field of Study: Massage Therapy*. *Program Name/Length:* 10 mos (1 day or 2 evenings per wk + 9 weekend seminars).
Degrees Offered: Diploma.
License/Certification Preparation: State: WI Licensed Massage Therapist; National Certification Board for Therapeutic Massage and Bodywork.
Admission Requirements: Min age: 18; High school diploma/GED.
Application Deadline(s): Fall: Aug 15 and Sep 15; Spring: Jan 15.
Tuition and Fees: $5675 + $500 books, supplies.
Financial Aid: VA approved.
Career Services: Career counseling; Career information; Internships.

Hudson

832. Saint Croix Center for the Healing Arts, Ltd
600 Hr Massage Therapy and Bodywork Program
411 County Hwy UU, Hudson, WI 54016
Phone: (715) 381-1402; *Fax:* (715) 381-1502
E-mail: sccha@spacestar.net *Internet:* http://www.sccha.com
Program Administrator: June Motzer-Trollen, Pres/Dir. *Admissions Contact:* June Motzer-Trollen.
Year Established: 1997.
Staff: Full-time: 1; Part-time: 9.
Avg Enrollment: 100. *Avg Class Size:* 12. *Number of Graduates per Year:* 20.
Wheelchair Access: Yes.
Field of Study: Acupressure; Aromatherapy; Massage Therapy*; Reflexology; Sports Massage. *Program Name/Length:* 600 hrs.
Degrees Offered: Certificate.
License/Certification Preparation: State: WI Licensed Massage Therapist; National Certification Board for Therapeutic Massage and Bodywork.

Admission Requirements: Min age: 18; High school diploma/GED.
Application Deadline(s): Fall; Winter; Spring; Summer.
Tuition and Fees: $5775 + $500 books, videos.
Financial Aid: Loans.
Career Services: Job information.

Madison

833. Capri College, Madison
Massage Therapy Program
6414 Odana Rd, Madison, WI 53719
Phone: (608) 274-5390; *Fax:* (608) 274-1215
Internet: http://www.capricollege.com
Year Established: 1994.
Staff: Full-time: 2; Part-time: 2.
Avg Enrollment: 48. *Avg Class Size:* 12. *Number of Graduates per Year:* 44.
Wheelchair Access: No.
Accreditation/Approval/Licensing: State board: WI Educational Approval Board; Accrediting Council for Continuing Education and Training; Accrediting Commission of Career Schools and Colleges of Technology.
Field of Study: Acupressure; Aromatherapy; Massage Therapy*; Reflexology; Reiki; Shiatsu; Swedish Massage*. *Program Name/Length:* 650 hrs, 7 mos.
Degrees Offered: Diploma; Certificate.
License/Certification Preparation: National Certification Board for Therapeutic Massage and Bodywork.
Admission Requirements: Min age: 17; High school diploma/GED; 2 professional massages; Interview with program director.
Financial Aid: Grants; Loans.
Career Services: Career information.

834. A SpiriTouch Institute, Inc
Massage Therapy Program
6225 University, Madison, WI 53705
Phone: (608) 236-9042; *Fax:* (608) 236-9570
E-mail: lynnzncmt@aol.com
Program Administrator: Lynn Zimmerman, Owner. *Admissions Contact:* Lori Hellenbrand, Admin Asst.
Year Established: 1997.
Staff: Part-time: 25.
Avg Enrollment: 100. *Avg Class Size:* 12 (day), 20 (night). *Number of Graduates per Year:* 100.
Wheelchair Access: No.
Accreditation/Approval/Licensing: State board: WI Educational Approval Board.
Field of Study: Energy Work; Massage Therapy*; Reiki. *Program Name/Length:* 700 hrs.
Degrees Offered: Diploma.
License/Certification Preparation: State: WI Licensed Massage Therapist; National Certification Board for Therapeutic Massage and Bodywork.

Admission Requirements: Min age: 18; High school diploma/GED; Interview.
Tuition and Fees: $5700 includes books.
Financial Aid: Scholarships; State government aid; Work study; Payment plan; Pending, VA approval.
Career Services: Career information; Job information.

Milwaukee

835. Lakeside School of Massage Therapy
1726 N 1st St, Ste 100, Milwaukee, WI 53212
Phone: (414) 372-4345; *Fax:* (414) 372-5350
E-mail: lakeschool@aol.com
Program Administrator: Claude Gagnon, Prog Dir. *Admissions Contact:* Susan Miller, Student Svcs Dir.
Year Established: 1985.
Staff: Part-time: 9.
Avg Enrollment: 75. *Avg Class Size:* 24. *Number of Graduates per Year:* 75.
Wheelchair Access: Yes.
Accreditation/Approval/Licensing: State board: WI Educational Approval Board; Commission on Massage Therapy Accreditation.
Field of Study: Acupressure; Massage Therapy*; Reflexology; Shiatsu. *Program Name/Length:* Certification, 600 hrs, 6-9 mos or 18 mos.
Degrees Offered: Certificate.
License/Certification Preparation: State: WI Dept of Regulation and Licensure; National Certification Board for Therapeutic Massage and Bodywork.
Admission Requirements: Min age: 18; High school diploma/GED.
Application Deadline(s): Fall: Aug; Spring: Mar.
Tuition and Fees: $5200 + $400 books.
Financial Aid: VA approved; Vocational rehabilitation; Payment plan.
Career Services: Career counseling; Career information.

836. Marquette University, College of Nursing
Nurse-Midwifery Program
PO Box 1881, Milwaukee, WI 53201-1881
Phone: (414) 288-3842
E-mail: leonavandevusse@marquette.edu
Program Administrator: Leona Vandevusse, CNM, PhD, Prog Dir. *Admissions Contact:* Leona Vandevusse.
Year Established: 1993.
Staff: Full-time: 3; Part-time: 1.
Avg Enrollment: 20. *Avg Class Size:* 10. *Number of Graduates per Year:* 10.
Wheelchair Access: Yes.
Accreditation/Approval/Licensing: American College of Nurse-Midwives, Division of Accreditation.

Field of Study: Midwifery*. *Program Name/Length:* 4 semesters/full-time (summers off), 2 yrs.
Degrees Offered: Certificate; MSN.
License/Certification Preparation: Certified Nurse-Midwife, American College of Nurse-Midwives.
Admission Requirements: Bachelor's degree in Nursing; Min GPA: 3.0; RN; Specific course prerequisites: statistics, physical assessment, nursing research; 1 yr maternal-child health-related experience.
Application Deadline(s): Fall: Feb 15.
Financial Aid: Fellowships; Federal government aid; Loans; Scholarships; State government aid; Work study.
Career Services: Career information.

837. Milwaukee School of Massage

600-Hour Swedish Massage Program
830 E Chambers St, Milwaukee, WI 53212
Phone: (414) 347-1151
Program Administrator: Wanda M. Beals, Chief Admin. *Admissions Contact:* Wanda M. Beals.
Year Established: 1995.
Staff: Part-time: 4.
Avg Enrollment: 25. *Avg Class Size:* 12. *Number of Graduates per Year:* 18.
Wheelchair Access: Yes.
Accreditation/Approval/Licensing: State board: WI Educational Approval Board.
Field of Study: Acupressure; Ayurvedic Medicine; CranioSacral Therapy; Energy Work; Feldenkrais; Massage Therapy*; Myofascial Release; Oriental Medicine; Reiki; Swedish Massage*. *Program Name/Length:* 600 hrs, 1 yr.
Degrees Offered: Diploma.
License/Certification Preparation: State: WI Licensed Massage Therapist; National Certification Board for Therapeutic Massage and Bodywork.
Admission Requirements: Min age: 18; High school diploma/GED.
Tuition and Fees: $5500.
Financial Aid: Loans.

Racine

838. Midwest Center for the Study of Oriental Medicine, Racine

6226 Bankers Rd, Ste 8, Racine, WI 53403
Phone: (414) 554-2010; *Fax:* (414) 554-7475
E-mail: dunbardoc@aol.com *Internet:* http://www.acupuncture.edu
Program Administrator: Dr. William Dunbar, Pres. *Admissions Contact:* Kris LaPoint.
Year Established: 1979.
Staff: Full-time: 10; Part-time: 10.
Avg Enrollment: 180. *Avg Class Size:* 30. *Number of Graduates per Year:* 30.
Wheelchair Access: Yes.

Accreditation/Approval/Licensing: Accreditation Commission for Acupuncture and Oriental Medicine.
Field of Study: Acupressure; Acupuncture*; Herbal Medicine; Oriental Medicine*; Traditional Chinese Medicine*. *Program Name/Length:* Acupuncture Therapist, 27 mos; Master of Science in Oriental Medicine, 3 yrs.
Degrees Offered: MS.
License/Certification Preparation: National Certification Commission for Acupuncture and Oriental Medicine.
Admission Requirements: Some college (2 yrs); Min GPA: 2.0.
Tuition and Fees: $2790 per qtr.
Financial Aid: Grants; Loans.

839. Wisconsin Institute of Chinese Herbology

6921 Mariner Dr, Racine, WI 53406
Phone: (414) 886-5858; *Fax:* (414) 886-5858
E-mail: herbalstudies@aol.com
Program Administrator: Arthur D. Shattuck, Dir. *Admissions Contact:* Arthur D. Shattuck.
Year Established: 1991.
Staff: Full-time: 3; Part-time: 3.
Avg Enrollment: 30. *Avg Class Size:* 18. *Number of Graduates per Year:* 19.
Wheelchair Access: Yes.
Field of Study: Animal Therapy; Herbal Medicine*; Oriental Medicine; Traditional Chinese Medicine*. *Program Name/Length:* Chinese Herbology, 1 yr.
Degrees Offered: Certificate.
License/Certification Preparation: National Certification Commission for Acupuncture and Oriental Medicine.
Admission Requirements: Min age: 21; High school diploma/GED.
Tuition and Fees: $2800.
Financial Aid: Scholarships.

840. Wisconsin Institute of Natural Wellness

6921 Mariner Dr, Racine, WI 53406
Phone: (414) 886-3344; *Fax:* (414) 632-9533
Program Administrator: Anne M. Frontier, Co-Dir; Arthur D. Shattuck, Co-Dir. *Admissions Contact:* Arthur D. Shattuck.
Year Established: 1995.
Staff: Full-time: 2; Part-time: 6.
Avg Enrollment: 36. *Avg Class Size:* 20. *Number of Graduates per Year:* 34.
Wheelchair Access: Yes.
Accreditation/Approval/Licensing: State board: WI Educational Approval Board.
Field of Study: Acupressure; Massage Therapy*; Reflexology; Reiki; Shiatsu; Tai Chi; Traditional Chinese Medicine. *Program Name/Length:* Professional Certification, 650 hrs, 1 yr.
Degrees Offered: Certificate.

License/Certification Preparation: National Certification Board for Therapeutic Massage and Bodywork; International Myomassethics Federation.
Admission Requirements: Min age: 18; High school diploma/GED.
Tuition and Fees: $5000.
Financial Aid: Scholarships.

Twin Lakes

841. Institute for Wholistic Education
33719 116th St, Twin Lakes, WI 53181

Phone: (414) 877-9396; *Fax:* (414) 889-8591
Program Administrator: Santosh Krinsky, Pres. *Admissions Contact:* Santosh Krinsky.
Year Established: 1988.
Staff: Part-time: 2.
Avg Enrollment: 12. *Number of Graduates per Year:* 10.
Wheelchair Access: No.
Field of Study: Ayurvedic Medicine*. *Program Name/Length:* Correspondence courses.
Degrees Offered: Certificate.
Admission Requirements: Min age: 15.
Tuition and Fees: $250 per course.

CANADIAN SCHOOLS

ALBERTA

Calgary

842. Calgary College of Holistic Health and Clinics, Inc

Massage Therapy; Holistic Reflexology
412 Silver Valley Rd NW, Calgary, AB T3B 4B9
Canada.
Phone: (403) 288-4511; *Fax:* (403) 288-0114
E-mail: neumannn@cadvision.com *Internet:* http://
www.cadvision.com/neumannn
Program Administrator: Dr. John Neumann, Dir.
Admissions Contact: Dr. John Neumann.
Year Established: 1986.
Staff: Full-time: 4; Part-time: 12.
Avg Enrollment: 120.
Wheelchair Access: Yes.
Accreditation/Approval/Licensing: State board: AB
Advanced Education and Career Development,
Licensed Private Vocational School; Accrediting
Commission of Career Schools and Colleges of
Technology.
Field of Study: Acupressure; Aromatherapy; En-
ergy Work; Hypnotherapy; Massage Therapy*;
Reflexology; Shiatsu. *Program Name/Length:*
Massage Therapy, 250 hrs, 7 wks or 15 week-
ends; Advanced Massage Techniques and
Reflexology, weekend seminars.
Degrees Offered: Certificate.
Admission Requirements: Min age: 16; High
school diploma/GED.
Tuition and Fees: $C1975 (Massage Therapy);
$C200 (Weekend seminars).
Financial Aid: Grants and loans for Alberta resi-
dents.
Career Services: Career counseling; Career infor-
mation.

843. Foothills College of Massage Therapy

7330 Fisher St SE, Ste 400, Calgary, AB T2H 2H8
Canada.
Phone: (403) 255-4445; *Fax:* (403) 255-4074
E-mail: info@fcomt.com *Internet:* http://www.
fcomt.com
Program Administrator: Beth Checkley, Dir. *Ad-
missions Contact:* Beth Checkley.
Year Established: 1994.
Staff: Part-time: 10.
Avg Enrollment: 75. *Avg Class Size:* 30. *Number
of Graduates per Year:* 70.
Wheelchair Access: Yes.
Accreditation/Approval/Licensing: Alberta Provin-
cial Government, Advanced Education and Ca-
reer Development.

Field of Study: Massage Therapy*. *Program
Name/Length:* 1000 hrs, 6 mos; 2200 hrs, 13
mos.
Degrees Offered: Diploma.
License/Certification Preparation: National Certification Board for Therapeutic Massage and
Bodywork; Alberta Registered Massage Therapists Society; Massage Therapists Association of
Alberta.
Admission Requirements: Min age: 18; High
school diploma/GED; Specific course prerequisites: grade 12 biology credit if under 23 yrs of
age.
Application Deadline(s): Fall: Aug 1; Spring: Feb
1.
Tuition and Fees: $C6500 (1000 hrs); $C13,760
(2200 hrs); includes books.
Financial Aid: Federal government aid; Employment Insurance Retraining Financing; Provincial
government aid.
Career Services: Resume service; Job information.

844. Mount Royal College Centre for Complementary Health Education

Faculty of Continuing Education and Extension
2204 2nd St SW, Calgary, AB T2S 1F5 Canada.
Phone: (403) 503-4886; *Fax:* (403) 503-4899
E-mail: aghani@mtroyal.ab.ca
Program Administrator: Sylvia Muiznieks, Prog
Admin. *Admissions Contact:* Attiya Ghani, Stu-
dent Advisor.
Year Established: 1982.
Staff: Full-time: 20.
Avg Enrollment: 80 full-time; 150 part-time. *Avg
Class Size:* 26. *Number of Graduates per Year:*
100.
Wheelchair Access: Yes.
Field of Study: Acupressure; Aromatherapy;
Herbal Medicine; Massage Therapy*;
Reflexology; Sports Massage. *Program
Name/Length:* Massage Therapy, 1000 hrs, 1
yr/full-time or 3 yrs/part-time; Holistic Certifi-
cates, 2 semesters.
Degrees Offered: Certificate.
License/Certification Preparation: Alberta Regis-
tered Massage Therapists Society.
Admission Requirements: Min age: 18; High
school diploma/GED.
Tuition and Fees: $C6250 per yr.
Financial Aid: Provincial student loans.
Career Services: Career counseling; Resume ser-
vice; Job information.

845. The School of Homeopathy-Devon, England

North American Flexible Learning Program, Administrative Office-Canada

4 Oakvale Pl SW, Calgary, AB T2V 1H4Canada
Phone: (403) 281-7976; *Fax:* (403) 281-7976
E-mail: stastnyp@cadvision.com *Internet:* http://www.homeopathyschool.com
Program Administrator: Misha Norland, Dir; Stuart Gracie, Course Mgr. *Admissions Contact:* Hana Stastny, MD, Canadian Representative.
Year Established: 1981.
Staff: Full-time: 3; Part-time: 12.
Avg Enrollment: 100.
Accreditation/Approval/Licensing: Council on Homeopathic Education.
Field of Study: Anatomy and Physiology; Homeopathy*; Pathology and Disease. *Program Name/Length:* Foundation Certificate, 1 1/2 yrs; Three Year Program + clinical practice and case supervision; Seminars given in various locations; Home study/Correspondence.
Degrees Offered: Diploma; Certificate.
License/Certification Preparation: Council for Homeopathic Certification; North American Society of Homeopaths.
Admission Requirements: Interview.
Tuition and Fees: $2690 (Foundation); $3695 (3-Yr Program) or $1595 per yr; $100 registration fee.
Financial Aid: Payment plan.

Career Services: Mentor program.

Edmonton

846. Yoga Association of Alberta

Teacher Training Program
Percy Page Centre, 11759 Groat Rd, Edmonton, AB T5M 3K6 Canada.
Phone: (403) 427-8776; *Fax:* (403) 427-0524
E-mail: yogaab@planet.eon.net *Internet:* http://www.geocities.com/Athens/Ithaca/5554
Program Administrator: Debbie Spence, Admin. *Admissions Contact:* Margo Balog; Debbie Spence.
Year Established: 1976.
Staff: Part-time: 3.
Avg Enrollment: 20. *Avg Class Size:* 15. *Number of Graduates per Year:* 8.
Wheelchair Access: Yes.
Field of Study: Yoga Teacher Training*. *Program Name/Length:* 300 hrs, 2 yrs.
Degrees Offered: Certificate.
License/Certification Preparation: AB Certification.
Admission Requirements: Min age: 18; High school diploma/GED; Specific course prerequisites: 2 yrs of yoga classes.
Tuition and Fees: $C1000-$C1500 per yr.
Financial Aid: Loans.
Career Services: Career information.

BRITISH COLUMBIA

Burnaby

847. Dominion Herbal College

7527 Kingsway, Burnaby, BC V3N 3C1 Canada.
Phone: (604) 521-5822; *Fax:* (604) 526-1561
E-mail: herbal@uniserve.com *Internet:* http://www.dominionherbal.com
Program Administrator: Judy Nelson, DC. *Admissions Contact:* Bernice Birzneck, RN, Registrar.
Year Established: 1926.
Staff: Full-time: 2; Part-time: 20.
Avg Enrollment: 200. *Avg Class Size:* 12. *Number of Graduates per Year:* 100.
Wheelchair Access: Yes.
Accreditation/Approval/Licensing: BC Private Postsecondary Ed Commission.
Field of Study: Aromatherapy*; Herbal Medicine*. *Program Name/Length:* Clinical Aromatherapy, 96 hrs, Saturdays; Chartered Herbalist, 1 yr, correspondence; Clinical Herbal Therapist, 3 yrs, Vancouver or Toronto classroom and correspondence; Clinical Herbal Medicine, 4 yr tutorial, home study and 500 hrs clinic; Clinical Herbal Medicine for Physicians, 2 yrs, home study and 150 hrs clinic; Phytomedicine for Pharmacists, 500 hrs clinic.
Degrees Offered: Diploma.
License/Certification Preparation: Canadian Herbalist Association of British Columbia.
Admission Requirements: High school diploma/GED; Specific course prerequisites: chemistry and biology for Aromatherapy and Clinical programs.
Application Deadline(s): Fall: Aug 15 for Clinical classroom.
Tuition and Fees: $C595 (Chartered); $C6500 per yr (3-yr Clinical); $C2500 per yr (4-yr Clinical).

Duncan

848. Meridian Institute
Certified Clinical Hypnotherapist
225 Canada Ave, Ste 105, Duncan, BC V9L 1T6
Canada.
Mailing Address: PO Box 753, Duncan, BC V9L
3Y1Canada
Phone: (250) 748-3588; *Fax:* (250) 748-3578
Program Administrator: Doris Gray, LPN, Exec
Dir/Head Instr. *Admissions Contact:* Doris
Gray.
Year Established: 1996.
Staff: Full-time: 1; Part-time: 5 guest speakers.
Avg Enrollment: 18. *Avg Class Size:* 18. *Number
of Graduates per Year:* 18.
Wheelchair Access: Yes.
Accreditation/Approval/Licensing: International
Medical and Dental Hypnotherapy Association.
Field of Study: Hypnotherapy*. *Program
Name/Length:* Master Hypnotist/Certified Clini-
cal Hypnotherapist, 200 hrs.
Degrees Offered: Certificate.
License/Certification Preparation: International
Medical and Dental Hypnotherapy Association.
Admission Requirements: Min age: 18; Interview.
Application Deadline(s): Winter: Aug.
Tuition and Fees: $2975.
Career Services: Referral service.

Vancouver

849. Vancouver Homeopathic Academy
Classical Homeopathy
PO Box 34095, Stn D, Vancouver, BC V6J
4M1Canada
Phone: (604) 708-9387; *Fax:* (604) 708-1547
Program Administrator: Murray Feldman, RSHom,
Dir. *Admissions Contact:* Kim Boutilier,
Admin.
Year Established: 1994.
Avg Enrollment: 25. *Avg Class Size:* 25. *Number
of Graduates per Year:* 15.
Wheelchair Access: No.
Accreditation/Approval/Licensing: State board: BC
Private Postsecondary Ed Commission; In pro-
cess, Council on Homeopathic Education.
Field of Study: Homeopathy*. *Program
Name/Length:* 4 yrs.
Degrees Offered: Diploma.
License/Certification Preparation: Council for Ho-
meopathic Certification; North American Soci-
ety of Homeopaths.
Admission Requirements: Min age: 21; High
school diploma/GED; Specific course prerequi-
sites: college-level anatomy and physiology;
Fluency in written and spoken English.
Application Deadline(s): Summer: Jul.

850. West Coast College of Massage Therapy
555 W Hastings St, 6th Fl, Vancouver, BC V6B
4N6 Canada.
Mailing Address: PO Box 12110, Vancouver, BC
V6B 4N6Canada
Phone: (604) 689-3854, (888) 449-2242; *Fax:*
(604) 689-9804
E-mail: dmahedyjr@aol.com *Internet:* http://www.
wccmt.edu
Program Administrator: Ron Garvock, RMT,
Dean. *Admissions Contact:* Christine Mullie,
Louise Morais, Admissions Officers.
Year Established: 1983.
Field of Study: Acupuncture*; Herbal Medicine*;
Humanistic Counseling*; Hydrotherapy; Massage Therapy*; Naturopathic Medicine*; Traditional Chinese Medicine*. *Program
Name/Length:* Diploma in Massage Therapy,
3150 hrs, 3 yrs; Diploma in Acupuncture/Tradi-
tional Chinese Medicine, 2250 hrs, 2 yrs; Diploma in Herbal Medicine, 1800 hrs, 2 yrs; Diploma in Humanistic Counseling Skills, 1350
hrs, 1 yr; Naturopathic Medicine, 4670 hrs, 4
yrs.
Admission Requirements: High school di-
ploma/GED; Some college (1 yr for Massage
Therapy, 3 yrs for Naturopathic Medicine); Specific course prerequisites: biology and grade 12
chemistry for Massage Therapy.
Application Deadline(s): Fall: Jul 31; Winter: Dec
1; Spring: Mar 31.
Tuition and Fees: $C25,100 + $C1500 books, supplies (Massage Therapy); $C15,450 + $C1250
books, supplies (Acupuncture); $C12,700 +
$C1000 books, supplies (Herbal Medicine);
$C9950 + $C750 books, supplies (Humanistic
Counseling); $C40,700 + $C2500 books, supplies (Naturopathic Medicine).
Financial Aid: Federal government aid; State government aid; Payment plan.
Career Services: Job information.

Victoria

851. Canadian College of Acupuncture and Oriental Medicine
4-Year Diploma Program in Traditional Chinese
Medicine
855 Cormorant St, Victoria, BC V8W 1R2 Canada.
Phone: (250) 384-2942; *Fax:* (250) 360-2871
E-mail: ccaom@islandnet.com *Internet:* http://
www.islandnet.com/~ccaom/
Program Administrator: David Rivers, MEd, Aca-
demic Dean. *Admissions Contact:* Diane St.
Hilair, Registrar.
Year Established: 1985.
Staff: Part-time: 12.
Avg Enrollment: 30. *Avg Class Size:* 26. *Number
of Graduates per Year:* 20.

Wheelchair Access: Yes.
Accreditation/Approval/Licensing: BC College of Acupuncturists; BC Private Postsecondary Ed Commission.
Field of Study: Acupressure; Acupuncture*; Herbal Medicine; Oriental Medicine*; Traditional Chinese Medicine*. *Program Name/Length:* Acupuncture and Traditional Chinese Medicine, 4 yrs.
Degrees Offered: Diploma.
License/Certification Preparation: British Columbia Provincial Certification; National Certification Commission for Acupuncture and Oriental Medicine.
Admission Requirements: Some college (2 yrs); Specific course prerequisites: human anatomy and physiology.
Application Deadline(s): Summer: Jun 30.
Tuition and Fees: $C6000 per yr.
Financial Aid: Government aid.

852. Dr. Vodder School, North America
PO Box 5701, Victoria, BC V8R 6S8Canada

Phone: (250) 598-9862; *Fax:* (250) 598-9862
E-mail: drvodderna@vodderschool.com *Internet:* http://www.vodderschool.com
Program Administrator: Robert Harris, Dir.
Year Established: 1994.
Staff: Full-time: 10.
Avg Enrollment: 500. *Avg Class Size:* 12. *Number of Graduates per Year:* 150.
Accreditation/Approval/Licensing: National Certification Board for Therapeutic Massage and Bodywork (CEUs).
Field of Study: Manual Lymph Drainage*. *Program Name/Length:* Dr. Vodder's Manual Lymph Drainage—Basic, 1 wk; Dr. Vodder's Manual Lymph Drainage—Therapy I, 1 wk; Therapy II and III, 2 wks; Review, 3 1/2 days; Seminars given in various locations.
Degrees Offered: Certificate.
Admission Requirements: Certified or licensed health care practitioner (500 hrs massage therapy training for massage therapists).
Tuition and Fees: $C550 per course.

MANITOBA

Winnipeg

853. Professional Institute of Massage Therapy, Winnipeg
570 Portage Ave, Winnipeg, MB R3C 0G4 Canada.
Phone: (204) 775-1642; *Fax:* (204) 775-1166
Program Administrator: Sue Mamer, Admin. *Admissions Contact:* Sue Mamer.
Year Established: 1994.
Staff: Part-time: 6.
Avg Enrollment: 36. *Avg Class Size:* 36. *Number of Graduates per Year:* 34.
Wheelchair Access: Yes.
Field of Study: Massage Therapy*. *Program Name/Length:* 2200 hrs, 2 yrs.

Degrees Offered: Diploma.
License/Certification Preparation: State: Manitoba; National Certification Board for Therapeutic Massage and Bodywork.
Admission Requirements: Min age: 18; High school diploma/GED; Specific course prerequisites: grade 13 biology.
Application Deadline(s): Fall: May.
Tuition and Fees: $6500 per yr.
Financial Aid: Federal government aid.
Career Services: Career counseling; Career information.

NOVA SCOTIA

Halifax

854. ICT Northumberland College
Massage Therapy Diploma Program
1660 Hollis St, Ste 301, Halifax, NS B3J 1V7 Canada.
Phone: (902) 425-2869; *Fax:* (902) 425-2858

E-mail: ncadmissions@ictschools.com *Internet:* http://www.ictschools.com
Program Administrator: Deborah M. Sherren, Executive Director. *Admissions Contact:* Dawn Schmidt, Admissions Officer.
Year Established: 1997.
Staff: Full-time: 8.

Avg Class Size: 65-100.
Wheelchair Access: Yes.
Accreditation/Approval/Licensing: Commission on Massage Therapy Accreditation.
Field of Study: Massage Therapy*. *Program Name/Length:* Massage Therapy Diploma Program, 2200 hrs, 2 yrs or 18 month accelerated program; Preadmission course.
Degrees Offered: Diploma.
License/Certification Preparation: National Certification Board for Therapeutic Massage and Bodywork.

Admission Requirements: High school diploma/GED.
Application Deadline(s): Fall; Winter.
Tuition and Fees: $C260 (Preadmission Course); $C7100 per yr (Massage Therapy Diploma).
Financial Aid: Scholarships.
Career Services: Career counseling; Career information; Internships.
Comments: Students who take preadmission course and successfully complete year one receive $C200 credit in year two.

ONTARIO

Gloucester

855. British Institute of Homeopathy
1445 St Joseph Blvd, Gloucester, ON K1C 7K9 Canada.
Phone: (613) 830-4759, (800) 579-4325 (Canada only); *Fax:* (613) 830-9174
E-mail: bih@aol.com *Internet:* http://www.homeopathy.com
Program Administrator: Rudi Verspoor, Dir. *Admissions Contact:* Patty Smith, Dean of Admissions and Student Affairs.
Year Established: 1988.
Staff: Full-time: 2; Part-time: 10.
Avg Enrollment: 100. *Avg Class Size:* 20. *Number of Graduates per Year:* 75.
Wheelchair Access: Yes.
Field of Study: Animal Therapy; Herbal Medicine; Homeopathy*; Midwifery; Naturopathic Medicine; Nutrition. *Program Name/Length:* Homeopathic Practitioner Diploma, 1200 hrs, 2-3 yrs; Postgraduate Practitioner Diploma, 1200 hrs, 2-3 yrs; Seminars given in various locations; Home study/Correspondence.
Degrees Offered: Diploma; Certificate.
License/Certification Preparation: Council for Homeopathic Certification; Homeopathic Academy of Naturopathic Physicians; North American Society of Homeopaths; National Board of Homeopathic Examiners.
Admission Requirements: Min age: 16 yrs; High school diploma/GED; Some college.
Financial Aid: Payment plan.
Career Services: Career counseling; Career information.

Jackson's Point

856. Artemisia Institute for Botanical and Preventive Health Care Education
PO Box 190, Jackson's Point, ON L0E 1L0 Canada
Phone: (905) 722-1074
E-mail: artemis@ils.net
Program Administrator: Christine E. DeVai, Dir. *Admissions Contact:* Christine E. DeVai.
Year Established: 1986.
Staff: Full-time: 1; Part-time: 2.
Avg Enrollment: 36. *Number of Graduates per Year:* 20.
Field of Study: Herbal Medicine*. *Program Name/Length:* Home study/Correspondence.
Degrees Offered: Certificate.
License/Certification Preparation: ON Herbalists Association.
Admission Requirements: High school diploma/GED.
Tuition and Fees: $US295 or $C440.
Financial Aid: Work study; Payment plan.
Career Services: Career counseling; Career information.

London

857. The D'Arcy Lane Institute, D'AL School of Equine Massage Therapy
Massage Therapy; Equine Massage Therapy
627 Maitland St, London, ON N5Y 2V7 Canada.
Phone: (519) 673-4420; *Fax:* (519) 673-0645
E-mail: darcyinc@serix.com *Internet:* http://www.serix.com/~darcyinc
Program Administrator: Rosemary Goyeau, CEO, Dir. *Admissions Contact:* Marnie Byloo, Registrar.
Year Established: 1983.
Staff: Full-time: 2; Part-time: 21.

Avg Enrollment: 100. *Avg Class Size:* 40.
Wheelchair Access: Yes.
Accreditation/Approval/Licensing: State board:
College of Massage Therapists of ON; ON Ministry of Education and Training.
Field of Study: Animal Therapy*; Equine Massage*; Massage Therapy*. *Program Name/Length:* Massage Therapy, 2200 hrs, 2 yrs; Equine Massage Therapy, 2200 hrs, 2 yrs.
Degrees Offered: Diploma.
License/Certification Preparation: College of Massage Therapists of ON.
Admission Requirements: Min age: 19; High school diploma/GED (grade 12).
Application Deadline(s): Fall: Aug 15; Winter: Dec 15.
Financial Aid: Federal government aid.
Career Services: Career information; Internships.

Newmarket

858. Canadian College of Massage and Hydrotherapy, Newmarket
543 Timothy St, Newmarket, ON L3Y 1R1 Canada.
Phone: (905) 853-5553; *Fax:* (905) 853-5324
E-mail: dmahedyjr@aol.com *Internet:* http://www. wccmt.edu
Program Administrator: Lee Kalpin, RMT, Dean. *Admissions Contact:* Kim Fountaine, Admissions/Financial Aid.
Year Established: 1946.
Staff: Full-time: 10; Part-time: 30.
Avg Enrollment: 650. *Avg Class Size:* 50. *Number of Graduates per Year:* 210.
Wheelchair Access: Yes.
Accreditation/Approval/Licensing: College of Massage Therapists of Ontario.
Field of Study: Acupuncture*; Herbal Medicine*; Humanistic Counseling*; Hydrotherapy; Massage Therapy*; Traditional Chinese Medicine*. *Program Name/Length:* Diploma in Massage Therapy, 2200 hrs, 2 yrs; Diploma in Acupuncture/Traditional Chinese Medicine, 2250 hrs, 2 yrs; Diploma in Herbal Medicine, 1800 hrs, 2 yrs; Diploma in Humanistic Counseling Skills, 1350 hrs, 1 yr.
Degrees Offered: Diploma.
License/Certification Preparation: ON Registered Massage Therapist.
Admission Requirements: Min age: 18; High school diploma/GED; Some college (1 yr); Specific course prerequisites: B in Biology.
Application Deadline(s): Fall: Jul 31; Winter: Dec 1; Spring: Mar 31.
Tuition and Fees: $C13,050 (Massage Therapy); $C15,450 (Acupuncture); $C12,700 (Herbal Medicine); $C9950 (Humanistic Counseling).
Financial Aid: Federal government aid; State government aid; Payment plan.
Career Services: Job information.

North York

859. Canadian College of Massage and Hydrotherapy, North York
5160 Yonge St, Ste 505, North York, ON M2N 6L7 Canada.
Phone: (416) 222-3586; *Fax:* (416) 222-9424
E-mail: dmahedyjr@aol.com *Internet:* http://www. wccmt.edu
Program Administrator: Ljubisa Terzic, MD, Dean. *Admissions Contact:* Margaret Ward, Admissions Officer.
Year Established: 1946.
Field of Study: Acupuncture*; Herbal Medicine*; Humanistic Counseling*; Hydrotherapy; Massage Therapy*; Traditional Chinese Medicine*. *Program Name/Length:* Diploma in Massage Therapy, 3150 hrs, 3 yrs; Diploma in Acupuncture/Traditional Chinese Medicine, 2250 hrs, 2 yrs; Diploma in Herbal Medicine, 1800 hrs, 2 yrs; Diploma in Humanistic Counseling Skills, 1350 hrs, 1 yr.
Admission Requirements: High school diploma/GED.
Application Deadline(s): Fall: Jul 31; Winter: Dec 1; Spring: Mar 31.
Tuition and Fees: $C13,050 + $C880 books, supplies (Massage Therapy); $C15,450 + $C1250 books, supplies (Acupuncture); $C12,700 + $C1000 books, supplies (Herbal Medicine); $C9950 + $C750 books, supplies (Humanistic Counseling).
Financial Aid: Federal government aid; State government aid; Payment plan.
Career Services: Job information.

Richmond Hill

860. Reaching Your Potential
Polarity Therapy Certification Training
11181 Yonge St, Rm 141, Richmond Hill, ON L4S 1L2 Canada.
Mailing Address: 40-646 Village Pkwy, Unionville, ON L3R 2S7Canada
Phone: (905) 944-8867; *Fax:* (905) 944-8869
E-mail: harrisw@internetfront.com
Program Administrator: Sher Smith, RN. *Admissions Contact:* Sher Smith.
Year Established: 1984.
Staff: Full-time: 1; Part-time: 5.
Avg Enrollment: 25. *Avg Class Size:* 10. *Number of Graduates per Year:* 15.
Wheelchair Access: Yes.
Accreditation/Approval/Licensing: American Polarity Therapy Association.
Field of Study: CranioSacral Therapy; Polarity Therapy*. *Program Name/Length:* Polarity Therapy Certification Level 1, 155 hrs; Polarity Therapy Certification Level 2, 615 hrs.
Degrees Offered: Certificate.

License/Certification Preparation: American Polarity Therapy Association.
Tuition and Fees: \$C1800 (Level 1); \$C4400 (Level 2).

Toronto

861. Canadian College of Naturopathic Medicine

2300 Yonge St, 18th Fl, Box 2431, Toronto, ON M4P 1E4 Canada.
Phone: (416) 486-8584; *Fax:* (416) 484-6821
Program Administrator: Cory Ross, DC, Academic VP. *Admissions Contact:* Catharine Shewell, Student Svcs Officer.
Year Established: 1978.
Staff: Full-time: 2; Part-time: 50.
Avg Enrollment: 125. *Avg Class Size:* 120. *Number of Graduates per Year:* 60.
Wheelchair Access: Yes.
Accreditation/Approval/Licensing: Candidacy, Council on Naturopathic Medical Education.
Field of Study: Acupuncture; Bodywork and Manipulation; Clinical Nutrition; Herbal Medicine; Homeopathy; Hydrotherapy; Naturopathic Medicine*; Traditional Chinese Medicine. *Program Name/Length:* Doctor of Naturopathic Medicine, 4000+ hrs, 4 yrs.
Degrees Offered: ND; Certificate in Naturopathic Medical Education.
License/Certification Preparation: ON Naturopathic Physician; Naturopathic Physicians Licensing Exam.
Admission Requirements: Some college (3 yrs); Min GPA: 3.0; Bachelor's degree recommended; Specific course prerequisites: general biology, biochemistry, general chemistry, organic chemistry, psychology.
Application Deadline(s): Fall: Feb; Winter: Apr.
Tuition and Fees: \$C12,000 (1st yr), \$C12,500 per yr (2nd-4th yrs).
Financial Aid: Loans.

862. Canadian Memorial Chiropractic College

1900 Bayview Ave, Toronto, ON M4G 3E6 Canada.
Phone: (416) 482-2340; *Fax:* (416) 482-9745
Internet: http://www.cmcc.ca
Program Administrator: Dr. Jean Moss, Pres. *Admissions Contact:* Dr. Stefan Pallister, Admissions Dir.
Year Established: 1945.
Staff: Full-time: 58; Part-time: 51.
Avg Enrollment: 150. *Number of Graduates per Year:* 150.
Wheelchair Access: Yes.
Accreditation/Approval/Licensing: Council on Chiropractic Education.
Field of Study: Chiropractic*. *Program Name/Length:* 4 yrs.

Degrees Offered: DC.
License/Certification Preparation: State and Provincial Boards; National Board of Chiropractic Examiners.
Admission Requirements: Some college (3 yrs); Min GPA: 2.25.
Application Deadline(s): Winter: Dec 31.
Financial Aid: Government aid; Loans; Provincial student aid; Scholarships.
Career Services: Career information.

863. Homeopathic College of Canada

280 Eglinton Ave E, Toronto, ON M4P 1L4 Canada
Phone: (416) 481-8816; *Fax:* (416) 481-4444
E-mail: info@homeopathy.edu *Internet:* http://www.homeopathy.edu
Program Administrator: Fernando Ania, ND, Pres. *Admissions Contact:* Luba Plotkin, MD, Registrar.
Year Established: 1991.
Staff: Full-time: 4; Part-time: 20.
Avg Enrollment: 50. *Avg Class Size:* 25. *Number of Graduates per Year:* 40.
Wheelchair Access: Yes.
Accreditation/Approval/Licensing: ON Homeopathic Association; Homeopathic Medical Council of Canada; Candidate, Council on Homeopathic Education.
Field of Study: Homeopathy*. *Program Name/Length:* Doctorate in Homeopathic Medicine and Science, 4 yrs; Doctorate in Homeopathic Medicine and Science for Health Professionals, 20 mos/part-time.
Degrees Offered: Diploma; DHMS.
License/Certification Preparation: Homeopathic Medical Council of Canada Board.
Admission Requirements: Some college (2 yrs); Bachelor's degree recommended; Medical degree required for advanced program.
Application Deadline(s): Fall: Jul 15.
Tuition and Fees: \$C6900 per yr.
Financial Aid: Loans; Scholarships.
Career Services: Career information.
Comments: Canadian college and university credits given for some courses.

864. ICT Kikkawa College

Massage Therapy Program
1678 Bloor St W, Toronto, ON M6P 1A9 Canada.
Phone: (416) 762-4857; *Fax:* (416) 762-5733
E-mail: kcadmissions@ictschools.com *Internet:* http://www.ictschools.com
Accreditation/Approval/Licensing: Commission on Massage Therapy Accreditation.
Field of Study: Massage Therapy*.

865. Institute of Traditional Chinese Medicine

Acupuncture and Chinese Herbal Medicine
368 Dupont St, Toronto, ON M5R 1V9 Canada.
Phone: (416) 925-6752; *Fax:* (416) 925-8920

Program Administrator: Dr. David Lam, ND, Dean. *Admissions Contact:* David Lam.
Year Established: 1970.
Staff: Part-time: 7.
Avg Enrollment: 40. *Avg Class Size:* 15. *Number of Graduates per Year:* 30.
Wheelchair Access: No.
Field of Study: Acupressure; Acupuncture*; Herbal Medicine*; Oriental Medicine; Qigong; Traditional Chinese Medicine*; Tui Na. *Program Name/Length:* Diploma of Traditional Chinese Medicine, 3 yrs.
Degrees Offered: Diploma; Certificate.
Admission Requirements: Some college (2 yrs).
Career Services: Referral service.

866. The Michener Institute for Applied Health Sciences

222 Saint Patrick St, Toronto, ON M5T 1V4 Canada.
Phone: (416) 596-3177; *Fax:* (416) 596-3180
E-mail: bbobb@staff.michener.on.ca *Internet:* http://www.michener.on.ca
Program Administrator: Liqun Zhang, Prog Dir. *Admissions Contact:* Angi Gallupe, Student Services.
Year Established: 1997.
Staff: Full-time: 2; Part-time: 4.
Avg Enrollment: 20. *Avg Class Size:* 20.
Wheelchair Access: Yes.
Field of Study: Acupuncture*; Traditional Chinese Medicine*. *Program Name/Length:* 4 yrs.
Degrees Offered: Diploma.
Admission Requirements: High school diploma/GED; Min GPA: 60%; Specific course prerequisites: biology, chemistry, English.
Application Deadline(s): Spring: Mar 1.
Tuition and Fees: $C8500 per yr.
Financial Aid: Fellowships; Provincial and national government aid.
Career Services: Career counseling; Career information.

867. Esther Myers Yoga Studio

Yoga Teacher Training
390 Dupont St, Ste 203, Toronto, ON M5R 1V9 Canada.
Phone: (416) 944-0838; *Fax:* (416) 944-9151
Program Administrator: Esther Myers, Dir. *Admissions Contact:* Linda Cherney, Teacher Training Admin.
Year Established: 1981.
Avg Enrollment: 20.
Wheelchair Access: No.
Field of Study: Yoga Teacher Training*. *Program Name/Length:* 2 yrs (part time).
Degrees Offered: Certificate.
Admission Requirements: Min age: 25; Specific course prerequisites: 2 yrs of yoga classes; Established daily practice.
Financial Aid: Scholarships.

868. Shiatsu Academy of Tokyo

320 Danforth Ave, Ste 206, Toronto, ON M4K 1N8 Canada.
Phone: (416) 466-8780; *Fax:* (416) 466-8719
E-mail: sait131@ibm.net *Internet:* http://www.toronto.com/shiatsuacademy
Program Administrator: Jan McClory, Admin. *Admissions Contact:* Jan McClory.
Year Established: 1990.
Staff: Part-time: 13.
Avg Enrollment: 20. *Avg Class Size:* 20. *Number of Graduates per Year:* 12.
Wheelchair Access: No.
Field of Study: Shiatsu*. *Program Name/Length:* Shiatsu Practitioner, 2 yrs.
Degrees Offered: Diploma.
License/Certification Preparation: National Certification Board for Therapeutic Massage and Bodywork.
Admission Requirements: Min age: 19; High school diploma/GED.
Application Deadline(s): Fall: Sep 1.
Tuition and Fees: $9900.
Career Services: Job information.

869. Shiatsu School of Canada, Inc/SSC Acupuncture Institute

Shiatsu Diploma Program; Acupuncture Diploma Program
547 College St, Toronto, ON M6G 1A9 Canada.
Phone: (416) 323-1818, (800) 263-1703; *Fax:* (416) 323-1681
E-mail: info@shiatsucanada.com *Internet:* http://www.shiatsucanada.com
Program Administrator: Kaz Kamiya, Dir. *Admissions Contact:* Euza Ierullo, Gen Mgr.
Year Established: 1986.
Staff: Part-time: 22.
Avg Enrollment: 48 (Shiatsu), 30 (Acupuncture). *Avg Class Size:* 32. *Number of Graduates per Year:* 32.
Wheelchair Access: No.
Accreditation/Approval/Licensing: Ontario Registered Private Vocational School.
Field of Study: Acupuncture*; Shiatsu*. *Program Name/Length:* Shiatsu Diploma Program, 2200 hrs; Acupuncture Diploma Program, 450 hrs.
Degrees Offered: Diploma.
License/Certification Preparation: Certification, Shiatsu Therapy Association of Ontario.
Admission Requirements: Min age: 18; High school diploma/GED; Audit 2 classes, for Shiatsu; Post-secondary anatomy course, for Acupuncture.
Application Deadline(s): Fall: Jun for Shiatsu; Winter: Dec for Acupuncture.
Financial Aid: Federal government aid; Payment plan; Provincial government aid.
Career Services: Career information; Job information; Referral service.

870. Sutherland-Chan School and Teaching Clinic

330 Dupont St, 4th Fl, Toronto, ON M6R 1K4 Canada.
Phone: (416) 924-1107; *Fax:* (416) 924-9413
E-mail: admissions@sutherland-chan.com *Internet:* http://www.sutherland-chan.com
Program Administrator: Debra Curties, Exec Dir. *Admissions Contact:* Marion Bishop, Student Svcs Dir.
Year Established: 1979.
Staff: Part-time: 45.
Avg Enrollment: 150. *Avg Class Size:* 60. *Number of Graduates per Year:* 140.
Wheelchair Access: Yes.
Field of Study: Massage Therapy*. *Program Name/Length:* 2 yrs (full-time).
Degrees Offered: Diploma.
License/Certification Preparation: ON Registration Examinations; National Certification Board for Therapeutic Massage and Bodywork.
Admission Requirements: High school diploma/GED; Specific course prerequisites: biology, physical and health ed; Sutherland-Chan Introductory Massage Course or 16 hr basic massage course.
Tuition and Fees: $7350 per yr.
Financial Aid: Provincial government aid; Ontario Student Assistance Program.
Career Services: Job information.

871. Toronto School of Homeopathic Medicine

17 Yorkville Ave, Ste 200, Toronto, ON M4W 1L1 Canada.
Phone: (416) 966-2350, (800) 572-6001; *Fax:* (416) 966-1724
E-mail: info@homeopathycanada.com *Internet:* http://www.homeopathycanada.com
Program Administrator: Raymond Edge, Pres. *Admissions Contact:* Shobhna Kapoor, Registar.
Year Established: 1995.
Staff: Full-time: 3; Part-time: 10.
Avg Enrollment: 90. *Avg Class Size:* 30. *Number of Graduates per Year:* 30.
Wheelchair Access: No.
Accreditation/Approval/Licensing: Council on Homeopathic Education; Ontario Federation of Homeopathic Practitioners.
Field of Study: Homeopathy*. *Program Name/Length:* Classical Homeopathy, 3- and 4-yr programs.
Degrees Offered: Diploma.
License/Certification Preparation: Council for Homeopathic Certification; North American Society of Homeopaths.
Admission Requirements: Some college (2 yrs); Mature applicants without prerequisites are also considered.
Application Deadline(s): Fall: Aug 1.
Tuition and Fees: $C4500.
Financial Aid: Scholarships.
Career Services: Career information.

QUEBEC

Montreal

872. Health Training Group

3789 Hampton Ave, Montreal, PQ H4A 2K7 Canada.
Phone: (514) 485-6373
Program Administrator: Howard Kiewe, Dir. *Admissions Contact:* Eastern Canada (514) 485-6373; Western Canada (604) 853-8963; Seattle (206) 527-0807; Hawaii (808) 322-0048.
Staff: Part-time: 5.
Avg Class Size: 15. *Number of Graduates per Year:* 30.
Accreditation/Approval/Licensing: American Polarity Therapy Association.
Field of Study: Polarity Therapy*. *Program Name/Length:* Associate Polarity Practitioner; Registered Polarity Practitioner; Seminars given in various locations.
Degrees Offered: Certificate.
License/Certification Preparation: APP, RPP; American Polarity Therapy Association.
Admission Requirements: Min age: 18.
Financial Aid: Government aid.
Career Services: Career counseling; Career information.

873. Polarity Associates of Montreal

5535 Beaucourt, Ste 10, Montreal, PQ H3W 2T7 Canada.
Phone: (514) 739-4673; *Fax:* (514) 440-0251
E-mail: aaxt@usa.net
Program Administrator: Andrea Axt, PhD, RPP. *Admissions Contact:* Andrea Axt.
Year Established: 1990.
Staff: Full-time: 1; Part-time: 4.
Avg Enrollment: 100. *Avg Class Size:* 10. *Number of Graduates per Year:* 30.

Accreditation/Approval/Licensing: Quebec Federation for Massage Therapists; American Polarity Therapy Association.
Field of Study: CranioSacral Therapy*; Polarity Therapy*. *Program Name/Length:* Association Polarity Practitioner, 6 mos; Registered Polarity Practitioner, 1 yr; CranioSacral Therapy, 2 mos.
Degrees Offered: Certificate.
License/Certification Preparation: Quebec Federation for Massage Therapists; APP and RPP; American Polarity Therapy Association.
Admission Requirements: Min age: 18.
Tuition and Fees: $C1000-$C2000 per yr.

874. Psychovisual Therapy Training
7306 Sherbrooke W, Montreal, PQ H4B 1R7 Canada.
Phone: (514) 489-6733; *Fax:* (514) 485-3828
E-mail: drknight@odyssee.net *Internet:* http://www.hypnosis.org
Program Administrator: Bryan M. Knight, PhD, Instr. *Admissions Contact:* Bryan M. Knight.
Year Established: 1995.
Staff: Full-time: 1.
Avg Enrollment: 25. *Avg Class Size:* 6. *Number of Graduates per Year:* 10.
Wheelchair Access: No.
Field of Study: Hypnotherapy*; Psychovisual Therapy*. *Program Name/Length:* Psychovisual Therapy, 3 mos.
Degrees Offered: Certificate.
Admission Requirements: Min age: 18; High school diploma/GED.
Tuition and Fees: $C350-$C500 per course.

Outremont

875. Canadian Academy of Homeopathy
1173 Boul Mont Royal, Outremont, PQ H2V 2H6 Canada.
Phone: (514) 279-6629; *Fax:* (514) 279-0111
E-mail: ya156112@alumnet.yorku.ca *Internet:* http://www.homeopathy.ca
Program Administrator: Francine Gauthier, Exec Dir. *Admissions Contact:* Francine Gauthier.
Year Established: 1986.
Staff: Part-time: 6.
Avg Enrollment: 35. *Avg Class Size:* 25. *Number of Graduates per Year:* 18.
Wheelchair Access: Yes.
Accreditation/Approval/Licensing: ON Naturopathic Association; Council on Homeopathic Education; Canadian College of Naturopathic

Medicine; Board of Drugless Therapists-Naturopathy.
Field of Study: Homeopathy*. *Program Name/Length:* Part I: Introduction to Acute Prescribing, 90 hrs, 6 mos, classroom or correspondence; Part II: Introduction to Chronic Prescribing, 160 hrs, 1 yr, classroom or correspondence; Part III: Advanced Chronic Prescribing, 504 hrs, 3 yrs, classroom or correspondence.
Degrees Offered: Diploma; FCAH, Fellow of the Canadian Academy of Homeopathy.
Admission Requirements: Health care professional or BScPharm required for Part I; Midwife, nurse practitioner, physician's asst, or medical degree required for Part III.
Tuition and Fees: $C2600 (Part I); $C7920 (Part III, classroom); $C9450 (Part III, correspondence).

Quebec

876. Centre Psycho-Corporel, Inc
Massotherapie et Soins Corporels
675 Marguerite Bourgeoys, Quebec, PQ G1S 3V8 Canada.
Phone: (418) 687-1165; *Fax:* (418) 687-1166
E-mail: opsante@mlink.net *Internet:* http://www.mlink.net/~opsante
Program Administrator: Yvon Dallaire, Pres/Dir. *Admissions Contact:* Aline Dumas, Coord.
Year Established: 1980.
Staff: Full-time: 6; Part-time: 10.
Avg Enrollment: 50. *Avg Class Size:* 20. *Number of Graduates per Year:* 50.
Wheelchair Access: No.
Accreditation/Approval/Licensing: Federation Quebecoise des Massotherapeutes.
Field of Study: Acupressure; Kinesiology; Manual Lymph Drainage*; Massage Therapy*; Qigong; Reflexology; Shiatsu*; Sports Massage*; Swedish Massage*. *Program Name/Length:* Level I, 400 hrs, 1 yr; Level I and II, 1000 hrs, 3 yrs; Home study/Correspondence.
Degrees Offered: Diploma.
License/Certification Preparation: Federation Quebecoise des Massotherapeutes.
Admission Requirements: Min age: 18; High school diploma/GED.
Tuition and Fees: $C10 per hr.
Financial Aid: Loans.
Career Services: Career counseling; Career information.

SASKATCHEWAN

Saskatoon

877. Professional Institute of Massage Therapy, Saskatoon

485 1st Ave N, Saskatoon, SK S7K 1X5 Canada.
Phone: (306) 955-5833; *Fax:* (306) 955-5864
E-mail: tracy.pimt@sk.sympatico.ca
Program Administrator: Tracy Bazylak, Admin.
   Admissions Contact: Tracy Bazylak.
Year Established: 1992.
Staff: Part-time: 8.
Avg Enrollment: 40. *Avg Class Size:* 40. *Number of Graduates per Year:* 37.
Wheelchair Access: Yes.
Field of Study: Massage Therapy*. *Program Name/Length:* 2200 hrs, 2 yrs.

Degrees Offered: Diploma.
License/Certification Preparation: State: Massage Therapy Association of Saskatchewan; National Certification Board for Therapeutic Massage and Bodywork.
Admission Requirements: Min age: 18; High school diploma/GED; Specific course prerequisites: grade 13 biology.
Application Deadline(s): Fall: May; Winter: Nov.
Tuition and Fees: $6600 per yr.
Financial Aid: Federal government aid.
Career Services: Career counseling; Career information.

RESOURCE INFORMATION

Selected Organizations, Publications, and Web Sites Dealing with Alternative and Complementary Health Care

ORGANIZATIONS, RESOURCES, AND ACCREDITING AGENCIES

General Information

Alternative & Complementary Medicine Center, HealthWorld Online
http://www.altmed.net
Guide to alternative medicine; professional referrals; resources; newsletter; global calendar.

Alternative Medicine-Health Care Information Resources
Http://www-hsl.mcmaster.ca/tomflem/altmed.html
Links to general and specific resources; information on alternative therapies.

The Alternative Medicine Home Page
http://www.pitt.edu/~cbw/altm.html
Databases and Internet resources. Information on modalities; links to practitioner directories and government resources.

American Holistic Health Association
PO Box 17400
Anaheim, CA 92817
(714) 779-6152
e-mail: ahha@healthy.net
http://www.healthy.net/ahha
Established 1989. Nonprofit, educational organization. Provides information on organizations, educational institutions, practitioners, and resource materials. Publishes quarterly newsletter AhHa! and booklet *Wellness from Within: The First Step*.

American Holistic Medical Association
6728 Old McLean Village Dr.
McLean, VA 22101
(703) 556-9728
http://www.holisticmedicine.org
Established 1978. Membership organization open to licensed DOs, MDs, and medical students with an interest in holistic health care. Publishes *National Referral Directory of Holistic Practitioners* and monthly journal *Holistic Medicine*. Annual conference, continuing education.

American Holistic Nurses Association
PO Box 2130
Flagstaff, AZ 86003-2130
(520) 526-2196; (800) 278-AHNA (2462); Fax (520) 526-2752
http://www.ahna.org
Established 1981. Membership organization; publishes monthly newsletter Beginnings and quarterly *Journal of Holistic Nursing*. Annual conference.

Dr. Bower's Complementary and Alternative Medicine Home Page
Http://galen.med.virginia.edu/~pjb3s/ComplementaryHomePage.html
Links to complementary medicine sites.

National Center for Complementary and Alternative Medicine
PO Box 8218
Silver Spring, MD 20907-8218
(888) 644-6226 (TTY access available); Fax (301) 495-4957
http://altmed.od.nih.gov/nccam
Established 1998; formerly National Institutes of Health, Office of Alternative Medicine. Facilitates and conducts research, evaluates modalities, and operates public information clearinghouse. Publishes newsletter and maintains calendar of events, including worldwide conferences and meetings.

NaturalHealers
Netstream
(206) 789-8289
e-mail: info@naturalhealers.com
http://www.naturalhealers.com
Common questions and answers about alternative therapies; listing of schools by state and subject.

New Age Journal Holistic Health Directory
http://www.newage.com
Directory of practitioners; Internet links.

The Rosenthal Center for Complementary & Alternative Medicine
Columbia University College of Physicians and Surgeons
630 W 168th St., Box 75
New York 10032
(212) 543-9550; Fax (212) 543-2845
http://cpmcnet.columbia.edu/dept/rosenthal
Provides information on medical schools offering courses on alternative and complementary medicine, and on legal and regulatory issues including state licensing laws. Maintains directory of databases and calendar of events.

Accreditation
(Accrediting agencies for specific modalities are listed under modality headings)

Accrediting Commission of Career Schools and Colleges of Technology
2101 Wilson Blvd., Ste. 302
Arlington, VA 22201
(703) 247-4212; Fax (703) 247-4533
e-mail: info@accsct.org
http://www.accsct.org
Established 1993, formerly the accrediting commission of the National Association of Trade & Technical Schools. Private, nonprofit accreditation agency recognized by the U.S. Department of Education.

Accrediting Council for Continuing Education and Training
1722 N St. NW
Washington, DC 20036
(202) 955-1113; Fax (202) 955-1118
http://www.accet.org
Voluntary affiliation of organizations, trade and professional associations, and private career schools. Establishes standards for evaluation and accreditation of noncollegiate postsecondary education and training.

Council for Higher Education Accreditation
1 Dupont Circle NW, Ste. 510
Washington, DC 20036-1136
(202) 955-6126; Fax (202) 955-6129
e-mail: chea@chea.org
http://www.chea.org
Nonprofit organization of colleges and universities; serves as the national advocate for accreditation.

Council on Occupational Education
41 Perimeter Center East NE, Ste. 640
Atlanta, GA 30346
(770) 396-3898; (800) 917-2081; Fax (770) 396-3790
e-mail: info@council.org
http://www.council.org
Nonprofit, voluntary membership organization; originally established 1971 as Commission on Occupational Education Institutions. National accrediting agency for postsecondary education and training.

Middle States Association of Colleges and Schools*
3624 Market St.
Philadelphia, PA 19104
(215) 662-5606; Fax (215) 662-5501
http://www.msache.org
Evaluates institutions as a whole rather than specific programs. Commission on Higher Education examines and accredits degree-granting colleges and universities in DE, DC, MD, NJ, NY, PA, PR, Panama, and U.S. Virgin Islands.

New England Association of Schools and Colleges, Inc.*
209 Burlington Rd.

---

*Regional accrediting organization that is recognized by the U.S. Department of Education.

Bedford, MA 01730
(617) 271-0022; Fax (617) 271-0950
http://www.neasc.org
Established 1885. Commission on Institutions of Higher Education and Commission on Technical and Career Institutions develops standards for postsecondary education in CT, ME, MA, NH, RI, and VT.

North Central Association of Colleges and Schools*
30 N LaSalle St., Ste. 2400
Chicago, IL 60602
(312) 263-0456; (800) 621-7440
e-mail: info@ncacihe.org
http://www.ncacihe.org
Established 1895. Membership organization for educational institutions. Commission on Institutions on Higher Education accredits degree-granting instititions in AK, AZ, CO, IA, IL, IN, KS, MI, MN, MO, ND, NE, OH, OK, NM, SD, WI, WV, and WY.

Northwest Association of Schools and Colleges*
1130 NE 33rd Pl., Ste. 120
Bellevue, WA 98004-1448
(425) 827-2005; Fax (425) 827-3395
e-mail: pjarnold@cocnasc.org
Accredits schools and colleges in AK, MT, ID, NV, OR, and WA.

Southern Association of Colleges and Schools*
1866 Southern Lane
Decatur, GA 30033
(800) 248-7701; Fax (404) 679-4558
http://www.sacs.org
Established 1895. Private, nonprofit, voluntary organization. Commission on Colleges sets standards for and accredits postsecondary degree-granting institutions in AL, FL, GA, KY, LA, MS, NC, SC, TN, TX, and VA.

U.S. Department of Education*
Accreditation & Eligibility Determination Division
ROB 3, Room 3915 7th & D St. SW
Washington, DC 20202-5244
(202) 708-7417
http://www.ifap.ed.gov/csb_html/agency.htm

Establishes criteria for accrediting agencies and associations, and recognizes those that meet national standards.

Western Association of Schools and Colleges*
Mills College, Box 9990
Oakland, CA 94613
(510) 632-5000; Fax (510) 632-8361
e-mail: wascsr@wasc.mills.edu
http://www.wascweb.org
Accredits schools and colleges in CA and HI.

Acupuncture and Oriental Medicine

Accreditation Commission for Acupuncture and Oriental Medicine
1010 Wayne Ave., Ste. 1270
Silver Spring, MD 20910
(301) 608-9680; Fax (301) 608-9576
e-mail: 73352,2467@compuserve.com
Established 1982; formerly the National Accreditation Commission for Schools and Colleges of Acupuncture and Oriental Medicine. Evaluates and accredits master's degree, master's level certificate, and diploma programs in Oriental medicine that meet accreditation criteria. Recognized by the U.S. Department of Education and the Council for Higher Education Accreditation.

Acupuncture.com
http://www.acupuncture.com
Frequently asked questions; information on research; practitioner referrals; student resources.

American Association of Oriental Medicine
433 Front St.
Catasaugua, PA 18032
(610) 266-1433; Fax (610) 264-2768
e-mail: aaom1@aol.com
http://www.aaom.org
Established 1981. Membership organization; advocates for licensing in all 50 states; operates national referral network. Provides information on training, licensing, and state associations. Publishes biannual newsletter *The American Acupuncturist*, and *Updates* on events and educational materials.

The American Foundation of Traditional Chinese Medicine
505 Beach St.
San Francisco, CA 94133
(415) 776-0502; Fax (415) 776-9053
Established 1982. Membership open to practitioners and interested individuals. Reference library; quarterly newsletter *Gateways*, includes research in Traditional Chinese Medicine.

American Oriental Bodywork Therapy Association
Laurel Oak Corporate Center, Ste. 408
1010 Haddonfield-Berlin Rd.
Voorhees, NJ 08043
(609) 782-1616; Fax (609) 782-1653
e-mail: aobta@prodigy.net
http://www.healthy.net/aobta
Established 1984. National nonprofit association, membership open to Certified Practitioners with 500 hours of approved training and Associates with 150 hours. Publishes quarterly *AOBTA Newsletter* and annual *AOBTA Directory*. Annual convention; practitioner referrals.

Council of Colleges of Acupuncture and Oriental Medicine
1010 Wayne Ave., Ste. 1270
Silver Spring, MD 20910
(301) 608-9175; Fax (301) 608-9576
e-mail: 77302,2436@compuserve.com
Established 1982; formerly National Council of Acupuncture Schools and Colleges. Organization of schools and colleges that offer programs with a minimum of 2 years of accredited training. Publishes *Guide to Accredited and Candidate Colleges*.

National Acupuncture and Oriental Medical Alliance
14637 Starr Rd. SE
Olalla, WA 93359
(253) 851-6896; Fax (253) 851-6883
http://www.acuall.org
Membership organization; referral service; information on schools and legislation. Publishes newsletter *The Forum*. Annual conference; workshops and seminars.

National Certification Commission for Acupuncture and Oriental Medicine
1424 16th St. NW, Ste. 501
Washington, DC 20036
(202) 232-1404; Fax (202) 462-6157
e-mail: info@nccaom.org
http://www.nccaom.org
Established 1982. Sets standards of competence for practitioners; administers semiannual national board examinations and certifies practitioners.

Alexander Technique

Alexander Technique International
1692 Massachusetts Ave., 3rd Fl.
Cambridge, MA 02138
(617) 497-2242
e-mail: ati@ati-net.com
http://www.ati-net.com
Established 1993. Nonprofit, membership organization. Provides information on training and practitioners; Internet links. Certifies practitioners through sponsorship.

American Society for the Alexander Technique (AmSAT)
Enterprise Bldg., 401 E Market St., #17
Charlottesville, VA 22902
(800) 473-0620; (804) 295-2840; Fax (804) 295-3947
e-mail: alexandertec@earthlink.net
http://www.alexandertech.org
Formerly North American Society of Teachers of the Alexander Technique. Provides information on training and practitioners. Approves teacher training courses, and certifies teachers who complete 1600 hours of approved training.

The Complete Guide to the Alexander Technique
http://www.alexandertechnique.com
Established and maintained by Alexander Technique—Nebraska, The Ontario Centre for the Alexander Technique and Robert Rickover. Information on Alexander Technique, courses and workshops, resources and Internet links.

Animal Therapy

Academy of Veterinary Homeopathy
751 NE 168th St.
North Miami, FL 33162-2427
(305) 652-1590; Fax (305) 653-7244
e-mail: avhlisth@naturalholistic.com
http://www.acadvethom.org
Established 1996. Offers accreditation training program for veterinarians; referral service; continuing education; conferences.

American Holistic Veterinary Medicine Association
2218 Old Emmorton Rd.
Bel Air, MD 21015
(410) 569-0795; Fax (410) 569-2346
e-mail: ahvma@compuserve.com
http://www.altvetmed.com
Membership organization; practitioner referrals. Publishes quarterly journal.

American Veterinary Chiropractic Association
623 Main St.
Hillsdale, IL 61257
(309) 658-2920; Fax (309) 658-2622
Established 1989. Membership organization; sponsors animal chiropractic certification course; reference library.

Association of Holistic Animal Practitioners
PO Box 500335
San Diego, CA 92150
(619) 223-0658
e-mail: animalsense@msn.com
Established 1997. International membership organization; referral service; continuing education; annual conference. Publishes quarterly newsletter *Association of Holistic Animal Practitioners*.

Aromatherapy (see also Herbal Medicine)

American Alliance of Aromatherapy
PO Box 309
Depoe Bay, OR 97341
(800) 809-9850; (800) 809-9808
e-mail: aaoa@wcn.net
Membership organization; publishes *International Journal of Aromatherapy* and *Aromatherapy Today*.

National Association for Holistic Aromatherapy
836 Hanley Industrial Court
St. Louis, MO 63144
(314) 963-2071; (888) ASK-NAHA (275-6242); Fax (314) 963-4454
e-mail: info@naha.org
http://www.naha.org
Established 1990. Membership organization; information on training; conferences and meetings. Publishes quarterly journal *Scentsitivity and Source/Practitioner Directory*.

Biofeedback

Association for Applied Psychophysiology & Biofeedback
10200 W 44th Ave., Ste. 304
Wheatridge, CO 80033-2840
(303) 422-8436; (800) 477-8892; Fax (303) 422-8894
e-mail: aapb@resourcenter.com
http://www.aapb.org
Established 1969, formerly Biofeedback Research Society. Membership organization; provides resource and research information; conducts conferences, meetings, and continuing education.

Biofeedback Certification Institute of America
10200 W 44th Ave., Ste. 304
Wheatridge, CO 80033
(303) 420-2902; Fax (303) 422-8894
e-mail: bcia@resourcenter.com
Established 1981. Accredits training providers; certifies individuals who pass written and practical competency examinations. Publishes *Register of Certificants* and *BCIA News*.

Chiropractic

American Chiropractic Association
1701 Clarendon Blvd.
Arlington, VA 22209
(703) 276-8800; Member services: (800) 986-4636; Fax (703) 243-2593
e-mail: amerchiro@aol.com
http://www.amerchiro.org

Professional organization of Doctors of Chiropractic. Provides information on training and practice, legislative issues, and research. Publishes *Journal of the American Chiropractic Association* and *ACA Today*.

Association of Chiropractic Colleges
4424 Montgomery Ave., Ste. 102
Bethesda, MD 20814
(301) 652-5066; (800) 284-1062; Fax (301) 913-9146
e-mail: obryonco@aol.com
http://www.chirocolleges.org
Membership organization for colleges of chiropractic. Continuing education; meetings.

Council on Chiropractic Education
7975 N Hayden Rd., Ste. A210
Scottsdale, AZ 85258
(602) 443-8877; Fax (602) 483-7333
e-mail: cceoffice@aol.com
Established 1971. Sets accreditation standards for chiropractic programs and institutions, also minimum admission requirements for prospective students. Recognized by the U.S. Department of Education.

International Chiropractors Association
1110 North Glebe Rd., Ste. 1000
Arlington, VA 22201
(800) 423-4690; (703) 528-5000
Established 1926. Publishes membership directory, bimonthly newsletter *ICA Today* and bimonthly *International Review of Chiropractic*. Annual conference; continuing education.

Feldenkrais

Feldenkrais Guild
PO Box 489
Albany, OR 97321-0143
(541) 926-0981; (800) 775-2118; Fax (541) 926-0572
e-mail: feldngld@peak.org
http://www.feldenkrais.com
Provides information on the Feldenkrais Method and professional training programs. Certifies practitioners and offers referrals. Publishes quarterly newsletter *SenseAbility*; conducts annual conference. Offers online lessons in Awareness through Movement.

Herbal Medicine

American Botanical Council
PO Box 144345
Austin, TX 78714-4345
(512) 926-4900; (800) 373-7105 subscriptions; Fax (512) 926-2345
e-mail: amebotcncl@aol.com
http://www.herbalgram.org
Established 1988. Nonprofit, educational organization; publishes *HerbalGram, The Journal of the American Botanical Council and the Herb Research* Foundation. Disseminates information on herbs and herbal research. Conferences; continuing education; calendar of events; Internet links.

American Herb Association
PO Box 1673
Nevada City, CA 95959
(916) 265-9552
Established 1981. Membership organization; provides information on research and educational programs, and sources for herb products and books. Publishes newsletter *The AHA Quarterly*, reports on clinical studies and legal issues.

American Herbalists Guild
PO Box 70
Roosevelt, UT 84066
(435) 722-8434; Fax (435) 722-8452
e-mail: ahgoffice@earthlink.net
http://www.healthy.net/herbalists
Membership organization; publishes membership referral directory and quarterly newsletter *The Herbalist*. Provides information on educational programs and conferences.

Herb Research Foundation
1007 Pearl St., Ste. 200
Boulder, CO 80302
(303) 449-2265
e-mail: info@herbs.org
http://www.herbs.org
Nonprofit research and educational membership organization. Conducts research and provides information; publishes *Herbs for Health*, and *HerbalGram* with the American Botanical Council.

Homeopathy

Council for Homeopathic Certification
PO Box 460190
San Francisco, CA 94146
(415) 789-7677; Fax (415) 695-8220
e-mail: homcert@igc.org
http://www.igc.org/~homcert
Administers certification examination for professional homeopaths; maintains directory of certified practitioners.

Council on Homeopathic Education
801 N Fairfax St., Ste. 306
Alexandria, VA 22314-1757
(518) 392-7975
e-mail: ched@igc.org
http://www.checu.org
Established 1982. Sets standards for training; evaluates and accredits programs on graduate and postgraduate levels.

Homeopathy Home
http://www.homeopathyhome.com
Directory of international organizations; practitioners in the United States and United Kingdom; information on training; reference library; Internet links.

National Board of Homeopathic Examiners
5663 NW 29th St.
Margate, FL 33063
(305) 974-3456
http://www.nbhe.com
Established 1987. Administers semiannual certification examinations for homeopathic practitioners who have earned a PhD, DC, MD, DO, AP, ND, OMD, or equivalent degree, and completed homeopathy training at an approved institution. Information on history and benefits of homeopathy; practitioner referrals.

National Center for Homeopathy
801 N Fairfax, Ste. 306
Alexandria, VA 22314
(703) 548-7790; Fax (703) 548-7792
e-mail: nchinfo@igc.apc.org
http://www.homeopathic.org
Established 1974. Provides information on training and licensing. Publishes *Directory of Practitioners, Study Groups, and Re-sources*, and *Homeopathy Today*. Annual conference offers workshops and seminars.

North American Society of Homeopaths
1122 E Pike St., Ste. 1122
Seattle, WA 98122
(541) 345-9815; (206) 720-7000; Fax (206) 329-5684
e-mail: nash@homeopathy.org
http://www.homeopathy.org
Established 1990. Membership organization; information on schools and training; conferences, meetings, and seminars. Publishes *Directory of Registered Homeopaths*, annual journal *The American Homeopath*, and quarterly newsletter *NASH News*.

Hypnotherapy

American Academy of Medical Hypnoanalysts
5628 Murray Rd. #4
Memphis, TN 38119-3876
(800) 344-9766; Fax (901) 683-1224
e-mail: info@aamh.com
http://www.aamh.com
Established 1977. Membership organization open to those with a master's-level degree in behavioral sciences, and clinical training, and practice in hypnoanalysis. Publishes newsletter and *Medical Hypnoanalysts Journal*; operates national professional referral service.

American Association of Professional Hypnotherapists
2443 Ash St., Ste. D
Palo Alto, CA 94306
(650) 323-3224
Established 1980. Membership organization open to professionals with designated training and experience. Publishes *National Register of Professional Hypnotherapists* and newsletter *Hypnotherapy Today*.

American Board of Hypnotherapy
16842 Von Karman Ave. #475
Irvine, CA 92714
(800) 872-9996; (714) 261-6400; Fax (714) 251-4632
e-mail: aih@hypnosis.com
http://www.hypnosis.com/abh

Registers and certifies professional hypnotists and hypnotherapists with required training and/or experience. Publishes *Journal of Hypnotherapy*; disseminates information on hypnosis; conducts continuing education programs.

American Council of Hypnotist Examiners
1147 E Broadway, Ste. 340
Glendale, CA 91205
(818) 242-1159; (818) 247-9379
Established 1980. Sponsors education programs; administers certification examinations for hypnotherapy practitioners. Publishes *Directory of Certified Members*, annual *American Hypnotherapy Report*, and quarterly *International Hypnotherapy Report*. Conducts annual International Hypnotherapy Conference.

American Society of Clinical Hypnosis
2200 E Devon Ave., Ste. 291
Des Plaines, IL 60018-4534
(847) 297-3317; Fax (847) 297-7309
e-mail: 70632.1663@compuserve.com
http://www.asch.net
Established 1957. Membership organization open to those with a medical degree or a master's degree in psychology, social work, or nursing. Sets standards for hypnotherapy training and conducts educational programs. Publishes quarterly *American Journal of Clinical Hypnosis* and *American Society of Clinical Hypnosis—Newsletter*. Annual meeting and workshop.

International Medical & Dental Hypnotherapy Association
4110 Edgeland, Ste. 800
Royal Oak, MI 48073
(800) 257-5467; (810) 549-5594; Fax (810) 549-5421
e-mail: aspencer@inst.com
http://www.infinityinst.com
Approves schools and certifies practitioners. Mentor program; Internet resources and links.

National Board for Certified Clinical Hypnotherapists, Inc.
8750 Georgia Ave., Ste. 142E
Silver Spring, MD 20910

(800) 449-8144; (301) 608-0123; Fax (301) 588-9535
e-mail: admin@natboard.com
http://www.natboard.com
Established 1991. Certifies individuals who meet training and experience requirements; promotes standards for national certification of clinical hypnotherapists; sponsors educational programs.

National Board for Hypnotherapy and Hypnotic Anaesthesiology
7841 W Ludlow Dr., Ste. A
Peoria, AZ 85381
(602) 843-2215; Fax (623) 878-3987
e-mail: nbhahypno@aol.com
http://www.nbha-medicine.com
Established 1984. Approves hypnotherapy instructors and certifies practitioners. Publishes quarterly *Adventures in Education*. Referral service; annual conference.

National Guild of Hypnotists
PO Box 308
Merrimack, NH 03054
(603) 429-9438; Fax (603) 424-8066
e-mail: nghhq@aol.com
http://www.ngh.net
Membership organization open to anyone with an interest in hypnosis. Publishes *The Journal of Hypnotism* and *Hypno-Gram* newsletter. Sponsors and approves training courses and continuing education programs; annual conference.

Massage and Bodywork

American Massage Therapy Association
820 Davis St., Ste. 100
Evanston, IL 60201-4444
(847) 864-0123; Fax (847) 864-1178
http://www.amtamassage.org
Established 1943. Membership organization; provides information on massage therapy and accredited schools; publishes quarterly newsletter *Hands On* and quarterly *Massage Therapy Journal*. Annual conferences; continuing education; practitioner referrals.

American Oriental Bodywork Therapy Association
Laurel Oak Corporate Center, Ste. 408
1010 Haddonfield-Berlin Rd.

Voorhees, NJ 08043
(609) 782-1616; Fax (609) 782-1653
e-mail: aobta@prodigy.net
http://www.healthy.net/aobta
Established 1984. National nonprofit association, membership open to Certified Practitioners with 500 hours of approved training and Associates with 150 hours. Publishes quarterly *AOBTA Newsletter* and annual *AOBTA Directory*. Annual convention; practitioner referrals.

Associated Bodywork & Massage Professionals
28677 Buffalo Park Rd.
Evergreen, CO 80439-7347
(800) 458-2267; (303) 674-8478; Fax (303) 674-0859
e-mail: expectmore@abmp.com
http://www.abmp.com
Established 1986. Membership organization; information on training programs; practitioner referrals; legislative information; Internet links to schools and associations. Accrediting division, International Massage and Somatic Therapies Certification Council, evaluates and accredits schools. Publishes *Massage & Bodywork* magazine, newsletter *Different Strokes, ABMP Touch Training Directory,* and *ABMP Massage and Bodywork Yellow Pages.*

Commission on Massage Therapy Accreditation
820 Davis St., Ste. 100
Evanston, IL 60201-4444
(847) 864-0123; Fax (847) 864-1178
http://www.comta.org
Sets standards for schools and training; evaluates and accredits programs that demonstrate compliance.

International Massage and Somatic Therapies Certification Council
28677 Buffalo Park Rd.
Evergreen, CO 80439-7347
(800) 458-2267; (303) 674-8478; Fax (303) 674-0859
e-mail: expectmore@abmp.com
http://www.abmp.com
Accreditation division of Associated Bodywork & Massage Professionals.

International Massage Association
3000 Connecticut Ave. NW, Ste. 308
Washington, DC 20008
(202) 387-6555
Established 1984. International membership association of massage practitioners and massage schools.

International Myomassethics Federation, Inc.
1720 Willow Creek Circle, Ste. 517
Eugene, OR 97402
(800) 433-4463; Fax (541) 485-7372
e-mail: myomasseth@aol.com
Established 1971. Information on research, employment, and continuing education. Annual international convention. Publishes newsletter, annual membership roster, and quarterly journal *Intramyomassethics Forum*.

National Certification Board for Therapeutic Massage and Bodywork
8201 Greensboro Dr., Ste. 300
McLean, VA 22102
(703) 610-9015; (800) 296-0664; Fax (703) 610-9005
http://www.ncbtmb.com
Independent, private nonprofit organization; administers national certification examination; establishes continuing education requirements for re-certification. Practitioner referrals; consumer information.

Midwifery

The American College of Nurse-Midwives
818 Connecticut Ave. NW, Ste. 900
Washington, DC 20006
(202) 728-9860; Fax (202) 728-9897
e-mail: info@acnm.org
http://www.acnm.org
Established 1955. Establishes educational requirements and clinical practice standards. Accredits education programs and administers national examination to certify practitioners. Publishes bimonthly *Journal of Nurse-Midwifery*. Continuing education; annual meeting.

Doulas of North America
1110 23rd Ave. East
Seattle, WA 98112

(206) 324-5440; Fax (206) 325-0472
e-mail: askdona@aol.com
http://www.dona.com
Established 1992. International membership organization; provides information about birth doulas and approved training courses. Certifies doulas and facilitates continuing education conferences and workshops. Publishes quarterly newsletter *The International Doula* and referral directory.

Midwifery Education Accreditation Council
220 W Birch, Ste. 5
Flagstaff, AZ 86001
(520) 214-0997; Fax (520) 773-9694
http://www.mana.org/meac/
Established 1991 by the National Coalition of Midwifery Educators. Evaluates programs and accredits those meeting established educational standards.

Midwives Alliance of North America
PO Box 175
Newton, KS 67114
(316) 283-4543; (888) 923-MANA (6262); Fax (316) 283-4543
e-mail: manainfo@aol.com
http://www.mana.org
Established 1982. Membership organization open to midwives, students, and interested individuals. Develops guidelines for education; publishes bimonthly *MANA News*. Legal and legislative information; annual conference.

North American Registry of Midwives
PO Box 1288
Nashville, TN 38483
(888) 84-BIRTH (842-4784)
http://www.mana.org/narm/
Established 1987. Sets standards for certification and practice; administers national examination for Certified Professional Midwife. Workshops, meetings.

Naturopathic Medicine

American Association of Naturopathic Physicians
601 Valley St., #105
Seattle, WA 98109
(206) 298-0126; Fax (206) 298-0129

e-mail: 74602.3715@compuserve.com
http://www.naturopathic.org
Established 1986. Membership organization; promotes standards for education and licensing. Conducts annual conference, annual convention, and continuing education programs. Publishes *AANP Quarterly Newsletter*.

Council on Naturopathic Medical Education
PO Box 11426
Eugene, OR 97440-3626
(541) 484-6028
e-mail: crest@clipper.net
http://www.cnme.org
Established 1978. National accrediting agency for naturopathic medical colleges, recognized by the U.S. Department of Education. Provides information on accredited colleges and programs, and candidates for accreditation. Publishes newsletter and quarterly Information Report.

Polarity Therapy

American Polarity Therapy Association
2888 Bluff St. #149
Boulder, CO 80301
(303) 545-2080; Fax (303) 545-2161
e-mail: hq@polaritytherapy.org
http://www.polaritytherapy.org
Approves trainings at Associate and Registered levels. Certifies graduates of approved trainings as Associate Polarity Practitioner and Registered Polarity Practitioner. Information on training and resources; practitioner referrals. Publishes quarterly newsletter *Energy*.

Reflexology

American Reflexology Certification Board
PO Box 620607
Littleton, CO 80162
(303) 933-6921; Fax (303) 904-0460
Established 1991. Administers national practitioner certification examination. Provides guidelines on selecting training and education, but does not accredit institutions or instructors. Provides practitioner referrals.

Home of Reflexology

http://www.reflexology.org
Information on reflexology and organizations; Internet links.

Reflexology Association of America

4012 S Rainbow Blvd., Box K585
Las Vegas, NV 89103-2059
(702) 871-9522
Membership organization; develops standards for practitioners and training. Provides information; publishes newsletter and holds biennial conference.

Reiki

International Center for Reiki Training

e-mail: center@reiki.org
http://www.reiki.org
Articles on Reiki; information on training and classes; practitioner referrals; Internet links.

The Reiki Alliance

PO Box 41
Cataldo, ID 83810
(208) 682-3535; Fax (208) 682-4848
e-mail: 74051.3471@compuserve.com
Established 1983. International membership organization of Reiki Masters practicing the Usui System of Reiki. Provides information on Reiki and Reiki practitioners.

Therapeutic Touch

Nurse Healers Professional Associates

1211 Locust St.
Philadelphia, PA 19107
(215) 545-8079; Fax (215) 545-8107
e-mail: nhpa@nursecominc.com
http://www.therapeutic-touch.com
Established 1977. Membership organization; provides information on therapeutic touch training programs; conducts research. Publishes quarterly *Cooperation Connection*. Annual conference.

Yoga

American Yoga Association

PO Box 19986
Sarasota, FL 34276
(941) 927-4977; Fax (941) 364-9153
Established 1968. Workshops and educational programs; publishes books, videos, and audiotapes. "Easy Does It Yoga Training Program" for people with physical limitations.

Himalayan International Institute

RR 1, Box 400
Honesdale, PA 18431
(800) 822-4547; (570) 253-5551; Fax (570) 253-9078
e-mail: hita@himalayaninstitute.org
http://www.himalayaninstitute.org
Established 1971. Worldwide classes and seminars. Himalayan Institute Teachers Association conducts Hatha Yoga Teachers Training and Certification Program. Referrals for teaching opportunities. Publishes *Yoga International* magazine.

International Association of Yoga Therapists

20 Sunnyside Ave., Ste A243
Mill Valley, CA 94941-1928
(415) 332-2478
e-mail: iayt@yoganet.com
Nonprofit membership organization; publishes *IAYT Journal* and *IAYT Newsletter*. Classes and seminars; international network & resource guide; referral service.

B.K.S. Iyengar Yoga National Association—U.S.

1420 Hawthorn Ave.
Boulder, CO 80304
(800) 889-YOGA (9642)
e-mail: laallard@aol.com
Membership organization; teacher referrals. Administers annual certification assessments. Magazine, books, and videos.

BOOKS

The growing interest in and access to alternative and complementary health care have prompted a proliferation of books on the topic. There is a wide range of information available on all aspects of alternative and complementary health care, including history, definitions and descriptions of modalities and therapies, principles, diagnosis and treatment of health conditions, case histories, research, and educational resources. The prospective practitioner can refer to books ranging from Cassileth's *The Alternative Medicine Handbook: The Complete Reference Guide to Alternative and Complementary Therapies,* Collinge's *The American Holistic Health Association Complete Guide to Alternative Medicine,* and Time-Life's *The Alternative Advisor: The Complete Guide to Natural Therapies and Alternative Treatments,* to Micozzi's textbook for physicians *Fundamentals of Complementary and Alternative Medicine.*

Overviews that offer basic information describing many different alternative therapies include Goldberg's *Alternative Medicine: The Definitive Guide,* Marti's *The Alternative Health & Medicine Encyclopedia* and Nash's *From Acupressure to Zen: An Encyclopedia of Natural Therapies.* Those focusing on one particular modality or health care approach include Beinfield's *Between Heaven and Earth: A Guide to Chinese Medicine,* Hoffman's *The Information Sourcebook of Herbal Medicine,* Murray and Pizzorno's *Encyclopedia of Natural Medicine,* and Ullman's *Discovering Homeopathy: Medicine for the 21st Century.*

The diverse licensing requirements for practitioners of alternative and complementary health care are addressed by Ashley's *Massage: A Career at Your Fingertips,* covering licensing requirements for the massage therapy profession, and Bianco's *Professional and Occupational Licensing Directory,* with information on state and federal licensing requirements and the government offices that oversee them.

For further bibliographical information, see Feuerman's *Alternative Medicine Resource Guide* and Page & Gotkin's *Health Inform's Resource Guide to Alternative Health.*

Selected Books on Alternative Health Care Annotated by Alan M. Rees*

Bratman, Steven. *The Alternative Medicine Sourcebook: A Realistic Evaluation of Alternative Healing Methods.* Los Angeles: Lowell House, 1997.

Bratman provides information and insights necessary to find a way through the maze of alternative possibilities prescribed by a licensed medical practitioner. Alternative medicine is defined broadly as "every available approach to healing that does not fall within the realm of conventional medicine." Most alternative practices provide treatment propelled by three ideas: the treatment must be natural, holistic, and promote wellness. A balanced explanation is given with respect to naturopathic medicine, herbal medicine, homeopathy, Chinese medicine, acupuncture, chiropractic, movement therapies, and spiritual approaches. A distinction is made between the scientific approaches to healing, such as naturopathy and homeopathy, and the healing arts, such as acupuncture. Specific guidance is given on how to use alternative

*Alan M. Rees is a medical information specialist, professor emeritus of library and information science at Case Western Reserve University, Cleveland, Ohio, and author of numerous reference works. The selected books are taken from *Consumer Health Information Source Book, 5th Edition* and *Consumer Health Information Source Book, 6th Edition,* both published by the Oryx Press, 1-800-279-6799, 1-800-279-4663 (fax), www.oryxpress.com.

medicine with recommended methods best suited to a number of common conditions. A largely successful attempt to provide a balanced approach to alternative medicine.

Cassileth, Barrie. *The Alternative Medicine Handbook: The Complete Reference Guide to Alternative and Complementary Therapies.* New York: Norton, 1998.

This is a serious and largely successful attempt to describe and evaluate over 50 alternative therapies such as Ayurveda, flower remedies, macrobiotics, Kirlian photography, chelation therapy, colon/detoxification therapies, Alexander technique, rolfing, light therapy, and faith healing. Each therapy is described in a standard format—what it is, what practitioners say it does, beliefs upon which it is based, research evidence to date, what the therapy can do for you, and where to go for treatment. Where no scientific evidence exists, this is so indicated, as in the case of nine unproved biological cancer therapies described. A balanced, analytical survey of alternative medicine by a founding member of the Advisory Council to the NIH Office of Alternative Medicine. Outstanding.

Collinge, William. *The American Holistic Health Association Guide to Alternative Medicine.* New York: Warner Books, 1996.

Attempts to provide a comprehensive and authoritative overview of the many alternative health care traditions available today. Collinge covers Chinese medicine, Ayurveda, naturopathic medicine, homeopathy, mind-body medicine, osteopathic medicine, chiropractic, and massage therapy. For each predominant medical tradition, Collinge explores the traditional roots, philosophy, and guiding principles for prevention, diagnosis, and treatment. Also included are comprehensive lists of organizations for alternative medicine, with phone numbers and addresses. Clearly written, with extensive bibliographic notes and documentation, this is a useful guide, although it presents comparatively little information on effectiveness, strengths, and limitations. Recommended.

Credit, Larry P., Sharon G. Hartunian, and others. *Your Guide to Complementary Medicine.* Garden City Park, NY: Avery, 1998.

An introduction to a number of complementary care approaches to a wide variety of ailments. Some 37 approaches are described including some lesser- known treatments such as lymphatic massage, polarity therapy, and Trager. Each approach is discussed in a standardized format—what it is, conditions that respond best, how it works, what to expect, costs/duration, credentials/education, how to find a practitioner, professional organizations, and recommended readings. The authors insist that, "these approaches are not viewed as alternatives but as complements. In part-

nership with conventional Western medicine, the treatments can bolster your potential for health and recovery." Interesting, informative, and easy to read.

Jacobs, Jennifer (ed.) *The Encyclopedia of Alternative Medicine: A Complete Family Guide to Complementary Therapies.* Boston: Journey Editions/Charles E. Tuttle, 1996.

This is a beautifully illustrated book with splendid color photographs, worthy of coffee table status. The book consists of several dozen contributed chapters covering a large number of alternative therapies. Part I of the book deals with natural healing; Part II, "The Power of Plants"; Part III, "Nutrition and Diet"; Part IV, "Mobility and Posture"; Part V, "The Mind"; Part VI, "Massage and Touch"; and Part VII, "Eastern Therapies." This book offers a most lucid and concise explanation of various alternative methods such as polarity therapy, flower essence therapy, naturopathic medicine, Rolfing, hypnotherapy, massage therapy, shiatsu, and so on. Also contains a glossary of terms, bibliography, and useful addresses. A valuable book for consumers to educate themselves about various treatment modalities so that they can make intelligent choices about their health care. Jacobs is a member of the Program Advisory Council of the National Institutes of Health Office of Alternative Medicine. A most attractive book that makes for easy reading. Highly Recommended

Lockie, Andrew, and Nicola Geddes. *The Complete Guide to Homeopathy.* New York: Dorling Kindersley, 1995.

Far from being just another sourcebook on homeopathy, this book (by two British homeopathists) is an oversized book worthy of coffee-table status. Like other Dorling Kindersley books, the photographs and illustrations are clear and colorful. Of particular value is the photographic index of 150 key and common remedies with details of their source, history, medicinal uses, and the factors that improve or worsen the symptoms treated. Included in the common remedies are 30 that are used extensively for minor, everyday complaints. Each remedy profiled includes common name, source, treatment, and key uses. Also of interest, is a section of the book that lists in tabulated form ailments, symptoms, cause, and onset, "you feel better with . . . ," "you feel worse from . . . ," remedy and dosage. An appealing, attractive, and highly readable source of information on homeopathy. More suitable for browsing than treatment applications.

Marti, James E. *The Alternative Health & Medicine Encyclopedia.* 2nd edition. Detroit: Visible Ink Press, 1997.

This is a second edition of a book originally published in 1995. The first edition presented more than 200 alternative therapies for more than 50 common medical disorders. This expanded and revised edition adds more than 100 new therapies for 20 additional disorders. The basic approach is the same in that, "while the old paradigm viewed the body basically as a machine, the new paradigm focuses on the interconnectivity of body, mind, emotions, social factors, and the environment in determining health status." Typical therapies covered include homeopathy, naturopathic medicine, and hydrotherapy. Separate chapters deal with the use of vitamins, minerals and trace elements, and botanical medicine. The alternative medicine approach to stress-related disorders, drug abuse and addiction, mental health, common male health problems, female health problems, cancer, heart disease, and aging is described. There are also detailed lists of resources. This is a highly readable, encyclopedic compilation of basic facts on a wide variety of alternative medicine therapies but with no attempt at the critical evaluation supplied by Barrie Cassileth's, *The Alternative Medicine Handbook,* (Norton, 1998).

Morton, Mary, and Michael Morton. *Five Steps to Selecting the Best Alternative Medicine: A Guide to Complementary and Interactive Health Care.* Novato, CA: New World Library, 1996.

This book starts with the premise that taking charge of your own health care can take both the courage to stand up to authority and a good deal of adeptness in sorting through the sometimes confusing information about the efficacy of various treatments. The Mortons outline in five basic steps how alternative medicine can work for you: learn your options, get good referrals, screen the candidates, interview the provider, and form a partnership. Overviews are provided for five licensed systems in alternative medicine—traditional Chinese medicine, naturopathic medicine, chiropractic, osteopathic, and the M.D. as alternate practitioner. Eminently readable, directive, and also informative.

Murray, Michael, and Joseph Pizzorno. *Encyclopedia of Natural Medicine.* Revised 2nd edition. Rocklin, CA: Prima, 1998.

This is an updated, revised edition of a book originally published in 1991. Murray and Pizzorno, naturopathic physicians and educators, define naturopathy as a system of health-oriented medicine that stresses maintenance of health and prevention of disease, in contrast with the traditional allopathic, disease-oriented system. Naturopathic physicians are trained to seek the underlying cause of a disease rather than simply to suppress the symptoms. Naturopathy draws upon nutritional therapy, natural diet, herbal medicine, Ayurveda, and Chinese medicine. Part One explains the cornerstones of good health; Part Two shows how key body systems can be enhanced

through detoxification, immune support, and stress management; and Part Three discusses how naturopathic medicine treats some 70 specific health problems. In each instance, the authors describe the condition and identify causes, therapeutic considerations, goals of therapy, and the use of dietary and lifestyle modification, nutritional supplements, and botanical medicines. The text is greatly enhanced by the liberal use of headings such as "Quick Review" and "Treatment Summary," together with informative diagrams and tables. This is a substantial contribution to the literature of alternative medicine in that it moves beyond simple description to a discussion of therapeutic approach and methods. Recommended.

Shealy, C. Norman. *The Illustrated Encyclopedia of Healing Remedies.* Boston: Element Books, 1998.

This book is a comprehensive discussion of the origins of eight alternative therapies—Ayurveda, Chinese herbal medicine, herbalism, aromatherapy, homeopathy, flower remedies, vitamins, and minerals. In each instance, coverage includes the background and history of the therapy together with how it works, information on visiting a practitioner, and data on specific remedies used with dosages and precautions. Part Two of the book consists of a description of 20 common ailments associated with body systems such as the digestive system, urinary system, and eyes. Each description indicates symptoms, treatment (herbalism, aromatherapy, homeopathy, etc.) and cautions. Part Three is a Reference Section that provides a glossary, list of further readings, and useful addresses. A short summary of the contents does not do justice to this book. The color photographs, diagrams and imaginative use of sidebars are of superlative quality. An excellent book worthy of coffee table status.

Stillerman, Elaine. *The Encyclopedia of Bodywork: From Acupressure to Zone Therapy.* New York: Facts on File, 1996.

The term "bodywork" includes "all the hands-on therapies, movement re-education systems, psychological techniques, and metaphysical and energetic modalities, which recognize the unity of body/mind/spirit/emotions." Two hundred alternative therapies are listed and described, many of which are quite rare and esoteric. Typical entries include body-mind centering, electrical current therapy, color therapy, moxibustion, heliotherapy, and short-wave diathermy. Entries range from several paragraphs in length to three or four pages. The text is clear and informative, while the value of the book is greatly enhanced by the inclusion of further readings at the end of most entries. This is a first-rate encyclopedic compilation of essential information on a wide variety of alternative therapies. Stillerman is a massage therapist.

Woodham, Anne, and David Peters. *Encyclopedia of Healing Therapies*. New York: Dorling Kindersley, 1997.

A highly attractive, coffee-table quality book that describes and illustrates the different approaches of complementary medicine. While introductory chapters describe holistic medicine, its rise in popularity, and the emphasis on wellness and well-being, the bulk of the book consists of a visual guide to over 90 widely used complementary therapies with information on their history and how they work, what to expect at a consultation, research and scientific evidence, self-help techniques, and compatibility with conventional medicine. Using high-quality photographs and illustrations, the book offers concise and informative descriptions of a wide variety of touch and movement therapies, medicinal therapies, mind and emotive therapies, and diagnostic techniques. A final section includes an extensive array of treatment options for over 200 mental, physical, and emotional health problems. Much of the content is readily available in other publications but is not presented in such an attractive manner.

Futher Books on Alternative Health Care Selected by Karen Rappaport

Albright, Peter. *The Complete Book of Complementary Therapies*. Allentown, PA: People's Medical Society, 1997.

Ashley, Martin. *Massage: A Career At Your Fingertips*. 3rd ed. Carmel, CA: Enterprise Publishing, 1998.

Beinfield, Harriet. *Between Heaven & Earth: A Guide to Chinese Medicine*. New York: Ballantine Books, 1991.

Bianco, David P., ed. *Professional and Occupational Licensing Directory: A Descriptive Guide to State and Federal Licensing, Registration & Certification Requirements*. 2nd ed. Detroit, MI: Gale Research, 1996.

Brown, Deni. *Encyclopedia of Herbs and Their Uses*. New York: Dorling Kindersly, 1995.

Feldenkrais, Moshe. *Awareness Through Movement*. San Francisco, CA: Harper San Francisco, 1972.

Feuerman, Francine. *Alternative Medicine Resource Guide*. Lanham, MD: Scarecrow Press, 1997.

Frawley, David. *Ayurvedic Healing: A Comprehensive Guide*. Salt Lake City, UT: Passage Press, 1989.

Freedman, Marilyn. *Mosby's Tour Guide to Alternative Medicine*. St. Louis, MO: Mosby-Year Book, Inc., 1997.

Goldberg, Burton. *Alternative Medicine: The Definitive Guide*. Tiburon, CA: Future Medicine Publishing, Inc., 1998.

Gordon, Rena. *Alternative Therapies: Exploring Options in Health Care*. New York: Springer, 1998.

Hoffman, David. *The Information Sourcebook of Herbal Medicine*. Freedom, CA: Crossing Press, 1994.

Jonas, Wayne B. *Essentials of Complementary & Alternative Medicine*. Baltimore, MD: Williams & Wilkins, 1998.

Juhan, Deane. *Job's Body: A Handbook for Bodywork*. Barrytown, NY: Station Hill Press, 1987.

Kaptchuk, Ted. *The Web That Has No Weaver: Understanding Chinese Medicine*. Chicago, IL: Contemporary Books, 1985.

Kastner, Mark. *Alternative Healing: The Complete A-Z Guide to 150 Alternative Therapies*. New York: Henry Holt, 1995.

Keville, Kathi. *Aromatherapy: A Complete Guide to the Healing Art*. Freedom, CA: The Crossing Press, 1995.

Lad, Vasant. *Ayurveda: The Science of Self-Healing*. Wilmot, CA: Lotus Light Publications, 1984.

Leibowitz, Judith. *Alexander Technique*. New York: Harper Perennial, 1990.

Micozzi, Marc. *Fundamentals of Complementary & Alternative Medicine*. New York: Churchill-Livingstone, 1995.

Morton, Mary. *Five Steps to Selecting the Best Alternative Medicines: A Guide to Complementary and Integrative Health Care*. Novato, CA: New World Library, 1996.

Nash, Barbara. *From Acupressure to Zen: An Encyclopedia of Natural Therapies*. Upland, PA: Diane Publishing Co., 1998.

O'Connor, Bonnie Blair. *Healing Traditions: Alternative Medicine and the Health Professions*. Philadelphia, PA: University of Pennsylvania Press, 1995.

Olsen, Kristin Gottschalk. *The Encyclopedia of Alternative Health Care.* New York: Pocket Books, 1990.

Page, Kate, and Janet Gotkin. *Health Inform's Resource Guide to Alternative Health.* Montrose, NY: Health Inform, 1997.

Price, Shirley, and Len Price. *Aromatherapy for Health Professionals.* New York: Churchill-Livingstone, 1995.

Segen, Joseph C. *Dictionary of Alternative Medicine.* Stamford, CT: Appleton & Lange, 1998.

Shafarman, Steven. *Awareness Heals: The Feldenkrais Method For Dynamic Health.* Reading, MA: Addison-Wesley Publishing Co., Inc., 1997.

Tappan, Frances. *Tappan's Handbook for Healing Massage Techniques: Classic, Holistic and Emerging Methods.* 3rd ed. Stamford, CT: Appleton & Lange, 1998.

Thomas, Richard. *The Complete Family Guide to Alternative Medicine: An Illustrated Encyclopedia of Natural Healing.* Rockport, MA: Element Books, 1996.

Time-Life Books Editors. *The Alternative Advisor: The Complete Guide to Natural Therapies and Alternative Treatments.* Alexandria, VA: Time-Life, Inc., 1997.

Ullman, Dana. *Discovering Homeopathy: Medicine for the 21st Century.* North Atlantic, 1991.

Weil, Andrew. *Health and Healing: Understanding Conventional and Alternative Medicine.* Boston, MA: Houghton Mifflin, 1983.

Weiss, Rudolf F. *Herbal Medicine.* Beaconsfield, England: Beaconsfield Publishers, Ltd., 1985.

PERIODICALS

Advances in Mind-Body Medicine
Fetzer Institute
9292 West KL Ave.
Kalamazoo, MI 49009
(616) 375-2000; Fax (616) 372-2163
e-mail: advances@fetzer.org
http://www.fetzer.org

*Alternative Health Practitioner: The Journal
of Complementary and Natural Care*
Springer Publishing Co.
536 Broadway
New York 10012
(212) 431-4370; Fax (212) 941-7842
e-mail: springer@springerpub.com
http://www.springerjournals.com
http://www.springerpub.com

*Alternative Therapies in Health and
Medicine*
Alternative Therapies
PO Box 627
Holmes, PA 19043
(800) 345-8112
http://www.alternativetherapies.com

The American Homeopath
North American Society of Homeopaths
1122 E Pike St., Ste. 1122
Seattle, WA 98122
(541) 345-9815; (206) 720-7000; Fax (206)
329-5684
e-mail: nash@homeopathy.org
Http://www.homeopathy.org

American Journal of Acupuncture
1840 41st Ave., Ste. 102
PO Box 610
Capitola, CA 95010
(831) 475-1700; Fax (831) 475-1439

American Journal of Clinical Hypnosis
American Society of Clinical Hypnosis
2200 E Devon Ave., Ste. 291

Des Plaines, IL 60018-4534
(847) 297-3317; Fax (847) 297-7309
e-mail: 70632.1663@compuserve.com
http://www.asch.net

*HerbalGram, The Journal of the American
Botanical Council and the Herb Research
Foundation*
American Botanical Council
PO Box 201660
Austin, TX 78720-2660
(512) 331-8868
http://www.herbalgram.org

Holistic Medicine
American Holistic Medical Association
6728 Old McLean Village Dr.
McLean, VA 22101
(703) 556-9728
http://www.holisticmedicine.org

Homeopathy Today
National Center for Homeopathy
801 N. Fairfax St., Ste 306
Alexandria, VA 22314
(703) 548-7790; Fax (703)548-7792
e-mail: ncinfo@igc.apc.org
http://www.homeopathic.org

Integrative Medicine
Elsevier Science
655 Avenue of the Americas
New York 10010
(212) 989-5800; (888) 437-4636
e-mail: usinfo-f@elsevier.com
http://www.elsevier.com

International Journal of Aromatherapy
American Alliance of Aromatherapy
PO Box 309
Depoe Bay, OR 97341
(800) 809-9850; Fax (800) 809-9808
e-mail: aaoa@wcn.net

Journal of Alternative and Complementary Medicine
Mary Ann Liebert, Inc.
2 Madison Ave.
Larchmont, NY 10538
(914) 834-3100
e-mail: info@liebert.com
http://www.liebertpub.com

Journal of Hypnotherapy
American Board of Hypnotherapy
16842 Von Karman Ave. #475
Irvine, CA 92714
(800) 872-9996; (714) 261-6400; Fax (714) 251-4632
e-mail: aih@hypnosis.com
http://www.hypnosis.com/abh

Massage & Bodywork
Associated Bodywork and Massage Professionals
28677 Buffalo Park Rd.
Evergreen, CO 80439-7347
(800) 458-2267; Fax (303) 674-0859
e-mail: expectmore@abmp.com
http://www.abmp.com

Massage Magazine
1315 W Mallon Ave.
Spokane, WA 99201
(509) 324-8117; (800) 533-4263

Massage Therapy Journal
American Massage Therapy Association
820 Davis St., Ste. 100, MTJ Subscription

Evanston, IL 60201-4444
(847) 864-0123; Fax (847) 864-1178
http://www.amtamassage.org

Medical Hypnoanalysts Journal
American Academy of Medical Hypnoanalysts
5628 Murray Rd. #4
Memphis, TN 38119-3876
(800) 344-9766; Fax (901) 683-1224
e-mail: info@aamh.com
http://www.aamh.com

Scentsitivity
National Association for Holistic Aromatherapy
836 Hanley Industrial Court
St. Louis, MO 63144
(314) 963-2071; (888) ASK-NAHA (275-6242); Fax (314) 963-4454
e-mail: info@naha.org
http://www.naha.org

Yoga International
Himalayan Institute
RR1, Box 407
Honesdale, PA 18431
(800) 253-6243; (570) 253-4929; Fax (570) 253-6360
e-mail: yimag@epix.com

Yoga Journal
PO Box 469088
Escondido, CA 92046-9088
(760) 796-6549; (800) 600-YOGA (9642)
e-mail: yoga@pcspublink.com

WORLD WIDE WEB SITES

This is a list of all the Web sites mentioned in the resource information sections of this book, condensed here for the convenience of Web users. Please see the specific subject areas in the resource information sections for brief annotations on these organizations and Web sites.

Academy of Veterinary Homeopathy
http://www.acadvethom.org

Acupuncture.com
http://www.acupuncture.com

Alexander Technique International
http://www.ati-net.com

Alternative & Complementary Medicine Center, HealthWorld Online
http://www.altmed.net

Alternative Medicine-Health Care Information Resources
http://www-hsl.mcmaster.ca/tomflem/altmed.html

The Alternative Medicine Home Page
http://www.pitt.edu/~cbw/altm.html

American Academy of Medical Hypnoanalysts
http://www.aamh.com

American Association of Naturopathic Physicians
http://www.naturopathic.org

American Association of Oriental Medicine
http://www.aaom.org

American Board of Hypnotherapy
http://www.hypnosis.com/abh

American Botanical Council
http://www.herbalgram.org

American Chiropractic Association
http://www.amerchiro.org

The American College of Nurse-Midwives
http://www.acnm.org

American Herbalists Guild
http://www.healthy.net/herbalists

American Holistic Health Association
http://www.healthy.net/ahha

American Holistic Medical Association
http://www.holisticmedicine.org

American Holistic Nurses Association
http://www.ahna.org

American Holistic Veterinary Medicine Association
http://www.altvetmed.com

American Massage Therapy Association
http://www.amtamassage.org

American Oriental Bodywork Therapy Association
http://www.healthy.net/aobta

American Polarity Therapy Association
http://www.polaritytherapy.org

American Society for the Alexander Technique
http://www.alexandertech.org

American Society of Clinical Hypnosis
http://www.asch.net

Associated Bodywork & Massage Professionals
http://www.abmp.com

Association for Applied Psychophysiology & Biofeedback
http://www.aapb.org

Association of Chiropractic Colleges
http://www.chirocolleges.org

Dr. Bower's Complementary and Alternative Medicine Home Page
Http://galen.med.virginia.edu/~pjb3s/ComplementaryHomePage.html

Commission on Massage Therapy Accreditation
http://www.comta.org

The Complete Guide to the Alexander Technique
http://www.alexandertechnique.com

Council for Homeopathic Certification
http://www.igc.org/~homcert

Council on Homeopathic Education
http://www.checu.org

Council on Naturopathic Medical Education
http://www.cnme.org

Doulas of North America
http://www.dona.com/

Feldenkrais Guild
http://www.feldenkrais.com

Herb Research Foundation
http://www.herbs.org

Home of Reflexology
http://www.reflexology.org

Homeopathy Home
http://www.homeopathyhome.com

Himalayan International Institute
http://www.himalayaninstitute.org

International Center for Reiki Training
http://www.reiki.org

International Medical & Dental Hypnotherapy Association
http://www.infinityinst.com

Midwifery Education Accreditation Council
http://www.mana.org/meac/

Midwives Alliance of North America
http://www.mana.org

National Acupuncture and Oriental Medical Alliance
http://www.acuall.org

National Association for Holistic Aromatherapy
http://www.naha.org

National Board for Certified Clinical Hypnotherapists, Inc.
http://www.natboard.com

National Board for Hypnotherapy and Hypnotic Anaesthesiology
http://www.nbha-medicine.com

National Board of Homeopathic Examiners
http://www.nbhe.com

National Center for Complementary and Alternative Medicine
http://altmed.od.nih.gov/nccam/

National Center for Homeopathy
http://www.homeopathic.org

National Certification Board for Therapeutic Massage and Bodywork
http://www.ncbtmb.com

National Certification Commission for Acupuncture and Oriental Medicine
http://www.nccaom.org

National Guild of Hypnotists
http://www.ngh.net

NaturalHealers
http://www.naturalhealers.com/

New Age Journal Holistic Health Directory
http://www.newage.com/

North American Registry of Midwives
http://www.mana.org/narm/

North American Society of Homeopaths
http://www.homeopathy.org

Nurse Healers Professional Associates
http://www.therapeutic-touch.com

The Rosenthal Center for Complementary & Alternative Medicine, Columbia University College of Physicians and Surgeons
http://cpmcnet.columbia.edu/dept/rosenthal/

INDEXES

SCHOOL NAMES INDEX

Numbers refer to entry numbers.

FIELDS OF STUDY INDEX

Numbers refer to entry numbers.

*Denotes schools where this field is a main program of study.

Acupressure *see also* **Jin Shin Do;
Reflexology; Shiatsu**
Academy of Chinese Healing Arts, Inc, 301
Academy of Healing Arts, Massage and Facial
  Skin Care, Inc, 283
Academy of Medical Arts and Business, 673
Academy of Natural Healing, 563
Academy of Natural Health Sciences, 527
Academy of Natural Therapies, 613
Academy of Natural Therapy, 236
Academy of Oriental Medicine, Austin, 723
Academy of Reflexology and Health Therapy
  International, 365
Acupressure-Acupuncture Institute*, 286
Acupressure Institute*, 30
Acupressure Institute of Alaska*, 4
Alexandria School of Scientific Therapeutics,
  Inc, 361
Alive and Well! Institute of Conscious Body-
  Work, 142
Alpha School of Massage, Inc, 272
American Institute of Massage Therapy, Costa
  Mesa, 48
American Institute of Massage Therapy, Kailua,
  333
American Taoist Healing Center*, 565
Arizona School of Integrative Studies, 5
The Asheville School of Massage, Inc*, 603
Atlanta School of Massage, 317
Bhumi's Yoga and Wellness Center, 629
Big Island Academy of Massage, Inc, 326
Big Sky Somatic Institute, 483
Blue Cliff School of Therapeutic Massage, Gulf
  Coast Campus, 473
Blue Cliff School of Therapeutic Massage,
  Kenner, 384
Blue Cliff School of Therapeutic Massage,
  Shreveport, 389
Blue Heron Academy of the Healing Arts and
  Sciences*, 446
Blue Ridge School of Massage and Yoga*, 783

Bluegrass Professional School of Massage
  Therapy, 381
BMSI Institute, LLC, 376
Boca Raton Institute, 260
Body Therapy Institute of Santa Barbara*, 168
Body Wellness Therapeutic Massage Academy,
  25
Calaveras College of Therapeutic Massage, 140
Calgary College of Holistic Health and Clinics,
  Inc, 842
California College of Physical Arts, Inc, 73
California Institute of Massage and Spa Ser-
  vices, 189
California Naturopathic College*, 53
Canadian College of Acupuncture and Oriental
  Medicine, 851
Capri College, Davenport, 370
Capri College, Madison, 833
Capri College of Massage Therapy, Cedar
  Rapids, 369
Career Training Academy, Monroeville, 680
Career Training Academy, New Kensington*,
  681
Caring Hands School of Massage*, 198
Karen Carlson International Academy of Holis-
  tic Massage and Science, 253
Carrie's Kadesh and School of Massage, 710
Cascade Institute of Massage and Body Ther-
  apies, 648
Cayce/Reilly School of Massotherapy, 796
Center for A Balanced Life, Inc, 472
Center for Human Integration, 685
Central California School of Body Therapy,
  165
Central Louisiana School of Therapeutic Mas-
  sage, Inc, 388
The Central Mass School of Massage and Ther-
  apy*, 429
Central Pennsylvania School of Massage, Inc,
  695
Centre Psycho-Corporel, Inc, 876

Thousand Oaks Healing Arts Institute, 196

The Touch Therapy Institute, 60

Touching for Health Center School of Professional Bodywork*, 192

Twin Lakes College of the Healing Arts, 176

Universal Center of Healing Arts, 488

Universal Institute of Healing Arts*, 778

University of Health Science*, 332

Utah College of Massage Therapy, 774

Utah College of Massage Therapy, Utah Valley Campus, 768

Vermont Institute of Massage Therapy*, 780

Virginia Academy of Massage Therapy*, 801

Vitality Training Center, 188

Wellspring Institute School of Therapeutic Bodywork, 455

Westbrook University, 536

White Mountain School of Applied Healing, 541

The Whole You School of Massage and Bodywork*, 615

Wisconsin Institute of Natural Wellness, 840

Acupuncture see also Oriental Medicine; Traditional Chinese Medicine

Academy for Five Element Acupuncture*, 271

Academy of Chinese Culture and Health Sciences*, 118

Academy of Chinese Healing Arts, Inc*, 301

Academy of Oriental Medicine, Austin*, 723

Acupressure-Acupuncture Institute*, 286

American College of Acupuncture and Oriental Medicine*, 745

American College of Traditional Chinese Medicine*, 150

American Taoist Healing Center*, 565

Atlantic Institute of Oriental Medicine*, 267

Bastyr University*, 810

Beijing School of Acupuncture and Oriental Medicine*, 741

Canadian College of Acupuncture and Oriental Medicine*, 851

Canadian College of Massage and Hydrotherapy, Newmarket*, 858

Canadian College of Massage and Hydrotherapy, North York*, 859

Canadian College of Naturopathic Medicine, 861

Classical Acupuncture Institute*, 275

Colorado School of Traditional Chinese Medicine*, 230

Dongguk Royal University*, 90

Emperor's College of Traditional Oriental Medicine*, 178

Five Branches Institute of Traditional Chinese Medicine*, 174

Florida College of Natural Health, Fort Lauderdale Campus*, 296

Florida College of Natural Health, Miami*, 288

Florida College of Natural Health, Orlando Campus*, 259

Florida College of Natural Health, Sarasota*, 303

Florida Health Academy, Naples*, 290

Florida Institute of Traditional Chinese Medicine*, 298

Hawaii College of Traditional Oriental Medicine*, 338

Inochi Institute, Inc.*, 481

Institute of Clinical Acupuncture and Oriental Medicine*, 330

Institute of Taoist Education and Acupuncture, Inc*, 214

Institute of Traditional Chinese Medicine*, 865

International Institute of Chinese Medicine*, 543

Kansas College of Chinese Medicine*, 378

Kyung San University USA School of Oriental Medicine*, 68

Maryland Institute of Traditional Chinese Medicine*, 397

Meiji College of Oriental Medicine*, 33

Mercy College*, 555

Meridian Institute*, 110

The Michener Institute for Applied Health Sciences*, 866

Midwest Center for the Study of Oriental Medicine, Chicago*, 346

Midwest Center for the Study of Oriental Medicine, Racine*, 838

Minnesota Institute of Acupuncture and Herbal Studies*, 471

The National College of Chiropractic, 353

National College of Oriental Medicine*, 292

New England School of Acupuncture*, 433

The New York College for Wholistic Health Education and Research*, 597

Northwest Institute of Acupuncture and Oriental Medicine*, 822

Northwestern College of Chiropractic*, 458

Oregon College of Oriental Medicine*, 661

Pacific College of Oriental Medicine, New York*, 582

Pacific College of Oriental Medicine, San Diego*, 146

Alexander Technique

Animal Medicine *see* Animal Therapy

Animal Therapy *see also* Equine Massage

Aston-Patterning Bodywork and Movement

Awareness Practices

Ayurvedic Medicine see also Maharishi Vedic Medicine

Colon Hydrotherapy

Connective Tissue Massage

CranioSacral Therapy

Deep Muscle Massage

Deep Tissue Massage

Doula *see also* Childbirth Education; Midwifery

Equine Massage *see also* Animal Therapy

Esalen Massage *see also* Swedish Massage

Exercise Therapy

Feldenkrais

Flower Essences *see also* Herbal Medicine; Homeopathy

Holistic Health *see also* **Mind-Body Medicine**

Holistic Nursing

Medical Massage

Midwifery see also Childbirth Education; Doula

Mind-Body Medicine *see also* **Ayurvedic Medicine; Body-Mind Centering; Body-Mind Clearing; Holistic Health; Holistic Nursing; Naturopathic Medicine; Traditional Chinese Medicine**

Myofascial Release

Myomassology see also Massage Therapy

Myotherapy see also Neuromuscular Therapy; Trigger Point Therapy

Naprapathy

Naturopathic Medicine

Neuro-Structural Bodywork

Neuromuscular Therapy see also Myotherapy; Trigger Point Therapy

On-Site Massage see also Chair Massage

Orgodynamics

Oriental Medicine see also Acupuncture; Traditional Chinese Medicine

Ortho-Bionomy

Orthopedic Massage

Pediatric Massage see also Infant Massage

Polarity Therapy

Postpartum Massage *see also* Pregnancy Massage; Prenatal Massage

Pregnancy Massage *see also* Postpartum Massage; Prenatal Massage

Prenatal Massage *see also* Postpartum Massage; Pregnancy Massage

MotherMassage: Massage During Pregnancy*, 576

Qigong *see also* Traditional Chinese Medicine

Rebirthing *see also* Breathwork

Reflexology *see also* Acupressure

Rosen Method Bodywork

Rubenfeld Synergy Method

Russian Massage

Shiatsu

Somatic Education *see also* Alexander Technique; Feldenkrais; Rubenfeld Synergy Method; Unergi Integrated Therapy

Spa Therapies

Sports Massage

Structural Integration

Yoga Therapy see also **Yoga Teacher Training**

Zero Balancing